The Fundamentals of Clinical Hematology

Third Edition

The Johns Hopkins Series in Hematology/Oncology

Jerry L. Spivak, M.D., and Martin D. Abeloff, M.D., Consulting Editors

The Fundamentals of Clinical Hematology

Third Edition

Edited by

Jerry L. Spivak, M.D.

*Professor and Director, Division of Hematology,
Department of Medicine, Johns Hopkins University School
of Medicine, Baltimore, Maryland*

and

Edward R. Eichner, M.D.

*Professor, Department of Medicine, University of
Oklahoma Health Sciences Center, Oklahoma City,
Oklahoma*

The Johns Hopkins University Press
Baltimore and London

The Johns Hopkins University Press
2715 North Charles Street
Baltimore, Maryland 21218-4319
The Johns Hopkins Press Ltd., London

Drug Dosage: The authors and publisher have exerted every effort to ensure that the selection and dosage of drugs discussed in this text accord with current recommendations and practice at the time of publication. However, in view of ongoing research, changes in governmental regulations, and the constant flow of information relating to drug therapy and drug reactions, the reader is urged to check the package insert of each drug for any change in indications and dosage and for warnings and precautions. This is particularly important when the recommended agent is a new and/or infrequently used drug.

ISBN 0-8018-4536-X

Library of Congress Cataloging-in-Publication Data

The Fundamentals of clinical hematology / edited by Jerry L. Spivak
    and Edward R. Eichner.—3rd ed.
        p.   cm.—(The Johns Hopkins series in hematology/oncology)
    Includes bibliographical references and index.
    ISBN 0-8018-4536-X (pbk. : alk. paper)
    1. Hematology.   I. Spivak, Jerry L.   II. Eichner, Edward R.
  III. Series.
    [DNLM: 1. Hematologic Diseases.   WH 100 F9802]
  RB145.F86   1993
  616.1′5—dc20
  DNLM/DLC
  for Library of Congress   92-1562
                                                     CIP

Contents

Preface to the Third Edition

The basic premise of *The Fundamentals of Clinical Hematology* is that diseases of the blood are best approached with a sound understanding of the physiology of hematopoiesis. A litany of clinical signs and symptoms rarely suffices to provide significant insight into either the pathophysiology of a particular disease process or the rationale for its treatment. Accordingly, contributors to this volume were asked, to the extent possible, to approach their topic from a physiologic perspective. Our intent was that this book be of particular value to those initiating their clinical training and also those whose training primarily involves the broad field of internal medicine without specialization in hematology.

Each edition of *The Fundamentals of Clinical Hematology* has undergone both extensive revision and expansion. With the information explosion created by recombinant DNA technology, this edition is no exception. In addition to expanded coverage of each topic, a chapter on bone marrow transplantation has been added, because the indications for this procedure have broadened to encompass a variety of hematologic disorders. A chapter on the porphyrias, lead intoxication, and sideroblastic anemias also has been added.

The editors wish to express their appreciation to the authors for their contributions to this textbook and to the Johns Hopkins University Press for undertaking its publication.

Contributors

Richard F. Ambinder, M.D., Ph.D.
Assistant Professor, Oncology Center, Johns Hopkins University, Baltimore, Maryland

William R. Bell, M.D.
Professor, Division of Hematology, Department of Medicine, Johns Hopkins University School of Medicine, Baltimore, Maryland

Sylvia S. Bottomley, M.D.
Professor, Department of Medicine, University of Oklahoma College of Medicine, and Staff Physician, VA Medical Center, Oklahoma City, Oklahoma

Hayden G. Braine, M.D.
Associate Professor, Department of Medicine, Johns Hopkins University School of Medicine, Baltimore, Maryland

Thomas P. Duffy, M.D.
Professor, Department of Medicine, Yale University School of Medicine, New Haven, Connecticut

Janice P. Dutcher, M.D.
Associate Professor, Department of Medicine, Albert Einstein College of Medicine, Bronx, New York

Edward R. Eichner, M.D.
Professor, Department of Medicine, University of Oklahoma College of Medicine, and Staff Physician, VA Medical Center, Oklahoma City, Oklahoma

William P. Hammond, M.D.
Associate Professor, Division of Hematology, Department of Medicine, University of Washington School of Medicine, Seattle, Washington

Richard J. Jones, M.D.
Associate Professor, Oncology Center, Johns Hopkins University, Baltimore, Maryland

Haig H. Kazazian, Jr., M.D.
Professor, Department of Pediatrics, and Director, Center for Medical Genetics, Johns Hopkins University School of Medicine, Baltimore, Maryland

Craig M. Kessler, M.D.
Professor and Director, Coagulation Laboratories, Division of Hematology-Oncology, Department of Medicine, George Washington University School of Medicine, Washington, D.C.

Thomas S. Kickler, M.D.
Associate Professor, Department of Laboratory Medicine, Johns Hopkins University School of Medicine, and Associate Director, Blood Bank and Transfusion Service, Johns Hopkins Hospital, Baltimore, Maryland

Robert A. Kyle, M.D.
Professor, Division of Hematology, Department of Internal Medicine, Mayo Medical School, Rochester, Minnesota

Richard D. Leavitt, M.D.
Director, Clinical Research, Genetics Institute, Cambridge, Massachusetts

Maura J. McGuire, M.D.
Instructor, Department of Medicine, Johns Hopkins University School of Medicine, Baltimore, Maryland

Patricia A. McIntyre, M.D.
Associate Professor Emerita, Department of Medicine, Johns Hopkins University School of Medicine, Baltimore, Maryland

Jeanette Mladenovic, M.D.
Associate Professor, Department of Medicine, State University of New York, Stony Brook, New York

Scott Murphy, M.D.
Professor, Department of Medicine, Thomas Jefferson Medical College, Philadelphia, Pennsylvania

Paul M. Ness, M.D.
Associate Professor, Department of Laboratory Medicine, Johns Hopkins University School of Medicine, and Director, Blood Bank and Transfusion Service, Johns Hopkins Hospital, Baltimore, Maryland

David S. Newcombe, M.D.
Professor, Department of Environmental Health
Sciences, Johns Hopkins University School of
Hygiene and Public Health, Baltimore, Maryland

Donald Pasquale, M.D.
Assistant Professor, Department of Medicine, Albany
Medical College, and Assistant Chief of Hematology,
Department of Veterans Affairs Medical Center,
Albany, New York

John A. Phillips III, M.D.
David T. Karzon Professor of Pediatrics and
Professor of Biochemistry, Department of Pediatrics,
Vanderbilt University School of Medicine, and
Director, Division of Genetics, Department of
Pediatrics, Vanderbilt University Medical Center,
Nashville, Tennessee

Peter J. Quesenberry, M.D.
Professor and Chief, Division of
Hematology/Oncology, Department of Internal
Medicine, University of Virginia Health Sciences
Center, Charlottesville, Virginia

G. David Roodman, M.D., Ph.D.
Professor, Department of Medicine, University of
Texas Health Sciences Center, San Antonio, Texas

Eric J. Seifter, M.D.
Assistant Professor, Oncology Center, Johns Hopkins
University, Baltimore, Maryland

R. Bradley Slease, M.D.
Professor, Hematology Section, Department of
Medicine, University of Oklahoma Health Sciences
Center, Oklahoma City, Oklahoma

Jerry L. Spivak, M.D.
Professor and Director, Division of Hematology,
Department of Medicine, Johns Hopkins University
School of Medicine, Baltimore, Maryland

Min-Fu Tsan, M.D., Ph.D.
Professor, Department of Medicine, Albany Medical
College, and Associate Chief of Staff for Research
and Development, Department of Veterans Affairs
Medical Center, Albany, New York

Peter H. Wiernik, M.D.
Gutman Professor and Chairman, Department of
Oncology, and Head, Division of Medical Oncology,
Albert Einstein College of Medicine, Bronx, New
York

Bruce A. Yirinec, M.D.
Fellow, Division of Hematology/Oncology,
Department of Internal Medicine, University of
Virginia Health Sciences Center, Charlottesville,
Virginia

The Fundamentals of Clinical Hematology

Third Edition

1

Hematopoietic Stem Cells and Clonal Disorders of Hematopoiesis

Bruce A. Yirinec, M.D., and Peter J. Quesenberry, M.D.

The regulation of human hematopoiesis employs a complex system of humoral and cellular interactions between numerous specialized cells to ensure the appropriate production of mature cellular elements for release into the peripheral blood. Bone marrow, the principle site of hematopoiesis, must continuously replenish the enormous numbers of circulating erythrocytes, leukocytes, and platelets that are lost to normal aging and utilization. It also must respond rapidly to stresses such as bleeding, inflammation, and infection by increasing the production of blood cells to meet increased demand.[1] Similarly, humoral and cellular immunity are dependent on the appropriate increased production of B and T lymphocytes in response to a continued barrage of antigenic stimuli. The understanding of the intricate control mechanisms over these processes has been advanced greatly by the identification of at least 14 hemolymphopoietic growth factors and the ongoing elucidation of their individual and collective roles in hematolymphopoiesis.[2]

A growth factor is a humoral substance defined by its ability to promote the growth, proliferation, and differentiation of receptive cells. It follows that a prerequisite for the identification of such a factor is the availability of an experimental system in which these effects can be demonstrated; erythropoiesis in animal models (mice and rabbit) provided such in vivo systems, from which the first support for humoral regulation of hematopoiesis came. In 1905, Carnot and Deflandre[3] reported that the infusion of serum from an anemic rabbit into a normal rabbit induced a rapid rise in hematocrit, suggesting the

transfer of an erythropoietic stimulatory substance. This humoral regulator of erythropoiesis was defined further by investigations with parabiotic rats and then polycythemic mice in whom erythropoiesis was suppressed by hypertransfusion;[4] the injection of a test substance into these animals, followed by measurement of the subsequent incorporation of radiolabelled iron into the red cells, provided an elegant bioassay of that substance's erythropoietic stimulatory capacity. This provided the basis for the initial characterization of a unique erythropoietic growth factor later termed *erythropoietin*.

Humoral influences on the myelopoietic and lymphoid lineages were not evaluated as easily.[1] In vivo models were inadequate, because these models lacked the internal control present in the hypertransfused mouse model of erythropoiesis. In addition, and in contrast to erythropoietin, there were no recognized disease states of excess or insufficient growth factors to direct the investigation. Therefore, characterization of these substances awaited the development of in vitro assays that would allow a direct observation of their effects on receptive hematopoietic cells that themselves had yet to be identified.

THE HEMATOPOIETIC STEM CELL

A basic tenet of hematology has been the existence of primitive hematopoietic cells from which mature erythrocytes, leukocytes, and platelets derive; relatively few

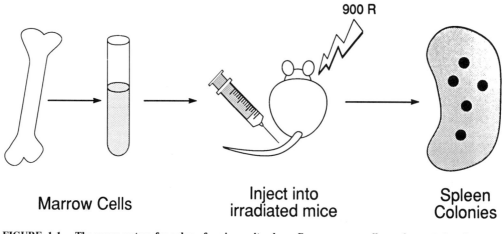

FIGURE 1.1.   The assay system for colony-forming unit-spleen. Bone marrow cells are harvested and injected into the tail vein of a "lethally" irradiated animal, and the subsequent formation of spleen colonies is assessed.

in number, these stem cells must possess extensive proliferative capacities to maintain the enormous cellular output of the bone marrow. In addition, their progeny must possess extensive differentiation capabilities that would result ultimately in the production of mature blood cells, and in the process, the stem cell pool must be sustained to assure the continuance of the hematopoietic process. These properties of high proliferative, differentiative, and self-renewal capabilities serve to define the stem cell.

In 1961, Till and McCulloch[5] provided the first experimental demonstration of the existence of these hematopoietic stem cells. Mouse marrow cells were injected into syngeneic mice that previously had received lethal radiation-induced ablation of their hematopoietic tissue; examination of the spleens 8 days later revealed the formation of discrete nodules consisting of erythroid, granulocytic, megakaryocytic, and undifferentiated cells in pure or mixed populations (Fig. 1.1). These nodules were termed *spleen colonies*. The majority of the spleen colonies were erythroid, with fewer granulocytic, megakaryocytic, and undifferentiated colonies. However, if the time to harvesting the spleen was extended, a majority of colonies were found to have mixed populations.

That the colonies each arose from single marrow cells and were thereby clonal in nature was supported by several observations. First, a linear relationship existed between the number of marrow cells injected and the number of spleen colonies formed.[5] In addition, radiation survival curves were compatible with the behavior of single cells. However, more definitive proof of the clonal nature of these nodules was provided by experi-

ments that utilized cells with radiation-induced chromosomal markers; in this situation, it was observed that the chromosomal marker was present in 95% to 99% of metaphases in some colonies.[6] Additional evidence for the clonality of these spleen colonies was provided by studies in which mixtures of normal and syngeneic cells with unique chromosomal markers were injected into irradiated assay animals and the karyotypes of the colonies determined; it was found that either all metaphases from individual colonies were normal or that all had the unique chromosomal marker. No mixed karyotypes were observed.[7]

These clonal colonies supported the existence of a murine marrow cell capable of extensive proliferation and differentiation, and this cell was termed the *colony-forming unit-spleen* (CFU-S). The self-renewal potential of the CFU-S was demonstrated by removing single-cell–derived colonies from the spleen 10 to 14 days after cell injection, then reinjecting a suspension of each into lethally-irradiated mice;[8] anywhere from 0 to 1000 new colonies per original colony were found. In addition, pure colonies of any one cell type were found to contain CFU-S that on retransplantation could form colonies of all cell types, suggesting that CFU-S is a pluripotential stem cell capable of differentiating along several lineage pathways.

Local environmental influences play an important role in determining the differentiation pathway the CFU-S takes.[9] Certain locations within the spleen appear to promote preferentially the formation of colonies with distinct cellular composition. Approximately 50% of spleen colonies are on the surface of the spleen, and 80% of these are erythroid or mixed. Erythroid colonies also tend to occur in the red pulp but not in the lymphoid follicles, and granulocytic colonies tend to grow along the trabeculae of the spleen or in subcapsular sheets and only occasionally beneath the capsule. Although this demonstration technically is more difficult, colonies of hematopoietic cells also are found in the marrow; unlike spleen colonies, these tend to differentiate along the granulocytic pathway.[9,10] The marrow microenvironment contains fibroblasts, endothelial cells, macrophages, and adventitial reticulum cells collectively called *stromal cells.* When irradiated marrow stroma devoid of hematopoietic cells is implanted in the spleens of lethally irradiated mice and marrow cells then injected into these same mice, the colonies that form in the marrow stroma are mostly granulocytic; those that form in the spleen mostly erythroid, again reflecting differential microenvironmental influences.[10]

CLONAL CULTURE TECHNIQUES

The development of techniques for in vitro cultures of marrow cells greatly facilitated the further characterization of hematopoietic stem cells, and the introduction of plasma clot[11,12] and methylcellulose[13] clonal culture techniques allowed in vitro study of erythropoiesis. Previous in vivo studies with erythropoietin suggested that the target cell of the hormone was a population of stem cells that were more differentiated than CFU-S and committed to erythropoiesis but that were morphologically distinct from erythroblasts.[14,15] This intermediate compartment of stem cells (termed the *erythropoietin-responsive cell compartment*) appeared to proliferate more rapidly than CFU-S and also recovered sooner after irradiation. Using the in vitro plasma clot culture technique, Axelrad et al.[11,12] further identified two separate classes of erythroid stem cells distinguished by their erythropoietin requirements and rapidity of growth. The burst-forming unit-erythroid (BFU-E) is a primitive erythroid stem cell that requires high levels of erythropoietin and a relatively long culture period to yield colonies; in contrast, a second stem cell, termed the *colony-forming unit-erythroid* (CFU-E), was found to give rise to small clusters of erythroid cells after several days of culture requiring relatively small amounts of erythropoietin. Evidence suggested that this second stem cell represented a mature descendant of the BFU-E. Hypertransfusion or actinomycin D selectively ablated the CFU-E compartment and led to increases in marrow BFU-E;[16] thus, erythropoietin appeared to both promote BFU-E differentiation to CFU-E and serve as a necessary factor for the in vivo survival of CFU-E.

Nonerythroid stem cell compartments were defined only after the development by Bradley and Metcalf[17] as

well as Pluznik and Sachs[18] of in vitro semisolid culture techniques that allowed for direct observation of the clonal growth of these cells under various environmental conditions. In this manner, it was discovered that a manipulation of the culture conditions, using various conditioned media or biologic fluids, could result in the preferential growth of colonies of specific cell types, including granulocytes, macrophages, erythrocytes, megakaryocytes, basophils, and eosinophils, as well as colonies of mixed cell population. Each type of colony required distinctly defined conditions for optimal growth.[19]

Combining in vitro clonal and liquid cultures and in vivo transplant models, investigators now have defined a number of stem/progenitor cells,[20,21] which are outlined in Table 1.1. Major points include the existence of an apparent stem cell hierarchy, including very primitive cells with extensive in vivo repopulating self-renewal, proliferative, and differentiative potential. These cells have been termed *long-term repopulating cells* and in general have not been found to express lineage-specific markers, that is, they are lineage negative and in the mouse express a limited number of specific antigenic markers (Sca, F*all*-3, c-*kit*). Their human counterpart also is lineage negative and expresses CD34 and low levels of HLA. These very primitive cells in general proliferate slowly, or in G_o, stain weakly for the mitochondrial dye rhodamine and adhere to marrow stromal cells in vitro. These "stem" cells may be responsible primarily for long-term in vivo marrow repopulation after marrow transplantation.

Another class of less primitive stem cells may account for short-term in vivo marrow repopulation.[20,21] This cell appears to have many surface characteristics of the long-term repopulating cells but stains brightly with rhodamine. In vitro models for these early cells include the blast colony-forming unit and high proliferative potential colony-forming cells. At varying time intervals (days 9 to 14), the CFU-S, which was the initial model for stem cell biology, in fact may represent a class of progenitor/stem cells overlapping with the short-term repopulating cells and more differentiated progenitor cells. In general, these more primitive stem cell classes appear to be responsive to multiple cytokines in regard to survival, proliferation, and differentiation.

More differentiated cells have been termed *progenitors,* and in vitro clonal assays have been described for colony-forming cell-megakaryocyte; granulocyte-macrophage; granulocyte; macrophage; eosinophil; mast cell; and a large number of bi, tri, quadra, penta, and hexa-lineage cells. In general, these progenitors have less renewal and proliferative responsiveness, and they respond to a more restricted number of cytokines[20] (discussed later) (Fig. 1.2). The work on in vitro cloning

TABLE 1.1. Hemopoietic Stem/Progenitor Cells

Stem/Progenitor Cell	Lineage	Growth Factor
Colony forming unit spleen, murine only, days 8 to 9 and 10 to 12	Erythroid, megakaryocyte, granulocyte/macrophage, and self-renewal	IL-3 and probably many others
Granulocyte-macrophage colony-forming cell	Granulocyte/macrophage	GM-CSF (to some extent G-CSF and CSF-1)
Macrophage colony-forming cell	Macrophage/monocyte	CSF-1 (to some extent GM-CSF and IL-3)
Granulocyte colony-forming cell	Granulocyte	G-CSF (to some extent GM-CSF and IL-3)
High proliferative potential colony-forming cell	Macrophage (potential for granulocyte, megakaryocyte)	CSF-1 and IL-3, and IL-1. Also GM-CSF and CSF-1, IL-3 and G-CSF, G-CSF and CSF-1, G-CSF and GM-CSF, IL-3 and GM-CSF, CSF-1 and IL-1 and IL-3 and combinations of three to six factors including c-*kit* ligand
Colony-forming unit-erythroid	Erythroid	Erythropoietin
Burst-forming unit-erythroid	Erythroid	Erythropoietin and G-CSF, IL-3, GM-CSF, or IL-4
Colony-forming unit-megakaryocyte	Megakaryocyte	IL-3, GM-CSF, G-CSF, IL-6, IL-4, IL-1, and thrombopoietin-like activities
Burst-forming unit-megakaryocyte	Megakaryocyte	IL-3, GM-CSF, thrombopoietin-like activity, and phorbol myristate acetate or cholera toxin, and various cytokine combinations
Colony-forming unit-granulocyte/erythroid/macrophage and megakaryocyte	Granulocyte/megakaryocyte/macrophage, and possibly T cell	IL-3 and GM-CSF
Blast colony	Blast cells renewal and multilineage differentiation	IL-3, G-CSF, IL-6, and possibly GM-CSF
Colony-forming unit-diffusion chamber	Granulocyte/macrophage, some megakaryocyte, erythroid	Not defined
Thy-1^{lo}Lin$^-$Sca-1$^+$ (murine only)	T, B, and myeloid cells	Multifactor responsive (not responsive to single factors)
CD34$^+$ HLA low lin$^-$ rhodamine dull and adherent to "stromal cells" (human only)	Multilineage	Multifactor responsive

Note: CSF = colony-stimulating factor; G-CSF = granulocyte colony-stimulating factor; GM-CSF = granulocyte-macrophage colony-stimulating factor; IL = interleukin; lin$^-$ = lineage negative.

indicated the existence of numerous regulatory hormones capable of stimulating stem cells or their immature progeny to form colonies of mature cells; these colony-stimulating factors (CSFs) were named for the morphology of the cells within the colonies each were stimulated to form, while other growth factors, termed *interleukins* (IL), were defined largely by in vitro liquid culture systems.

GENERAL CHARACTERISTICS

The hemolymphopoietic growth factors are glycoproteins ranging in size from 18,000 to more than 90,000 kd. Most are monomeric proteins, but CSF-1 and IL-5 exist as homodimers. These two also have membrane-based and excreted forms. The biologic activity of each cytokine is derived from the native nonglycosylated protein, and the carbohydrate moieties attached via posttranslational glycosylation appear to protect each hormone from degradation. In addition, these carbohydrate moieties may influence the biodistribution of some cytokines by affecting their binding affinities to extracellular matrix proteins such as proteoglycans. Evidence from studies using long-term cultures suggests that such interactions between cytokines and extracellular matrix proteins may facilitate the presentation of growth factors to their receptors on target cells.[23]

A unique gene encodes for each growth factor.[22] There is little sequence homology among the genes for the various human cytokines, with the exception of IL-6 and granulocyte colony-stimulating factor (G-CSF), which share several nearly identical coding sequences. However, some cross-species sequence homology exists, as evidenced by the erythropoietin gene, which is

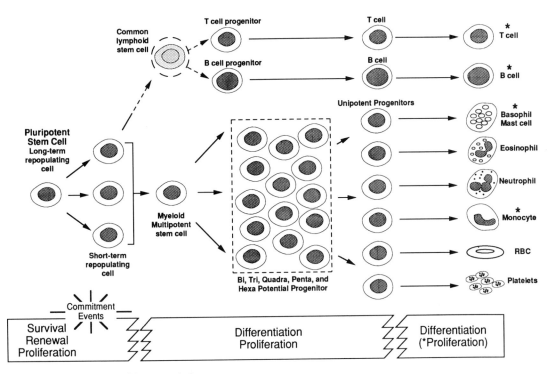

FIGURE 1.2. A model of hematopoiesis.

identical in mouse, monkey, and human; nevertheless, the final protein products display less similarity, with 79% (mouse) and 94% (monkey) homologies with the human gene product. Several growth factors demonstrate cross-species activity as well; for example, murine cells respond to human erythropoietin, G-CSF, CSF-1, IL-5, and IL-6. Such examples of the relative conservation of structure and function of these cytokines across species attest to the importance of their biologic roles in ensuring the survival of the organism.

The chromosomal locations for the genes encoding many of the human growth factors have been identified,[22] and those for granulocyte-macrophage colony-stimulating factor (GM-CSF), CSF-1, IL-3, platelet-derived growth factor, and endothelial cell growth factor are clustered on the long arm of chromosome 5. This area also contains genes for several receptors, including the CSF-1 receptor, glucocorticoid receptor, and β_2-adrenergic receptor. Interestingly, a deletion of this portion of the genome (5q$^-$) is found in subsets of patients with a myelodysplastic syndrome and secondary acute myeloid leukemia, and it is associated with a poor prognosis. Whether this hemizygous state may contribute in the pathogenesis of these diseases is still under investigation.

The processes involved in regulating the expression of the cytokine genes are not well understood. A variety

of stimuli, including bacterial infection, endotoxin, tumor necrosis factor, IL-1, interferon, hypoxia, phorbol esters, and various lectins, can induce the production of growth factors. In the homeostatic state, growth factors, excluding erythropoietin, generally are present in low concentrations in the peripheral circulation; in the setting of acute stress, as with infection or tissue injury, cytokine levels rapidly rise. IL-1, IL-6, and G-CSF demonstrate the most pronounced increases in concentration. A wide variety of cells are capable of producing cytokines, including T cells, B cells, monocytes, macrophages, endothelial cells, fibroblasts, vascular smooth muscle cells, mesothelial cells, microglial cells, astrocytes, polymorphonuclear cells, keratinocytes, thymic epithelial cells, synoviocytes, mesangial cells, osteoblasts, and natural killer cells; G-CSF, GM-CSF, and CSF-1 are produced most commonly.[24] These may constitute a network of peripheral sentinel cells that respond to noxious stimuli by releasing growth factors, which in turn promote increased hematopoiesis and marrow stromal cytokine production (Fig. 1.3).

The hemolymphopoietic growth factors share several other important properties as well. All exert biologic activity at extremely low concentrations, and minor perturbations in the hormonal microenvironment may have dramatic effects on the growth and differentiation of cells. Although initially defined by their abilities to

Cytokine Emergency Response

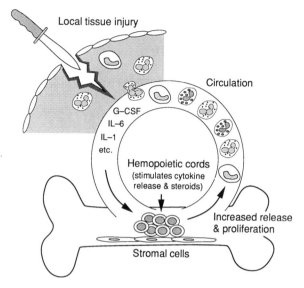

FIGURE 1.3.   A model of the response to inflammatory stimulus for the regulation of myeloid cell production.

effect discrete changes in the proliferation, differentiation, or function of specific cells, these cytokines have broad activity on multiple target cells. Within a cell lineage, they may induce the proliferation and differentiation of the immature progenitors while promoting functional changes such as chemotaxis in their mature progeny. In addition, each usually displays varying effects on multiple cell lineages, as illustrated by the actions of IL-6 on B cells, myeloma cells, megakaryocytes, granulocytes, monocytes, and early stem cells. Only two factors appear to have lineage specificity: erythropoietin for the erythroid pathway, and CSF-1 for the macrophage pathway.

The consequence of this schema is that target cells may be stimulated simultaneously by multiple cytokines. In general, these growth factor interactions are synergistic or additive, and up to (or over) seven factor synergies exist.[1] This may be an important mechanism by which these factors exert local influences at extremely low concentrations within the marrow microenvironment. Stromal cells could modulate the proliferation, differentiation, and survival of early stem cells by secreting low levels of a variety of cytokines, thereby creating a complex hormonal milieu; in this setting, differentiation pathways could be determined by either the relative local concentrations of growth factors, the sequence of growth factor-receptor interactions, or the actual configuration of a series of growth factors pre-

sented to a target stem cell. In situations of physiologic stress such as infection, the highly elevated levels of circulating cytokines could override these normal local regulatory mechanisms.

ERYTHROPOIETIN

Although the existence of erythropoietin (epo) was first demonstrated experimentally in 1906, the protein was not biochemically defined until 1977, when Miyake et al., utilizing purified hormone from human urine, determined a partial amino acid sequence. In 1985, the human erythropoietin gene was cloned simultaneously by Lin et al. and Jacobs et al., thus allowing mass production of the first recombinant hematopoietic growth factor.

Erythropoietin is relatively unique among the hemopoietins in that it most closely behaves as a classic hormone in the physiologic sense. It is produced largely in the kidneys, and more than 90% of circulating levels in adult mammals is secreted by the kidneys.[19] A peritubular interstitial cell is responsible, as evidenced by studies of the in situ expression of erythropoietin mRNA.[26,27] The liver, the principal producer of erythropoietin in utero, supplies less than 10% in adults. Hepatocytes are the principal source.[28] Tissue hypoxia secondary to anemia, hypoxemia, ischemia, or high oxygen-affinity hemoglobins is the stimulus for the increased production of epo[29] although the mechanism by which this occurs remains unclear. An oxygen-sensing heme protein may be involved, because there is evidence that carbon monoxide can inhibit hypoxemia-induced production of erythropoietin.[30]

Erythropoietin promotes erythropoiesis by a poorly understood mechanism.[25] Studies have demonstrated the induction of rapid increases in intracellular calcium concentrations following ligand-receptor binding, suggesting that calcium may be involved in the second message. Although relatively lineage specific, erythropoietin has in vitro stimulatory effects on megakaryocytic lineages;[31] the in vivo importance of this is unclear as neither platelet nor white blood cell counts are elevated in patients with secondary polycythemia and increased endogenous erythropoietin levels. Similarly, transgenic mice given an extra erythropoietin gene demonstrate isolated erythrocytosis without alterations in other cell counts. Erythropoietin also interacts with other growth factors, such as IL-3, IL-4, G-CSF, and GM-CSF, to stimulate early erythroid progenitors. In addition, a number of hormones that have no intrinsic erythropoietin activity appear to be capable of potentiating the effects of erythropoietin on the in vitro growth of erythroid clones; these include growth hormone,[32] thyroid hormones,[33] and androgens.[34] These studies may explain the erythropoietic effect of exogenous androgens in vivo in humans as well as the anemias seen in posthypophysectomy or hypothyroidism.

COLONY-STIMULATING FACTOR-1

Colony-stimulating factor-1 was the first CSF to be defined biochemically.[25] As its alternate name, macrophage colony-stimulating factor, suggests, CSF-1 was characterized initially by its effects on the monocyte–macrophage lineage during in vitro agar colony assays. The original sources of CSF-1 were human urine and murine L-cell conditioned media; subsequently, the murine and human genes were identified and cloned. CSF-1 demonstrates relative lineage specificity by primarily stimulating the proliferation and differentiation of macrophage colonies. However, it does appear to display some stimulatory activity on neutrophil progenitors in culture as well. GM-CSF greatly enhances the proliferative effects of CSF-1 on the formation of human macrophage colonies, and such synergistic activity is common among the hematopoietic cytokines. Indeed, CSF-1 acts in combination with GM-CSF, G-CSF, IL-1, and IL-3 to affect the colony formation of early hematopoietic progenitors, including those of high proliferative potential colony-forming cells.

The hemopoietins commonly effect changes in the functional status of their target cells. CSF-1 enhances the ability of mature macrophages to partake in antibody-dependent cell-mediated cytotoxicity and tumor-cell killing. It also increases macrophage phagocytic capabilities while promoting increased intracellular killing of candida. In addition, CSF-1 induces human monocyte migration. At low concentrations, CSF-1 has the capacity to decrease macrophage protein catabolism and increases in vitro survival; at higher concentrations, it promotes protein synthesis and stimulates cell proliferation. CSF-1 also stimulates the production and/or release of a variety of substances by monocytes and macrophages, including G-CSF, IL-1, interferon, tumor necrosis factor, plasminogen activator, ferritin, superoxide dismutase, and prostaglandin E.

GRANULOCYTE-MACROPHAGE COLONY-STIMULATING FACTOR

Granulocyte-macrophage colony-stimulating factor was defined by its ability to promote the in vitro colony formation of pure granulocytes, monocytes, or mixed granulocyte-monocyte populations.[25] GM-CSF was isolated originally from murine lung-conditioned medium and later from a human T-cell leukemic line. Both human and murine genes have been cloned, and recombinant DNA technology has provided commercial production of the human cytokine. Unlike CSF-1, GM-CSF demonstrates greater lineage promiscuity, with proliferative/differentiative effects on several cell types; these include normal human promyelocytes and myelocytes in the granulocyte pathway, monocytes, eosinophils, basophils, and progenitors of megakaryocytes and eosinophils. Myeloid leukemic cells possess GM-CSF receptors and demonstrate proliferative responses to the cytokine both in vitro and in vivo. In addition, GM-CSF stimulates the growth of several nonhematopoietic cells, including fibroblasts, endothelial cells, and certain neoplastic cell lines including small-cell and colon carcinomas. Several synergistic actions have been identified as well. GM-CSF amplifies in vitro erythropoietin-induced erythroid colony formation, and in concert with CSF-1, IL-3, or G-CSF, it supports the proliferation of the murine high proliferative potential colony-forming cells. Similarly, GM-CSF supports the in vitro proliferation of primitive human stem cells. GM-CSF also has direct effects on the lymphoid system, as evidenced by its augmentation of the IL-2–induced proliferation of T cells.

A multitude of alterations in the functional capabilities of mature neutrophils are affected by GM-CSF, and both cytotoxic and phagocytic activities against bacteria, yeast, parasites, and antibody-coated tumor cells are enhanced. Superoxide anion production is increased, and leukotriene B_4 synthesis is promoted. GM-CSF inhibits the motile and migratory capabilities of neutrophils and enhances the cell–cell adhesion capacity of mature granulocytes by increasing the expression of adhesion-promoting glycoproteins on the cell surface. GM-CSF also enhances human eosinophil cytotoxicity and leukotriene synthesis, and it promotes human basophil histamine release.

GRANULOCYTE COLONY-STIMULATING FACTOR

Granulocyte colony-stimulating factor initially was characterized by its ability to stimulate the in vitro formation of pure granulocyte colonies,[25] and it has been demonstrated since to have a broader spectrum of activity. Like GM-CSF, G-CSF was purified first from mouse lung culture media. Both murine and human G-CSF genes have been cloned, and recombinant human G-CSF is now available for clinical use. G-CSF stimulates some granulocyte-macrophage progenitors *in vitro* as well as some human myeloid leukemia cells. Endothelial cells, fibroblasts, and some small-cell carcinoma cell lines are sensitive to its proliferation effects, and G-CSF demonstrates synergistic activity with several cytokines. In combination with IL-3, it stimulates *in vitro* both megakaryocyte colony and blast colony formation; it also induces pre-B–cell generation in liquid culture systems. G-CSF interacts with GM-CSF to promote granulocyte-macrophage colonies and with GM-CSF, IL-3, or CSF-1 to stimulate high proliferative potential colony-forming cells; therefore, it may exert significant influence on primitive marrow stem cells. Among G-CSF's qualitative effects on mature progeny are increased chemotactic abilities of both neutrophils and monocytes as well as enhanced antibody-dependent cell-mediated cytotoxicity, phagocytosis, and superoxide anion release by granulocytes. The ability of G-CSF to stimulate neutrophilic leukocytosis via increased marrow production and release of granulocytes into circulation has led to its clinical use in various neutropenic states.

INTERLEUKIN-3

Interleukin-3, or multi-colony-stimulating factor, is a testament to the diverse spectrum of activity of most hematopoietins.[25] Progenitors of virtually all the myeloid lineages, including megakaryocytes, granulocytes, macrophages, eosinophils, basophils, and mast cells, as well as erythrocytes and the lymphoid lineages of B cells, T cells, and natural killer cells exhibit variable degrees of responsiveness to this cytokine. Initially purified from the WEHI-3B murine myelomonocytic leukemic line, IL-3 was characterized by its ability to induce 20-α-hydroxy steroid dehydrogenase activity in splenic lymphocytes and thus was defined as a T-lymphocyte stimulator and, hence, an interleukin. Both murine and human IL-3 genes have been cloned, and recombinant human IL-3 is available for clinical trials.

Interleukin-3 has synergistic activity with several growth factors. It acts in concert with erythropoietin to stimulate erythroid stem cells, and in combination with CSF-1, GM-CSF, and G-CSF, IL-3 stimulates high proliferative potential colony-forming cells as well as the proliferation of blood monocytes and peritoneal macrophages. In murine models, IL-3 with GM-CSF and CSF-1 induces progenitor cells into cell cycle; in primate models, sequential IL-3 followed by GM-CSF synergistically increases the levels of neutrophils, monocytes, lymphocytes, and eosinophils. IL-3 augments megakaryocytic colony proliferation induced by GM-CSF and has prominent proliferative effects on the eosinophilic and mast cell lineages. Additional biologic activities include the promotion of increased neutrophil, monocyte, eosinophil, mast cell, and platelet counts.

IN VIVO ACTION AND CLINICAL UTILITY

Recombinant erythropoietin, G-CSF, GM-CSF, CSF-1, and IL-3 have now been extensively tested in both animal species and humans, and the first three have been approved by the Food and Drug Administration for various clinical indications.[35,36] In general, they have been found to stimulate in vivo the lineages that would have been predicted from their in vitro actions. Erythropoietin reproducibly stimulates the production of red cells in the mouse and human and has been found to be highly effective in correcting the anemia of renal failure as well as the anemia associated with rheumatoid arthritis, cancer, and HIV infection. Its utility in other disease states continues to be evaluated. The administration of G-CSF in vivo predominantly stimulates neutrophil production but also has variable effects on lymphocyte and platelet levels. It has been shown to be extraordinarily effective in raising neutrophil levels and in preventing infections in most patients with chronic neutropenias, including those with cyclic neutropenia, chronic idiopathic neutropenia, and Kostmann syndrome; it also has been shown to lessen the severity of neutropenia and its accompanying morbidity in patients treated with cytotoxic anticancer drugs. GM-CSF stimulates a broader range of cell types in vivo, including neutrophils, monocytes, eosinophils, basophils, and variably, lymphocytes and platelets; paradoxically, the latter sometimes fall with the administration of GM-CSF. As with G-CSF, GM-CSF lessens the neutropenia seen after cancer chemotherapy, but as yet, neither agent has been shown to increase survival in cancer patients. CSF-1 predominantly increases macrophages, and IL-3 has multilineage effects in humans with more predominant effects on platelet levels than the other cytokines tested.

THE OTHER INTERLEUKINS

A number of other cytokines have been described, some of which are now entering or already in clinical trials.[25] IL-1 has many effects on many systems, such as inducing other cytokines from a number of cells; stimulating T and B cells; and directly stimulating relatively early stem cells, especially when in combination with other cytokines such as CSF-1, G-CSF, or GM-CSF. Especially when in concert with other cytokines, IL-1 also has been shown to lessen neutropenia after irradiation or cytoxic drugs in animals and humans. IL-2 is a T-cell growth factor and has been used widely in vitro for possible antitumor effects. IL-4 was characterized first as a B-cell factor, but IL-4 clearly has effects on myeloid lineages when combined with other cytokines. IL-5 is a B-cell factor and has eosinophil-stimulating activity, and it also stimulates mast cells. IL-6 is a very pleiotropic agent that stimulates B cells, T cells, neutrophils, monocytes, and megakaryocytes, has impressive platelet-stimulating effects in primates, and is entering clinical trials. IL-7 was defined as a pre-B-cell factor and has particularly prominent effects when in combination with c-*kit* ligand; it also has stimulatory effects in vivo on platelet recovery in irradiated mice. IL-8 and IL-10 are not growth factors, or at least have not been fully characterized as such. IL-8 is an inflammatory mediator, while IL-10 inhibits the secretion of various cytokines. IL-9 is both a T-cell factor and a cytokine that synergizes with erythropoietin. IL-11 is a cytokine with a spectrum of biologic activity virtually identical to that of IL-6.

c-*Kit* Ligand and Receptor

There are two murine models of marrow deficiency states, the W/W^v and S1/S1^d mice. In the former, a deficiency of marrow stem cells leads to a macrocytic anemia with lesser defects in other myeloid lineages; the S1/S1^d mouse has an identical phenotype but normal stem cells and a defective microenvironment. Both mice also have germ cell and melanocyte defects. Elegant studies showed that the macrocytic anemia and stem cell deficit in W/W^v mice could be corrected by stem cells from the S1/S1^d mouse, and the microenvironmental defect in S1/S1^d mice could be corrected by "stroma" (irradiated spleen tissue) from W/W^v mice. In a similar vein, the melanocyte and, to a lesser extent, the germ cell defects in these mice showed cross-complementation.

The discovery that the W/W^v defect mapped to the c-*kit* oncogene and was caused by point mutations affecting the tyrosine kinase receptor coded for by c-*kit* eventually was followed by the characterization of the ligand for this receptor, termed *c-kit ligand, stem cell factor, mast cell factor,* or *steel factor*.[37] The abnormalities in S1/S1^d mice were found to be based on a deficiency of this factor, a cytokine with a secreted and stromally based form; this cytokine appears to be a potent growth factor for very primitive stem cells that acts synergistically with many other growth factors to stimulate erythroid, granulocyte-macrophage, mast cell, megakaryocyte, and lymphoid lineages. In vivo activity has been demonstrated, and clinical trials are beginning.

RECEPTORS AND SECOND MESSENGER SIGNALING

The receptors on which cytokines act have been divided into several receptor families, characterized by either structure or enzyme activity. One receptor family, termed the *hemopoietin receptor family*, is characterized in its extracellular domain by having four cysteines and a Trp-Ser-X-Trp-Ser motif near the transmembrane region of the receptor. This characteristic structure is evidenced by receptors for prolactin, erythropoietin, GM-CSF, G-CSF, and IL-2 through IL-7.[38]

Another receptor family is coded for by oncogenes; and expresses tyrosine kinase activity. Included in this family are receptors for CSF-1 (the c-*fms* receptor), platelet-derived growth factor, and c-*kit* ligand or steel factor.

Interleukin-1α and IL-1β, although sharing only a 25% homology, interact with some receptors with the same biologic results. Recently, an IL-1 receptor antagonist was defined and genetically cloned, and this shows 25% homology with IL-1α and -β. However, it blocks the action of both at the receptor.

Recent work also has indicated that high-affinity receptors exist for GM-CSF, IL-5, and IL-3 consisting of dimer pairs of α- and β-chains. The α-chains are specific for each cytokine and constitute low-affinity receptors; they also share a common β-chain. Competition between these cytokines for receptor binding on specific cell classes (monocyte for GM-CSF and IL-3; or basophil, and eosinophil for GM-CSF, IL-3, and IL-5) appears to be explained by the limited availability of the β-chain. Differences in these receptor families may determine in part differences in second messenger signaling.

The mechanism by which cytokine-receptor interactions signal a cell to survive, proliferate, or differentiate still are not well understood. A number of Ser-Thr or tyrosine kinases have been implicated, along with a specific calmodulin-binding protein, and Raf-1 and MAP-1 kinases may be specific entities involved in cytokine signaling. The nuclear mechanisms also are just being worked out, but cytokines clearly alter various transcription factors and CSF-1 was shown recently to induce cell-cycle progression by modulating cyclins.

INHIBITORS

Inhibitors of hematopoiesis or stem cells have been relatively poorly characterized in the past, but with the availability of serum-free systems and purified progenitors (stem cell populations), a fuller understanding of the importance of inhibitors is developing. A number of substances, including lactoferrin, interferons, and acidic isoferritins, have been implicated as inhibitors of hemopoiesis. More recently, transforming growth factor-beta and macrophage inflammatory protein-1α have been found to be potent inhibitors of relatively early hematopoietic progenitor/stem cells.

CLINICAL DISORDERS OF CYTOKINES AND STEM CELLS

Chronic Myelogenous Leukemia

A number of disorders of hematopoietic stem cells have been defined, and chronic myelogenous leukemia (CML) is perhaps the prototypic clonal stem cell disease. Studies in the 1960s showed that the Philadelphia chromosome (9;22 translocation) was present in erythroid, granulocytic, and megakaryocytic cells. The Philadelphia chromosome was not found in fibroblasts or lymphocytes. However, other studies[39,40] have indicated the origin of at least some B and T cells from CML progenitors; these data indicate that CML is a clonal disorder involving the myeloid pluripotent stem cell. We now know that this translocation places the breakpoint cluster region adjacent to the oncogene *abl* and results in a characteristic breakpoint cluster region–*abl* fusion protein.

Further evidence of the clonality of CML has been derived from a study of persons heterozygous for the X-linked glucose-6-phosphate dehydrogenase (G6PD) locus.[41] The Lyon hypothesis states that X chromosomes are randomly inactivated early in embryogenesis. Thus, individuals heterozygous for an X-linked characteristic such as G6PD isoenzymes A and B will have cells either positive for isoenzyme A or isoenzyme B; no cells will have both isoenzymes.[42] If a cell population is derived from multiple cells, both isoenzymes should be present, but if the cell population is derived from a single progenitor cell, that is, the cell population is clonal, then it will contain only one isoenzyme. Because G6PD isoenzymes can be detected from extracts of as few as 50 cells, this method permitted a determination of whether cell populations from a number of different disease states are either clonal (contain one isoenzyme type) or derived from multiple cells (contain both isoenzymes). Studies in black patients with CML who were heterozygous for G6PD isoenzymes A and B have revealed that platelets, red cells, and granulocytes contain one isoenzyme type, while fibroblasts and lymphocytes contain both isoenzymes;[43,44] studies by Fialkow[45] also showed that while lymphoid cells do not appear to have the Philadelphia chromosome, subpopulations of B lymphocytes appear to have a clonal origin based on G6PD markers. Not all B or T lymphocytes are derived from the clone, but it appears clear that some are, suggesting that the neoplastic transformation in CML may indeed involve a stem cell common to the hematopoietic stem cell and the lymphocytic progenitors. The speculation that CML may involve a stem cell common to both the myeloid and lymphoid lines is supported further by observations that a significant proportion of patients with CML who undergo blast transformation (approximately 20%) have blasts with a lymphoid morphology and respond to chemotherapy that is ordinarily most effective for acute lymphocytic leukemia, that is, regimens containing vincristine and prednisone.[46,47]

Terminal deoxynucleotidyl transferase (TdT) is a unique DNA synthetic enzyme whose expression is restricted under ordinary conditions to primitive cells in the thymus and prothymocytes in the bone marrow, and its presence in blasts from a relatively large percentage of patients with CML in blast crisis also suggests a lymphoid-type transformation in some of these cases.[48] TdT activity of blasts seems to be a good discriminator between lymphoblasts, which are positive, and myeloblasts, which are negative, in the acute leukemias. Thus, the finding of TdT-positive blasts in patients with CML in blast crisis suggests that the blast transformation in these cases may occur in lymphoid cells. However, it should be noted that there is a poor correlation between the morphology of the blasts and whether they are TdT positive.[48]

Chronic myelogenous leukemia stem cells are cytokine responsive. Juvenile CML appears to be related to a selective hypersensitivity of the neoplastic progenitors to GM-CSF.[49]

Polycythemia Vera

Polycythemia vera is a disease that involves neoplastic transformation of the hematopoietic stem cell. Studies utilizing G6PD isoenzyme markers have shown that red cells, platelets, and granulocytes are clonal in this disorder, whereas lymphocytes and fibroblasts are not.[50] However, there are early, conflicting studies regarding the involvement of lymphocytes;[51] studies by Prchal et al.[52] showed that in vitro erythroid colonies (CFU-E) from patients with polycythemia vera grew without added erythropoietin, indicating that either growth was autonomous or that the CFU-E were responding to extremely low concentrations of erythropoietin present in the fetal calf serum used in the culture media.[52] Studies that utilized G6PD isoenzyme markers for the erythroid clones demonstrated that all the "autonomous" clones had only one type of isoenzyme, but when exogenous erythropoietin was added to the culture wells, increasing numbers of colonies formed that contained both isoenzyme types. This latter observation strongly suggests there is a coexistent normal clone of stem cells in polycythemia vera that probably is suppressed in vivo because of low to absent erythropoietin production associated with the erythrocytosis. More recent studies suggest that polycythemia vera erythroid progenitors have only a single, low-affinity receptor, indicating that the progenitor cells in polycythemia vera are not more sensitive to erythropoietin than are normal progenitors. Other studies have indicated the production of mitogenic factors from peripheral blood mononuclear cells of patients with polycythemia vera as well.[53]

Myelofibrosis and Myeloid Metaplasia

Along with CML and polycythemia vera, myelofibrosis and myeloid metaplasia have been classified as myeloproliferative disorders. Controversy has existed as to whether the marrow myelofibrosis was a primary feature of this disease or a secondary reactive phenomenon. One female patient with myelofibrosis and myeloid metaplasia was studied utilizing the G6PD isoenzyme marker system,[54] and in this case, the red cells, platelets, and granulocytes were clonal while skin- and marrow-derived fibroblasts had both isoenzyme types. These data indicate that the marrow fibrosis is a secondary phenomenon in at least some cases of myelofibrosis and myeloid metaplasia and suggest chemotherapy may have a place in the treatment of this disease. Regression of fibrosis after marrow transplantation also suggests that the fibrosis is secondary, and speculation has linked the fibrosis in some cases to the production of platelet-derived growth factor by the neoplastic clone. In addition, the data on the myeloproliferative diseases suggest that the marrow fibrosis occasionally seen in polycythemia vera and CML may be a secondary reactive event as well.

Preleukemic Disorders

One group of disorders is related in certain ways to the myeloproliferative syndromes and probably represents neoplastic transformations at the level of the hematopoietic stem cell; these disorders include the myelodysplastic syndromes and paroxysmal nocturnal hemoglobinuria (PNH). The evidence that these are clonal disorders of the hematopoietic stem cells is not as definitive as the evidence in CML, polycythemia vera, and myelofibrosis and myeloid metaplasia, but it is suggestive nevertheless. Some patients with myelodysplastic syndromes will develop acute myelogenous leukemia (AML), and at presentation, there are frequent dysplastic features in all three cell lines.

Paroxysmal nocturnal hemoglobinuria is characterized by abnormal sensitivity of the red cells to complement lysis.[55] However, it has been demonstrated that both platelets and granulocytes also have an abnormal sensitivity to lysis by antibodies and complement;[56,57] furthermore, in one female patient heterozygous for the A and B isoenzymes of G6PD, the complement-sensitive red blood cells contained only the B isoenzyme,

indicating a clonal origin.[58] A number of proteins are absent or decreased on PNH cells, including acetylcholinesterase, FCRγIII, DAF, or CD59. It now has been established that patients with PNH have cells that lack proteins anchored by glycosyl-phosphatidylinositol (GPI) linkages.[59] This defect in GPI-anchored proteins may underlie the complement sensitivity of both differentiated and progenitor cells. The observations that aplastic anemia precedes some cases of PNH and that some cases of PNH evolve into AML are additional clues suggesting this disease may involve primarily an abnormality at the hematopoietic stem cell level. It also is intriguing that a number of patients with myelofibrosis and myeloid metaplasia or aplastic anemia have a population of red cells having abnormal complement sensitivity.[60,61]

The myelodysplastic syndromes appear to involve a neoplastic derangement at the hematopoietic stem cell level. The preleukemic state presents as chronic refractory anemia, neutropenia, thrombocytopenia, and dysplastic abnormalities of all three cell lines in the bone marrow, usually with increased levels of immature myeloid elements; however, it cannot be diagnosed as overt AML. Studies using restriction fragment length polymorphisms have recently shown that seven of eight patients with myelodysplastic syndromes had a clonal process involving myeloid and lymphoid series; other studies using G6PD analysis have indicated that red cells, platelets, and granulocytes in myelodysplastic syndromes are clonal.[62] Bone marrow cells from individuals with myelodysplastic syndromes usually, but not always, show defective in vitro CFU-C growth, frequently with abnormal differentiation, and myelodysplastic syndromes cells are sensitive to a number of cytokines, GM-CSF producing more proliferation and G-CSF more differentiation. Clinical studies have indicated that the administration of GM-CSF to patients with myelodysplastic syndromes can result in both the progression of the neoplastic clone to overt AML and increased cycling status of the clone; this latter result has been used to try to prime the neoplastic blasts for cell cycle–specific chemotherapy with cytosine arabinoside.

Acute Myelogenous Leukemia

Approximately half the patients with AML in relapse have an abnormal karyotype, and the same chromosomal abnormality may reappear with relapse in individual patients after having disappeared during remission.[63] In one patient, both blasts and red cells appeared to be clonal as determined by G6PD markers;[64] these observations suggest that AML is a clonal neoplasm of the hematopoietic stem cell.

The observation of the coexistence of both abnormal and normal karyotypes in patients with AML, with normal karyotypes predominantly during the overt stages of the disease and becoming either rare or undetectable during complete remission, suggests that there may be two populations of cells in some patients, a neoplastic clone and a normal hematopoietic cell population. This situation would be analogous to that in polycythemia vera, that is, a clone of malignant cells with suppression of the normal cells, and studies utilizing the clonal soft agar culture system have shown that the great majority of patients with AML have grossly abnormal growth patterns in vitro. In general, these cells show poor colony formation, abnormal differentiation, an abnormally light and buoyant density, and other evidence of defective growth;[65] the leukemic cells, however, retain their growth factor dependence. AML cells virtually always are dependent on one or a combination of the following growth factors: GM-CSF, G-CSF, CSF-1, IL-6, and c-*kit* ligand.[66] When remission is induced in patients with AML, most of the noted abnormalities in vitro, with some notable exceptions, tend to normalize; however, it is possible that some remission states may represent not the emergence of a normal, coexistent population of cells but rather an induced differentiation of the neoplastic clone.[67,68]

The mechanism for the suppression of normal hematopoiesis in patients with AML is not defined clearly. A number of studies have suggested that leukemic cells may elaborate substances inhibitory to normal coexistent stem cells, but there is no uniform agreement on this point.[69] In some cases, especially when there has been a precedent hematologic disorder (i.e., preleukemia), it appears there may be no coexistent normal hematopoietic cells; this may explain why these patients do so poorly with cytotoxic chemotherapy.

Recently, the M3 (FAB classification) subset of AML, acute promyelocytic leukemia, was shown to be characterized by a translocation of the retinoic acid receptor α-gene that maps to chromosome 17q21, close to translocation (15;17) that characterizes acute promyelocytic leukemia and results in the synthesis of a fusion MYL/RAR protein.[70] Acute promyelocytic leukemia cells also differentiate with exposure to all-*trans*-retinoic acid, and the treatment of patients with this leads to complete, albeit transient, remissions in most cases.[71]

In summary, AML is a neoplastic disease of the hematopoietic stem cell that is still responsive to regulatory factors. Furthermore, both normal and neoplastic hematopoietic cells may coexist in some cases, whereas there may be only a neoplastic clone present in others.

Also, and although not the thrust of this chapter, several well-characterized clonal lymphoid diseases provide models for the study of clonal hematopoietic diseases. Multiple myeloma and chronic lymphocytic leukemia are clonal neoplasms of B lymphocytes in which normal lymphopoiesis or immune function appears to be suppressed and clonality of the neoplastic cells has been established definitively. Diseases that appear to be neoplastic clonal disorders of the hematopoietic stem cell include CML, polycythemia vera, myelofibrosis and myeloid metaplasia, paroxysmal nocturnal hemoglobinuria, acute myelogenous leukemia, and idiopathic refractory sideroblastic anemia.

APLASTIC ANEMIA

An absolute deficiency of hematopoietic stem cells also probably underlies a number of chronic cytopenic states that are not neoplastic, and the most dramatic disease characterized by an apparent deficiency of hematopoietic stem cells is aplastic anemia. Theoretically, aplastic anemia could be caused by either an absolute deficiency of stem cells, a defect in the stromal microenvironment (such as is seen in $S1/S1^d$ mouse), a defect in helper lymphocytes, a deficiency of cellular or humoral regulators, or inhibitors directed at the stem cell or regulator level. The majority of patients with aplastic anemia who have received bone marrow transplants from identical twins without any other therapy have been cured of their aplasia,[72] and this strongly suggests that most cases are secondary to a deficiency of marrow stem cells or possibly marrow "helper" lymphocytes. The minority of cases, in which patients with aplastic anemia have received transplants of isogeneic marrow from a normal twin and have not had normal marrow reconstitution, along with the small subset of patients having well-documented aplastic anemia who have recovered after treatment with cytotoxic drugs or antilymphocyte globulin, suggests that some instances of aplastic anemia may be mediated by a cellular or humoral immune attack against bone marrow precursor cells.[72–75] However, other studies have indicated that cytotoxic drugs or antilymphocyte globulin could exert these effects by the release of hematopoietic cytokines.[76] The majority of patients with aplastic anemia have a marked deficit in bone marrow CFU-C, but some very intriguing studies have presented evidence to implicate a population of lymphocytes as growth inhibitors of CFU-C and CFU-E in certain patients with aplastic anemia.[77–79] There is little convincing evidence for the existence of humoral inhibitors in patients with aplastic anemia, and a deficit in normal regulators has not been found. Thus, most cases probably represent an absolute deficiency of hematopoietic stem cells. In some, this appears to be caused by drug- or toxin-induced damage of stem cells, whereas in others, a virus-induced lesion seems to underlie the aplasia. Hepatitis virus has been implicated most prominently in aplastic anemia, but multilineage marrow hypoplasias, especially in the setting of immune deficiency, have been seen with Epstein-Barr virus, cytomegalovirus, human immunodeficiency virus, and parvovirus. In the case of parvovirus, there is evidence that early marrow progenitor/stem cells might be infected. In many cases, of course, no inciting event is obvious.

The primary treatment of severe aplastic anemia is marrow transplantation, although cyclosporine, cytotoxic drugs, antithymocyte globulin, and acyclovir are used as well. Recent trials of IL-3[80] and GM-CSF[81] showed some increases in neutrophils but found little impact on the production of platelets or red cells. Both GM-CSF and G-CSF selectively raise the level of neutrophils in patients with moderately severe aplastic anemia, but thus far, studies trying to implicate various cytokines such as IL-1 or interferon-γ in the etiology of aplastic anemia have produced conflicting results.

Cyclic Neutropenia

Cyclic neutropenia, or more properly, cyclic hematopoiesis, appears to represent another state in which there is an absolute deficiency of hematopoietic stem cells.[82] Studies in animal models have suggested that this disorder may represent a moderate deficiency of stem cells, in contrast to aplastic anemia where a severe deficiency exists. Cyclic neutropenia in humans is characterized by a cyclic recurrence of profound neutropenia (usually every 3 weeks) frequently associated with fever and infections; the onset usually occurs in infancy but may occur at any age. Also, detailed studies have revealed that monocytes, lymphocytes, reticulocytes, and platelets all cycle in this disorder. The cycle length is approximately the same for each cell type (3 weeks), but the cycles themselves are out of phase with each other.[82] Fluctuations of erythropoietin and CSA levels have been demonstrated in both animals and humans with this disorder, and humans respond to G-CSF by a rise in neutrophil count and becoming essentially asymptomatic.[83] In general, however, cycling persists. Both humans and gray collie dogs can be cured by bone marrow transplantation, and taken altogether, these data indicate that cyclic neutropenia probably is a disease of pluripotent stem cells. However, one study indicated that the adult form of cyclic neutropenia may be a clonal proliferation of large granular lymphocytes of T-cell origin;[84] the studies showing that humans and gray collie dogs with this disorder can be cured with allogeneic bone marrow transplantation suggest, but do not prove, that this disease represents a simple quantitative deficiency of hematopoietic stem cells.

The use of chromosomal markers and isoenzymes in conjunction with in vitro clonal assays has permitted the recognition of some diseases that involve the pluripotent hematopoietic stem cell. Less is known about disorders that involve committed hematopoietic progenitor cells (BFU-E, CFU-E, CFU-C, and CFU-megakaryocyte); candidate disorders include congenital and acquired red cell aplasia, granulocytopenia, and megakaryocytic aplasia.

Disorders of Cytokines

We are just entering the era of hematopoietic cytokine diseases; perhaps the first to be defined were the secondary polycythemias due to an excess production of erythropoietin either in response to tissue hypoxia or by neoplastic cells and the anemia of renal failure. More recently, Castleman disease[85] and atrial myxoma have been associated with an overproduction of IL-6. Neoplastic production of G-CSF probably accounts for some cases of neutrophilic leukocytosis in cancer patients, and there has been one case of cyclic thrombocytopenia apparently caused by an antibody to the GM-CSF receptor.[86] A possible relationship between G-CSF and Sweet syndrome (neutrophilic dermatosis) has been suggested as well, and osteopetrosis in mice, but probably not humans, appears to be due to a mutation in the *CSF-1* gene with defective production of CSF-1.[87]

REFERENCES

1. Quesenberry PJ. Granulocyte-macrophage growth factors. In: Fisher JW, ed. Handbook of Experimental Pharmacology, Volume 101: Biochemical Pharmacology of Blood and Bloodforming Organs. Berlin: Springer-Verlag, 1992:449–91.
2. Williams ME, Quesenberry PJ. Hematopoietic growth factors. In: Stass SA, ed. Hematologic Pathology. New York: Marcel Dekker, 1992.
3. Carnot P, Deflandre G. Sur l'activite hemopoietique du serum encours de la regeneration du sang. Comptes Rendus de l'Academie des Sciences, Serie Generale, La Vie des Sciences (Paris) 1905;143:384–6.
4. Erslev AJ. Humoral regulation of red cell production. Blood 1953;8:349.
5. Till JE, McCulloch EA. A direct measurement of radiation sensitivity of normal mouse bone marrow cells. Radiat Res 1961;14:213.
6. Becker AJ, McCulloch EA, Till JE. Cytological demonstration of the clonal nature of spleen colonies. J Cell Physiol 1967;69:65.
7. Welshons WJ. Detection and use of cytological anomalies in the mouse. In: Pauen C. Magas C, Frota-Pessoa O, Caldas LR, eds. Mammalian Cytogenetics and Related Problems in Radiobiology. Oxford: Pergamon Press, 1964:233.
8. Siminovitch L, McCulloch EA, Till JE. The distribution of colony-forming cells among spleen colonies. J Cell Comp Physiol 1963;62:327.
9. Curry JL, Trentin JJ. Hemopoietic spleen cell colony studies. I: Growth and differentiation. Dev Biol 1967;15:395.

10. Wolf NS, Trentin JJ. Hemopoietic colony studies. V: Effect of hemopoietic organ stroma on differentiation of pluripotent stem cells. J Exp Med 1968;127:205.

11. Axelrad AA, McLeod DL, Shreeve MM, Health DS. Properties of cells that produce erythrocytic colonies in vitro. In: Robinson WA, ed. Hemopoiesis in Culture. DHEW publication No. (NIH) 74-205. Washington, D.C.: US Government Printing Office, 1974:226.

12. McLeod DL, Shreeve MM, Axelrad AA. Improved plasma culture system for production of erythrocytic colonies in vitro: quantitative assay method for CFU-E. Blood 1974;44:519.

13. Iscove NN, Sieber F. Erythroid progenitors in mouse bone marrow detected by macroscopic colony formation in culture. Exp Hematol 1975;3:32.

14. Schooley JC. The effect of erythropoietin on the growth and development of spleen colony-forming cells. J Cell Physiol 1966;68:249.

15. Gurney CW, Fried W. The regulation of numbers of primitive hemopoietic cells. Proc Natl Acad Sci U S A 1965;54:1148.

16. Zuckerman KS, Sullivan R, Quesenberry PJ. Effects of actino-mycin in vivo on murine erythroid stem cells. Blood 1978;51:957.

17. Bradley TR, Metcalf D. The growth of mouse bone marrow cells in vitro. Aust J Exp Biol Med Sci 1966;44:287–99.

18. Pluznik DH, Sachs L. The cloning of normal "mast" cells in tissue culture. J Cell Comp Physiol 1965;66:319–24.

19. Metcalf D. The colony stimulating factors: discovery, develop-ment and clinical applications. Cancer 1990;65:2185–95.

20. Quesenberry PJ. The blueness of stem cells. Exp Hematol 1991;19:725–8.

21. Quesenberry PJ. Stroma-dependent hematolymphopoietic stem cells. In: Muller-Sieburg C, ed. Current Topics in Microbiology and Immunology, Volume 177: Hematopoietic Stem Cells. New York: Springer-Verlag, 1992.

22. Robinson BE, Quesenberry PJ. Hematopoietic growth factors: overview and clinical applications, part 1. Am J Med Sci 1990;300:163–70.

23. Gordon MY, Riley GP, Watt SM, Greaves MF. Compartmental-ization of a haematopoietic growth factor (GM-CSF) by gly-cosaminoglycans in the bone marrow microenvironment. Nature 1987;326:403.

24. Kittler LW, Quesenberry PJ. Stromal growth factor production. In: Long MW, Wicha M, eds. The Hematopoietic Microenviron-ment. Baltimore: The Johns Hopkins University Press, in press. (1993)

25. Robinson BE, Quesenberry PJ. Hematopoietic growth factors: overview and clinical applications, part 2. Am J Med Sci 1990;300:237–44.

26. Koury ST, Bondurant MC, Koury MJ. Localization of erythro-poietin, synthesizing cells in murine kidneys by in situ hybridiza-tion. Blood 1988;71:425.

27. Lacombe C, DaSilva JL, Bruneval P. Peritubular cells are the site of erythropoietin synthesis in the murine hypoxic kidney. J Clin Invest 1988;81:620.

28. Koury ST, Bondurant MC, Koury MJ, Semenza GL. Localiza-tion of cells producing erythropoietin in murine liver by *in situ* hybridization. Blood 1991;77:2497.

29. Cotes PM, Spivak JL. Erythropoietin in health and disease. In: Erslev AJ, Adamson JW, Eschbach JW, Winearls CG, eds. Erythropoietin: Molecular, Cellular, and Clinical Biology. Balti-more: The Johns Hopkins University Press, 1991:184–207.

30. Goldberg MA, Dunning SP, Bunn HF. Regulation of the eryth-ropoietin gene: Evidence that the oxygen sensor is a heme protein. Science 1988;242:1412.

31. Berridge MV et al. Effects of recombinant human erythropoietin on megakaryocytes and on platelet production in the rat. Blood 1988;72:970.

32. Golde DW, Bersch N, Li CH. Growth hormone: Species specific stimulation of erythropoietin in vitro. Science 1977;196:1112.

33. Golde DE, Bersch N, Chopra IJ, Cline MJ. Thyroid hormones stimulate erythropoiesis in vitro. Br J Haematol 1977;37:173.

34. Singer JW, Adamson JW. Steroids and hematopoiesis. II: The effect of steroids on in vitro erythroid colony growth: evidence for different classes of steroids. J Cell Physiol 1976;88:135.

35. Erickson N, Quesenberry PJ. Regulation of erythropoiesis: the role of growth factors. In: Wheby MS, ed. Medical Clinics of North America. Philadelphia: W. B. Saunders, 1992;76:745.

36. Grosh WW, Quesenberry PJ. Hemopoietic regulation. In: Semin Oncol 1992. In press.

37. Witte ON. Steel locus defines new multipotent growth factor. Cell 1990;63:5.

38. Nicola NA. Structural and functional characteristics of receptors for colony-stimulating factors. In: Quesenberry PJ, Asano S, Saito K. eds. Hematopoietic Growth Factors: Molecular Biology to Clinical Applications of rG-CSF. Tokyo: Excerpta Medica, 1991:101–20.

39. Fauser AA, Kanz L, Bross KJ, Lohr GW. T cells and probably B cells arise from the malignant clone in chronic myelogenous leukemia. J Clin Invest 1985;75:1080.

40. Schuh AC, Sutherland DR, Horsfall W, et al. Chronic myeloid leukemia arising in a progenitor common to T cells and myeloid cells. Leukemia 1990;4:631.

41. Beutler E, Collins Z, Irwin LE. Value of genetic variants of glucose-6-phosphate dehydrogenase in tracing the origin of ma-lignant tumors. N Engl J Med 1967;276:389.

42. Fialkow PJ. Clonal origins of human tumors. Biochem Biophys Acta 1976;458:283.

43. Fialkow PJ, Jacobson RJ, Papayannopoulou T. Chronic myelog-enous leukemia: clonal origin in a stem cell common to the granulocyte, erythrocyte, platelet and monocyte/macrophage. Am J Med 1977;63:125.

44. Fialkow PJ, Gartler SM, Yoshida A. Clonal origin of chronic myelocytic leukemia in man. Proc Natl Acad Sci U S A 1967;58:1468.

45. Fialkow PJ. Use of glucose-6-phosphate dehydrogenase markers to study meyloproliferative and lymphoproliferative disease. In: Neth R, Hofschneider PH, Mannweiler K, eds. Modern Trends in Human Leukemia, 3rd Edition. New York: Springer-Verlag, in press.

46. Boggs DR. Hematopoietic stem cell theory in relation to possible lymphoblastic conversion of chronic myeloid leukemia. Blood 1974;44:449.

47. Canellos GP, DeVita VT, Wang-Peng J, Carbone PP. Hemato-logic and cytogenetic remission of blast transformation in chronic granulocytic leukemia. Blood 1971;38:671.

48. Marks SM, Baltimore D, McCaffrey R. Terminal transferase and response to vincristine-prednisone in blastic chronic myeloge-nous leukemia. N Engl J Med 1978;298:812.

49. Emanuel PD, Bates LJ, Castleberry RP, Gualtieri RJ, Zuckerman KS. Selective hypersensitivity to granulocyte-macrophage col-ony stimulating factor by juvenile chronic myeloid leukemia hematopoietic progenitors. Blood 1991;77:924–9.

50. Adamson JW, Fialkow PJ, Murphy S, Prchal JF, Steinmann L. Polycythemia vera: stem cell and probably clonal origin of disease. N Engl J Med 1976;295:913.

51. Raskind WH, Jacobson R, Murphy S, Adamson JW, Fialkow PJ. Evidence for the involvement of B lymphoid cells in poly-cythemia vera and essential thrombocythemia. J Clin Invest 1985;75:1388.

52. Prchal JF, Adamson JW, Murphy S, Steinmann L, Fialkow PJ.

Polycythemia vera: demonstration of normal and abnormal stem cell and characterization of the in vitro response to erythropoietin. J Cell Physiol 1976;89:489.

53. Eid J, Ebert RF, Gesell MS, Spivak JL. Intracellular growth factors in polcythemia vera and other myeloproliferative disorders. Proc Natl Acad Sci U S A 1987;84:532.

54. Jacobson RJ, Salo A, Fialkow PJ. Agnogenic myeloid metaplasia: a clonal proliferation of hematopoietic stem cells with secondary myelofibrosis. Blood 1978;51:189.

55. Rosse WF. Phosphatidylinositol-linked proteins and paroxysmal nocturnal hemoglobinuria. Blood 1990;75:1595.

56. Aster RH, Enright SE. A platelet and granulocyte defect in paroxysmal nocturnal hemoglobinuria: usefulness for detecting platelet antibodies. J Clin Invest 1969;48:1199.

57. Dixon RH, Rosse WF. Mechanism of complement mediated activation of human platelets in vitro. J Clin Invest 1977;59:360.

58. Oni SB, Osunkoya BO, Luzzatto L. Paroxysmal nocturnal hemoglobinuria: evidence for monoclonal origin of abnormal red cells. Blood 1970;36:145.

59. Rosse WF. Phosphatidylinositol-linked proteins and paroxysmal nocturnal hemoglobinuria. Blood 1990;75:1595–601.

60. Lewis SM, Dave JV. The aplastic anemia-paroxysmal nocturnal haemoglobinuria syndrome. Br J Haematol 1967;13:236.

61. Hansen NE, Kollman SA. Paroxysmal nocturnal hemoglobinuria in myelofibrosis. Blood 1970;36:428.

62. Janssen JWG, Buschle M, Layton M, et al. Clonal analysis of myelodysplastic syndromes: evidence of multipotent stem cell origin. Blood 1989;73:248–54.

63. Sandberg AA, Hossfeld DK. Chromosomal abnormalities in human neoplasia. Annu Rev Med 1970;21:379.

64. Wiggans RG, Jacobson RJ, Fialkow PJ, Wooley PV III, MacDonald JS, Schein PS. Probable clonal origin of acute myeloblastic leukemia following radiation and chemotherapy of colon cancer. Blood 1978;52:659.

65. Moore MSS, Spitzer G, Williams N, Metcalf D, Buchley J. Agar culture studies in 127 cases of untreated acute leukemia: the prognostic value of reclassification of leukemia according to in vitro growth characteristics. Blood 1974;44:1.

66. Metcalf D, Moore MAS, Sheridan JW, Spitzer G. Responsiveness of human granulocytic leukemic cells to colony-stimulating factor. Blood 1974;43:847.

67. Fibach E, Hayoshi M, Sachs L. Control of normal differentiation of myeloid leukemia cells to macrophages and granulocytes. Proc Natl Acad Sci U S A 1973;70:343.

68. Davies AR, Schmitt RG. Auer bodies in mature neutrophils. JAMA 1968;203:895.

69. Quesenberry PJ, Rappaport JM, Fountebuoni A, Sullivan R, Zuckerman K, Ryan M. Inhibition of normal murine hematopoiesis by leukemic cells. N Engl J Med 1978;299:71.

70. De The H, Chomienne C, Lanotte M, Degos L, Dejean A. The t(15;17) translocation of acute promyelocytic leukaemia fuses the retinoic acid receptor α gene to a novel transcribed locus. Nature 1990;347:558–61.

71. Castaigne S, Chomienne C, Daniel MT, et al. All-trans retinoic acid as a differentiation therapy for acute promyelocytic leukemia. I: Clinical results. Blood 1990;76:1704–9.

72. Thomas ED, Rudolph RH, Fefer A, Storb R, Slichter S, Buckner CD. Isogeneic marrow grafting in man. Exp Hematol 1974;21:16.

73. Jeannet M, Rubinstein A, Pelet B, Kummer H. Prolonged remission of severe aplastic anemia after ALG pretreatment and HLA-semi-incompatible bone marrow cell transfusion. Transplant Proc 1974;6:359.

74. Thomas ED, Storb R, Giblett R, et al. Recovery from aplastic anemia following attempted marrow transplantation. Exp Hematol 1976;4:97.

75. Baran DT, Griner PF, Klemperer MR. Recovery from aplastic anemia after treatment with cyclophosphamide. N Engl J Med 1976;295:1522.

76. Barbano GC, Schenone A, Ronchella S, et al. Anti-lymphocyte globulin stimulates normal human T cells to proliferate and to release lymphokines in vitro: a study at the clonal level. Blood 1988;72:956–63.

77. Kurnick JE, Robinson W, Dickery CA. In vitro granulocytic colony-forming potential of bone marrow from patients with granulocytopenia and aplastic anemia. Proc Soc Exp Biol Med 1971;137:917.

78. Kagan WA, Ascensao JA, Pahua RN, et al. Aplastic anemia: presence in human bone marrow of cells that suppress myelopoiesis. Proc Natl Acad Sci U S A 1976;73:2890.

79. Hoffmann R, Zanjani ED, Lutton JD, Zalusky R, Wasserman LR. Suppression of erythroid colony formation by lymphocytes from patients with aplastic anemia. N Engl J Med 1977;296:10.

80. Ganser A, Lindemann A, Seipelt G, et al. Effects of recombinant human interleukin-3 in aplastic anemia. Blood 1990;76:1287–92.

81. Guinan EC, Sieff CA, Oette DH, Nathan DG. A phase I/II trial of recombinant granulocyte-macrophage colony stimulating factor for children with aplastic anemia. Blood 1990;76:1077–82.

82. Guerry D, Dale LV, Omine DC, Perry S, Wolff SM. Periodic hematopoiesis in human cyclic neutropenia. J Clin Invest 1973;52:3220.

83. Hammond WP IV, Price TH, Souza LM, Dale DC. Treatment of cyclic neutropenia with granulocyte colony stimulating factor. N Engl J Med 1989;320:1306–11.

84. Loughran TP Jr, Hammond WP IV. Adult-onset cyclic neutropenia is a benign neoplasm associated with clonal proliferation of large granular lymphocytes. J Exp Med 1986;164:2089–94.

85. Yoshizaki K, Matsuda T, Nishimoto N, et al. Pathogenic significance of interleukin-6 (IL-6/BSF-2) in Castleman's disease. Blood 1989;74:1360–7.

86. Hoffman R, Briddell RA, van Besien K, et al. Acquired cyclic amegakaryocytic thrombocytopenia associated with an immunoglobulin blocking the action of granulocyte-macrophage colony-stimulating factor. N Engl J Med 1989;321:97–102.

87. Kodama H, Yamasaki A, Nose M, et al. Congenital osteoclast deficiency in osteopetrotic (op/op) mice is cured by injections of macrophage colony stimulating factor. J Exp Med 1991;173:269–72.

2

Iron Deficiency

Thomas P. Duffy, M.D.

Iron is the most precious metal of the body: as the core of the oxygen-delivering hemoglobin molecule, it is essential to life. The metabolism of iron is dominated by its role in the synthesis of hemoglobin, and a remarkable system exists within the body to ensure a constant supply of iron for the maintenance of an optimal red cell mass.[1] The major portion of iron required for the daily synthesis of hemoglobin (20 to 30 mg) is not dependent on external sources but is acquired by a recycling of iron from the breakdown of senescent red blood cells. Only a small amount of iron (1 to 2 mg) needs to be absorbed each day from the diet, which normally contains a surplus of foodstuffs containing iron. Any acute demands or excess losses are provided for by additional reserves of iron present in various storage forms throughout the body (500 to 1000 mg). Iron metabolism is, therefore, tailored to meet the critical needs of hemoglobin production by a combination of conservation and recycling, with a backup reserve of storage depots of iron (Fig. 2.1). Any reduction in the delivery of iron for hemoglobin synthesis represents a major breakdown in this beautifully modulated system.

Such breakdowns do occur, and iron deficiency is the most common form of nutritional deficiency in the world as well as the most common organic disorder seen in clinical medicine.[2] Iron deficiency anemia represents the most exaggerated form of iron depletion and occurs only after the storage forms of iron have been mobilized. An earlier stage of iron deficiency exists when the stores are absent but anemia has not yet developed; this poses a threat to maintenance of the hemoglobin mass if the daily needs are overwhelmed by additional demands (e.g., pregnancy or gastrointestinal bleeding). Iron de-

ficiency represents a spectrum of disorders, with anemia the last but potentially most threatening development. The implications of this sequence are important in both the investigation and the therapy of iron deficiency, with or without attendant anemia.

THE INGESTION AND ABSORPTION OF IRON

To provide sufficient iron for normal synthesis of hemoglobin and other iron-containing proteins, the body absorbs small amounts of iron through the intestinal mucosa, most effectively within the duodenum and upper portions of the jejunum. The acid medium of the stomach solubilizes iron complexes contained in food, and there is enhancement of absorption in the small intestine. The amount and success of absorption are dependent on many factors, one of the most important being the amount of iron in the diet.[3,4]

The normal American diet provides 10 to 20 mg of iron each day; each 1000 calories in food usually contains approximately 5 to 6 mg of iron. The ease with which iron in food can be absorbed varies. When iron is present as part of a heme ring in the animal proteins hemoglobin or myoglobin, the iron is absorbed directly as heme, with subsequent enzymatic degradation of the heme and liberation of free iron within intestinal cells.[5] Iron contained in vegetable protein exists as ferric hydroxide complexes; this trivalent form of iron requires reduction to the divalent ferrous form before absorption can maximally occur. The presence of reducing substances such as ascorbate, succinate, and lactate in the diet increases the amount of the divalent ferrous form and facilitates absorption; other substances such as

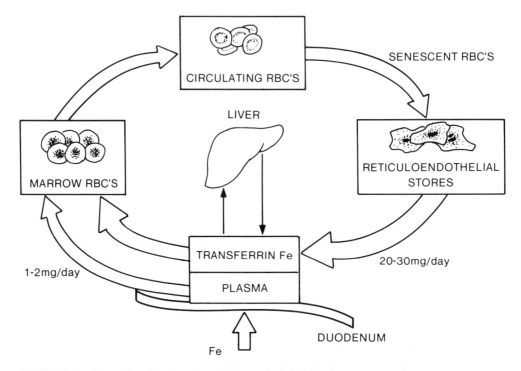

FIGURE 2.1.   Normal iron kinetics. *Note:* **RBCs = red blood cells; Fe = iron.**

phytates, tannates, phosphates (antacids), and antibiotics (e.g., tetracycline) may form complexes with iron and inhibit its absorption.

Usually, only 5% to 10% of dietary iron is absorbed to provide the daily dietary requirement of 1 to 2 mg, but this percentage can increase three to five times if iron stores are depleted. This control of iron balance by absorption is unique; the control of other substances within the body is usually by some form of elimination. The mechanism or mechanisms controlling the absorption of iron are not completely understood, but there is evidence that the initial entry of iron across the brush border of the human intestine is an active transport process.[6] A capacity for regulating iron absorption resides in the mucosa of the proximal small intestine, with an inverse relationship between serum transferrin saturation or ferritin levels and mucosal uptake of iron.[7] However, such entry into the mucosal cell does not guarantee transit through the lining cell for participation in the body's iron metabolism. The intestinal mucosa not only is the gateway for iron but also determines how much iron enters the body under physiologic conditions. If body iron stores are depleted, there is little trapping of iron within the intestinal cell and iron is rapidly transported to the plasma. With adequate iron stores and little need for additional absorption of iron, dietary iron is not

rapidly transported to plasma but remains stored in the intestinal cell; such iron is lost from the body when the epithelial cell is sloughed at the villus tip. The mechanism that instructs the mucosal cell of the body's iron needs is not known;[8] saturation of iron-transport proteins, serum or intestinal cell levels of ferritin, and plasma iron turnover all have been attributed a central role,[9] but definitive proof of the mechanism is still lacking. Evidence that hypoxemia, hemolytic anemias, and states of ineffective erythropoiesis are characterized by increased iron absorption, even in the face of adequate to increased iron stores,[10] is a complicating factor.

The body's mechanism of control is again evident in another facet of iron metabolism. The total iron content of the body normally remains fixed within relatively narrow limits; otherwise, siderosis or iron deficiency would occur. Several contingency mechanisms exist to modulate the amount of iron absorbed, ensuring a constant and adequate supply for the hemoglobin needs of the body.

THE TRANSPORT AND UPTAKE OF IRON

Iron is absorbed from the small intestine in the ferrous form and is transported as ferric iron to other iron-containing proteins and to hemoglobin-synthesizing sites within the marrow.[11] Iron travels linked to the transport protein transferrin, a β_1-globulin with a molecular weight of approximately 80,000. Pickup of iron from the intestinal mucosal cell requires that oxidation of ferrous iron has occurred, a reaction in which the oxidants ceruloplasmin and xanthine oxidase may participate. Transferrin also conveys iron from its storage sites in the reticuloendothelial cells of the bone marrow, liver, and spleen, and from the parenchymal cells of the liver to cells engaged in hemoglobin production.

Transferrin consists of a single polypeptide chain that is folded into two globular domains, each containing a binding site for one trivalent form of iron. The binding of iron to transferrin is accompanied by simultaneous bicarbonate ion attachment, which increases the binding affinity of the transferrin iron complex and facilitates uncoupling of iron. Controversy previously existed regarding the equivalency of the two binding sites of transferrin; some investigators had demonstrated nonidentity of the binding sites with different affinities for absorbed, intestinal or "anabolic" iron and degraded, reticuloendothelial or "catabolic" iron. Splitting of the symmetric transferrin molecule into the two globular fragments has resolved the controversy, because each half of the molecule is identical in its transport properties.[12]

Transferrin is a true transport protein: it is not destroyed in the process of transport but is recycled to scavenge for free iron. The protein is synthesized by the liver in inverse proportion to the iron content of hepatic parenchymal cells; more transferrin is produced in iron deficiency states. It is usually present in amounts of 300 mg/100 ml and normally is only one-third saturated with iron. The perturbations in iron levels and saturation of transferrin in various disease states are used as diagnostic tools.[13]

Transferrin performs several facilitating roles in iron metabolism. It increases the solubility of iron in plasma, protects the body against elemental iron toxicity, and imparts a direction of flow to iron molecules. The flow of iron is dictated by the presence of numerous transferrin receptor sites on the surface of red blood cells engaged in hemoglobin production, and the density of such receptor sites is directly proportional to the hemoglobin-synthesizing capacities of the cell.[14] Mono- or diferric transferrin attaches to transferrin receptors present in the red blood cell membrane. Endocytosis of the receptor and its ligand occurs with subsequent separation of iron from the complex within vesicles derived by invagination of the red blood cell membrane. After the iron is unloaded, free transferrin or apotransferrin is released from the cell to repeat its role in iron transport; apotransferrin has a weaker binding affinity to red blood cells than does the iron-laden transferrin complex. If the need for iron or hemoglobin synthesis is filled, saturated transferrin will deliver its iron, derived from intestinal absorption, to the parenchymal cells of the liver. This direction of iron flow makes the hepatic parenchymal cells the receptacle for any excessive, absorbed iron as occurs in conditions such as primary hemochromatosis.

The transport of iron across the intestinal mucosa is tailored to body needs; the transport of iron into developing red blood cells is also controlled by a feedback inhibitor system regulating the supply of iron according to the cell's need for hemoglobin synthesis. Once inside the cell, 80% to 90% of iron is taken up by mitochondria, the sites of protoporphyrin synthesis and, following iron incorporation, of heme synthesis. Heme is released to join with globin, a product of cytoplasmic-based ribosomal activity, and any excess free heme over and above its counterpart in globin synthesis down regulates the rate of iron uptake by inhibiting the endocytosis of any further iron.[15] The cell has no need for additional iron once free heme is present. This represents another example of the body's remarkable coordination of iron needs and iron supply: adequate amounts are delivered, but wastage is avoided.

A small amount of iron (10% to 20%) in excess of the hemoglobin needs of the red blood cell is diverted to a storage form by incorporation into ferritin molecules.[16] The role of such storage iron within the red blood cells is uncertain, although it probably serves as a source of iron for ongoing hemoglobin synthesis, a surfeit for the all-important hemoglobin metabolism. Red blood cells containing ferritin granules constitute 20% to 30% of erythrocyte precursors in iron-repleted marrow; such iron-containing cells are called *sideroblasts* and are a normal finding in the marrow, with their granules distributed homogeneously throughout the cytoplasm. These granules are actively extruded from the red blood cells to surrounding reticuloendothelial cells before the red blood cell leaves the marrow or the granules are removed in their passage through the spleen,[17] and their iron contents reenter the recyclable stores of the body.

THE STORAGE OF IRON

After a life-span of approximately 90 to 120 days in the peripheral blood, senescent red blood cells are broken down by the reticuloendothelial cells of the body. Hemoglobin is degraded into its constituent parts, with liberation of bilirubin; iron and the amino acids of globin reenter the body pool for reutilization in hemoglobin and protein synthesis, respectively. Any iron in excess of immediate needs is stored as either ferritin or hemosiderin.[13] Ferritin is a submicroscopic, water-soluble substance, consisting of a protein shell (apoferritin) surrounding a core of hydrated iron-oxide-phosphate complexes;[18] the hepatic synthesis of apoferritin is induced by exposure to iron. Hemosiderin is a larger molecule than ferritin; it is microscopic and water insoluble and is composed of aggregates of ferritin and variable amounts of protein, lipids, and carbohydrates. As excess iron accumulates, hemosiderin is present in larger amounts than ferritin. As iron is mobilized, ferritin is utilized initially and is released from the reticuloendothelial system. The size of the iron storage pool varies; it is normally 800 to 1000 mg in adult males, 300 to 500 mg in adult females, and often absent in young children and most adolescents.

Examination of the bone marrow provides an easy assessment of body iron stores.[19] Prussian blue staining of marrow aspirates reveals the characteristic blue-green iron deposits within the reticuloendothelial cells of the marrow. This storehouse provides the reserve for any increased iron demands; iron-deficient hematopoiesis will not supervene until this pool has been mobilized. The absence of iron in marrow reticuloendothelial cells is a hallmark of iron deficiency anemia, and its presence in those cells indicates some basis for anemia other than iron deficiency.

Release of iron from storage sites is accomplished by linkup with transferrin. In the rare cases of congenital atransferrinemia,[20] mobilization of iron from storage sites is not possible and markedly iron-deficient hematopoiesis exists in the presence of the reticuloendothelial iron overload. A similar but not quite as severe defect in hemoglobinization of red blood cells may occur when there is defective liberation or transport of iron from reticuloendothelial cells; this occurs in association with a variety of inflammatory and infectious disorders and is classified under the category of the anemia of chronic disease.[21] Here again, the marrow is replete with iron at a time when iron-deficient erythropoiesis exists.

Ferritin has usually been considered a tissue-storage form of iron but sensitive immunoradiometric methods are available now which quantitate the small amounts of ferritin that circulate in plasma.[22] The specific role of plasma ferritin is unknown but its measurement provides a most important tool, because plasma ferritin levels provide a gauge of total body iron stores. In iron-deficiency states, the reduction in plasma ferritin temporally and quantitatively parallels the reduction in marrow iron.[23] However, since ferritin is an acute phase reactant the presence of intercurrent conditions such as liver disease, infection, inflammation, neoplastic disease, or tissue necrosis will independently elevate plasma ferritin. Therefore, determination of the plasma

ferritin level can substitute for marrow assessment of iron only in the absence of such conditions.[24]

The storage pool is the principal source of iron to the plasma and provides 20 to 30 mg of iron for daily erythropoiesis. This contrasts with the 1 to 2 mg of iron that needs to be absorbed from the diet each day. Recognition of this conservation system permits a logical approach to the problem of iron deficiency.

LABORATORY DIAGNOSIS

In the early stage of iron deficiency, iron stores are first depleted and plasma ferritin levels fall; absence of iron within the bone marrow and low plasma ferritin levels are the initial occurrences with iron loss. It is only after iron stores are exhausted that the serum iron level falls; with the reduction in storage and circulating iron, more transferrin is freed up, with an absolute increase in its level. This second temporal manifestation of iron deficiency results in the classic pattern of a low serum iron level and a high iron-binding capacity, with a transferrin saturation of less than 15%.[25] It is at this level that iron delivery to the marrow is inadequate for hematopoiesis and decreased numbers of red blood cells are produced.[26] At this stage, the protoporphyrin linkup with iron does not occur efficiently, resulting in elevated levels of free erythrocyte protoporphyrin.

Anemia develops once iron stores have been mobilized and plasma iron has fallen. Initially, the anemia is normochromic, normocytic, and with normal iron indices. The red blood cells then become microcytic with a mean corpuscular volume (MCV) of less than 80 μm^3;[27] the microcytosis is attributed to additional red blood cell divisions before arrival at some critical hemoglobin concentration. The final manifestation of iron deficiency is the classic hypochromic, microcytic anemia with reduced numbers of red blood cells bearing a low MCV and mean corpuscular hemoglobin concentration (MCHC).[28]

Such a stepwise progression in the development of iron deficiency has important diagnostic implications. One can be iron depleted and still not be anemic. Hypochromic, microcytic anemia is the final stage of severe iron depletion; it occurs only if marrow iron stores are exhausted. Iron deficiency anemia can be confirmed by marrow examination, but performance of a bone marrow examination is a painful and moderately costly procedure. Reduction of plasma ferritin to levels of less than 12 $\mu g/L$ is also diagnostic and provides an easy means for determining total body iron stores.[29]

Before the availability of means for determining plasma ferritin levels, serum iron levels and transferrin saturation were utilized most frequently to diagnose iron deficiency; as stated previously, a saturation of less than 15% is characteristic for iron deficiency. However, many factors that determine the plasma levels of iron and transferrin are independent of erythropoiesis; the level of transferrin parallels the serum albumin level and is depressed in several disease states. Pregnancy or ingestion of oral contraceptives or medicinal iron may affect also these measurements and distort their interpretation. Therefore, one must recognize that although the lowered saturation of transferrin ($<$ 15%) is diagnostic of iron deficiency it is not specific for it, and there also may be iron deficiency in the absence of these findings. This is likely to occur when iron deficiency is complicated by infection or malignancy, which leads to independent reduction of transferrin levels. Unfortunately, plasma ferritin levels also may be altered in the same situation, because ferritin, as an acute phase reactant, is elevated in most systemic illnesses. The plasma ferritin ceiling of 12 µg/L as an index of iron deficiency must be elevated to 60 or 100 µg/L when iron deficiency is accompanied by other systemic diseases; these criteria have been established by studying patients with rheumatoid arthritis, an inflammatory condition frequently complicated by aspirin-induced iron deficiency.[30]

Elevated levels of free erythrocyte protoporphyrin (FEP) in red blood cells coincide with the reduction in transferrin saturation.[31] Major elevations of FEP occur in lead poisoning, and screening programs in children may capitalize on this easy determination to discover iron deficiency and/or lead poisoning.[32] Determination of FEP levels also permits an assessment of antecedent iron metabolism after a patient has been started on iron therapy, because a major complement of cells with elevated FEP levels remains and provides evidence of the previously inadequate iron incorporation into the protoporphyrin ring. Red blood cell ferritin measurements also may offer the same retrospective examination of iron metabolism.[33]

The last development in iron deficiency is anemia. This anemia is initially normochromic, normocytic anemia, but later there is an increasing population of microcytic cells. These findings have led to the important clinical observation that a reduced MCV in the presence of modest anemia is suggestive of iron deficiency. A red cell distribution width (RDW) curve permits graphic demonstration of this population of microcytic cells and earlier recognition of iron deficiency anemia.[34] The unfolding of the total picture of iron deficiency produces the peripheral smear evidence of hypochromic, microcytic cells and Coulter counter documentation of a low MCV and MCHC (Table 2.1).

There are other conditions that may produce hypochromic, microcytic blood smears (Table 2.2). Defective hemoglobin synthesis may arise from many

TABLE 2.1. Temporal Stages in the Development of Iron Deficiency Anemia

Absent marrow iron stores
Serum ferritin $<$ 12 µg/L

$\downarrow$ Serum iron and $\uparrow$ iron-binding capacity

Transferrin saturation $<$ 15%
$\uparrow$ FEP:hemoglobin ratio

Normochromic, normocytic anemia
Abnormal red blood cell distribution width

Microcytic (MCV $<$ 80 µm^3) anemia

Hypochromic (MCHC $<$ 30 g%), microcytic anemia

abnormalities other than simple iron deficiency; iron is only one part of the hemoglobin molecule. Abnormal globin synthesis in thalassemia results in hypochromic, microcytic red blood cells, many of which are target forms, and hemoglobin electrophoresis is indicated in the appropriate ethnic populations to make this diagnosis. A helpful clue (correct in approximately 70% of such cases) is the Mentzer index, which capitalizes on the fact that iron deficiency creates reduced numbers of moderately microcytic red blood cells, whereas there are larger numbers of severely microcytic red blood cells in β-thalassemia.[35] The ratio of MCV to red blood cell count is greater than 13 in iron deficiency and less than 13 in patients with β-thalassemia trait according to the Mentzer index.

The anemia of chronic disease is usually normochromic and normocytic, although hypochromic, microcytic changes may occur.[36] Defective hemoglobin synthesis in these conditions is attributable to faulty iron transport. The diagnosis is suggested by a low or low-normal serum level of iron associated with a low or low-normal iron-binding capacity, a constellation resulting in a normal transferrin saturation. This is not foolproof, and marrow documentation of iron-filled storage cells may be necessary. The performance of a bone marrow examination may uncover another cause of hypochromic red blood cells, that is, the presence of ringed sideroblasts, which are evidence of defective heme synthesis with iron pathologically distributed in mitochondria.[37] The hypochromic cells in this disorder are more frequently associated with normal or increased cell size (MCV).

Copper deficiency has been described as a cause of hypochromic, microcytic anemia; this is attributed to the role of copper-containing oxidants in iron transport.[38] This deficiency is associated with leukopenia and hair changes, which may suggest the diagnosis.

TABLE 2.2. **The Differential Diagnosis of Hypochromic Anemias**

Cause	Marrow Iron	Plasma Ferritin	Transferrin Saturation
Iron deficiency	Absent	$<12 \mu g/L$	$<15\%$
Anemia of chronic disease	Present	Normal	Normal
Thalassemia	Present	Normal to elevated	Normal to elevated
Sideroblastic anemia	Ringed sideroblasts	Elevated	Normal to elevated
Aluminum overload	Present	Normal to elevated	Normal to elevated
Copper deficiency	Present	—	Normal to elevated

Aluminum accumulation, especially in patients hemodialized for renal failure, is a more recently recognized cause of a hypochromic, microcytic anemia.[39] Aluminum, a trivalent metal, travels in linkage to transferrin and likely interferes with iron metabolism via this pathway. Mobilization of the aluminum with an iron-chelating agent such as desferrioxamine leads to reversal of this lesion.

Numerous tests are available to make the laboratory diagnosis of iron deficiency and to differentiate it from other causes of hypochromic, microcytic anemia; the choice is usually dictated by the clinical circumstances surrounding each case. In the hospitalized patient with many factors possibly affecting iron metabolism, it is often simpler, more rapid, and more productive to proceed directly to bone marrow examination to assess marrow stores of iron. In an outpatient population with uncomplicated anemia (young women with metrorrhagia or men with a clinical history suggestive of gastrointestinal bleeding), determination of plasma ferritin, serum iron and iron-binding capacity, or even a diagnostic–therapeutic trial of iron may suffice to make the diagnosis. Large screening programs of schoolchildren might better use FEP levels. If one recognizes the pitfalls in interpreting such laboratory data and keeps in mind the temporal sequence in laboratory abnormalities in iron-deficiency states, the diagnosis of iron deficiency anemia should not present any major challenge.

CLINICAL DIAGNOSIS

The clinical manifestations of iron deficiency may be suggested by the appearance of anemia in certain age groups. Inadequate dietary-iron intake is almost wholly restricted to infants on milk diets. The menstruating adolescent girl on a marginal diet is at double jeopardy because of the demands of an expanding blood pool and the blood losses incurred with menstruation.[40] The latter averages 40 to 60 ml of blood each menstrual period; this amounts to 20 to 30 mg of iron or 0.6 to 1.0 mg/day of iron over the baseline needs of 1 mg/day. In a menstruating female, iron deficiency usually can be attributed to menstrual blood loss.

The pregnant female is a special candidate for the development of iron deficiency;[41,42] she requires 2.5 to 3.0 mg/day of iron in a situation where iron stores already may be reduced or absent. The iron-transferrin complex preferentially binds to placental cells; this accounts for normal hematocrits in infants born to mothers who have iron-deficiency anemia. This large demand for iron leads to the recommendation that all pregnant women receive supplemental iron.

An adult male or postmenopausal female requires only 1 mg/day of iron, and these individuals should easily absorb such amounts from their diet. Malabsorption of iron may occur with sprue or celiac disease, but this is a rare cause of iron deficiency. In adult males and postmenopausal females, blood loss must be considered as the etiology of the iron deficiency and the source of blood loss as gastrointestinal until proven otherwise. The implications of this dictum are that all such individuals require an evaluation of their gastrointestinal tract (sigmoidoscopy; colonoscopy; barium enema; esophageal, stomach, and small bowel contrast studies) even though there is no evidence of gastrointestinal bleeding. In the majority of cases, iron deficiency anemia may result from peptic ulcers, large hiatal hernias, esophageal varices, aspirin- or alcohol-induced gastritis, regional enteritis, hemorrhoids, benign or malignant tumors, or vascular lesions;[43] partial gastrectomies are followed frequently by the development of iron deficiency anemia.[44] An abdominal workup with normal findings does not necessarily exclude pathology, and there should be a repeat evaluation in a few weeks to months, especially if anemia recurs or any evidence of gastrointestinal bleeding is documented. The impetus for a vigorous approach to discover the etiology of anemia is the real possibility that patients with iron deficiency anemia and normal gastrointestinal evaluations will prove subsequently to have a malignancy.

Sources other than gastrointestinal bleeding may produce excessive blood loss. The gross hematuria that occurs in patients with sickle cell trait may lead to iron deficiency anemia. Iron also may be lost through the kidneys in forms other than blood, namely as free hemoglobin or hemosiderin in association with intravascular hemolysis, as seen in patients with paroxysmal nocturnal hemoglobinuria or with prosthetic heart valves. All patients with artificial heart valves are candidates for the "Waring blender" syndrome, with traumatic hemolysis of their red blood cells. The iron loss in such conditions may amount to 10 to 20 mg/d, and the supervention of iron deficiency anemia will exacerbate the hemolysis and further compromise the cardiovascular status of these patients. Monitoring lactate dehydrogenase levels, haptoglobin saturation, and hemosiderin excretion in the urine is a good means of documenting the presence and severity of this complication.[45]

Loss of iron into the lung may lead to the paradoxic situation of iron deficiency anemia in the presence of iron overload of the lung parenchyma.[46] Pulmonary hemosiderosis may be a component of cardiopulmonary disease (mitral stenosis), Goodpasture syndrome with pulmonary hemorrhage and glomerulonephritis, vasculitis, or idiopathic. Prussian blue staining of alveolar macrophages may reveal prominent hemosiderin granules in exfoliated pulmonary cells; such iron is not available for the body's needs since it cannot be mobilized from the pulmonary tissue. Chest radiographs are usually abnormal in these patients; however, in rare cases, chest radiographs have been normal but the presence of iron was documented on lung biopsy.

A newer aspect of iron deficiency anemia has been unmasked by the employment of erythropoietin for the treatment of the anemia of renal failure. Many of these patients have borderline iron stores as they embark on erythropoietin stimulation of erythropoiesis; the average iron loss attributable to hemodialysis is 2 g/year. The failure of erythropoietin to elicit a response should suggest iron deficiency as a cause of the erythropoietin refractory state.[47]

The diagnosis of iron deficiency anemia, therefore, is only the beginning of the diagnostic evaluation; one must accept the responsibility for discovering the cause. Iron deficiency is evidence of some underlying, excessive demand on the iron storehouse of the body. It can occur in all age groups, and it may have a cause as benign as the "Good Samaritan" syndrome (too many blood donations) or as threatening as an occult malignancy. Treatment of iron deficiency with attention to the red blood cell count alone overlooks the major therapeutic implications of this diagnosis, viz, the cause must be discovered and eliminated.

The clinical signs and symptoms of iron deficiency are interesting and varied.[48] Many of the symptoms can be attributed to the underlying anemia, although depletion of essential energy-producing, iron-containing tissue enzymes may contribute to the frequently present malaise, fatigue, and muscular weakness;[49,50] alter-

ations in thermoregulation and thyroid function also have been described in iron-deficiency states.[51] Changes in the surface epithelium of the body result in complaints of sore tongue (glossitis) and breakdown of the corners of the mouth (angular stomatitis); achlorhydria and atrophic gastritis occur with iron deficiency and may decrease the efficiency of absorption of iron in foodstuffs. The achlorhydria resolves with iron repletion, but the atrophic gastritis is not reversible with iron therapy. Spooning of the nails occurs, and this koilonychia is a peripheral clue to iron deficiency.[52]

Dysphagia resulting from an esophageal web infrequently develops in elderly women with iron deficiency anemia; this condition has received the eponyms *Patterson-Kelly* and *Plummer-Vinson syndromes*. Its rareness in American women with iron deficiency anemia suggests that its cause may be something other than iron deficiency. The web has a premalignant potential, and its importance derives as much from this specter as from its multiple eponyms.[53]

The many alterations in the surface epithelium may account for one of the most fascinating symptoms of iron deficiency, that is, the development of perverse appetites, or pica.[54] This is the compulsive eating of a single item of food or ice, dirt, or something else which is within easy reach of the victim. The ingestion of abnormal quantities of laundry starch, ice, or leaded paint is not the cause but a symptom of iron deficiency. Treatment with iron results in correction of the compulsion.

TREATMENT

The basic principle in the treatment of iron deficiency is simple: supply the missing ingredient in amounts adequate to correct any anemia and to restock the storage reserves. This task is made difficult by several factors, the major one being the occurrence of gastrointestinal irritation in approximately 30% of subjects who ingest a prescribed dose of oral iron. Patient noncompliance is related to this gastrointestinal toxicity (constipation, diarrhea, dyspepsia) and to the prolonged period of iron ingestion. The problem is further compounded by a dazzling array of iron preparations of mounting chemical complexity and escalating costs.

The cheapest preparation of iron is ferrous sulfate (300 mg), containing 60 mg of elemental iron in each tablet. Ferrous gluconate contains only 30 mg of elemental iron per tablet but may be tolerated better simply because of the reduced quantity of iron in each tablet. All iron tablets are better absorbed on an empty stomach and should be prescribed for ingestion between meals and at bedtime; however, iron tablets may be taken with meals, trading off lesser absorption for a decrease in gastrointestinal irritation. The practice of ingesting antacids with iron is to be discouraged, because the phosphates contained in antacids will form complexes with the iron.

Iron is prescribed as one 300-mg ferrous sulfate tablet daily, with gradual increase to one tablet three or four times daily as tolerated. On this regimen, there should be reticulocytosis within 1 to 2 weeks, although not to the extent seen with responses in megaloblastic anemias, and the hemoglobin level will correct at a rate of 1 to 2 g/week. The return of the hemoglobin level to normal obviously is not the endpoint of treatment; iron is administered for a period two to three times as long as the period initially required to normalize the hemoglobin. Because ferritin determinations can be used to assess iron stores, such levels may allow a more quantitative administration of iron to reestablish the stores.

There is a group of patients who do not tolerate or absorb the usual iron medications. In patients who have undergone a gastrojejunostomy (frequently complicated by iron deficiency anemia), iron tablets will bypass the major area of iron absorption in the upper small intestine; a solution of ferrous sulfate (taken by straw to avoid staining the teeth) will obviate the breakdown of tablets and may be an acceptable substitute in this group of patients. Individuals with malabsorption syndromes or intolerable gastrointestinal side effects from oral iron as well as patients who require large amounts of iron because of continuing, significant blood loss (vascular lesions of the gastrointestinal tract as in hereditary hemorrhagic telangiectasia or patients on long-term hemodialysis) are candidates for parenteral iron administration. An unusual but helpful role for parenteral iron administration is in those patients with recurrent gastrointestinal bleeding of undetermined cause. Melena may alert the patient to the need for hospitalization; oral iron may mask this important sign because of the black color imparted to the stool with iron therapy.

Iron dextran[55] is the most frequently used parenteral iron preparation. Calculation of the necessary dose is based on the fact that each gram of hemoglobin contains 3.4 mg of iron; an additional 500 to 1000 mg should be administered to compensate for storage iron needs. It had been suggested formerly that an excess of 25% to 30% over the calculated dose was necessary because of the poor utilization and longer processing of the larger molecule of iron dextran, but this theory has been discarded. There is no need to give any extra parenteral iron.

Iron dextran is associated with local and systemic reactions. Febrile reactions and local irritation at intramuscular sites are common. Anaphylaxis may occur, although this is feared more with intravenous administration than with intramuscular injection. A test dose of 0.5 ml (50 mg/ml) is administered intramuscularly; within 2 or 3 days this dosage may be increased to 2.5 ml/day given until replacement has been completed. The preparation will stain body tissues even if given by a Z-track technique (i.e., displacement of the skin laterally before injection).

In individuals who require more rapid replacement of iron (noncompliance, poor muscle mass, large iron needs), the iron dextran preparation may be administered intravenously.[56] The calculated amount is administered slowly in 250 to 500 ml of saline over a period of approximately 1 hour. Life-threatening, immediate anaphylactic reactions may occur in a small number of individuals (3 of 481 patients) receiving intravenous iron. Severe delayed reactions consisting of lymphadenopathy, myalgias, fever, and headache occur more frequently (8 of 481 patients) with a special proclivity for individuals with underlying collagen vascular disease.[57] Because of these reactions, there should be a strong indication for choosing intravenous iron over other preparations.

REFERENCES

1. Worwood M. The clinical biochemistry of iron. Semin Hematol 1977;14:31.
2. DeMaeyer E, Adiels-Tegman M. The prevalence of anaemia in the world. World Health Stat Q 1985;38:302.
3. Charlton RW, Bothwell TH. Iron absorption. Ann Rev Med 1983;34:55–68.
4. Martinez-Torres C, Layrisse M. Nutritional factors in iron deficiency: Food iron absorption. Clin Haematol 1973;2:339.
5. Turnbull AL, Cleton F, Finch CA. Iron absorption. IV. The absorption of hemoglobin iron. J Clin Invest 1962;41:1897–1907.
6. Aisen P, Brown E. The iron-binding function of transferrin in iron metabolism. Semin Hematol 1977;14:31.
7. Huebers H, Finch C. The physiology of transferrin and transferrin receptors. Physiol Rev 1987;67:520.
8. Osterloh KRS, Simpson RJ, Peters TJ. The role of mucosal transferrin in intestinal iron absorption. Br J Haematol 1987;65:1–3.
9. Finch CA, Huebers H, Eng M, et al. Effect of transfused reticulocytes on iron exchange. Blood 1982;59:364–69.
10. Pootrakul P, Kitcharoen K, Yansukon P, et al. The effect of erythroid hyperplasia on iron balance. Blood 1988;71:112.
11. Brock JH. The biology of iron. In: de Sousa M, Brock JH, eds. Iron in Immunity, Cancer and Inflammation. New York: John Wiley, 1989:35–53.
12. Brown E. Transferrin—iron-binding sites. Blood 1977;50:1151.
13. Arosio P, Cairo G, Levi S. The molecular biology of iron-binding proteins. In: de Sousa M, Brock JH, eds. Iron in Immunity, Cancer and Inflammation. New York: John Wiley, 1989:55–79.
14. Muta K, Nishimura J, Ideguchi H, et al. Erythroblast transferrin receptors and transferrin kinetics in iron deficiency and various anemias. Am J Hematol 25:155–63, 1987;25:155–63.
15. Egyed A, Fodor I, Lelkes G. Coated pit formation: a membrane function involved in the regulation of cellular iron uptake. Br J Haematol 1986;64:263.
16. Hodgetts J, Hoy TG, Jacobs A. Iron uptake and ferritin synthesis in human erythroblasts. Clin Sci 1986;70:53–7.

17. Cartwright G, Deiss A. Sideroblasts, siderocytes and sideroblastic anemia. N Engl J Med 1975;292:185.

18. Harrison P. Ferritin: an iron storage molecule. Semin Hematol 1977;14:55.

19. Fong TP, Okafor L, Thomas W Jr, et al. Stainable iron in aspirated and needle biopsy specimens of marrow. Am J Hematol 1977;2:47.

20. Goya N, Miyazaki S, Kodata S, et al. A family of congenital atransferrinemia. Blood 1972;40:239–45.

21. Konijn A, Hershkot C. The anaemia of inflammation and chronic disease. In: de Sousa M, Brock JH, eds. Iron in Immunity, Cancer and Inflammation. New York: John Wiley, 1989:55–79.

22. Worwood M. Serum ferritin. Clin Sci 1986;70:215–20.

23. Jacobs A, Worwood M. Ferritin in serum: clinical and biochemical implications. N Engl J Med 1975;292:951.

24. Cazzola M, Ascari E. Red cell ferritin as a diagnostic tool. Br J Haematol 1986;62:209.

25. Cook J. Clinical evaluation of iron deficiency. Semin Hematol 1982;119:6–18.

26. Hillman RS, Henderson PA. Control of marrow production by relative iron supply. J Clin Invest 1969;48:454–60.

27. Okuno T, Chon A. The significance of small erythrocytes. Am J Clin Pathol 1975;64:48.

28. England J, Ward S, Down M. Microcytosis, anisocytosis and the red cell indices in iron deficiency. Br J Haematol 1976;34:589.

29. Jacobs A, Worwood M. The clinical use of serum ferritin estimation. Br J Haematol 1975;31:1.

30. Vreugdenhil G, Baltus CA, van Eijk HG, et al. Anaemia of chronic disease: diagnostic significance of erythrocyte and serological parameters in iron deficient rheumatoid arthritis patients. Br J Rheumatol 1990;29:105–10.

31. Piomelli S, Brickman A, Carlos E. Rapid diagnosis of iron deficiency by measurement of free erythrocyte protoporphyrin and hemoglobin. Pediatrics 1976;57:136.

32. Labbe R, Rettmer R. Zinc protoporphyrin: a product of iron deficient erythropoiesis. Semin Hematol 1989;26:40.

33. Cazzola M, Ascari E. Red blood cell ferritin. Br J Haematol 1986;62:209.

34. Thompson WG, Meola T, Lipkin M Jr, et al. Red cell distribution width, mean corpuscular volume, and transferrin saturation in the diagnosis of iron deficiency. Arch Intern Med 1988;148:2128–30.

35. Mentzer WC. Differentiation of iron deficiency from thalassemia trait. Lancet 1973;i:882.

36. Cartwright GE. The anemia of chronic disorders. Semin Hematol 1966;3:351.

37. Bottomley SS. Sideroblastic anaemia. Clin Haematol 1982;11:389–409.

38. Williams DM, Lee GR, Cartwright GE. Ferrioxidase activity of rat ceruloplasmin. Am J Physiol 1974;227:1094.

39. Rosenlof K, Fyhrquist F, Tenhunen R. Erythropoietin, aluminum, and anaemia in patients on haemodialysis. Lancet 1990;335:247–9.

40. Rowland TW. Iron deficiency in the young athlete. Pediatr Clin North Am 1990;37:1153–63.

41. De Leeuw NK, Lowenstein L, Hsieh YS. Iron deficiency and hydremia in normal pregnancy. Medicine 1966;45:291.

42. Pritchard JA, Scott DE, Iron demands during pregnancy. In: Hallberg L, Harwerth HG, Vannetti N, eds. Iron Deficiency. New York: Academic Press, 1970:173–92.

43. Beveridge BR, Bannerman RM, Evanson JM, et al. Hypochronic anaemia: a retrospective study and follow-up. Q J Med 1965;34:145.

44. Hines JD, Hoffbrand AV, Miller DL. The hematologic complications following partial gastrectomy. Am J Med 1967;43:555.

45. Kloster F. Diagnosis and management of complications of prosthetic heart valves. Am J Cardiol 1975;35:872.

46. Donald KJ. Alveolar capillary basement membrane lesions in Goodpasture's syndrome and idiopathic pulmonary hemosiderosis. Am J Med 1975;59:642.

47. Van Wyck DB. Iron management during recombinant human erythropoietin therapy. Am J Kidney Dis 1989;14:9–13.

48. Dallman P. Manifestations of iron deficiency. Semin Hematol 1972;19:19–30.

49. Willis WT, Gohil K, Brooks GA, et al. Iron deficiency: improved exercise performance within 15 hours of iron treatment in rats. J Nutr 1990;120:909–16.

50. Davies KJA, Maguire JA, Brooks CA, et al. Muscle mitochondrial bioenergetics, oxygen supply and work capacity during dietary iron deficiency and repletion. Am J Physiol 1984;242:E418–27.

51. Beard JL, Borel MJ, Derr J. Impaired thermoregulation and thyroid function in iron-deficiency anemia. Am J Clin Nutr 1990;52:813–19.

52. Chisholm M. Tissue changes associated with iron deficiency. Clin Haematol 1973;2:303.

53. Bredenkamp JK, Castro DJ, Mickel RA. Importance of iron repletion in the management of Plummer-Vinson syndrome. Ann Otol Rhinol Laryngol 1990;99:51–4.

54. Crosby W. Pica: a compulsion caused by iron deficiency. Br J Haematol 1976;34:341.

55. Kernoff L. Utilization of iron dextran in recurrent iron deficiency anemia. Br J Haematol 1975;30:419.

56. Auerbach M, Witt D, Toler W, et al. Clinical use of the total dose intravenous infusion of iron dextran. J Lab Clin Med 1988;111:566.

57. Hamstra R, Block M, Schocket A. Intravenous iron dextran in clinical medicine. JAMA 1980;243:1726.

3

Macrocytic Anemia

Edward R. Eichner, M.D.

The routine use of automated blood counters has increased our awareness of macrocytosis, an abnormality that can be clinically significant whether or not anemia is present. Two studies[1,2] showed that mild to moderate macrocytosis is relatively common, at least in hospitalized patients, and is not always associated with the disorders that cause megaloblastic anemia. In one study, approximately 25% of patients with moderate macrocytosis were not deficient in folate or vitamin B_{12} and had no alcoholism or liver disease.[1] In another study, moderate macrocytosis without megaloblastic hematopoiesis was seen in patients with sideroblastic anemia, aplastic anemia, hypothyroidism, and neoplasms.[2] Therefore, macrocytosis and macrocytic anemia can be divided arbitrarily into anemia associated with normoblastic marrow (nonmegaloblastic macrocytic anemia) and anemia associated with megaloblastic marrow.

NONMEGALOBLASTIC MACROCYTIC ANEMIA

The main causes of nonmegaloblastic macrocytic anemia are:

Chronic hemolytic anemia (reticulocytosis)
Acquired sideroblastic anemia
Hypothyroidism
Aplastic anemia
Neoplasms*

Alcoholism†
? Liver disease

Reticulocytes are approximately 20% larger than mature red cells, so any anemia with brisk reticulocytosis, such as chronic hemolytic anemia or major hemorrhagic anemia, will be macrocytic. Acquired idiopathic sideroblastic anemia is often macrocytic; in a classic study, approximately 80% of patients had an elevated mean corpuscular volume (MCV). The macrocytosis and poikilocytosis (the morphologic hallmark of ineffective erythropoiesis) in the peripheral smear of these patients can resemble that of the megaloblastic anemias, and clues for underlying sideroblastic anemia include a population of hypochromic, stippled cells and the lack of hypersegmented neutrophils. Alcohol, perhaps the most common cause of reversible, drug-induced sideroblastic anemia, has been indicted in Great Britain as a cause of nonmegaloblastic macrocytosis;[3] the effects of alcohol are considered later.

More than one half of the patients with uncomplicated anemia of hypothyroidism have mild macrocytosis on diagnosis. In almost all patients with hypothyroidism, the MCV decreases during the first weeks of thyroid replacement. The mechanism of macrocytosis in uncomplicated hypothyroidism remains unclear. Up to 10% of patients with hypothyroidism develop pernicious anemia. Folate deficiency has been described in selected patients with severe hypothyroidism, but it is uncommon in the general hypothyroid population.

---

*Neoplasms most often result in a normocytic anemia.

†Megaloblastic marrow is usually associated with alcoholism.

Mild to moderate macrocytosis is common in patients with hypoplastic and aplastic anemia. The mechanism is unknown but may relate to the high levels of erythropoietin in these disorders. One of erythropoietin's alleged effects is to accelerate the delivery of erythrocytes to the peripheral blood by reducing the number of mitoses between the pronormoblastic and late polychromatic stages; this results in a macrocytic red cell.

Although the literature is replete with references to macrocytosis in liver disease, the concept that macrocytosis with liver disease is a distinct etiologic entity is debated. The red cell membrane in liver disease may take up excess cholesterol from the plasma to increase its surface area and thereby "spread out" on smear to form a thin macrocyte. True macrocytosis, however, as defined by an MCV over 100 μm^3, is probably rare in liver disease without folate deficiency, alcoholism, the reticulocytosis of hemolysis, or blood loss.

Macrocytosis occurs in diverse hematologic malignancies and solid tumors, especially those treated with drugs that inhibit the synthesis of purine or pyrimidine. Macrocytosis is common in patients with renal allografts treated with azathioprine, and it also has been reported in patients with connective tissue diseases who are treated with azathioprine and even in those treated with cyclophosphamide, an alkylating agent. The mechanism of macrocytosis in untreated neoplasms remains unclear; that seen in multiple myeloma may conceivably be due in part to rouleau formation if it persists to any degree in the diluted blood specimen run through the automated counter. Artifactually high MCVs (with low red-cell counts) can occur in patients with mycoplasmal pneumonia and high titers of cold agglutinins, and this temperature-dependent aggregation of red cells and elevated MCV can be returned to normal by warming the tube of blood to body temperature and repeating the determination. Rare causes of nonmegaloblastic macrocytosis are some of the congenital dyserythropoietic anemias; these disorders are marked by striking multinucleation of the erythroblasts.

Minimal macrocytosis is so common in hospitalized patients that an elevated MCV probably does not warrant further investigation unless it is at least 10% above the upper limit of normal recognized in a given laboratory. Moderate macrocytosis, however, even without anemia, is usually significant. In a hospital study of 100 consecutive patients with MCVs over 115 μm^3, 40% of whom were not anemic, 50 had a deficiency of folate, vitamin B_{12}, or both, and another 26 had alcoholism or liver disease (usually alcoholic).[1] Thirteen patients had other disorders, mainly neoplasms or refractory anemia, which could explain their macrocytosis, and only 11 patients had unexplained macrocytosis. In an interesting extension of this concept, 3% of 8000 employees of an insurance company were found on routine screening to have elevated MCVs; the majority occurred in nonanemic persons, and further investigation of the first 17 such subjects showed that 16 were abusing alcohol.[4] Work in France showed a direct relationship between the MCV and the amount of alcohol consumed,[5] and work in Great Britain showed that smoking, per se, slightly increases the MCV.[6] Thus, even in nonanemic patients, macrocytosis should not be ignored, as it is associated with a variety of nonmegaloblastic and megaloblastic disorders. In general, the higher the MCV, the more likely it is that the underlying disorder will be megaloblastic. Investigating all patients with moderate macrocytosis has a high diagnostic yield, especially for a folate or vitamin B_{12} deficiency and for alcoholism.

Alas, recent studies suggest that physicians sometimes ignore the MCV. In one prospective study of hospital patients, anemia was seldom diagnosed in the traditional way, that is, by ordering diagnostic tests after perusing the complete blood count and peripheral blood smear. The diagnosis was more "situational" than analytic, and the treatment more empiric than specific. Physicians examined the peripheral smear less than 10% of the time, and macrocytic anemia was even misclassified occasionally as "dilutional" or microcytic.[7]

Another study investigated how physicians in primary care respond to macrocytosis in clinic patients. Nearly 4% of over 3800 patients had macrocytosis, which was usually mild. This macrocytosis, however, was often overlooked or incompletely evaluated. It appeared that the physicians "reacted in a shotgun fashion" rather than by working through the differential diagnosis, and it was concluded that when physicians fail to act on macrocytosis, they may miss treatable diseases such as vitamin B_{12} deficiency, folate deficiency in pregnancy, hypothyroidism, or occult alcoholism.[8]

For optimal diagnosis, macrocytosis should be heeded. To be sure, a recent study suggested that mild macrocytosis, taken in isolation, is too nonspecific for precise diagnosis in today's hospitalized patients, who tend to have complex illnesses and multifactorial anemias. That study, however, was retrospective and did not analyze the utility of the peripheral smear.[9] Suffice it to say that the MCV today is alive, well, and helpful.[10]

MEGALOBLASTIC ANEMIA

The megaloblast is the morphologic hallmark of impaired formation of deoxyribonucleic acid (DNA); the ultimate biochemical basis for the megaloblast is inadequate conversion of deoxyuridylate to thymidylate, which leads to a slowing of the DNA synthesis per unit of time in affected cells. The abnormal synthesis of

DNA delays the maturation of the nucleus, whereas the normal synthesis of ribonucleic acid (RNA) and protein allows normal formation of hemoglobin. The result is the characteristic "cytonuclear dissociation" of the megaloblast.

Etiology

The causes of megaloblastic anemia include:

Folate deficiency
Vitamin B_{12} deficiency
Erythroleukemia
Orotic aciduria
Thiamine dependency*
Arsenic poisoning*
Chronic ingestion of an analgesic*

In more than 90% of cases, the cause is either folate or vitamin B_{12} deficiency. The megaloblastoid erythropoiesis of erythroleukemia (Di Guglielmo syndrome) accounts for some cases, and a morphologic clue to erythroleukemia is multinucleation of the megaloblastoid erythroid precursors, along with the leukemic myeloblasts that are usually present in small numbers at diagnosis and inevitably increase with time. The term *erythroleukemia* is a misnomer in that the red cell series is not leukemic; its production can be abrogated and its appearance changed to normoblastic when these patients are transfused to a normal hemoglobin level. Apparently, the erythropoietic machinery is deranged in this smoldering monomyelocytic leukemia. The mechanism is unknown but is apparently unrelated to folate or vitamin B_{12} metabolism. Moderate macrocytosis with megaloblastoid precursors often is a hallmark of the *preleukemic syndrome,* a constellation of ineffective hematopoiesis, peripheral blood cytopenias, and a hypercellular marrow that precedes by months to years the classic findings of acute myelogenous leukemia in elderly patients.[11] Erythroleukemia and preleukemia are now usually considered myelodysplastic syndromes.

The remaining cases of megaloblastic anemias are confined to a few rare syndromes or case reports. Megaloblastic anemia occurs in Lesch-Nyhan syndrome; in this syndrome, characterized by hyperuricemia and a failure of cells to salvage hypoxanthine, increased purine synthesis occurs and presumably diverts folate to this need, creating folate deficiency. Approximately 10 children with megaloblastic anemia and orotic aciduria also have been reported. In this

disorder, an enzyme deficiency inhibits the synthesis of pyrimidine; the megaloblastic marrow does not respond to folate or vitamin B_{12} but reverts to normoblastic with large quantities of nucleosides, especially uridine. There also are isolated case reports of megaloblastic anemia responsive to thiamine, megaloblastic anemia from arsenic poisoning, and megaloblastic anemia associated with chronic ingestion of an analgesic. Finally, certain drugs, especially antifolates, cause megaloblastic anemia.

Megaloblastic changes not only occur in the bone marrow but also in all reproducing cells and are therefore found throughout the intestinal tract and even in the cervicovaginal epithelium. It is impossible to tell morphologically whether folate or vitamin B_{12} deficiency is the cause of the megaloblastosis. It is imperative, however, to differentiate between these two deficiencies, because each has many possible underlying causes that need therapy.

THE METABOLIC INTERRELATIONSHIPS OF FOLATE AND VITAMIN B_{12}. Clinical and biochemical evidence suggests that the metabolism of folate is intertwined with that of vitamin B_{12}. Pharmacologic doses of folic acid almost invariably cause a hematologic remission, albeit partial and temporary, in patients with deficient vitamin B_{12}. Pharmacologic doses of vitamin B_{12} produce reticulocytosis in some patients with folate-deficient megaloblastic anemia, although this reticulocytosis is delayed, is accompanied by little morphologic change in megaloblastosis, and has not been seen by all investigators. The urinary excretion of formiminoglutamic acid is increased in both folate and vitamin B_{12} deficiency; thus, the morphologic identity, therapeutic responses, and biochemical similarities suggest interrelated roles of these vitamins in the pathogenesis of megaloblastic anemia.[12]

Only two enzymatic reactions dependent on vitamin B_{12} have been demonstrated unequivocally in humans. One, the methylation of homocysteine to methionine, links vitamin B_{12} and folate metabolism and provides evidence that folate deficiency is the final common pathway leading to the formation of megaloblasts in both folate and vitamin B_{12} deficiency. The second, the methylmalonate–succinate isomerization, involves only vitamin B_{12} and forms a link between lipid and carbohydrate metabolism, resulting in speculation about its possible role in the synthesis of myelin, which is deranged in vitamin B_{12} but not in folate deficiency.

The methylation of homocysteine to methionine is catalyzed by the enzyme 5-methyltetrahydrofolate (MTHF)-homocysteine transmethylase, which requires methyl B_{12} as a cofactor. Because methionine also is

---

*Isolated case reports.

available from the diet, the main importance of this reaction is probably the regeneration of tetrahydrofolate from 5-MTHF. Thus, MTHF is the main circulating and transport form of folate, but it must donate its methyl group to homocysteine to form tetrahydrofolate and then receive a one-carbon unit from serine to become 5,10-methylenetetrahydrofolate, which donates its one-carbon unit to deoxyuridylate to form thymidylate and thus contributes to DNA (Fig. 3.1). There is now much evidence that MTHF becomes "trapped" in the serum of patients with vitamin B_{12} deficiency and that the ultimate block in DNA synthesis in vitamin B_{12} deficiency is a block in folate metabolism.

The initial clues to the "methylfolate trap" in vitamin B_{12} deficiency were the findings of the accumulation of MTHF in the serum of vitamin B_{12}–deficient patients and, on injection, its delayed clearance from their plasma.[12,13] Subsequent clinical and biochemical observations solidified the concept of the methylfolate trap. For example, the uptake of MTHF by phytohemagglutinin (PHA)-stimulated lymphocytes and by bone marrow cells of vitamin B_{12}–deficient patients is impaired and can be corrected by the addition of vitamin B_{12}. Thus, MTHF is trapped both outside and inside cells, because vitamin B_{12} deficiency limits its conversion to

tetrahydrofolate. The morphologic identity of the megaloblast in vitamin B_{12} and folate deficiency is thus explained by an underlying biochemical identity: both disorders are characterized by an abnormal metabolism of folate.

The second enzymatic reaction, the methylmalonate–succinate isomerization, does not involve folate and may explain in part the specificity of the neurologic lesion, subacute combined degeneration, to vitamin B_{12} deficiency. One source of methylmalonyl coenzyme A (CoA) is propionate, a short-chain fatty acid. Propionyl CoA undergoes carboxylation to the D isomer of methylmalonyl CoA, which is then racemized to its L isomer. L-Methylmalonyl CoA is metabolized to succinyl CoA by an intramolecular change: it is catalyzed by the enzyme methylmalonyl-CoA mutase, which requires 5′-deoxyadenosyl-B_{12} as an essential cofactor. Succinyl CoA enters the citric acid cycle. This vitamin B_{12}–dependent pathway thus links lipid to carbohydrate metabolism and may explain in part the neurologic deficit in vitamin B_{12} deficiency. Thus, patients with deficient vitamin B_{12} are unable to metabolize propionate normally, and the defective myelin in vitamin B_{12} neuropathy has been shown to have an abnormal composition of fatty acid.[14] It should be stressed, however,

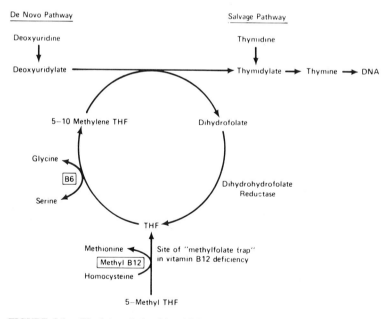

FIGURE 3.1. **The interrelationship of folate and vitamin B_{12} in DNA synthesis. The principal circulating form of folate is MTHF, whereas 5,10-methylenetetrahydrofolate is the folate that donates a one-carbon unit to deoxyuridylate to form thymidylate. Vitamin B_{12} deficiency causes the accumulation of MTHF and the depletion of other folates, that is, the "methylfolate trap." Several drugs cause megaloblastosis by inhibiting dihydrofolate reductase.**

that the ultimate lesion in vitamin B_{12} neuropathy remains unknown.

THE METABOLISM OF FOLATE. Folic acid (pteroylglutamic acid [PGA]) does not exist in the human body. Humans are unable to synthesize folic acid and depend on the absorption of dietary folate in the form of reduced derivatives of PGA linked to one to six L-glutamic acid residues in γ-carboxy linkages (folyl polyglutamate). The minimum daily requirement is estimated to be 50 μg of PGA, and surveys have indicated that many normal diets contain only 200 to 250 μg of PGA equivalents. The preparation of food can further limit the folate content, because folate is heat labile and water soluble. Excessive heating of food, or boiling and discarding the water, will substantially reduce dietary folate. Thus, there is little margin of error for the increased folate need of pregnancy, hemolytic anemia, or malabsorption. This explains the high prevalence of folate deficiency during pregnancy in general and the 50% prevalence in pregnant women who exclusively eat finely divided, well-boiled foods. These facets are compounded by the minimal body stores of folate; folate deficiency anemia has been induced in 4 months in a normal volunteer on a folate-deficient diet and has been seen within 5 weeks in subjects receiving hyperalimentation with a folate-free parenteral preparation.[15]

Dietary folate is absorbed, probably by an active process, primarily in the duodenum and jejunum. The enzyme "conjugase" (γ-L-glutamylcarboxy-peptidase) strips the glutamates off the nonabsorbable polyglutamates to leave the absorbable monoglutamates. During absorption, the folate is methylated and reduced to appear in the portal blood as MTHF, the principal transport of folate.[16] MTHF is removed by the liver and other cells, where it is again polyglutamated, and research indicates that polyglutamates rather than monoglutamates are the principal folate coenzymes.[17]

FOLATE-BINDING PROTEINS. Approximately 40% of serum folate is loosely bound to serum proteins, primarily albumin. In addition, a small percentage (perhaps 10%) of serum folate is bound to a specific folate-binding protein. The nature, specificity, and physiologic roles of folate binders have been the subject of increasing research, and Rothenberg and da Costa[18] reported an intracellular and serum folate binder in patients with chronic myelocytic leukemia and later in pregnant women or in those taking oral contraceptives. This binder consists in part of a 30,000 to 35,000 molecular weight glycoprotein that shows reversible binding with partially and fully reduced folates but irreversible binding with oxidized folates; these features suggest a role in the transport or intracellular metabolism of certain folates.

Low titers of unsaturated folate-binding protein are found in the serum of many normal subjects, and elevated levels of this protein have been reported in uremia and liver disease.[19] One group reported that the elevated serum levels of folate-binding protein in uremia withhold folate from the tissues to produce megaloblastic anemia in the face of a normal serum folate level. In our study of uremic patients, however, we could not support this theory; we found that elevated levels of serum folate-binding protein in uremia do not retard the delivery of folate to the tissues.[20]

In a general hospital population, we found elevated serum levels of unsaturated folate-binding protein in patients with metastatic cancer, active granulomatous disease, and alcoholic liver disease.[21] It seems likely that this specific folate-binding protein is an intracellular protein involved with the regulation of folate metabolism and that it appears in the serum as an index of the activity of certain cells, such as leukocytes and liver cells. Elevated serum levels of unsaturated folate-binding protein, which can be measured easily by radioassay, should alert clinicians to the possibility of certain diseases and may stimulate investigators to pursue possible abnormalities of folate metabolism in such cases.

DRUG-INDUCED MEGALOBLASTOSIS. Drugs that cause megaloblastosis can be divided into three main groups:

1. those that interfere with folate metabolism by inhibiting dihydrofolate reductase or by unknown mechanisms,
2. those that interfere with the absorption of vitamin B_{12}, and
3. those that interfere with DNA synthesis by inhibiting purine or pyrimidine synthesis.

Examples of drugs that inhibit dihydrofolate reductase (Fig. 3.1) are methotrexate, pyrimethamine, triamterene, and trimethoprim. Triamterene, a potassium-sparing diuretic, is a mild dihydrofolate reductase inhibitor that has a lower affinity for the enzyme than does methotrexate or pyrimethamine. The possibility of megaloblastosis with the use of this drug would occur in patients with low folate stores. Trimethoprim, a folate antagonist with a high affinity for bacterial dihydrofolate reductase but a low affinity for human marrow dihydrofolate reductase, also is unlikely to produce megaloblastosis if patients have normal folate stores. Alcohol, phenytoin, and oral contraceptives are examples of drugs that interfere with folate metabolism by unknown mechanisms; these agents are considered later. Drugs that interfere with the absorption of vitamin B_{12} include *p*-aminosalicylic acid (PAS), neomycin, colchicine, cholestyramine, and ethanol. Drugs that interfere with DNA synthesis by inhibiting purine synthesis include 6-mercaptopurine, azathioprine, and thioguanine. Drugs that interfere with DNA synthesis by inhibiting pyrimidine synthesis are 5-fluorouracil, hydroxyurea, and cytarabine.[22] A new mechanism is the inactivation of cellular vitamin B_{12} by the prolonged administration of nitrous oxide,[23] and the marrow depression and megaloblastoid change can be prevented by the administration of folinic acid before surgery for patients who are to receive nitrous oxide for 24 hours or longer.[24]

FOLATE DEFICIENCY. The main causes of folate deficiency include:

> Dietary lack of folate
> Malabsorption of folate
>> Sprue
> Increased need of folate
>> Pregnancy
>> Chronic hemolytic anemia
>> Chronic hemodialysis
>> Exfoliative dermatitis
>> Neoplasms
> Drugs
>> Dihydrofolate reductase inhibitors (methotrexate, pyrimethamine, triamterene, trimethoprim)
>> Alcohol
>> Phenytoin
>> Oral contraceptives

A poor diet can lead in weeks or months to folate deficiency anemia. The malabsorption of dietary folate is a common cause of folate deficiency. There is usually a history of diarrhea, weight loss, and steatorrhea, but these signs may be lacking or unimpressive in some cases of celiac sprue (gluten-induced enteropathy). In fact, a study of 57 patients with celiac sprue documented the frequent lack of classic malabsorption features and the unreliability of the routine malabsorption screening tests. More than 80% of these patients, however, had subnormal serum folate levels, and one third had macrocytosis. It was concluded that a random serum folate level is a valuable screening test for celiac disease in adults.[25]

Folate deficiency is almost invariably present in tropical sprue. Research with jejunal perfusion of simple and conjugated folates in this disorder has shown that both monoglutamates and polyglutamates are malabsorbed. This folate malabsorption is due to a yet-unexplained defect in folate transport by the abnormal

mucosa rather than to a deficiency in folate conjugase as was formerly thought.[26]

An increased need for folate occurs in pregnancy, lactation, hemolytic anemia, hyperthyroidism, rapidly growing cancers, agnogenic myeloid metaplasia, chronic exfoliative dermatitis, and chronic hemodialysis. Patients with any of these conditions have an increased risk of folate deficiency anemia unless their diets are rich in folate. The most common example of this imbalance between the supply of and demand for folate is the patient with sickle cell anemia who develops a worsening of anemia, reticulocytopenia, and megaloblastosis, which are all reversible with folic acid therapy.

Rare causes of folate-deficient megaloblastic anemia include congenital malabsorption of folate and congenital deficiencies of various folate enzymes, such as dihydrofolate reductase deficiency.

Alcohol. The most common drug that causes folate deficiency is alcohol. Up to 50% of alcoholics have megaloblastic anemia associated with folate deficiency. Alcohol has several direct effects on the bone marrow and also has multiple adverse effects on folate metabolism.[27] Large amounts of alcohol daily can produce vacuolated pronormoblasts in the marrow, elevated serum iron levels, and mild thrombocytopenia in those eating an otherwise optimal diet. The intake of 15 ounces of alcohol daily prevents or aborts a reticulocyte response to physiologic amounts of folic acid, and alcohol accelerates the onset of folate-deficient megaloblastic anemia in subjects on low-folate diets. The antifolate action of alcohol is complex; the combination of dietary folate deficiency and prolonged alcohol intake results in intestinal malabsorption of several water-soluble substances, including folic acid. Also, the ingestion or infusion of alcohol acutely lowers the serum folate level by a yet-unknown mechanism.[28] Folate deficiency in alcoholics is, of course, also related to poor nutrition.

The macrocytic anemia of alcoholism apparently is not caused by folate deficiency in all cases. Research in Great Britain indicated that although folate deficiency is relatively common among alcoholics there, these patients more frequently have macrocytosis, sometimes with mild megaloblastosis, without folate deficiency. This finding emphasizes an apparently direct, toxic effect of alcohol in the developing erythroblast.[3,29]

The macrocytic anemia of alcoholism can be complicated by the formation of ring sideroblasts. Although this was attributed originally to the reduced levels of pyridoxal phosphate from ethanol-induced suppression of pyridoxine kinase, it is now suggested that a defect in the formation of pyridoxal phosphate is not involved in most cases of alcoholic sideroblastic anemia.[30] Other investigators have suggested that acetaldehyde, a degradation product of ethanol, enhances the breakdown of pyridoxal phosphate by displacing it from a cellular protein binder to enhance its degradation by a phosphate enzyme. In any case, the appearance of ring sideroblasts in alcoholic subjects often correlates with coexistent folate deficiency.[31] It seems possible that the high serum iron induced by the ineffective erythropoiesis of folate deficiency, along with the mitochondrial damage induced by ethanol, produces the ring sideroblast in these patients.

The anemias of alcoholism seem diverse, but differences in the timing of the medical evaluation rather than in etiology may yield different patterns of anemia in alcohol patients. The evolution of anemia in many alcoholics proceeds through predictable stages:

1. negative vitamin balance, which begins when the patient reduces dietary intake and ingests large amounts of alcohol and in which the serum folate level sharply falls with no abnormality in erythropoiesis;
2. megaloblastic conversion, which may occur as early as 1 week after the initiation of alcohol intake and a poor diet;
3. sideroblastic conversion, which may occur soon after the megaloblastic change;
4. early resolution, a recovery stage in which a rapid disappearance of megaloblastic change with a persistence of ring sideroblasts gives the appearance of a pure sideroblastic anemia; and
5. late resolution, occurring 7 to 10 days after admission to the hospital, in which the bone marrow erythroid hyperplasia and reticulocytosis in response to folate simulate a hemolytic state.

Thus, the type of anemia in alcoholic patients depends, in part, on the timing of the medical evaluation of that anemia.[19]

Phenytoin. Long-term anticonvulsant therapy also is associated with folate-deficient megaloblastic anemia. Phenytoin has been the prime offender and the most studied agent, although megaloblastosis has been described with phenobarbital and primidone as well. The incidence of megaloblastic anemia in patients on continuous, long-term phenytoin therapy is less than 1%, but the incidence of macrocytosis has ranged up to 30% in some studies. Pregnancy and poor diet are additional precipitating factors in some cases; more than 50% of patients on long-term anticonvulsant therapy have significantly lower values of serum red cell folate than do comparable controls. The megaloblastic anemia always responds to treatment with even low doses of folic acid.

The mechanism by which phenytoin produces folate deficiency remains unknown. Early reports indicated that phenytoin caused a malabsorption of dietary polyglutamates by inhibiting intestinal conjugates; later reports have not confirmed this finding. Mechanisms under investigation are:

1. a competitive interaction between folate coenzymes and phenytoin,
2. a malabsorption of folic acid by the intestinal cell either because of a direct effect of phenytoin or an alkalinization of jejunal contents,
3. an induction by phenytoin of hepatic enzymes that catabolize folate,
4. an increased demand for folate as a coenzyme for the metabolism of anticonvulsants, and
5. a displacement of folate from plasma proteins by phenytoin.

In light of the relatively low prevalence of folate-deficient megaloblastic anemia in patients taking long-term phenytoin, it seems likely that the changes in folate metabolism induced by this agent, whether they be related to mild malabsorption, subtle metabolic changes, or merely displacement from plasma albumin, are not major enough to induce folate deficiency in the presence of optimal dietary folate.[32]

Oral Contraceptives. Oral contraceptives have been associated with folate deficiency anemia, but this is a very rare occurrence. Less than 50 cases have been reported. In some series, serum or red cell folate concentrations have been reduced in women using oral contraceptives. Early research suggested that oral contraceptives interfered with polyglutamate folate absorption, but more recent research has failed to support this concept. One group found that women on oral contraceptives have increased urinary excretion of folate, and the investigation of some cases of megaloblastic anemia in woman taking oral contraceptives revealed that these women have subclinical malabsorption, usually celiac sprue. The consensus is that the subtle abnormality in folate metabolism induced by oral contraceptives, whether it be a mild malabsorption of dietary folate, increased urinary loss of folate, or a yet-unknown mechanism, is not severe enough to cause folate deficiency in the otherwise normal woman.[33]

Research has suggested that the increased use of folate induced by oral contraceptive agents is greatest at the end-organ level, that is, oral contraceptives locally deplete folate enzymes, leading to folate deficiency in the uterus. Thus, almost 20% of 115 women taking oral contraceptives had mild megaloblastic change in Papanicolaou cervicovaginal smear, whereas none had a subnormal serum folate level, macrocytosis, or anemia. Supplemental folate given to eight such women caused the reversion of cervical smears to normal within 3 weeks. Fifty control women had no megaloblastic change in cervical smear.[33] These data raise interesting questions regarding differential local effects of folate deficiency in humans; furthermore, they are of practical importance. Although the nuclear changes in megaloblastic cervical smears differ from those in patients with dyskaryosis or dysplasia, it is possible that, on cursory examination, a megaloblastic Papanicolaou smear might be mislabeled as premalignant.[33]

In light of the consensus that oral contraceptives do not induce folate deficiency in otherwise normal women and the apparent benign nature of the mild megaloblastic changes in Papanicolaou smears, it is believed that women on oral contraceptives need not take supplemental folic acid. It should be noted, however, that one group reported subnormal levels of serum vitamin B_{12} in healthy young women taking oral contraceptive agents. The mechanism for this abnormality remains unknown, and their findings await confirmation.

FOLATE AND THE NERVOUS SYSTEM. Although progress has been made toward understanding the metabolic basis of megaloblastosis, the metabolic nature of the nervous system complications of vitamin B_{12} deficiency has eluded explanation. Folate deficiency classically has not been thought to produce neurologic damage. However, there has been increasing interest in the role of folate in nervous system metabolism, neuropsychiatric illness, and antiepileptic and convulsant mechanisms.[34] The brain contains relatively high concentrations of folate, and it has long been known that cerebrospinal fluid (CSF) has concentrations of folate approximately three times higher than serum concentrations. Furthermore, it has been shown that MTHF, but not folic acid, is actively transported across the choroid plexus into the CSF. Although the brain may lack dihydrofolate reductase, it contains several other folate enzymes, and it is speculated that MTHF is involved in central nervous system (CNS) events. Folate may be a physiologic methyl donor in the brain and may interact with the metabolism of monoamines; in addition, folic acid is a convulsant in certain animal studies, although the evidence for the exacerbation of epilepsy in humans by folic acid is conflicting. Some studies report exacerbation, but most fail to confirm this. Nevertheless, that folate compounds can be convulsant in animal models and that the three major anticonvulsants—phenytoin, phenobarbital, and primidone—have antifolate properties continue to fuel speculation. One study further

complicated this area: patients on long-term anticonvulsant therapy with no hematologic abnormality were found to have a lower mean CSF vitamin B_{12} level than did normal subjects. Also, nine patients with anticonvulsant-associated megaloblastic anemia had the expected low levels of serum and CSF folate but, in addition, had strikingly low levels of CSF vitamin B_{12}. This study suggested that the neuropsychiatric syndromes ascribed to folate deficiency during anticonvulsant therapy in fact may be secondary to the depletion of vitamin B_{12} in the CNS.[35]

Reports of neurologic damage from folate deficiency[36] should be viewed with caution. In contrast to vitamin B_{12} deficiency, in which the depletion of body stores takes years, low levels of serum folate develop in weeks or months on deficient diets. Folate deficiency is common in elderly patients (especially those with mental symptoms), is probably accompanied by other deficiencies from general malnutrition, and is sometimes complicated by alcoholism. Also in contrast to vitamin B_{12} deficiency, it is extremely rare to encounter pure folate deficiency. Then, too, the full interrelationship between folate and vitamin B_{12} metabolism remains unknown. Although folate deficiency may alter nervous system function, much research remains to be done before this concept becomes firmly entrenched.

THE METABOLISM OF VITAMIN B_{12}. Vitamin B_{12} is modified porphyrin with a ribonucleotide side chain and a central cobalt atom. Humans cannot synthesize vitamin B_{12} and are dependent on the absorption of dietary vitamin B_{12}, which is synthesized exclusively by microorganisms. The main sources of vitamin B_{12} in the human diet are liver, animal tissues, and dairy products. Normal American diets contain 15 to 30 $\mu g/d$ of vitamin B_{12}, whereas the minimum daily requirement is 1 to 3 μg. Body stores of vitamin B_{12} are large (2 to 4 mg), and there is an efficient enterohepatic circulation of vitamin B_{12} by way of the bile. Therefore, in contrast to folate deficiency, it takes 3 to 9 years to develop vitamin B_{12} deficiency after the absorption of dietary vitamin B_{12} ceases.

Vitamin B_{12} is absorbed actively in the distal ileum and passively, probably by diffusion, throughout the small intestine. The passive route becomes important only with pharmacologic amounts of vitamin B_{12}; approximately 1% of the administered dose is absorbed. The active absorption of dietary vitamin B_{12} depends on intrinsic factor, a carrier glycoprotein secreted by the parietal cells of the stomach that binds and protects vitamin B_{12} after it is released from foods. Intrinsic factor has two polypeptide chains and a molecular weight of approximately 60,000; one molecule binds one molecule of vitamin B_{12} very avidly and protects it from proteolytic digestion and utilization by intestinal bacteria. The complex passes into the small intestine, where it attaches to receptors on the brush border of the ileal mucosa cell in the presence of ionic calcium and a pH of 6.6 or greater. The nature of the ileal receptor remains unknown. Once attached to the receptor, intrinsic factor probably is not absorbed, whereas vitamin B_{12} enters the epithelial cell where it apparently attaches to unknown transport proteins. Vitamin B_{12} then enters the portal blood bound to a specific transport protein, transcobalamin II (TC II), which carries the vitamin to cells and facilitates cellular uptake.

VITAMIN B_{12}–BINDING PROTEINS. In the plasma, vitamin B_{12} is handled by at least two binding proteins: TC II, the delivery protein; and TC I, the intracellular and serum storage protein for vitamin B_{12}, which binds the vitamin avidly and accounts for the endogenous serum vitamin B_{12} level but does not deliver vitamin B_{12} to cells. Although intrinsic factor and TC II are vitally important to normal metabolism of vitamin B_{12}, the role of TC I is relatively unimportant. This is evidenced by the lack of a hematologic disorder, despite a low level of serum vitamin B_{12}, in people devoid of TC I. Conversely, the congenital lack of TC II leads to severe megaloblastic anemia in infancy despite normal levels of serum vitamin B_{12}; the only successful treatment is large parenteral doses of vitamin B_{12}.

Most of the TC I in plasma derives from granulocytes. TC I is an α-globulin with a molecular weight of approximately 150,000; TC II is a β-globulin with a molecular weight of approximately 38,000. Research using isoelectric focusing and affinity chromatography has made it possible to isolate, characterize, and compare other vitamin B_{12}–binding proteins from different materials. These all closely resemble TC I, and whether there is basically only one such protein (termed *R protein* or *cobalophilin*) or many functionally and chemically different proteins within the α-globulin family, is controversial. The growing consensus seems to be that the R proteins similar to TC I, found in milk, saliva, amniotic fluid, tears, and granulocytes, are all related in that they have a common peptide backbone and differ only in carbohydrate structure, probably mainly in sialic acid content.

This point of view would argue that the "new" vitamin B_{12}–binding protein discovered in 1972 (TC III) is actually just a partially separated fraction of the microheterogenous plasma cobalophilin family and that it should not be artificially distinguished from TC I. In fact, on isoelectric focusing, the border between TC I and TC III is diffuse and arbitrary, and there are not two but at least five subcompartments of this family of binding proteins. Thus, it seems that the cobalophilin

proteins consist of several components, that is, isoproteins, which have slightly variable carbohydrate composition and therefore differ slightly, especially in their catabolic rate. The function of these cobalophilin proteins is unknown, but it is speculated that they may act as antimicrobial agents by tightly binding vitamin B_{12} and withholding it from microorganisms.[37]

Abnormalities in serum levels of vitamin B_{12} and its binding proteins can help in the diagnosis of certain diseases (Table 3.1). Because TC I derives mainly from granulocytes, marked serum elevations are noted in chronic myelocytic leukemia and occasionally have been reported in leukemoid reactions. In addition, patients with metastatic cancer occasionally have extremely high levels of serum vitamin B_{12} and TC I (greater than those in even the most intense granulocytic proliferation and unexplained by leukocytosis).[38] Elevated serum levels of TC III are found in polycythemia vera and certain other myeloproliferative disorders. Elevated serum levels of TC II are a newly described finding in Gaucher disease, and extraordinary elevations of serum vitamin B_{12}–binding protein have been reported in three young patients with hepatoma. All had normal white cell counts and no evidence of megaloblastosis; the cobalophilin in these patients was slightly smaller than other members of this group and may represent a new vitamin B_{12} binder. Tumor tissue from one of the patients was rich in this binder, and secretion by the tumor seems to be the cause of the elevated serum levels.[39] Elevated serum levels of vitamin B_{12} are also seen in acute hepatitis. Finally, there are also reports of a patient with metastatic carcinoma of the lung in whom most of the circulating vitamin B_{12} was bound in a macromolecular complex containing a polyclonal immunoglobulin as well as reports of an acquired antibody to TC II, causing markedly elevated serum levels of vitamin B_{12} in an alcoholic patient with recurrent lung abscesses.[40]

TABLE 3.1. **Disorders Causing an Elevated Level of Serum Vitamin B_{12}**

Disorder	Main Binder Responsible
Chronic myelocytic leukemia	TC I
Leukemoid reaction	TC I
Metastatic cancer	TC I
Polycythemia vera	TC III
Gaucher disease*	TC II
Adolescent hepatoma	R binder
Acute hepatitis	TC I

*The level of serum vitamin B_{12} is normal, but the serum unsaturated B_{12} binding capacity is markedly elevated because of increased levels of TC II.

VITAMIN B_{12} DEFICIENCY. The main causes of vitamin B_{12} deficiency include:

Dietary lack of vitamin B_{12}
   Vegetarians; vegans
Lack of intrinsic factor
   Pernicious anemia
   Gastrectomy
Competition for vitamin B_{12}
   Diphyllobothrium latum (in Scandinavia)
   Blind loops; jejunal diverticula
Impaired ileal absorption of vitamin B_{12}
   Regional ileitis; ileal resection
   Sprue, especially tropical
   Defective receptors (Imerslund-Grasbeck syndrome)
   Chronic pancreatitis
Lack of transport protein
   Congenital deficiency of TC II

In light of the availability of vitamin B_{12} in meat and dairy products, its efficient absorption, and its large body stores, dietary deficiency of vitamin B_{12} is rare. It is limited essentially to vegetarians and vegans (who do not drink milk), and even strict vegetarians generally do not develop vitamin B_{12} deficiency unless they also begin to omit dairy products, as when they adopt a low-cholesterol diet.[41] Even in these groups, vitamin B_{12} deficiency takes years to develop. Vegetarians, with adequate intrinsic factor, resorb endogenous biliary vitamin B_{12} and are seemingly protected against vitamin B_{12} deficiency longer than are patients with pernicious anemia who lack intrinsic factor and are unable to resorb vitamin B_{12} in the bile. In fact, new evidence suggests that some vegans do not become overtly deficient in vitamin B_{12} until subtle vitamin B_{12} malabsorption occurs with the onset of gastric atrophy late in life.[42] A report from Great Britain stressed that Hindu Asian patients in that country, 15% of whom have the trait for β-thalassemia, can develop vitamin B_{12} deficiency from their strict vegetarianism without macrocytosis because of the coexisting β-thalassemia. The demonstration of severe megaloblastic anemia and other abnormalities from vitamin B_{12} deficiency in the infant of a vegan mother points out the need for vitamin B_{12} supplementation for vegan women who breast-feed their infants or for supplementation for the infants themselves.[43]

The classic example and most common cause of vitamin B_{12}–deficient anemia is pernicious anemia, which results from an impaired or complete lack of gastric secretions of intrinsic factor. The usual adult type of pernicious anemia affects middle-aged or elderly persons, probably because of genetic susceptibility and an associated, age-related chronic gastritis. Pernicious anemia is most frequent in persons of northern European ancestry but is not uncommon in blacks. In fact, evidence now suggests that pernicious anemia in American blacks may equal that in white's of all origins other than northern European and that, compared with whites, black women with pernicious anemia develop it at a significantly younger age and have a significantly greater prevalence of circulating antibody to intrinsic factor.[44]

The etiology of the impaired intrinsic factor production in pernicious anemia remains unknown, but there are interesting immunologic abnormalities and associations with other diseases. Most patients with pernicious anemia have antibodies directed against intrinsic factor; cell-mediated immunity to intrinsic factor has also been demonstrated in pernicious anemia. Antibodies against intrinsic factor are found in the serum, gastric juice, and even saliva of many of these patients. The two most common antibodies are type I, or blocking antibody, which prevents vitamin B_{12} from binding to intrinsic factor, and type II, or binding antibody, which reacts with the intrinsic factor–vitamin B_{12} complex. The blocking antibody has been found in the serum of 75% of patients and the binding antibody in the serum of 50%, but not without blocking antibody. The significance of this difference remains unexplained, but it may represent a greater immunogenicity of the intrinsic factor antigen that stimulates the blocking antibody. The presence of circulating intrinsic factor antibodies is almost pathognomonic of pernicious anemia, although there are rare exceptions.[45]

The serum of 90% of patients with pernicious anemia contains an antibody directed against the microvilli of the canalicular system of the gastric parietal cell. However, this antibody, also found in the gastric juice in 75% of patients and gastric mucosal plasma cells in 60%, is not specific for pernicious anemia. It also is seen in 30% to 60% of persons with idiopathic chronic atrophic gastritis without pernicious anemia, in 60% of persons with gastritis associated with iron deficiency, and in 25% of relatives of patients with pernicious anemia. The finding of serum parietal canalicular antibodies in the presence of a megaloblastic anemia, however, makes the diagnosis of pernicious anemia likely, and if intrinsic factor antibodies are present, this diagnosis is almost certain.[45]

Although there is evidence that both arms (B cells and T cells) of the immunoresponse may be involved in the production of pathologic changes in the stomach in pernicious anemia, an argument against B cell–mediated "autoimmune" phenomena being the primary cause of pernicious anemia is that pernicious anemia occurs in association with immunoglobulin deficiency. More than 20 such patients have been described; the immunodeficiency may be the isolated IgA type or panhypogammaglobulinemia. Ten patients with idiopathic, adult-onset immunoglobulin deficiency and pernicious anemia were reported in 1969; all had atrophic gastritis, achlorhydria, and no intrinsic factor. Unusual features were the early onset of pernicious anemia (mean age, 34 years) and the lack of antibodies to parietal cells and intrinsic factor. Delayed cell-mediated immunomechanisms were intact in these patients. It thus seems likely that gastric atrophy in such patients results from cellular immune hyperactivity and, in this sense, could be "autoimmune." However, isolated IgA deficiency occurs in approximately 1 of every 500 adults, and although the prevalence of acquired panhypogammaglobulinemia is not known, the putative link between pernicious anemia and dysgammaglobulinemia may be a chance association.[45]

Pernicious anemia, however, is associated with other endocrinologic or "autoimmune" diseases. Thyroid disease, especially primary hypothyroidism and Hashimoto thyroiditis, is often associated with pernicious anemia, Addison disease, and hypoparathyroidism. In women, there are statistically significant associations among three "autoimmune" diseases: pernicious anemia, vitiligo, and Graves disease. The evidence for a link between pernicious anemia and the histocompatibility antigens remains controversial; some studies find and others refute a link between pernicious anemia and certain HLA antigens.

A rare cause of vitamin B_{12} deficiency is congenital pernicious anemia, probably inherited as an autosomal recessive disorder, in which the child lacks intrinsic factor but has normal gastric mucosa and secretion of gastric acid. Any damage to parietal cells may reduce their secretion of intrinsic factor. Thus, any condition leading to chronic gastritis, such as chronic alcoholism, may produce vitamin B_{12} malabsorption, which is reversible. Vitamin B_{12} deficiency will, of course, follow total gastrectomy, although usually not for 5 years or more. Partial gastrectomy, particularly for gastric ulcer, also may be followed by a decrease in the secretion of intrinsic factor and, in time, pernicious anemia. The ingestion of corrosive toxicants and, rarely, extensive scirrhous carcinoma may impair the secretion of intrinsic factor.

Vitamin B_{12} deficiency may result from the destruction of vitamin B_{12} en route to or from malabsorption at the distal ileum. The fish tapeworm, *Diphyllobothrium latum*, when in the proximal jejunum, splits vitamin B_{12} from intrinsic factor and uses the vitamin. In time, it causes vitamin B_{12} deficiency and megaloblastic anemia (in 3% of carriers in Scandinavia), but this is not seen in the United States. Bacteria in intestinal diverticular or "blind loops" may also use vitamin B_{12} and cause vitamin B_{12} deficiency. This disorder is usually apparent because of gastrointestinal symptoms; the absorption of radioactive vitamin B_{12} should return to normal after 10 days of tetracycline therapy. The mucosa of the distal ileum may be damaged from diseases such as regional ileitis or drugs such as PAS, colchicine, neomycin, or alcohol, with resultant malabsorption of vitamin B_{12}. Also, florid megaloblastosis from folate deficiency has caused megaloblastic change of the small bowel, with reversible vitamin B_{12} malabsorption.[46] Approximately 50 cases of familial, selective vitamin B_{12} malabsorption syndrome in children, usually associated with proteinuria (Imerslund-Graesbeck syndrome), have been described; this defect may be due to a lack of or defective ileal receptors for the intrinsic factor–vitamin B_{12} complex and, when combined with proteinuria, may reflect a defect in membrane translocation of large molecules by the intestine and kidney. Intraluminal factors such as low pH with the Zollinger-Ellison syndrome or lack of an unknown pancreatic factor in chronic pancreatic insufficiency may produce vitamin B_{12} malabsorption at the distal ileum.[47] Approximately 40% of patients with chronic pancreatitis malabsorb vitamin B_{12}, and malabsorption of crystalline vitamin B_{12} has also been reported in cystic fibrosis. Evidence now suggests that vitamin B_{12} is preferentially bound to salivary R protein as opposed to gastric intrinsic factor and that the etiology of the vitamin B_{12} malabsorption in pancreatic insufficiency is the lack of pancreatic proteases that normally degrade R protein, thus releasing vitamin B_{12} for binding by intrinsic factor.[48] Both tropical and nontropical sprue (celiac disease) are reversible causes of vitamin B_{12} deficiency from damage to the ileal mucosa. Vitamin B_{12} deficiency also has been reported rarely owing to secretion of a biologically inert intrinsic factor.

Vitamin B_{12} deficiency can also occur from a congenital deficiency of TC II, the protein that picks up vitamin B_{12} from the distal ileum and delivers it to the liver and other cells. This severe megaloblastic anemia occurs early in infancy and can remain undiagnosed if the physician is unaware that serum vitamin B_{12} levels are normal in this condition, because the level of TC I, the vitamin B_{12} binder that carries most of the circulating vitamin B_{12}, is normal.

It has been suggested that large daily doses of vitamin C may destroy vitamin B_{12} in food and in serum. This theory has been carefully investigated, and it currently appears that "megadose" vitamin C may cause artificially low levels of serum vitamin B_{12} in some assays by increasing the cyanide requirement. Vitamin B_{12} destruction by vitamin C *in vivo*, however, probably does not occur.[49]

Diagnosis

The initial diagnosis of megaloblastic anemia is usually suspected when the MCV is elevated and the peripheral smear shows the characteristic macrocytes

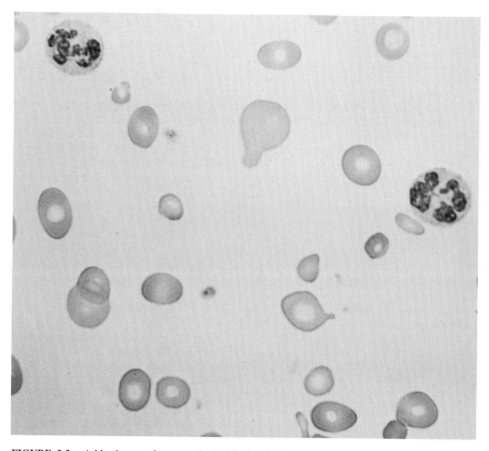

FIGURE 3.2. A blood smear from a patient with vitamin B$_{12}$ deficiency, demonstrating macrocytosis with oval macrocytes, poikilocytosis, and hypersegmented neutrophils.

and hypersegmented neutrophils. The classic oval mac-rocytes are always mixed with other abnormal shapes, such as "teardrop cells" and various other small, dis-torted cells; this poikilocytosis reflects the underlying ineffective erythropoiesis (Fig. 3.2). Other findings include large red cells with two areas of central pallor (twinning defect, probably from a failure to make the final cell division), Howell-Jolly bodies (nuclear rem-nants), and large platelets. When the anemia is severe, nucleated red cells may be seen in the smear, and the characteristic cytonuclear dissociation is apparent even in the peripheral smear.

Hypersegmentation (mean lobe count, 3.5 or greater) of the polymorphonuclear leukocytes in the smear is a clue for underlying megaloblastic hematopoiesis, even without macrocytosis or anemia. In a study of 58 patients with hypersegmentation without macrocytic anemia, 45 had a deficiency of folate, vitamin B$_{12}$, or both; 7 were uremic; and only 6 had hypersegmentation of deficiency by an unexplained cause.[50] Hypersegmen-tation has long been associated with uremia (probably some patients are folate deficient) and also apparently occurs as a rare familial trait. Despite the hypersegmen-tation, neutrophil function has been shown to be rela-tively normal in folate and vitamin B$_{12}$ deficiency.

The diagnosis of megaloblastic anemia is confirmed by megaloblastic changes in the aspirated bone marrow (Fig. 3.3). The marrow is typically hypercellular with many mitotic figures. The erythroid series shows young, nonpyknotic nuclei with normal hemoglobin; this be-comes easier to recognize in the later red cells, which have abundant hemoglobin, whereas the nucleus re-mains reticular and immature. In the myeloid series, the metamyelocytes and bands are often very large with huge "horseshoe" nuclei (Fig. 3.4). Rarely (4 of 129 cases in one report), erythroid hypoplasia with a great preponderance of myeloid precursors and a scarcity of megaloblasts is seen; this may be especially common in pregnancy and has been misdiagnosed as acute myelo-cytic leukemia.[51] Concomitant iron deficiency masks

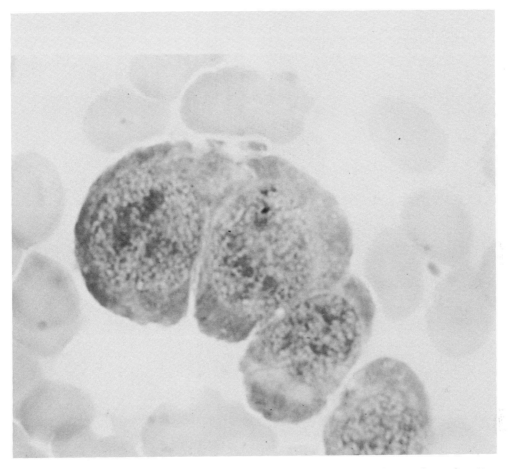

FIGURE 3.3. Four megaloblastic erythroid precursors showing the characteristic open chromatin pattern.

the megaloblastic features in the erythroid series by limiting the formation of hemoglobin. This brings the nuclear and cytoplasmic development more into balance and minimizes the distinctive cytonuclear dissociation. This situation is suggested by a dimorphic peripheral smear with both hypochromia and macrocytosis. The serum transferrin remains relatively saturated, but the marrow iron stores are less plentiful than in an uncomplicated case of megaloblastic anemia. If the patient is treated with only folate or vitamin B_{12}, the iron deficiency soon becomes readily apparent; conversely, treatment with iron alone will soon lead to florid megaloblastic erythropoiesis. Combined deficiencies of folate and iron are most common in pregnant women, patients with small bowel disease, and alcoholics who frequently donate blood; combined deficiencies of vitamin B_{12} and iron are most common after gastrectomy.

The Clinical Picture

Once megaloblastosis has been confirmed, its cause must be defined. The clinical setting will provide clues as to folate versus vitamin B_{12} deficiency. One third of patients with pernicious anemia have a family history of megaloblastosis, and pernicious anemia is most common in persons of northern European ancestry (fair skin, blond hair, premature graying, blue eyes, and large ears). The dietary history is usually normal in vitamin B_{12} deficiency, although anorexia and diarrhea may appear as late features. Vegetarians and vegans, however, are prone to nutritional vitamin B_{12} deficiency. Folate-deficient patients usually have poor diets, often associated with alcoholism or bizarre food habits; foods boiled excessively lose most of their folate. A history of gastric or ileal resection favors vitamin B_{12} deficiency,

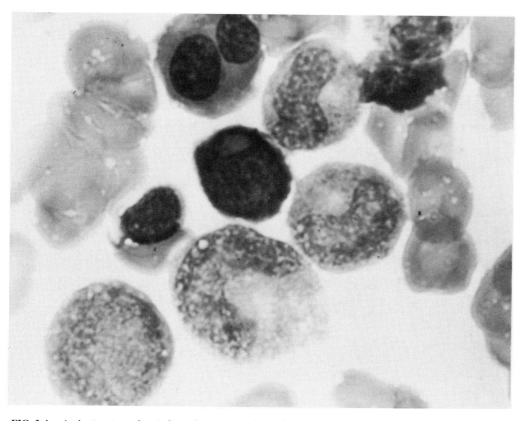

FIG 3.4. A giant metamyelocyte from the marrow of a patient with vitamin B_{12} deficiency. A binucleate megaloblast showing cytoplasmic dissociation is present.

and symptoms of malabsorption favor folate deficiency even though vitamin B_{12} deficiency may coexist or even predominate in small bowel disease, especially tropical sprue. The patient also must be questioned carefully about the use of drugs that may inhibit the metabolism of folate or vitamin B_{12}.

Neurologic symptoms, especially paresthesias, abnormal gait or fine coordination, or mental deterioration, favor vitamin B_{12} deficiency, as do the physical findings of disease in the long tracts of the posterior and lateral columns of the spinal cord (subacute combined degeneration). Such findings include impaired vibratory and position sense, changes in reflexes, ataxic or spastic gait, and impaired bladder or bowel function. Occasionally, a psychosis ("megaloblastic madness") will be the dominant feature of vitamin B_{12} deficiency and will be cured by timely therapy.[52]

Recent research suggests that the clinical picture of vitamin B_{12} deficiency can be more varied and subtle than was formerly thought. This stems from the wide availability of the serum vitamin B_{12} test in clinical practice and the consequent detection of many people

with subnormal values on this test. When such people are studied, it seems that subtle neurologic signs and symptoms—paresthesias, sensory changes, ataxia, memory loss, weakness, and changes in personality or mood—are the only features of the vitamin B_{12} deficiency in many of them. Contrary to common belief, then, neurologic pathophysiology is not always a consequence of late or severe vitamin B_{12} deficiency but can occur as an early feature, before the patient has clear-cut anemia or macrocytosis. For example, in one noted study of 141 consecutive patients with "neuropsychiatric abnormalities due to vitamin B_{12} deficiency," 40 of them (28%) had no anemia or macrocytosis, and many had only modest depression (100 to 200 pg/ml) of the serum vitamin B_{12} level. In some of these patients, who remained undiagnosed because of a low index of suspicion, megaloblastic anemia failed to develop even after years without treatment.[53] Upon perusal, many such patients had either a high-normal MCV or a low-normal hemoglobin level, and more than 90% had clues in the peripheral smear (hypersegmentation of neutrophils and/or macroovalocytes). Such clues, however, were often subtle and had been overlooked on routine laboratory analysis.

Similar trends toward the underdiagnosis of subtle vitamin B_{12} deficiency were noted in a recent analysis of 300 patients with serum vitamin B_{12} levels of less than 200 pg/ml[54] as well as an analysis of 70 consecutively diagnosed patients with pernicious anemia, wherein anemia was absent in 19% and macrocytosis was absent in 33% of the patients.[55] The new message here is that a low level of serum vitamin B_{12} should be taken seriously, even in patients with little or no obvious hematologic evidence of deficiency, and that the diagnosis of vitamin B_{12} deficiency should be pursued in any patient with subtle hematologic or neuropsychiatric abnormalities of the kind seen in vitamin B_{12} deficiency.

How best to establish that diagnosis is controversial and discussed later. Various authorities favor assaying for serum methylmalonic acid and total homocysteine[54] or using the deoxyuridine suppression test,[56] but these tests are not yet widely accepted or available. The Schilling test (discussed later) can be used, but it is becoming recognized that subtle vitamin B_{12} deficiency can sometimes occur despite a normal Schilling test.[57] Subtle vitamin B_{12} deficiency with a normal Schilling test occurs, it seems, in a patient with evolving gastric atrophy who loses gastric acid and enzymes before losing gastric intrinsic factor; when this happens, the patient can no longer split off and absorb the vitamin B_{12} in food but can still absorb the free, unbound vitamin B_{12} used in the classic Schilling test.

This new research says that, more often than we once thought, low levels of serum vitamin B_{12} are clinically important. In a recent study of 250 patients with low vitamin B_{12} levels, the management was deemed adequate only about one third of the time. In fact, the physician seemingly ignored the report of a low serum vitamin B_{12} level about 40% of the time.[58] Low levels of serum vitamin B_{12} can no longer be ignored.[59]

Aside from the neurologic signs, the physical examination is no help in differential diagnosis, because it shows only the signs of chronic anemia and perhaps the icterus and minimal splenomegaly of ineffective erythropoiesis and extravascular hemolysis. A study of 40 consecutive patients hospitalized for pernicious anemia showed a common failure by physicians to suspect the disease from clinical examination, even though most cases were advanced and the anemia was frequently recognized.[60] The triad of weakness, paresthesias, and sore tongue was rare. Only weakness was common, and sore tongue was present in only 10% of the patients. Many had angina, dyspnea, or edema, which often led to the diagnosis of coronary artery disease. Another sizable group was thought to have cancer; this was suspected because of anemia, weakness, and weight loss, and the anorexia and bowel disturbances pointed to the gastrointestinal tract as the possible site of malignancy. Several patients also were thought to have nonmalignant abdominal diseases. The neurologic signs present in 40% were not widely appreciated, and mental symptoms were often ascribed to cerebral arteriosclerosis. Some physicians thought the presence of pancytopenia excluded pernicious anemia as a possibility.

To have the proper "image" of pernicious anemia, one must remember that it is a systemic deficiency of vitamin B_{12} that may involve three blood cell lines (pancytopenia is common in severe cases), the brain, spinal cord, peripheral nerves, and gastrointestinal tract from the tongue to the colon.[60] Ancillary laboratory abnormalities include an elevated indirect bilirubin level and a normal-to-high serum iron level from the ineffective erythropoiesis and the extravascular hemolysis of megaloblastic anemia. Serum lactic dehydrogenase (LDH) levels may be extremely elevated, especially in severely anemic patients, and the source apparently is the megaloblast. Intriguingly, serum LDH is said to be normal in the megaloblastoid anemia of erythroleukemia. Serum muramidase is also elevated, and because muramidase derives mainly from granulocytes, the elevation in this enzyme suggests that the neutropenia in megaloblastic anemia results primarily from increased, probably ineffective granulocytic turnover. Serum gastrin is elevated in pernicious anemia because the gastrin-producing cells in the antrum of the stomach are uninhibited in the face of achlorhydria.

LABORATORY INVESTIGATION. The main diagnostic tests are:

> Tests of choice for diagnosis:
>   Serum and red cell folate levels
>   Serum vitamin B_{12} level
> Tests to support a diagnosis of vitamin B_{12} deficiency:
>   Gastric achlorhydria (in adult pernicious anemia)
>   Schilling test (establishes the type of vitamin B_{12} malabsorption)
>   Urinary excretion of methylmalonic acid (rarely needed)
> Special test:
>   Therapeutic trial (when vitamin assays are unavailable)

The laboratory tests of choice are the serum and red cell folate level and the serum vitamin B_{12} level determinations. These can be assayed either microbiologically or radioisotopically. A commercial radioassay kit measures both vitamins simultaneously, and preliminary comparative studies have verified its accuracy. False-low radioassay results due to contamination of the serum by intravenous administration of the radioisotope can occur within 1 week after diagnostic scans, and microbiologic assays are invalidated by certain antibiotics, especially penicillin, tetracycline, and chloramphenicol.

The serum folate level is a very sensitive index of negative folate balance; it falls within days of beginning a folate-free diet. It is the first laboratory sign of folate deficiency and may precede hematologic changes by weeks to months. Borderline low values are very common, however, and many such patients still have adequate tissue stores of folate. Also, common drugs, such as aspirin, displace folate from albumin. This accounts for the common finding of subnormal serum folate levels without hematologic abnormalities in patients with rheumatoid arthritis. Fortunately, because of the methylfolate trap discussed earlier (Fig. 3.1), serum folate levels tend to be high-normal or elevated in vitamin B_{12} deficiency and when accompanied by a low serum vitamin B_{12} level suggest vitamin B_{12} deficiency.

Mature red cells are relatively impermeable to folate, so their content of folate reflects the marrow folate status at the time they were generated. Therefore, subnormal red cell folate levels in conjunction with subnormal serum folate levels suggest tissue folate deficiency and generally correlate with the degree of hematologic abnormality. Red cell folate can, of course, still be normal in megaloblastic anemia of especially rapid onset, but this situation is rare. The red cell folate alone cannot be used to diagnose folate deficiency, because the values in two thirds of patients with vitamin B_{12} deficiency are subnormal. The folate in red cells is mainly polyglutamate, and because of the methylfolate trap in vitamin B_{12} deficiency, MTHF is unable to be converted to tetrahydrofolate (Fig. 3.1), the substrate of choice for the formation of polyglutamate.[17]

Urinary excretion of formiminoglutamic acid after 15 g of oral histidine is no longer used to diagnose folate deficiency. It is cumbersome, and it cannot be used in differential diagnosis because it is often positive in vitamin B_{12} deficiency. Tests of folate absorption are not clinically practical and are not really needed in the differential diagnosis of megaloblastic anemia. They serve to measure small bowel absorption, which can be better assessed by other tests.

The measurement of the serum vitamin B_{12} level is the most useful test to diagnose vitamin B_{12} deficiency. The

radioassay has replaced the microbiologic assay in most centers, but the false-normal values in some patients with pernicious anemia call for careful hematologic assessment and sound clinical judgment by the physician. Low serum levels of vitamin B_{12} with apparently normal tissue stores have been reported in pregnancy and multiple myeloma (possibly dilutional), and recent radioisotopic scans can cause false-low serum vitamin B_{12} (and folate) radioassay results unless the laboratory runs a serum blank to detect the contaminating radioisotope.[61]

The value of the serum vitamin B_{12} level as a diagnostic tool depends on the physician's attitude: a study of the utility of routine vitamin B_{12} determinations in the workup of anemia revealed that when pernicious anemia was suspected, physicians carried out extensive evaluations for vitamin B_{12} malabsorption before receipt of the low vitamin B_{12} level. Also, when vitamin B_{12} deficiency was not suspected, physicians largely ignored the return of a low value.[62] As mentioned earlier, this mode of thinking is no longer valid: new research suggests that low levels of vitamin B_{12} cannot be ignored safely.

Table 3.2 summarizes the characteristic diagnostic patterns of the vitamin assays, and Table 3.3 summarizes the most common causes of false-low serum vitamin B_{12} and folate results. The disorders that might cause a false-high serum vitamin B_{12} level are listed in Table 3.1. The two most common causes of a false-high serum folate level are the intake of dietary or vitamin folate before the specimen is drawn and hemolysis of the specimen, because the red cell folate content greatly exceeds the serum content.

Once the serum vitamin B_{12} level is found to be deficient, it is necessary to establish the physiologic cause by testing the absorption of vitamin B_{12}. Although whole-body counting methods are becoming available, the most widely used test is still the urinary excretion test of Schilling. In this test, 0.5 to 2 µg of radioactive vitamin B_{12} is given orally, followed 2 hours later by an intramuscular injection of 1000 µg of nonradioactive vitamin B_{12} to saturate tissue binders for vitamin B_{12} and thereby allow the absorbed, radioactive vitamin B_{12} to be excreted in the urine. Normal subjects excrete 10% to 35% of the administered dose in the urine over the next 24 hours, although congestive heart failure or renal disease may slow excretion. Patients with severe malabsorption of vitamin B_{12}, from either lack of intrinsic

TABLE 3.2.   Diagnostic Patterns of Vitamin Assays

Characteristic Diagnostic Profiles	Serum Vitamin B_{12}	Serum Folate	Red Cell Folate
Folate deficiency	Normal	Low	Low
Vitamin B_{12} deficiency	Low	Normal or high	Low or normal
Combined deficiency	Low	Low	Low

TABLE 3.3. **The Most Common Causes of Falsely Low Results on Vitamin Assays**

Serum Vitamin B_{12}	Serum Folate
Late pregnancy	Antibiotics or antimetabolites
Multiple myeloma	Improper handling of specimen (heat-labile)
Megadoses of vitamin C	Aspirin (high-dose)
Recent radioisotopic scan	Recent radioisotopic scan

factor or intestinal malabsorption, excrete less than 3%. The test is then repeated with commercial intrinsic factor given with the radioactive vitamin B_{12}; in pernicious anemia, the absorption is normalized, whereas in intestinal malabsorption, the excretion remains low. Misleading results of second-stage Schilling tests can occur in pernicious anemia when the intrinsic factor used is encapsulated, outdated, or otherwise inactive. When bacterial competition is suspected, as with blind loops, the test will revert to normal after 10 days of tetracycline therapy. Prior therapy with vitamin B_{12} does not alter the diagnostic pattern of the Schilling test in a patient with pernicious anemia.

Commercial kits simplify the Schilling test by giving two isotopes of vitamin B_{12} simultaneously: one free and one bound to intrinsic factor. Normal persons absorb both isotopes equally, whereas those with pernicious anemia absorb more of the intrinsic factor–bound isotope. There may be some exchange between the free and the bound vitamin B_{12}, however, and these kits require more investigation before being accepted. A common problem is that the value for the absorption of the free vitamin B_{12} is spuriously high, whereas the value for the absorption of the intrinsic factor–bound vitamin B_{12} is spuriously low, thus narrowing the difference and making it more difficult to diagnose vitamin B_{12} malabsorption with certainty.[63]

Because of the common problem of inadequate urine collection, many physicians prefer to obtain a 10-hour plasma radioactivity level during the Schilling test; a significant elevation of this value signifies normal absorption of vitamin B_{12}. Megaloblastic abnormality of the small bowel mucosa in advanced cases of either vitamin B_{12} or folate deficiency can blunt the expected response in the Schilling test, but therapy with the appropriate vitamin for several weeks restores the mucosa to normal and normalizes the Schilling test.[46,64] It must be stressed that an abnormal Schilling test diagnoses only vitamin B_{12} malabsorption, not pernicious anemia; tissue stores of vitamin B_{12} last for several years after the absorption of vitamin B_{12} ceases.

Gastric achlorhydria is present in virtually all adults with pernicious anemia, so the lack of free acid after maximal histamine stimulation supports the diagnosis of pernicious anemia. The gastric juice can also be assayed for its intrinsic factor content by a modification of the vitamin B_{12} radioassay; this test is not yet widely available and is not needed in most cases. The urinary excretion of methylmalonic acid is increased in vitamin B_{12} but not in folate deficiency. Therefore, the measurement of the urinary excretion of methylmalonic acid after an oral valine or isoleucine load can be used to diagnose vitamin B_{12} deficiency, but it is not a sensitive test. It is cumbersome, and it is not really needed for diagnosis.

The use of a therapeutic trial to establish the cause of megaloblastic anemia is rarely necessary now that serum vitamin assays are widely available. When properly done, however, a therapeutic trial is reliable. The patient should not be critically ill; should be free of infection, inflammation, or renal disease; and must be kept on a constant basal diet low in folate and vitamin B_{12}. The patient is then given daily physiologic doses of vitamin B_{12} (2 μg parenterally) or folic acid (100 μg orally or parenterally) for 10 days and observed for a hematologic response.

The clinical setting provides clues to the cause of a megaloblastic anemia that is usually first suspected because of macrocytosis, hypersegmented neutrophils, and elevated serum bilirubin and LDH and is confirmed by the demonstration of a megaloblastic marrow. The cause is identified by assays of the levels of serum and red cell folate and serum vitamin B_{12}. If these tests are unavailable, a therapeutic trial can yield the diagnosis. In vitamin B_{12} deficiency, absorption tests are necessary to pinpoint the physiologic cause. In folate deficiency, information about the intake of food, alcohol, and certain drugs will often establish the probable physiologic cause, but some patients will require additional tests to document the underlying small bowel malabsorption.

Management

FOLATE DEFICIENCY. Patients with anemia caused by folate deficiency respond well to folic acid, even in the presence of small bowel disease. Responses to as little as 25 to 50 μg of folic acid daily have been seen. However, daily doses of 300 μg in pregnancy and 500 μg in chronic hemolytic anemias may be necessary because of increased need. Because the normal daily requirement is less than 100 μg, a daily oral dose of 0.1 mg will gradually correct folate deficiency; larger doses will correct it faster. Because the bulk of larger doses is lost in urine and larger doses may mask the hematologic aspects of B_{12} deficiency while allowing the neurologic damage to progress, the Food and Drug Administration set the upper limit on commercial dosage of folic acid at 1 mg. Thus, 0.1-mg, 0.15-mg, and 1-mg folic acid tablets are now available in the United States. The therapy of choice for most patients is 1 mg daily for 2 weeks to replenish body folate stores; some physicians advocate treatment of up to 4 months for small bowel disease.

The patient should be instructed in basic nutrition. In many patients, the cause of the deficiency is reversible by improved intake of foods high in folate, such as liver, greens, and yeast; in patients with celiac sprue, a gluten-free diet is indicated. For alcoholic patients, sobriety is the key.

Prophylactic folic acid therapy is indicated in pregnancy, because the fetus uses maternal folate stores to such a degree that severe megaloblastic anemia may occur in the mother. Some multivitamin preparations do not contain any folic acid; it was taken out of these vitamins years ago to prevent inadvertent masking of vitamin B_{12} deficiency. Thus, a pregnant woman should take folate-containing vitamins or should receive 0.3 mg of folic acid daily throughout the pregnancy. Chronic prophylactic therapy is also indicated for patients with sickle cell anemia, thalassemia major, tropical or nontropical sprue, and agnogenic myeloid metaplasia; for infants on goat's milk; for children with protein-calorie malnutrition; and for patients being chronically dialyzed. In megaloblastic anemia caused by anticonvulsant drugs, folate therapy is given without withdrawal of the anticonvulsant. It has been suggested that folic acid increases the frequency of seizures, but this has not been substantiated by controlled trials.

VITAMIN B_{12} DEFICIENCY. Because patients with pernicious anemia, lacking gastric intrinsic factor, are unable to absorb standard doses of vitamin B_{12}, parenteral injection is the therapy of choice in the United States. Oral therapy using huge daily doses (1000 μg/d), however, is popular in Sweden and—as gauged by serum vitamin B_{12} levels and the hematologic response—seems to work.[65]

Cyanocobalamin is the preferred preparation. It is stable, inexpensive, and nontoxic, and the body converts it to physiologic forms. It suffices to treat any clinical feature of vitamin B_{12} deficiency, with the possible exception of the rare tobacco amblyopia, for which some recommend the more expensive and physiologic hydroxycobalamin.

Body stores are easily replenished by several injections of large doses of cyanocobalamin. The actual schedule of injections is not critical as long as 15 to 20 are given over a few weeks. It is convenient to give daily injections of 1000 μg while the patient is in the hospital and then one or two injections every week for several weeks. Although a larger fraction (80% to 85%) of a 1000-μg dose is lost in the urine than that from a smaller dose, the absolute amount retained is greater, thus justifying the larger dose. Twenty injections will provide about 3 mg of vitamin stores. There is no proof that patients with neuropathy benefit from larger doses.

Maintenance therapy must continue for life; 1000 μg once a month suffices. Occasionally, the patient will stop the injections, and the pernicious anemia will relapse. In one recent study, this occurred in about 10% of 333 patients. The mean interval before relapse was about 5 years, and the features were mimetic, that is, the relapse mimicked the first episode.[66]

Prophylactic B_{12} therapy should be given after total gastrectomy or ileal resection and to those patients with partial gastrectomy who have impaired B_{12} absorption and low levels of serum B_{12}.

Unfortunately, vitamin B_{12} is still used too often as a placebo. A recent study in the United States found that of 1222 patients in a rural health clinic, 120 (10%) got regular cyanocobalamin injections. Only 4 of these patients, however, met accepted criteria for its use.[67]

GENERAL COMMENTS. There is a notable mortality among elderly patients with severe megaloblastic anemia. A review of 108 patients with severe megaloblastic anemia (hematocrit under 25%) admitted to one hospital in Scotland showed that 14% died, whereas only 1.6% of similar patients with severe iron deficiency anemia died.[68] In a study of the mortality of 128 patients with severe megaloblastic anemia, over one half the deaths occurred during the first week of hospitalization, and one third were unexpected. Blood transfusion, usually whole blood, had been given to over one half of the patients. The predominant cause of death was congestive heart failure.

The most difficult management decision is whether to transfuse a severely anemic patient. In most cases, the heart has adapted to the slowly progressive anemia, and the benefit of rapidly increasing the hemoglobin level is outweighed by the danger of precipitating congestive heart failure and perhaps death. If, however, the anemia is extreme and the patient elderly and critically ill, one unit of packed red cells should be given slowly over 12 hours along with a diuretic, and the patient should be watched closely for signs of congestive heart failure. Such a patient is usually pancytopenic; after blood is obtained for vitamin assays, he or she should be treated with both folate and vitamin B_{12}. The final diagnosis can be sorted out later when the patient is less ill.

A single report suggested that hypokalemia during the early response to vitamin therapy may contribute to death in severe megaloblastic anemia.[68] A sharp fall in the serum potassium level occurred in 31 of 34 severely anemic patients, usually within the first 2 days of therapy, just before reticulocytosis. Hypokalemia was attributed to the uptake of potassium by rapidly proliferating marrow cells, along with a cessation of the release of potassium for dying marrow cells as ineffective erythropoiesis was reversed. Other groups, however, find relatively minor falls in potassium among similar patients, and the clinical importance of this phenomenon is uncertain. Until more information is available, it may be wise to monitor potassium during early therapy and to give oral potassium supplements for borderline or low levels of serum potassium.

The response to therapy should be monitored in all patients. The serum iron falls to subnormal levels within 24 hours and may remain low for weeks; the serum LDH level begins to fall within 2 days. Reticulocytosis begins on day 2 and reaches a peak proportional to the initial severity of the anemia on day 6. The hemoglobin usually begins to rise within 10 days and continues at an ever-slowing rate to normal within 8 weeks. Leukopenia and thrombocytopenia also are readily corrected by therapy; a transient rebound thrombocytosis may occur during the second week of therapy. The hypersegmentation of neutrophils persists for about 2 weeks and, thus, may be a valuable clue to the previous existence of a megaloblastic state in the patient seen after recent therapy with vitamin B_{12} or folic acid, or after the withdrawal of alcohol.[69] A delayed hematologic response suggests concomitant iron deficiency, infection, inflammation, or malignancy.

The epithelial changes also respond rapidly. Gastrointestinal symptoms are usually gone within 2 weeks, but the reversal of neurologic damage is considerably slower and related to the extent and duration of the disease. Psychosis of several weeks' duration has been dramatically reversed with vitamin B_{12} therapy.[52] The patient presenting with severe ataxia and an inability to walk for several months may eventually walk again, but the patient presenting with paraplegia and loss of sphincter control from advanced combined degeneration will probably remain bedridden even though the neurologic damage is arrested by vitamin B_{12} therapy.

Benign gastric polyps occur in 7% of patients with pernicious anemia. Gastric carcinoma may eventually develop in 6% to 8% of these patients, but the frequency of gastric carcinoma in pernicious anemia, as in the general population, is decreasing. Early recognition of gastric carcinoma, however, remains a vexing problem. Routine annual gastroscopy or roentgenographic study of the upper gastrointestinal tract is probably not warranted, but the patient with pernicious anemia should be checked at least annually for occult blood in the stool and for early hematologic signs of iron deficiency. The patient should report promptly any dyspepsia, change in bowel habits, or weight loss. Early diagnosis of gastric carcinoma may save a life.

Finally, a new study shows that patients with pernicious anemia may have an increased risk for colorectal adenocarcinoma in the 5 years after the diagnosis of their anemia.[70]

REFERENCES

1. McPhedran P, Barnes MG, Weinstein JS, et al. Interpretation of electronically determined macrocytosis. Ann Intern Med 1973;78:677.
2. Chanarin I, England JM, Hoffbrand AV. Significance of large red blood cells. Br J Haematol 1973;25:351.
3. Wu A, Chanarin I, Levi AJ. Macrocytosis of chronic alcoholism. Lancet 1974;i:829.
4. Ungar KW, Johnson D. Red blood cell mean corpuscular volume: a potential indicator of alcohol usage in a working population. Am J Med Sci 1974;267:281.
5. Papoz L, Warnet JM, Pequignot G, et al. Alcohol consumption in a healthy population: relationship to gamma-glutamyl transferase activity and mean corpuscular volume. JAMA 1981;245:1748.
6. Chalmers DM, Levi AJ, Chanarin I, et al. Mean cell volume in a working population: the effects of age, smoking, alcohol and oral contraception. Br J Haematol 1979;43:631.
7. Self KG, Conrady MM, Eichner ER. Failure to diagnose anemia in medical inpatients. Am J Med 1986;81:786–90.
8. Wymer A, Becker DM. Recognition and evaluation of red blood cell macrocytosis in the primary care setting. J Gen Intern Med 1990;5:192–7.
9. Seward SJ, Safran C, Marton KI, Robinson SH. Does the mean corpuscular volume help physicians evaluate hospitalized patients with anemia? J Gen Intern Med 1990;5:187–91.
10. Hillman RS. After sixty years: the MCV is alive and well. J Gen Intern Med 1990;5:264–5.
11. Koeffler HP, Golde DW. Human preleukemia. Ann Intern Med 1980;93:347.
12. Das KC, Herbert V. Vitamin B_{12}-folate interrelationships. Clin Haematol 1976;5:697.
13. Nixon PF, Bertino JR. Impaired utilization of serum folate in pernicious anemia: a study with radiolabeled 5-methyltetrahydrofolate. J Clin Invest 1972;51:1431.
14. Frenkel EP. Abnormal fatty acid metabolism in peripheral nerves of patients with pernicious anemia. J Clin Invest 1973;52:1237.
15. Ballard HS, Lindenbaum J. Megaloblastic anemia complicating hyperalimentation therapy. Am J Med 1974;56:740.
16. Rosenberg IH. Folate absorption and malabsorption. N Engl J Med 1975;293:1303.
17. Hoffbrand AV. Synthesis and breakdown of natural folates (folate polyglutamates). Prog Hematol 1975;9:85.
18. Rothenberg SP, da Costa M. Folate binding proteins and radioassay for folate. Clin Hematol 1976;5:569.
19. Colman N, Herbert V. Total folate binding capacity of normal human plasma, and variations in uremia, cirrhosis, and pregnancy. Blood 1976;48:911.
20. Paine CJ, Hargrove MD Jr, Eichner ER. Folic acid binding protein and folate balance in uremia. Arch Intern Med 1976;136:756.
21. Eichner ER, McDonald CR, Dickson VL. Elevated serum levels of unsaturated folate binding protein: clinical correlates in a general hospital population. Am J Clin Nutr 1978;31:1988.
22. Stebbins R, Bertino JR. Megaloblastic anemia produced by drugs. Clin Haematol 1976;5:619.

23. Amess JAL, Burman JF, Rees GM, et al. Megaloblastic hae-mopoiesis in patients receiving nitrous oxide. Lancet 1978;ii:339.
24. Scott JM, Weir DG. Drug-induced megaloblastic change. Clin Haematol 1980;9:587.
25. Roberts RK, Cowen AE. The changing clinical presentation of coeliac disease in adults. Med J Aust 1977;1:89.
26. Corcino JJ, Reisenauer AM, Halstead CH. Jejunal perfusion of simple and conjugated folates in tropical sprue. J Clin Invest 1976;58:298.
27. Eichner ER. The hematologic disorders of alcoholism. Am J Med 1973;54:621.
28. Waldrop CAJ, Heatley RV, Tennant GB, et al. Acute folate deficiency in surgical patients on amino acid/ethanol intravenous nutrition. Lancet 1975;ii:640.
29. Wu A, Chanarin I, Slavin G, et al. Folate deficiency in the alcoholic: its relationship to clinical and haematological abnor-malities, liver disease and folate stores. Br J Haematol 1975;29:469.
30. Chillar RK, Johnson CS, Beutler E. Erythrocyte pyridoxine kinase levels in patients with sideroblastic anemia. N Engl J Med 1976;195:881.
31. Pierce HI, McGuffin RG, Hillman RS. Clinical studies in alco-holic sideroblastosis. Arch Intern Med 1976;136:283.
32. Weber TH, Sakari K, Tammisto P, et al. Long-term use of phenytoin: effects on whole blood and red cell folate and haema-tological parameters. Scand J Haematol 1977;18:81.
33. Lindenbaum J, Whitehead N, Reyner F. Oral contraceptive hormones, folate metabolism, and the cervical epithelium. Am J Clin Nutr 1975;28:346.
34. Reynolds EH. Neurological aspects of folate and vitamin B_{12} metabolism. Clin Haematol 1976;5:661.
35. Frenkel EP, McCall MS, Sheehan RG. Cerebrospinal fluid folate and vitamin B_{12} in anti-convulsant-induced megaloblastosis. J Lab Clin Med 1973;81:105.
36. Manzoor M, Runcie J. Folate-responsive neuropathy: report of 10 cases. BMJ 1976;1:1176.
37. Stenman UH. Intrinsic factor and the vitamin B_{12} binding pro-teins. Clin Haematol 1976;5:473.
38. Carmel R. Extreme elevation of serum transcobalamin I in patients with metastatic cancer. N Engl J Med 1975;292:282.
39. Waxman S, Gilbert HS. A tumor-related vitamin B_{12}-binding protein in adolescent hepatoma. N Engl J Med 1973;289:1053.
40. Carmel R, Tatsis B, Baril L. Circulating antibody to transcobal-amin II causing retention of vitamin B_{12} in the blood. Blood 1977;49:987.
41. Murphy MF. Vitamin B_{12} deficiency due to a low-cholesterol diet in a vegetarian. Ann Intern Med 1981;94:57.
42. Carmel R. Nutritional vitamin-B_{12} malabsorption: possible con-tributory role of subtle vitamin-B_{12} malabsorption. Ann Intern Med 1978;88:647.
43. Higginbottom MC, Sweetman L, Nyhan WL. A syndrome of methylmalonic aciduria, homocystinuria, megaloblastic anemia and neurologic abnormalities in a vitamin B_{12}-deficient breast-fed infant of a strict vegetarian. N Engl J Med 1978;299:317.
44. Carmel R, Johnson CS. Racial patterns in pernicious anemia: early age at onset and increased frequency of intrinsic-factor antibody in black women. N Engl J Med 1978;298:647.
45. Taylor KB. Immune aspects of pernicious anemia and atrophic gastritis. Clin Haematol 1976;5:497.
46. Hermos JA, Adams WH, Liu YK, et al. Mucosa of the small intestine in folate-deficient alcoholics. Ann Intern Med 1972;76:957.
47. Toskes PP, Hansell J, Cerda J, et al. Vitamin B_{12} malabsorption in chronic pancreatic insufficiency: studies suggesting the pres-ence of a pancreatic "intrinsic factor." N Engl J Med 1971;284:627.
48. Allen RH, Seetharam B, Allen NC, et al. Correction of cobalamin malabsorption in pancreatic insufficiency with a cobalamin ana-logue that binds with high affinity to R protein but not to intrinsic factor: in vivo evidence that a failure to partially degrade R protein is responsible for cobalamin malabsorption in pancreatic insuffi-ciency. J Clin Invest 1978;61:1628.
49. Marcus M, Prabhudesai M, Wassef S. Stability of vitamin B_{12} in the presence of ascorbic acid in food and serum: restoration by cyanide of apparent loss. Am J Clin Nutr 1980;33:137.
50. Hettersley PG, Engels JL. Neutrophilic hypersegmentation with-out macrocytic anemia. West J Med 1974;121:179.
51. Pezzimenti JF, Lindenbaum J. Megaloblastic anemia associated with erythroid hypoplasia. Am J Med 1972;53:748.
52. Hart RJ Jr, McCurdy PR. Psychosis in vitamin B_{12} deficiency. Arch Intern Med 1971;128:596.
53. Lindenbaum J, Healton EB, Savage D, et al. Neuropsychiatric disorders caused by cobalamin deficiency in the absence of anemia or macrocytosis. N Engl J Med 1988;318:1720–8.
54. Stabler SP, Allen RH, Savage DG, Lindenbaum J. Clinical spectrum and diagnosis of cobalamin deficiency. Blood 1990;76:871–81.
55. Carmel R. Pernicious anemia: the expected findings of very low serum cobalamin levels, anemia, and macrocytosis are often lacking. Arch Intern Med 1988;148:1712–4.
56. Carmel R, Karnaze DS. The deoxyuridine suppression test iden-tifies subtle cobalamin deficiency in patients without typical megaloblastic anemia. JAMA 1985; 253:1284–7.
57. Carmel R, Sinow RM, Siegel ME, Samloff IM. Food cobalamin malabsorption occurs frequently in patients with unexplained low serum cobalamin levels. Arch Intern Med 1988;148:1715–9.
58. Carmel R, Karnaze DS. Physician response to low serum cobal-amin levels. Arch Intern Med 1986;146:1161–5.
59. Herbert V. Don't ignore low serum cobalamin levels. Arch Intern Med 1988;148:1705–7.
60. Hall CA. The nondiagnosis of pernicious anemia. Ann Intern Med 1965;63:951.
61. Carmel R. Artifactual radioassay results due to serum contamina-tion by intravenous radioisotope administration: falsely low se-rum vitamin B_{12} and folic acid results. Am J Clin Pathol 1978;70:364.
62. Pierce HI, Hillman RS. The value of the serum vitamin B_{12} level in diagnosing B_{12} deficiency. Blood 1974;43:915.
63. Carmel R. The Schilling test. Ann Intern Med 1980;92:570.
64. Lindenbaum J, Pezzimenti JF, Shea N. Small-intestinal function in vitamin B_{12} deficiency. Ann Intern Med 1974;80:326.
65. Lederle FA. Oral cobalamin for pernicious anemia: medicine's best kept secret? JAMA 1991;265:94–5.
66. Savage D, Lindenbaum J. Relapses after interruption of cyanoco-balamin therapy in patients with pernicious anemia. Am J Med 1983;74:765–72.
67. Lawhorne L, Ringdahl D. Cyanocobalamin injections for patients without documented deficiency. JAMA 1989;261:1920–3.
68. Lawson DH, Murray RM, Parker JLW. Early mortality in the megaloblastic anaemias. Q J Med 1972;41:1.
69. Nath BJ, Lindenbaum J. Persistence of neutrophil hypersegmen-tation during recovery from megaloblastic granulopoiesis. Ann Intern Med 1979;90:757.
70. Talley NJ, Chute CG, Larson DE, et al. Risk for colorectal adenocarcinoma in pernicious anemia: a population-based cohort study. Ann Intern Med 1989;110:738–42.

4

Hemoglobinopathies and Thalassemias

John A. Phillips III, M.D., and Haig H. Kazazian, Jr., M.D.

The biosynthesis of hemoglobin in the erythrocyte is one of the most striking examples of cellular specialization known in nature. Inherited disorders of hemoglobin synthesis, such as the hemoglobinopathies and the thalassemia syndromes, are common and significant clinical conditions. This chapter briefly summarizes current knowledge of the structure, function, and biosynthesis of normal hemoglobin and discusses clinical diseases resulting from qualitative (hemoglobinopathies) or quantitative (thalassemia syndromes) defects in globin synthesis.

NORMAL HUMAN HEMOGLOBIN

Hemoglobin is a tetramer with a molecular weight of 64,500. It consists of two α- and two non-α-globin polypeptide chains, each having a single covalently bound heme group. Each of these four heme groups consists of an iron atom bound within a protoporphyrin-IX ring.[1]

In humans, the six known different globin polypeptide chains are designated α, β, γ, δ, ϵ, and ζ. Each chain consists of a specified sequence of amino acids linked by peptide bonds. The α-chains contain 141 amino acids, while the β-, γ-, δ-, and ϵ-chains have 146 residues. The ϵ-, γ-, and δ-chains are more similar to β- than to α-chains, differing from β-chains at 36, 39, and 10 positions, respectively.[1,2] The ϵ- and ζ-globins are found in embryonic erythrocytes. The ϵ sequence encodes an embryonic β-like chain, and the ζ sequence encodes an embryonic α-like chain.

The hemoglobin composition of erythrocyte lysates can be quantified by zone electrophoresis. Table 4.1 shows the different hemoglobin tetramers, their structure, percentage in normal adult lysate, and conditions in which levels are increased.[1] Hemoglobin A ($\alpha_2\beta_2$) is usually 92% of the total hemoglobin in normal adults. Hemoglobin A_2 ($\alpha_2\delta_2$) constitutes approximately 2.5% and is distributed evenly in normal red cells; it may be increased in β-thalassemias and megaloblastic anemia and decreased in iron deficiency and sideroblastic anemias.

Hemoglobin A_{1c} differs from hemoglobin A by the posttranslational addition of a glucose at the NH_2-terminal of the β-chain; hence, this tetramer's structure is α_2 (β-N-glucose)$_2$. The proportion of hemoglobin A_{1c} (5% in normal patients) is related to the intracellular glucose concentration and the red cell lifespan. In patients with diabetes, the concentration of hemoglobin A_{1c} is increased approximately twofold because of the elevated glucose concentration in their red cells.[1]

While hemoglobin F ($\alpha_2\gamma_2$) comprises the bulk of hemoglobin in newborn humans (50% to 85%) it declines rapidly after birth, reaching concentrations of 10% to 15% by 4 months of age. Subsequently, the decline is slower, and adult levels of less than 1% are reached by 3 to 4 years of age. Fetal hemoglobin may be increased in β- and $\delta\beta$-thalassemia, hereditary persistence of fetal hemoglobin, trisomy 13, some cases of thyrotoxicosis, megaloblastic and aplastic anemia, leukemia and various malignancies involving marrow,

An earlier version of this chapter appeared as "Haemoglobinopathies and Thalassaemias," in Emery AH, Rimoin DL, eds. *Principles and Practice of Medical Genetics*, 2nd ed. London: Churchill Livingstone, 1990:1315–42.

TABLE 4.1. Human Hemoglobins

Hb Name	Synonym	Structure	Percentage in Adults	Conditions in Which Increased
A	Adult Hb	$\alpha_2\beta_2$	92	
A_{1c}		$\alpha_2(\beta\text{-N-glucose})_2$	5	Diabetes mellitus
A_2		$\alpha_2\delta_2$	2.5	β-Thalassemia
F	Fetal Hb	$\alpha_2\gamma_2$	<1	Newborn, β-thalassemia, and marrow stress
H		β_4	0	Some α-thalassemias
Barts		γ_4	0	Some α-thalassemias
Gower 1	Embryonic Hb	$\zeta_2\epsilon_2$	0	Early embryos (<8 weeks)
Gower 2	Embryonic Hb	$\alpha_2\epsilon_2$	0	Early embryos (<8 weeks)
Portland	Embryonic Hb	$\zeta_2\tau_2$	0	Early embryos (<8 weeks) and α°-thalassemia (hydrops fetalis)

Source: Bunn et al. 1986.[3]
Note: Hb = hemoglobin.

sickle cell anemia, and during pregnancy.[4] Hemoglobin F is measured by resistance to alkali, electrophoresis, or column chromatography.

Hemoglobins Gower 1 ($\zeta_2\epsilon_2$), Gower 2 ($\alpha_2\epsilon_2$), and Portland ($\zeta_2\gamma_2$) are embryonic hemoglobins found in fetuses before 7 to 10 weeks of gestation. At 4 to 5 weeks of gestation, a simultaneous decrease in the production of ζ- and ϵ-chains and an increase in the production of α- and γ-chains occur.[5] β-Chain synthesis in reticulocytes accounts for 4% of non-α synthesis at 5 weeks of gestation and gradually increases thereafter.[6] While the time of the decrease in ϵ- and ζ-chains coincides with the switch from yolk sac to hepatic-derived erythrocytes, the restriction of embryonic chain synthesis to yolk sac cells and the converse restriction of γ- and β-chains to hepatic cells have not been proven.

Hemoglobins H and Barts are tetramers of β- and γ-chains, respectively, and both function very poorly in transporting oxygen. These two hemoglobins may be increased in some types of α-thalassemia.

Primary and Secondary Structures

The primary structure of each globin chain is its amino acid sequence: 141 amino acids in the α-chains and 146 in the β-, γ-, δ-, and ϵ-chains. Figure 4.1 shows the primary structure of the α- and β-chains.

The relationship between adjacent amino acids along the chain enables interactions that can result in one of the two basic configurations of the secondary structure: the α-helix or the β-pleated sheet. The α-helix, stabilized by hydrogen bonding between carbonyl and amino groups, has 3.6 amino acid residues per turn. Approximately 75% of hemoglobin in its native state is in the α-helix form, as shown in Figure 4.1. The β-pleated-sheet configuration predominates in other molecules such as immunoglobulins and chymotrypsin.

At specific locations in the hemoglobin subunits, the rodlike α-helix is interrupted by nonhelical segments that allow folding. On x-ray crystallography, the conformations of the α- and β-hemoglobin subunits are seen to be similar. The β-globin chain has eight helical segments, A through H, and the secondary structure of the α-globin corresponds to that of the β-globin except for the absence of residues forming the D helical region (Fig. 4.1). The histidine residue at position 8 of the F helical segment (F8) is linked covalently to the heme iron molecule. This histidine residue is located at position 87 in the α- and 92 in the β-chain, and mutations altering it have important pathologic consequences. Amino acids with charged side groups (e.g., lysine, arginine, and glutamic acid) lie on the external surface, while uncharged residues tend to be oriented toward the interior of the molecule.[7]

Tertiary and Quaternary Structures

Tertiary structure refers to the configuration of a protein subunit in three-dimensional space, while *quaternary structure* refers to the relationships of the four hemoglobin subunits to each other. The hemoglobin tetramer has been shown by x-ray crystallography to be an oblate spheroid with a diameter of 5.5 nm and a single axis of symmetry. The globin chains are folded, so the four heme groups are in surface clefts equidistant from each other. The four subunits forming the tetramers are labeled α_1, α_2, β_1, and β_2. While there is no contact between the two β-chains, each α-chain touches both β-chains. Bonds across the α_1–β_1 interface are firmer than those at the α_1–β_2 interface, and changes from oxy-

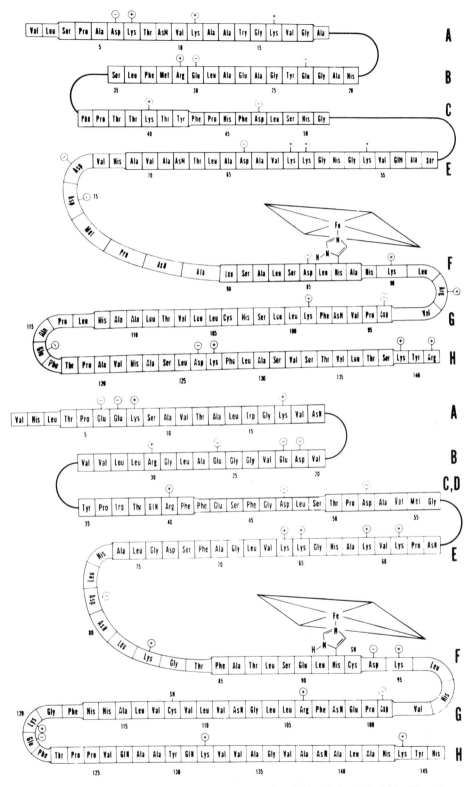

FIGURE 4.1. The primary and secondary structures of α-globin (*Top*) and β-globin (*Bottom*) chains. Residues in α-helix configuration are in squares; nonhelical residues are in rectangles. (*Source:* Murayama 1971.[9] Courtesy of Charles C. Thomas, Springfield, Ill.)

to deoxyhemoglobin involve more extensive movement at the α_1–β_2 interface. The quaternary structure changes markedly when changing from oxy- to deoxyhemoglobin, and this accounts for many of the observed changes in physical properties. Hemoglobin mutations resulting in amino acid substitutions at these points can alter markedly specific functional properties.[7]

FUNCTIONAL PROPERTIES

For hemoglobin to fulfill its physiologic role, it must bind oxygen with a certain affinity. One measure of oxygen affinity is P_{50} (the partial pressure of oxygen in mm Hg that is required for 50% saturation of hemoglobin): a hemoglobin with increased P_{50} has decreased oxygen affinity (Fig. 4.2). Oxygen affinity also is affected by a number of environmental factors, including temperature, pH, concentration of organic phosphate, and P_{CO_2} (Fig. 4.2).[8]

The sigmoid shape of the oxyhemoglobin dissociation curve reflects heme–heme interaction, that is, successive oxygenation of each heme group in the tetramer increases the oxygen affinity of the remaining unoxygenated heme groups. The basis of the heme–heme interaction is the decrease in the atomic radius of the heme iron that occurs with oxygenation, allowing the iron atom to fit into the plane of the porphyrin ring. A series of conformational changes that affect the other heme groups amplifies this alteration.[8] The resulting sigmoid oxyhemoglobin dissociation curve has great

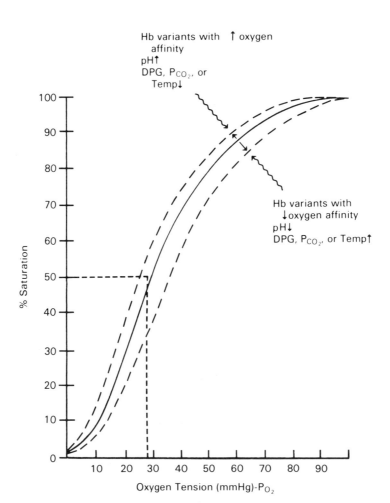

FIGURE 4.2. The oxyhemoglobin dissociation curve and the effect of different factors on oxygen affinity. *Note:* Hb = hemoglobin. (*Source:* Phillips and Kazazian 1990, p. 1318.)

physiologic importance, because it enables large amounts of oxygen to be bound or released with a small increase or decrease in oxygen tension. In contrast to hemoglobin A, hemoglobins H (β_4) and Barts (γ_4) lack subunit interaction and have a hyperbolic rather than sigmoid oxyhemoglobin dissociation curve, which prevents the release of oxygen at physiologic oxygen tensions.

The Bohr effect is a change in the oxygen affinity of hemoglobin with a change in pH. This effect is beneficial at the tissue level, where the lower pH decreases the oxygen affinity and promotes the release of oxygen (Fig. 4.2). The uptake of oxygen in the lungs is enhanced by the opposite changes in pH and P_{CO_2}.

Red cells have unusually high concentrations of 2,3-diphosphoglycerate (2,3-DPG). One molecule of 2,3-DPG sits in a pocket in deoxyhemoglobin bound to specific β-chain residues (1, 2, 82, and 143 of both β-chains). The importance of the binding is that 2,3-DPG stabilizes the deoxygenated form of hemoglobin in preference to the oxygenated form, thereby lowering the oxygen affinity of the molecule. The γ-chain of hemoglobin F lacks the β^{143}-histidine residue, and the resultant decrease in the binding of 2,3-DPG to hemoglobin F accounts for the increased oxygen affinity of fetal red cells compared to that of adult red cells.[8,9]

THE BIOSYNTHESIS OF HEMOGLOBIN

Genetics

In humans, eight different genetic loci code for the six globin genes.[2,10–14] In addition, at least three pseudogenes have sequences similar to other globin genes but differ in that they are not expressed into globin proteins.[15,16] Normally, globin tetramers are formed of two α- or α-like chains and two non-α-chains; Figure 4.3 provides a schematic representation of the interaction of the products of these genes. Because humans are diploid (i.e., have one pair of each nonsex chromosome or autosome), they have two genes for each autosomal locus. For example, two loci encode the structure of the α-chain, thus there are four α-chain genes. In contrast, there is only a single β-globin locus and, therefore, two β-genes (Fig. 4.3). The relative numbers of α- and β-loci are important in understanding the different inheritance patterns of α- and β-thalassemia as well as the different relative amounts of variant hemoglobin in individuals carrying a variant α- or β-globin gene. These quantitative differences directly correlate with the clinical severity of the various disorders.

The region of chromosome 11 (11p15.5) containing the β-like genes (ϵ, $^G\gamma$, $^A\gamma$, δ, β) has been mapped thoroughly by restriction endonuclease analysis (Fig.

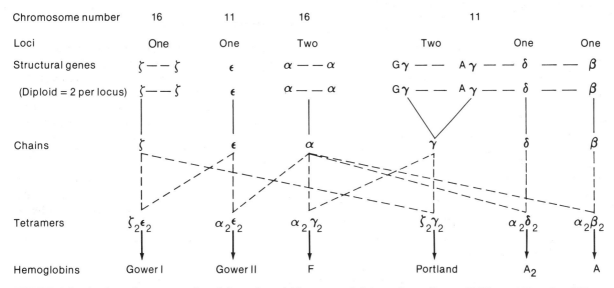

FIGURE 4.3. A schematic representation of the various globin genes and their products. (*Source:* Phillips and Kazazian 1990, p. 1318.)

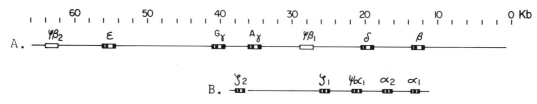

FIGURE 4.4. **Globin-gene complexes.** *A*, β-Gene complex on chromosome 11. *B*, α-Gene complex on chromosome 16. Distances along both chromosomes are measured in kilobases (*kb*) at the top. (*Source:* Phillips and Kazazian 1990, p. 1319.)

4.4) and sequenced.[2,17–20] Each of these genes contains two intervening sequences (IVSs) that interrupt the coding sequence at the junctions of the codons for amino acids 30 and 31 as well as 104 and 105. The first IVS is 122 to 130 base pairs (bp) and the second 850 to 904 bp in length. The entire β-gene cluster spans about 50 kilobases (kb) and contains one ε-, two γ-, one δ-, and one β-locus, plus one pseudogene locus.[15]

The pseudogene (ψβ) has sequences that are similar to β-gene sequences, but it differs in having altered sequences that prevent the production of functional globin chains. Pseudogenes comprise a minority of the single-gene sequences in both the α- and β-gene regions. Single-gene sequences, in turn, comprise only about 7 kb of the 50 kb of DNA in the β-gene region, while the remaining 43 kb are flanking sequences that presumably have some unknown regulatory role. In this regard, nucleotides within the 4-kb 5′ to the δ-locus have been suggested to be important in regulating the τ-gene, because their deletion in some forms of hereditary persistence of fetal hemoglobin (HPFH) is associated with increased γ-gene expression.[21] Also, more recently, sequences in the 20-kb upstream of the ε-globin gene have been shown to be critical for position-independent expression of the β-globin gene in transgenic mice.[22]

The α-gene complex contains two α-loci that have 3.6 kb between their centers, one ζ-locus, one pseudo-α-locus (ψα₁), and one pseudo-ζ-locus. The pseudo-ζ-locus results from a single nucleotide substitution that is polymorphic in some populations; thus, some individuals have a ψζ₁ locus and others a second functional ζ-gene at that site. Figure 4.4*B* depicts this complex, which is on chromosome 16; it should be noted that in each case about 4 kb separate the ζ₁-, ψα₁-, α₂-, and α₁-loci, suggesting the existence of discrete duplication units in the DNA.[16] α-Genes have smaller intervening sequences than the β-like genes; IVS 1 contains 114 bp, while IVS 2 contains 132 bp.

Ontogeny

The globin genes are expressed at different times and in different relative amounts during human development (Fig. 4.5). The sequence of appearance of the various globin chains is helpful in understanding the timing of the onset of clinical manifestations of the hemoglobinopathies and thalassemias. For example, a deficiency of α- or γ-chain synthesis and α- or γ-variants with abnormal functions should be observed at birth, while a deficiency of β-chains may not cause symptoms until several months of age. Levels of β-chain variants, such as hemoglobin S, also progressively increase during the first months of life, so the onset of clinical manifestations may be delayed until the latter half of the first year.

The Biosynthesis of Globin

The genetic information for every normal and abnormal globin chain is encoded in the nucleotide sequence of the DNA. These sequences, or genes, are located at specific loci on chromosomes 16 and 11.[23–26]

As mentioned earlier, IVSs reside between the portions of the globin genes that are translated into protein. These IVSs are present in the gene and the RNA transcribed from the gene, which is called messenger RNA precursor (pre-mRNA) (Fig. 4.6). Pre-mRNA undergoes excision of the intervening sequences and splicing of the translated portions.[27] Studies of the function of hybrid SV-40-β-globin genes in cultured monkey kidney cells suggest that the excision of IVS is crucial to mRNA transport from the nucleus to the cytoplasm.[28]

Further processing occurs at each end of this RNA molecule.[29] At the 5′ end, guanosine is added in a special triphosphate linkage, and this guanosine as well as the next two nucleotides are then methylated. These

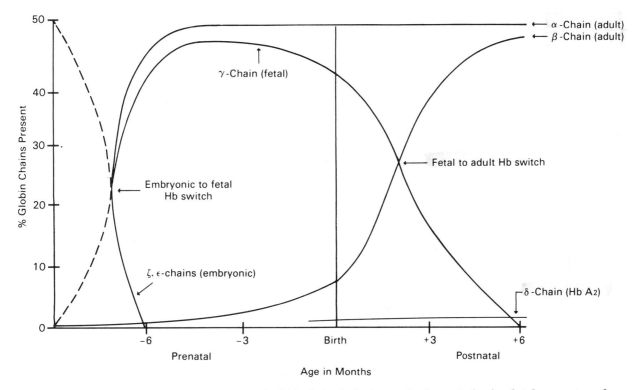

FIGURE 4.5. Qualitative and quantitative changes in globin chains during human development, showing that the percentage of β-chains accumulated in early fetal development is much less than the percentage synthesized during fetal development. (*Source:* Bunn, Forget, and Ranney 1977.[1])

5'-end modifications are called *capping* and *methylation,* and while their function is not completely known, they have been shown to be vital for initiating the translation of many mRNAs, including globin mRNAs. The 3'-end modification involves the addition of about 150 adenylic acid nucleotides (poly[A]); the addition of poly(A) also may be important for transporting mRNA to the cytoplasm and its subsequent stability. With the aging of the mRNA, the poly(A) "tail" shortens.[30]

Once the processed mRNA has been transported to the cytoplasm, it binds to ribosomes. The first step in the translation (initiation) requires the binding of mRNA to the two ribosome subunits, amino acyl-transfer (t)RNA, guanosine triphosphate, and protein initiation factors. The initiation occurs at the 5', or capped, end of the mRNA, which corresponds to the NH$_2$-terminal end of the globin chain. Protein synthesis then proceeds toward the COOH-terminal end. Four to six chains of varying length (nascent chains) undergo translation on the same mRNA simultaneously, and when these nascent chains attain full length, a termination codon is reached. Because no tRNA is available for decoding this codon, the synthesis of polypeptide stops and, with the assistance of protein termination factors, the polypeptide chain is released from the ribosome and its mRNA. About one third of the mature mRNA sequence is not used for translation, but these untranslated nucleotides (which are located at both ends of the molecule) may have other regulatory functions.[29]

The protein chain assumes its secondary and tertiary structures due to interactions resulting from its amino acid sequence. Next, heme is bound, and in combination with other polypeptide subunits, the quaternary hemoglobin molecule is formed. Figure 4.6 shows these steps.

VARIANTS OF HUMAN HEMOGLOBIN

Molecular Etiology

Abnormal hemoglobins result from either mutations that change the sequence or number of nucleotides within the globin gene involved or a mispairing during meiosis that fuses two different genes. Mutation can cause the substitution, addition, or deletion of one or more amino acids in the polypeptide sequence of the affected globin (Table 4.2).

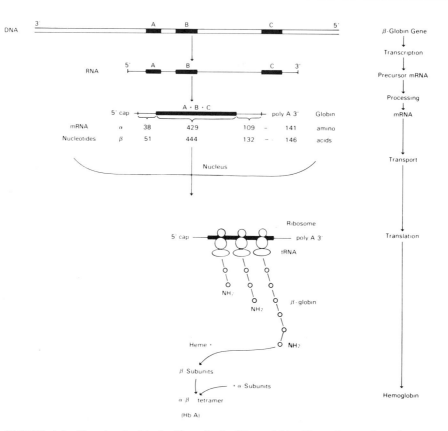

FIGURE 4.6. **Steps involved in the biosynthesis of hemoglobin. The understanding of the order and function of various steps is incomplete. (*Source:* Phillips and Kazazian 1990, p. 1320.)**

Single-base changes can result in single amino acid substitutions (e.g., hemoglobin S [$\beta^{6 \text{ Glu}\rightarrow\text{Val}}$]), shortened chains due to premature termination of translation (e.g., hemoglobin McKees Rock [$\beta^{145 \text{ Tyr}\rightarrow\text{Termination}}$]), or elongated chains. Elongated chains result when the terminator codon undergoes mutation to a codon for an amino acid, such as UAA→CAA in hemoglobin Constant Spring. Two other elongated chains are hemoglobin Icaria and hemoglobin Koya Dora, both of which also have 31 additional residues and differ from hemoglobin Constant Spring only at residue 142.[3]

Single-base deletions or additions can cause a frameshift in the normal reading process.[31] For example, in the α^{Wayne}-variant, a single-base deletion (A) causes the following codons to be read out of phase:

Deletions of three or multiples of three nucleotides in the DNA cause deletions of one or more amino acids. It is interesting that of 13 examples of this type, all are β-chain variants, including hemoglobin Leiden ($\beta^{6 \text{ or } 7}_{\text{Glu}\rightarrow 0}$) and hemoglobin Gun Hill ($\beta^{91-95 \text{ [Leu-His-Cys-Asp-Lys]}\rightarrow 0}$). Deletions of segments of genes may be due to nonhomologous crossing over after mispairing in meiosis. This mechanism accounts for the Lepore (δβ-fusion chains) and anti-Lepore globins (βδ-fusion chains) as well as Kenya globin (γβ-fusion chain).[29]

Known Variants

Table 4.3 shows the numbers of known hemoglobin variants resulting from changes in the nucleotide base

Lys	Tyr	Arg	Term	Asn	Thr	Val	Lys
(AAA	– UAC	– CGU)	– UAA ⟶	(AAU	– ACC	– GUU)	– AAG

TABLE 4.2. The Molecular Basis of Hemoglobinopathies

Mutation	Example	Clinical Manifestation
Nucleotide base substitutions to a codon for another amino acid	Hb S ($\beta^{6\ Glu\ \rightarrow\ Val}$)	Sickling
	Hb C$_{Harlem}$ ($\beta^{6\ Glu\ \rightarrow\ Val} + \beta^{73\ Asp\ \rightarrow\ Asn}$)	Sickling
Termination	Hb McKees Rock ($\beta^{145\ Tyr\ \rightarrow\ Termination}$)	Increased oxygen affinity and polycythemia
Amino acid instead of termination	Hb Constant Spring ($\alpha^{Termination\ \rightarrow\ Gln}$)	Decreased synthesis (thalassemia-like)
Nucleotide base deletions		
Single base deletion → frameshift	Hb Wayne ($\alpha^{139-141\ [Lys-Tyr-Arg]\ \rightarrow\ [Asn-Thr-Val...]}$)	Normal
Triplet deletion → single amino acid	Hb Leiden ($\beta^{6\ or\ 7\ Glu\ \rightarrow\ 0}$)	Unstable
Multiple codon	Hb Gun Hill ($\beta^{91-95\ [Leu-His-Cys-Asp-Lys]\ \rightarrow\ 0}$)	Unstable
Cross-over	Hb Lepore ($\delta\beta$-fusion with segments of δ and β lost)	Decreased synthesis (thalassemia-like)
Whole gene	α-Thalassemia$_1$ and α-thalassemia$_2$ combination	Hb H disease
Nucleotide base additions		
Two bases added → frameshift	Hb Cranston ($\beta^{144\ [Tyr-His]\ \rightarrow\ [Ser-Ile-Thr]}$)	Unstable
Multiple codon	Hb Grady (9 bases → 3 additional amino acids)	Normal

Source: Phillips and Kazazian 1990, p. 1321.
Note: Hb = Hemoglobin.

number or sequence in DNA. Most of these were detected by zone electrophoresis, which separates hemoglobins on the basis of charge differences resulting from the amino acid substitutions. Because many mutations that do not change the protein's charge are not detected by this method, many undetected hemoglobin variants must still exist in the population. The number of β-variants (232) is approximately twice that of the α-variants (126), even though there are two α-loci and a single β-locus. Also, the percentage of β-chain variants that have abnormal physical properties (47%) is twice that of the α-chain variants (19%). The great majority of these mutants arise from a single-base substitution that results in a single amino acid substitution; many of these substitutions, even some of those that produce abnormal physical properties in the variant hemoglobin, are clinically silent and were detected only by population screening. Other substitutions cause:

1. instability of the tetramer;
2. deformity of the three-dimensional structure;
3. inhibition of ferric iron reduction;
4. alteration of the residues that interact with heme, 2,3-DPG, or at the $\alpha\beta$-subunit contact site; or
5. abnormality of other properties of the molecule, resulting in a variety of clinical phenotypes (Table 4.4).

TABLE 4.3. Known Variants of Hemoglobin

Globin Chain	Total Variants, *n*	Abnormal Properties			
		Clinically Silent, *n (%)*	Unstable, *n (%)*	Abnormal Oxygen Affinity, *n (%)*	Ferric Hemoglobin, *n (%)*
α	126	102 (81)	16 (12)	6 (5)	2 (2)
β	232	122 (52)	68 (30)	39 (16)	3 (1)
γ	38	36 (95)	1 (3)	—	1 (3)
δ	15	15 (100)	—	—	—
Total	411	275 (66)	85 (22)	45 (11)	5 (1)

Source: International Hemoglobin Information Center 1984[32] and Bunn and Forget 1986.[33]
Note: The percentages may be greater than 100, because some variants have more than one abnormal property. Also, fusion variants are not included.

TABLE 4.4. The Clinical Manifestations of Hemoglobin Mutant

Type	Example	Clinical Manifestation
Sickling	Hb S	Sickling due to decreased solubility
Unstable	Hb Bristol	Anemia with Heinz body formation
Abnormal oxygen affinity		
Decreased	Hb Kansas	Mild anemia possible
Increased	Hb Chesapeake	Polycythemia due to decreased oxygen transport
M hemoglobin	Hb M$_{Boston}$	Cyanosis due to ferric hemoglobin
Decreased synthesis	Hb Lepore	Thalassemia

Source: Phillips and Kazazian 1990, p. 1322.
Note: Hb = Hemoglobin.

The location of the amino acid changed by the mutation often can be correlated with the resultant phenotype. Unstable hemoglobin variants are caused by several types of change in the primary sequence that affect the secondary, tertiary, or quaternary structure. These substitutions tend to be at residues in the molecule's interior, at contact points between chains, at residues that interact with the heme groups,[7] or when a proline residue replaces another amino acid within an α-helical region (hemoglobins Genova [$\beta^{28}(B10)^{Leu \to Pro}$] and Abraham Lincoln [$\beta^{32}(B14)^{Leu \to Pro}$]) resulting in a disruption of the helix. Hemoglobin Philly [$\beta^{35}(C1)^{Tyr \to Phe}$] is also unstable, secondary to a missing α-hydrogen bond normally found between the α_1- and β_1-subunits. Many other unstable hemoglobins are the result of mutations affecting residues that bind heme or are in the hydrophobic heme cleft (e.g., hemoglobins Gun Hill [$\beta^{91-95 \ (Leu-His-Cys-Asp-Lys) \to 0}$] and Hammersmith [$\beta^{42 \ Phe \to Ser}$]).

Substitutions on the surface of the molecule usually do not affect the tertiary structure or heme–heme interaction, but they may permit molecular interactions that decrease solubility under certain conditions (hemoglobin S [$\beta^{6 \ Glu \to Val}$]). The substitution of tyrosine for either of the histidines that bind the iron molecule (E7 or F8) results in increased stability of the ferric (oxidized) iron state seen in M hemoglobins, M$_{Boston}$ [$\alpha^{58}(E7)^{His \to Tyr}$] and M$_{Iwate}$ [$\beta^{87}(F8)^{His \to Typ}$]. Substitution at an $\alpha_1\beta_1$-subunit contact point, such as β^{99}, can disturb heme–heme interactions, causing increased oxygen affinity and polycythemia, as with hemoglobin Kempsey [$\beta^{99}(G1)^{Asp \to Asn}$].[7]

The Inheritance of Hemoglobinopathies

Variants of α-, β-, γ-, or δ-globins result from mutations affecting their respective genes. All the variants for β-chains, for example, are coded by alleles, because they result from different genes found at the single β-chromosomal locus. Heterozygotes for a hemoglobin containing an abnormal β-globin have an abnormal as well as a normal β-gene at that locus, and their status often is described by the term *trait*. Because most variants are rare, they usually occur in the heterozygous state and, if they cause clinical symptoms, are examples of autosomal dominant conditions. When both alleles code for the same common β-variant, the individual is then homozygous and is said to have the "disease" state. However, the term *sickle cell disease* often is used to describe a similar phenotype that is seen when any of several genotypes (SS, SC, S/β-thal, SD$_{Punjab}$, or SO$_{Arab}$) is exposed to a certain environment (hypoxia). Furthermore, under conditions of severe hypoxia, a person with the AS genotype or "trait" can also manifest symptoms of the sickle cell disease phenotype. This distinction between the genotype (homozygous and heterozygous) and the phenotype (trait and disease) is an important one, and it should be noted that the patterns of inheritance of hemoglobin variants are expressed more precisely in terms of genotypes and not phenotypes.

Table 4.5 shows the inheritance risks from matings of individuals who are normal, heterozygous, or homozygous for variant hemoglobins. Because there are multiple alleles for each locus, a person who is heterozygous for two alleles at the same locus (usually referred to as a genetic compound) may be seen (e.g., an individual with two different hemoglobins). A mating between an AA and an SC individual can result in AS or AC but not AA or SC offspring; however, a mating of an AS and an AC individual can result in offspring who are AA, AS, AC, or SC. This pattern of Mendelian inheritance is called *codominant inheritance*.

SICKLE CELL ANEMIA AND RELATED DISORDERS
Molecular Basis

The sickle cell gene results from a point mutation that causes the amino acid substitution $\beta^{6 \ Glu \to Val}$; therefore, hemoglobin S is $\alpha_2^A\beta_2^{6 \ Glu \to Val}$. The frequency of sickle trait (hemoglobin AS) among blacks in the United States at birth is approximately 8%, and the incidence of sickle cell anemia at birth should be approximately 0.16%, or 1 per 625 births.[34] This contrasts with the higher carrier frequencies (up to 30%) seen in some areas of Africa, that are due to the protective advantage conferred by the

TABLE 4.5. The Risks of Inheriting a Hemoglobin Variant

Parents	Offspring		
	Homozygous Normal, %	Heterozygous, %	Homozygous Affected, %
Both normal	100	0	0
Normal/Heterozygous	50	50	0
Normal/Homozygous	0	100	0
Both heterozygous	25	50	25
Heterozygous/Homozygous	0	50	50
Both homozygous	0	0	100

Source: Phillips and Kazazian 1990, p. 1323.

carrier state against falciparum malaria. As expected, the prevalence of sickle cell anemia differs in these two populations. The prevalence of sickle cell anemia among all blacks in the United States is about 1 per 1875, considerably lower than expected from the incidence at birth. It is still lower in some underdeveloped regions of Africa, despite the higher incidence of this trait, due to higher mortality in infancy.[34] The β^S gene is also found in Italy, Greece, the Middle East, and India.

The Pathophysiology of Sickling

The substitution of valine for glutamic acid at the β^6 residue causes a change on the surface of the deoxygenated β^s-chain, which allows it to interact in a special way with other β-chains. This interaction results in the formation by $\alpha_2{}^A\beta_2{}^S$ tetramers of a 14-stranded helical polymer with a diameter of 15 to 17 nm. The parallel alignment of these rodlike polymers, in turn, causes the deformation seen in sickled erythrocytes. In sickle cell anemia, the sickling process may begin when the oxygen saturation of hemoglobin S is decreased to 85%, but it does not occur in heterozygotes (hemoglobin AS) until the oxygen saturation of hemoglobin is decreased to 40%.[35] In addition to a decrease in oxygen tension, a reduction in pH or increase in 2,3-DPG also promotes sickling. These factors probably interact in patients with sickle cell anemia, because their blood normally has an increased concentration of 2,3-DPG.

The viscosity of oxygenated sickle cell blood is increased primarily due to irreversibly sickled cells but also to increased levels of γ-globin. When the blood becomes deoxygenated, viscosity increases further due to the cellular rigidity that occurs with sickling. This increases the exposure time of erythrocytes to a hypoxic environment, and the lower tissue pH decreases the oxygen affinity, which further promotes sickling. The end result is the occlusion of capillaries and arterioles and infarction of the surrounding tissues. Hemolysis

probably occurs secondary to increased mechanical fragility of deformed cells and membrane damage.

Clinical Aspects of Sickle Cell Disease

As Figure 4.5 shows, β-chain production usually does not reach sufficient levels to cause symptoms until the second half of the first year of life. As higher concentrations of hemoglobin S are reached in erythrocytes, the cells become susceptible to hemolysis and a progressive hemolytic anemia with splenomegaly is seen. The increased rate of erythropoiesis leads to erythroid marrow expansion and increased folic acid requirements. However, the two major problems for young children with sickle cell disease are infections and vaso-occlusive crises.

Children with sickle cell anemia have an increased susceptibility to potentially life-threatening bacterial infections, including sepsis and meningitis caused by *Streptococcus pneumoniae* and *Haemophilus influenzae*. The relative risk of sickle cell anemia patients compared with that of normal individuals for pneumococcal *H. influenzae* and all bacterial meningitis is 579:1, 116:1, and 309:1, respectively.[36] These patients also are susceptible to bacterial pneumonia (often pneumococcus), osteomyelitis (*Salmonella* and *Staphylococcus*) (Fig. 4.7), and urinary tract infections (*Escherichia coli* and *Klebsiella*). Increased susceptibility also is seen for *Shigella* and *Mycoplasma pneumoniae*. Several factors that contribute to this susceptibility are functional hyposplenism, impaired antibody response, decreased opsonization, impaired complement activation in the properdin pathway, and abnormal chemotaxis.

Bacterial infection is the most common reason for the hospitalization of pediatric patients with sickle cell anemia and often leads to the diagnosis.[36] Serious bacterial infections are seen in approximately one third of children with sickle cell anemia before 4 years of age.

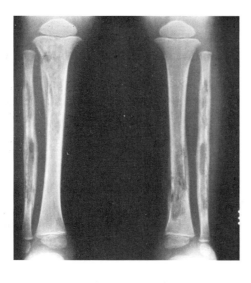 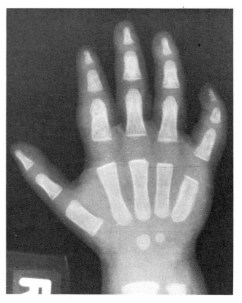

FIGURE 4.7. Radiographic changes in sickle cell anemia. A, Changes in the tibias and fibulas secondary to *Salmonella* osteomyelitis. B, Hand-and-foot syndrome with soft-tissue swelling and focal areas of cortical destruction and periosteal new bone formation. (*Source:* Courtesy of Dr. John Dorst.)

Infection, not crisis, is the most common cause of death in these children, although infections often precipitate crises.

Vaso-occlusive crises begin in infancy with dactylitis, or hand-and-foot syndrome (Fig. 4.7). Later crises may involve the periosteum, bones, or joints, resulting in infarction that must be differentiated from osteomyelitis and septic arthritis. Vaso-occlusive crises and sepsis are difficult to differentiate and often co-exist in younger children.

Pulmonary crises with pleural pain and fever may be due to infection, in situ thrombosis, or embolism. Other clinical manifestations include splenic sequestration, abdominal and aplastic crises, cholelithiasis, hepatic infarcts, occlusion of cerebral vessels, ocular changes, hematuria, hyposthenuria, hyponatremia, priapism, and skin ulcers.[4,35]

Diagnosis

The peripheral blood smear of patients with sickle cell anemia may have normal, irreversibly sickled, target, and nucleated red cells. Howell-Jolly bodies and red cell fragments are also present, especially after functional asplenia develops (Fig. 4.8A). The clinical history of crises or severe infections with anemia, abnormal red cell morphology on peripheral smear with a normal or elevated mean corpuscular volume, positive sickling test, and hemoglobin S (> 80%) and F on hemoglobin electrophoresis makes the diagnosis of sickle cell anemia probable. However, family studies indicating that both parents have the sickle cell trait are helpful to exclude S/β-thalassemia and S/HPFH. In addition, siblings should be tested to identify and treat previously undiagnosed cases.

Treatment

At present, there is no safe drug to ameliorate this condition, but a number of antisickling agents are undergoing trials.[37] Hydroxyurea has been given experimentally to patients with sickle cell anemia. This drug increases the production of fetal hemoglobin, presumably through its effect of speeding erythroid precursors through their maturation steps. Hydroxyurea appears to reduce painful crises and hemolysis in uncontrolled studies with a small number of patients,[38] but it is not yet in general use.

Infections should be treated promptly with antibiotics, and some centers advocate prophylactic antibiotic treatment. A polyvalent pneumococcal polysaccharide has been shown to afford some protection against systemic infections due to *Streptococcus pneumoniae* in sickle cell disease and in patients who have undergone

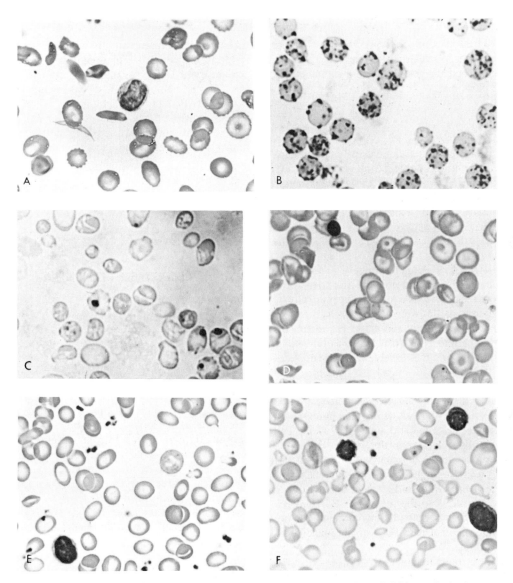

FIGURE 4.8. Peripheral blood smears from patients with various disorders of globin synthesis. A, Homozygous sickle cell anemia. B, Unstable hemoglobin Zurich with Heinz bodies. C, Hemoglobin H disease. D, Sickle/β-thalassemia. E, β-Thalassemia trait. F, Homozygous β-thalassemia. B and C were prepared as follows: whole blood with ethylenediaminetetraacetic acid was incubated at 41°C for 3 to 6 hours, then a 1:1 mixture of blood and 0.5% rhodanile blue in 0.9% saline was made and immediately smeared. Hemoglobin precipitates formed secondary to heating are seen. (*Source:* Courtesy of Dr. William Zinkham.)

splenectomy.[39] However, multiple clinical failures as well as side effects have been reported.[40,41]

The associated anemia is usually tolerated well, but if folate deficiency occurs, the anemia becomes more severe and is associated with macrocytosis, hyperseg- mented granulocytes, and a decrease in the percentage of reticulocytes. Folate deficiency is easily prevented by daily folic acid supplement. Transfusions are seldom indicated for uncomplicated anemia, but exchange transfusions can be effective for life-threatening vaso-occlusive crises (e.g., cerebral) or in preparation for surgery. Crises should be managed with vigorous hydration because of the patient's increased blood viscosity and inability to concentrate urine. Acidosis and hypoxia should be treated and analgesics given for the accompanying severe pain.

Prevention

During genetic counseling, couples where both partners are heterozygous for the sickle cell gene (they have sickle cell trait) are advised of their 25% risk for having children with the disease, and certain couples may request prenatal diagnosis. In the past several years, methods for the prenatal detection of sickle cell anemia have improved to the point where they are now available to all couples at risk.

Between 1975 and 1979, approximately 50 couples at risk for sickle cell anemia had prenatal diagnosis using fetal blood obtained by fetoscopy or placental aspiration.[42,43] Synthetic studies were used to detect the types of β-chain produced in fetal red cells. However, the significant risk of fetoscopy (6% fetal mortality), its limited availability, and the variable clinical course of the disease limited the widespread use of these methods.[44]

In 1978, Kan and Dozy discovered that restriction endonuclease studies of DNA from fetal amniocytes also could enable the prenatal diagnosis of sickle cell anemia in a substantial proportion of cases.[45] The applicability of this test was expanded through use of polymorphic restriction endonuclease sites near the β-locus, and when family studies were carried out to assign DNA "markers" to the respective β^A- and β^S-bearing chromosomes of both parents, prenatal diagnosis could be accomplished in 90% of pregnancies by amniocentesis alone.[46]

In 1982, it was found that the restriction enzyme *Mst* II (or *Cvn* I) cut the β^A-globin gene at codons 5–7 of the gene but failed to cut the β^S-globin gene at this point (the mutation site). Prenatal diagnosis could then be accomplished without family studies in all couples at risk. Now, gene-amplification techniques (polymerase chain reaction)[47] in conjunction with *Mst* II allow prenatal diagnosis of sickle cell anemia in a few days without Southern blotting.[48]

Interactions with Sickle Hemoglobin

Heterozygotes for hemoglobin S (AS) are generally asymptomatic; however, severe hypoxia (oxygen saturation <40%) can induce sickling. The loop of Henle provides an environment in which both the pH and oxygen tension are decreased sufficiently to cause sick-

ling, resulting in microinfarctions, hematuria, and hyposthenuria. Exposure to hypoxia also can cause splenic and other organ infarcts in individuals with sickle trait.

In the United States, hemoglobin C trait is found at birth in about 3% of blacks, hemoglobin SC disease in 1 per 833, and hemoglobin C disease in approximately 1 per 1250.[34] Patients with hemoglobin SC disease tend to have a variable course, with most complications occurring less frequently than in sickle cell disease. Other hemoglobin variants that interact with hemoglobin S are D_{Punjab}, O_{Arab}, C_{Harlem}, and β-thalassemia. Clinical manifestations tend to be severe in patients with hemoglobins SS, D_{Punjab}, and SO_{Arab}; moderate in those with hemoglobins SC, S/β-thalassemia, and CC; and mild or absent in those with hemoglobin AS and hemoglobin AC trait.

VARIANTS OF UNSTABLE HEMOGLOBIN

Molecular Basis

At least 85 unstable hemoglobin variants are known (Table 4.3). Among these, β-variants are four times more frequent than α-variants (68:16), a discrepancy that may be due to the smaller percentage of unstable hemoglobin and, hence, milder clinical symptoms associated with the α-chain variants. An individual with a single variant α-gene has three normal α-genes, so the proportion of unstable hemoglobin in the red cells is very small (5% to 20%). In contrast, an individual with a single variant β-gene has only one normal β-gene, so the unstable hemoglobin containing the variant β-chain comprises a greater proportion of the total cellular hemoglobin synthesized (20% to 40%).[49] Because the gene frequencies for these variants are extremely low, almost all the affected individuals seen are heterozygotes.

The increased propensity of unstable hemoglobins to denature can result from several types of mutation. As mentioned previously, the α-helix of α- or β-globin can be disrupted by proline replacing another amino acid within the helix. There are at least 10 examples of this type of disruption of primary and secondary structure, including hemoglobin Bibba ($\alpha^{136\ Leu\rightarrow Pro}$) and hemoglobin Genova ($\beta^{28\ Leu\rightarrow Pro}$).[7] Deletions of amino acid residues alter the primary and secondary structures as well as the conformation of the hemoglobin molecules, and 8 of the 10 variants of this type are unstable (e.g., hemoglobin Leiden [$\beta^{6\ or\ 7\ Glu\rightarrow 0}$] and hemoglobin Gun Hill [$\beta^{91-95\ (Leu-His-Cys-Asp-Lys)\rightarrow 0}$]).[49] Interference with interchain contacts permits the αβ-dimers to dissociate into monomers; for example, hemoglobin Philly ($\beta^{35\ Tyr\rightarrow Phe}$) and hemoglobin Tacoma ($\beta^{30\ Arg\rightarrow Ser}$) lack the hydrogen bonds normally linking the α- and β-subunits. Substitutions that affect heme binding or disturb the hydrophobic heme pocket (certain nonpolar residues in the CD, E, F, and FG regions) decrease the molecule's stability (Fig. 4.1). There are more than 30 such mutations, and most result in unstable hemoglobins such as hemoglobin Bristol ($\beta^{67\ Val \rightarrow Asp}$) and hemoglobin Köln ($\beta^{98\ Val \rightarrow Met}$).[7] Finally, globin chain elongation can result in instability due to the hydrophobic properties of the extended chain (e.g., hemoglobin Cranston [$\beta^{144-151}$]).[49]

These variant hemoglobins tend to denature spontaneously, and the globin subunits precipitate in the red cell, forming aggregates or Heinz bodies. The Heinz bodies adhere to the red cell membrane and result in decreased pliability of the cell, and inflexible erythrocytes are then selectively trapped by the reticuloendothelial system.

Clinical Aspects of Unstable Hemoglobins

Patients often present in infancy or early childhood with a hemolytic anemia, jaundice, and splenomegaly, or later with cholelithiasis. Some variants also cause cyanosis due to their abnormal properties (i.e., propensity to form methemoglobin or decreased oxygen affinity). The clinical severity varies with different unstable variants; for β-variants, symptoms appear after the γ-to-β transition in hemoglobin synthesis (Fig. 4.5).

Diagnosis

The peripheral smear may be normal or hypochromic. Staining with a supravital stain, such as 1% methyl violet, demonstrates preformed Heinz bodies (Fig. 4.8B). The formation of a hemoglobin precipitate when a hemolysate is incubated at 50°C or higher, or at 37°C in 17% isopropanol demonstrates the heat instability of the variant hemoglobin. Hemoglobin electrophoresis by the usual methods may detect only about one half of the unstable variants, because the charge of these variants is often unaltered by the substitutions. Oxygen saturation curves of whole blood may indicate normal (20% of the unstable variants), decreased (30%), or increased (50%) oxygen affinity.[49]

Treatment

Treatment is generally supportive. If hemolysis is severe, prophylactic folate may be indicated. Oxidant drugs such as sulfonamides increase hemolysis in some patients and should be avoided, and transfusions are indicated only in the treatment of aplastic crises. While splenectomy may result in improvement of the anemia, it also increases the risk of septicemia, especially in young patients. Because of the mortality associated with septicemia in patients who undergo this procedure, the physician should reserve splenectomy for selected patients, and it should be postponed until the patient is at least 6 years of age. Administration of pneumococcal vaccine and prophylactic antibodies also should be considered.[49]

VARIANTS OF HEMOGLOBIN WITH ALTERED OXYGEN AFFINITY

Molecular Basis

The oxygen dissociation curve shown in Figure 4.2 is sigmoid shaped because of heme–heme interactions. Mutations that affect heme–heme interaction, the Bohr effect, or deoxyhemoglobin–2,3-DPG interaction can change the shape or position of the oxygen dissociation curve. Mutations affecting the $\alpha_1\beta_2$-subunit contact point also can alter heme–heme interaction by causing the deoxyhemoglobin conformation to be less stable. These mutations result in increased stability of the oxyhemoglobin conformation and increased oxygen affinity (hemoglobin Kempsey [$\beta^{99\ Asp \rightarrow Asn}$]); alternatively, the oxyhemoglobin conformation can be destabilized by mutations affecting the $\alpha^{94}\beta^{102}$ contact point, resulting in decreased oxygen affinity (hemoglobin Kansas [$\beta^{102\ Asn \rightarrow Thr}$]). Substitutions at the COOH-terminal ends of globin chains can lead to instability of the deoxyhemoglobin conformations and increased oxygen affinity (hemoglobin Bethesda [$\beta^{145\ Tyr \rightarrow His}$]) as well as reduction in the Bohr effect. 2,3-DPG binds to residues β^1, β^2, β^{82}, and β^{143} in the deoxygenated form, and substitutions altering these residues tend to have increased oxygen affinity (hemoglobin F [γ-globin has a serine for histidine substitution at position 143]).[8]

The variants with increased oxygen affinity shift the oxygen dissociation curve to the left (Fig. 4.2), resulting in less oxygen delivery per gram of hemoglobin. To compensate, the hemoglobin concentration, blood flow, or both increase to partially restore oxygen delivery to the tissues.[8] Some variants with increased oxygen affinity do not cause polycythemia because of the small fraction of the total hemoglobin they comprise or because of compensatory changes in the shape of the oxygen dissociation curve. Variants with decreased oxygen affinity have a shift to the right and increased oxygen delivery per gram of hemoglobin; as a result, the hemoglobin concentration is normal or decreased (hemoglobin Beth Israel [$\beta^{102\ Asn \rightarrow Ser}$]).[50]

Clinical Aspects and Diagnosis

Because gene frequencies for nearly all variant hemoglobins are very low, patients are nearly always heterozygotes. β-Chain variants outnumber α-chain variants by 2 to 1 (Table 4.3). The great majority of patients are asymptomatic, and when oxygen affinity is increased, the major finding is polycythemia with erythrocytosis, normal white blood cell and platelet counts, and absence of splenomegaly. Because approximately half of these variants cannot be detected on routine electrophoresis, whole-blood oxygen affinity studies are required for diagnosis. Some concern has been raised about risk to the fetuses of mothers who have variants with increased oxygen affinity, but the little data available regarding the outcome of such pregnancies do not, in general, seem to indicate increased fetal mortality.[8]

Treatment

The condition is generally considered benign. It is important to avoid chemical treatment of the compensatory polycythemia unless hematocrit levels are high enough to cause increased viscosity.

VARIANTS OF M HEMOGLOBIN
Molecular Basis

There are five known variants of M hemoglobin, four of which result from the substitution of tyrosine for histidine at positions α^{58}, α^{87}, β^{63}, and β^{92} (M_{Boston} [$\alpha^{58 His \rightarrow Tyr}$], M_{Iwate} [$\alpha^{87 His \rightarrow Tyr}$], $M_{Saskatoon}$ [$\beta^{63 His \rightarrow Tyr}$], and $M_{Hyde Park}$ [$\beta^{92 His \rightarrow Tyr}$]). The substituted tyrosine may form a stable bond with the ferric form of the heme iron. This bond prevents interaction of the affected α- or β-chain's ferric iron with oxygen, but it does not render the globin–heme unit unstable. Both α-variants (M_{Boston} and M_{Iwate}) have decreased oxygen affinity, two of the β-variants ($M_{Hyde Park}$ and $M_{Saskatoon}$) have normal affinity, and the final β-variant ($M_{Milwaukee}$) has decreased oxygen affinity.[8,51]

Clinical Aspects

M hemoglobin variants, like other rare hemoglobin disorders, are inherited in an autosomal dominant pattern, and the age of onset of cyanosis differs depending on whether the α- or β-chain is affected. With α-chain variants, cyanosis is seen at birth, while β-chain variants develop cyanosis at about 6 months of age, when γ-to-β switching is nearly complete (Fig. 4.5).

Diagnosis

The blood is chocolate brown and does not change color on exposure to oxygen. Usually, there is no anemia, and routine electrophoresis may be normal.

Spectral analysis allows the differentiation of M hemoglobins from methemoglobin secondary to diaphorase-I deficiency; the latter is a red cell enzyme deficiency inherited in an autosomal recessive pattern.[51] Because the modes of inheritance for M hemoglobins and diaphorase deficiency differ, one parent of a patient with the former is usually affected, while both parents of a patient with diaphorase deficiency are unaffected.

Treatment

No treatment is indicated. However, the diagnosis should be made so that extensive cardiac and pulmonary evaluations can be avoided.

THALASSEMIAS: QUANTITATIVE DISORDERS OF GLOBIN SYNTHESIS

The thalassemia syndromes are genetic disorders characterized by absent or deficient synthesis of one or more of the normal globin chains. The absence of globin synthesis is designated by an "o" superscript (e.g., β° thalassemia), while the presence of an insufficient amount of the gene product is noted by a "+" superscript (e.g., β⁺ thalassemia). When there is partial synthesis of the affected globin chain, it usually is structurally normal; therefore, the defect is a quantitative one secondary to unbalanced globin synthesis. This contrasts with the hemoglobinopathies, in which the variant hemoglobins are qualitatively or structurally abnormal. Thalassemia is distributed primarily among peoples of Mediterranean, African, Middle Eastern, Indian, Chinese, and Southeast Asian descent, but sporadic cases have been reported in many other ethnic groups.[52,33]

Molecular Basis

As discussed previously and shown in Figure 4.6, the biosynthesis of globin has many steps, each of which has the potential for regulating the amount of globin chains produced. The thalassemia syndromes provide examples of defects at essentially every step. First, the deletion of the DNA sequences coding for the structural gene occurs in most α-thalassemias (Fig. 4.9) and in certain rare types of β-thalassemia, one of which is common in Indians[33] (Table 4.6). Evidence has accumulated that the chromosome in most blacks, Filipinos, and some Chinese, which has one of the two α-genes deleted, arose by a mispairing of the 5' α-gene of one chromosome 16 with the 3' α-gene of its homologue and subsequent unequal crossing over.[54,55] The reciprocal chromosome, one containing three α-genes, has been observed in Mediterraneans and blacks.[56] In Chinese,

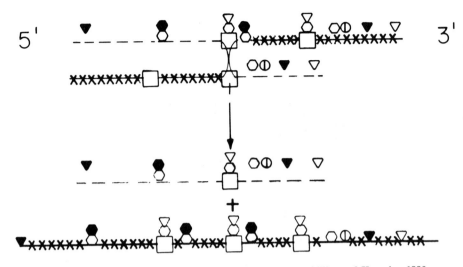

FIGURE 4.9. Deletions in the α-globin gene cluster. (*Source:* Phillips and Kazazian 1990, p. 1330.)

about one third of chromosome 16s containing a single functional α-globin gene originated from a simple deletion of the 5' α-gene, while another one third have a nondeletion defect.[57] Chromosomes lacking both α-genes have been studied in Asians, and they have large deletions that remove $\psi\zeta_1$, $-\psi\alpha-$, and both α-genes

TABLE 4.6. The Characteristics of Certain Thalassemia States

Condition	Parents	Inheritance Risk, %	Hemoglobin Electrophoresis	DNA Sequences	mRNA
Heterozygotes					
Silent carrier (α-thalassemia$_2$)	α-Thalassemia, normal	50	1% to 2% γ_4 (birth)	3α	Slight ↓ α
α-Thalassemia trait (α-thalassemia$_1$)	Both α-thalassemia$_2$ or α-thalassemia$_1$, normal	25 50	5% γ_4 (birth)	2α	↓↓ α
Hemoglobin H	α-Thalassemia$_1$, α-thalassemia$_2$	25	4% to 30% β_4 (adults) 20% to 40% γ_4 (birth)	1α	↓↓↓ α
β$^+$-Thalassemia	β$^+$/β, normal	50	Hb A$_2$ ↑, slight ↑ F, or 5% to 12% F	2β	↓ β
β°-Thalassemia	β°/β, normal	50	Hb A$_2$↑, slight ↑ F	2β	0 or ↓β
δβ°-Thalassemia	δβ°/δβ, normal	50	5% to 20% Hb F	1β and 1δ	↓ δ and β
δβ-Lepore	Lepore/β, normal	50	Slight ↑ Hb F, normal or ↓A$_2$, and 5% to 15% Lepore	1δ, 1β, and 1δβ-Lepore	↓ δβ-Lepore
Hemoglobin Constant Spring (CS)	Hemoglobin CS heterozygote, normal	50	1% to 2% γ_4 (birth), 0.5% to 1% Hb CS	3α α^{CS}	↓ CS
Homozygotes					
Hydrops fetalis (α°-thalassemia$_1$)	Both α-thalassemia$_1$	25	80% γ_4 (birth) 10% $\delta_2\gamma_2$, 10% β_4	0α	0α
β°-Thalassemia	Both β°/β	25	↑Hb F + A$_2$, OA	2β	0 or ↓β
β$^+$-Thalassemia	Both β$^+$/β, or one β$^+$/β and one β°/β	25	↑Hb F + A$_2$, ↓ A	2β	↓ β
δβ°-Thalassemia	Both δβ°/δβ	25	100% Hb F OA, and OA$_2$	0 β, 0 δ	0 δ and 0 β
δβ-Lepore	Both Lepore/β	25	75% Hb F, 25% Lepore	2δβ-Lepore	↓ δβ-Lepore
Hemoglobin Constant Spring (CS)	Both Hb CS heterozygotes	25	5% to 6% Hb CS	2α 2α^{CS}	↓ CS

Source: Orkin and Nathan 1976[52] and Weatherall 1976.[53]

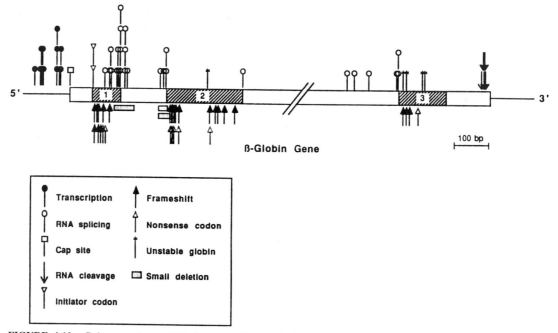

FIGURE 4.10. Point mutations in β-thalassemia. The *hatched bars* indicate exons 1, 2, and 3. (*Source:* Kazanian 1990[60].)

while leaving the ζ-gene intact.[58] A large number of different deletions in the α-globin gene complex have been observed[33] (Fig. 4.9).

In 1991, we knew of roughly 100 point mutations in the β-globin gene and five deletions affecting only the β-globin gene that produce "simple" β-thalassemia.[59] Figure 4.10 and Table 4.7 show the location of 90 of these abnormalities in the gene and their effect on gene expression. The mutations produce defects in transcription, RNA splicing and modification, translation via frameshifts and nonsense codons, and may produce a highly unstable β-globin.

Transcription mutations are all relatively mild and commonly observed in β-thalassemia intermedia. They are single nucleotide substitutions in the TATA box at −30 from the transcription start site, in the ACACCC distal promoter region at −90, but none has yet been observed in the CCAAT box at −70. RNA splicing mutations occur at splice junctions, in consensus sequences around splice junctions, introns to produce new donor and acceptor splice sites, and cryptic splice sites in exons. These latter mutations alter sequences that are similar to donor splice sites at the 5′ ends of introns but that normally are not used for splicing. By making these sequences resemble more closely the consensus sequence for a donor splice site, these mutations activate the cryptic site, and its use leads to the production of abnormal RNA and slowed normal splicing. Regarding

splice site mutations, it is worth noting the marked discrepancy between the number of different alleles in the consensus donor sequence of intron-1 (9) and the consensus donor sequence of intron-2 (1).

RNA modification defects are found at both the 5′ end (or cap site) and the 3′ end in the RNA cleavage and polyadenylation signal. The cap site mutation that changes the first A residue to a C may work either by reducing the transcription itself or by slowing the 5′ capping process, which may reduce the stability of mRNA. The mutations in the AATAAA signal at the 3′ end of the transcript markedly reduce the RNA cleavage and lead to elongated mRNA molecules that are probably unstable.

Frameshift mutations are deletions or additions of 1, 2, or 4 nucleotides that change the ribosome reading frame and cause a premature termination of translation. Likewise, nonsense codon mutations directly stop translation. Missense mutations may rarely produce β-thalassemia when they lead to a highly unstable β-globin, and this is the case with β[Indianapolis] and β[Houston]. These mutations are generally found in exon 3, affect the formation of αβ-dimer, and are dominant (that is, they produce thalassemia intermedia in the heterozygous state).

Most deletions in the β-globin gene cluster affect more than the β-globin gene and produce δ β-thalassemia, γ δ β-thalassemia, or HPFH syndromes. One 619-bp deletion affects the β-globin gene and is the most common β-thalassemia allele in Indians; rarely, four other small deletions of the β-globin gene have been seen. The Lepore deletions, which produce fusion δβ-globins due to unequal crossing over between mispaired δ- and β-globin genes, are also causes of a β-thalassemia phenotype. A β-thalassemia gene unassociated with mutation in the β-globin gene and with the β-globin gene cluster has been reported, but no further information or substantiation has appeared. The mutations themselves are population specific, as summarized in Table 4.8.

Rare deletions that eliminate the locus activating region 5' to the ε-globin gene also produce β-thalassemia trait by blocking expression of the β-globin gene on the chromosome carrying the deletion.

Pathophysiology

In the thalassemia syndromes, there is reduced or absent synthesis of the affected globin chain, and the unaffected chain continues to be synthesized at relatively normal levels. An imbalance results that causes the aggregation and precipitation of excess unpaired chains. In β-thalassemia, free α-chains aggregate. These aggregates are highly insoluble and form inclusions in nucleated erythroid precursors in the bone marrow, and the inclusion bodies cause intramedullary hemolysis (ineffective erythropoiesis). In contrast, the γ_4 (hemoglobin Barts) and β_4 (hemoglobin H) tetramers that form in α-thalassemia are more soluble. Thus, in severe α-thalassemias, inclusions are seen in mature erythrocytes and the ineffective erythropoiesis of β-thalassemia is absent. In any severe thalassemia, removal of these inclusions from erythrocytes by the reticuloendothelial system damages the cells and produces "teardrop" forms. Splenomegaly can be secondary to splenic congestion or hypersplenism, and after the spleen is removed, cell destruction continues at a decreased rate in the liver and the number of red cell inclusions may increase greatly. The large number of erythroid precursors expands the marrow cavities, resulting in bone deformities, thinning, and occasional pathologic fractures (Fig. 4.11).[61]

The accumulation of iron results from increased gastrointestinal absorption stimulated by the anemia, blood transfusions, and decreased utilization for hemoglobin synthesis. The deposition of excess iron causes damage to the heart, pancreas, and other tissues.

Also, the requirements for folic acid are increased in thalassemia. If deficiencies develop, they may worsen the anemia.

Clinical Features

α-THALASSEMIA. These patients are often of Mediterranean or Oriental descent, but the frequency of mild α-thalassemia is also high in blacks. When the mutation affects both α-loci on the same chromosome 16, the genotype is called α-thalassemia₁ (--). When a single locus on only one chromosome 16 is affected, the genotype is α-thalassemia₂ (α-).

Four clinical types are seen, depending on the number of α-genes affected. The most severe form is α°-thalassemia (α-thalassemia₁ homozygote) (--/--), or hydrops fetalis with hemoglobin Barts. This condition is usually found in Oriental infants who are spontaneously aborted or die of severe hydrops shortly after birth. In the usual case, more than 80% of the hemoglobin is hemoglobin Barts (γ_4), which has a very high affinity for oxygen, causing severe tissue hypoxia; the remainder is hemoglobin Portland ($\zeta_2\gamma_2$) and hemoglobin H (β_4). Both parents carry the α-thal₁ trait.[62]

The frequency of hemoglobin H disease (--/α-) is high in Southeast Asians, Greeks, and Italians. The anemia varies, with an average of 8 to 10 g of hemoglobin per 100 ml of blood, and reticulocytes comprise 5% to 10% of red cells. Splenomegaly and, occasionally, hepatomegaly are found. The red cells are microcytic (decreased mean corpuscular volume [MCV]) and their hemoglobin content (mean corpuscular hemoglobin [MCH]) decreased, but the concentration of hemoglobin per cell (mean corpuscular hemoglobin concentration [MCHC]) is normal. On the peripheral smear, poikilocytosis, polychromasia, and target cells are seen. The β_4-tetramer (hemoglobin H) inclusions are seen easily following incubation with 1% brilliant cresyl blue, or after splenectomy, they can be seen occasionally with methylene blue reticulocyte or Wright's stains (Fig. 4.8C).[62] Studies of the synthesis of the globin chain suggest an α/β ratio of 0.3:0.4 rather than 1, and most individuals have a genotype comprised of α-thalassemia₁ and α-thalassemia₂ (--/α-) (Fig. 4.12). This imbalance causes 20% or higher levels of hemoglobin Barts at birth and 4% to 30% levels of hemoglobin H after the switch from γ- to β-chain synthesis is complete. Both tetramers precipitate, causing an inclusion-body hemolytic anemia. Deficient synthesis of the α-chain causes a drop in hemoglobin A_2 ($\alpha_2\delta_2$) levels to 1% to 1.5%; deficient α-chain synthesis is secondary to a deficiency of α-globin mRNA, caused by a deletion of three of the four α-genes. Usually, one of the parents of such a patient has α-thalassemia₁ (--), and the other has α-thalassemia₂ (α-). The risk of offspring from such matings inheriting hemoglobin H disease is 25% with each pregnancy (Table 4.6).[63]

Individuals with heterozygous α-thal₁ (Fig. 4.12) are usually of Oriental or Mediterranean descent. They arerelatively asymptomatic but have a mild microcytic anemia (10 to 12 g of hemoglobin/100 ml of blood) and mild poikilocytosis and anisocytosis. The diagnosis of α-thal trait should be considered seriously when the

TABLE 4.7. Point Mutations in β-Thalassemia

Mutant Class	Type*	Origin
Nonfunctional mRNA		
Nonsense mutants		
Codon 17 (A→T)	0	Chinese
Codon 39 (C→T)	0	Mediterranean, European
Codon 15 (G→A)	0	Asian Indian
Codon 121 (G→T)	0	Polish, Swiss
Codon 37 (G→A)	0	Saudi Arabian
Codon 43 (G→T)	0	Chinese
Codon 61 (A→T)	0	Black
Codon 35 (C→A)	0	Thai
Codon 22 (G→T)	0	Reunion Islander
Frameshift mutants		
−1: codon 1 (−G)	0	Mediterranean
−2: codon 8 (−AA)	0	Turkish
−1: codon 16 (−C)	0	Asian Indian
−1: codon 44 (−C)	0	Kurdish
+1: codon 47 (+A)	0	Surinamese black
+1: codon 8/9 (+G)	0	Asian Indian
−4: codons 41/42 (−CTTT)	0	Asian Indian, Chinese
−1: codon 6 (−A)	0	Mediterranean
+1: codons 71/72 (+A)	0	Chinese
+1: codons 106/107 (+G)	0	American black
−1: codons 76 (−C)	0	Italian
−2: codon 5 (−CT)	0	Mediterranean
−1: codon 11 (−T)	0	Mexican
−1: codon 35 (−C)	0	Indonesian
−2, +1: codon 114 (−CT, +G)	+	French
+1: codons 14/15 (+G)	0	Chinese
−7: codons 37–39	0	Turkish
+2: codon 94 (+TG)	0	Italian
−1: codon 64 (−G)	0	Swiss
−1: codon 109 (−G)	+	Lithuanian
−1: codons 36–37 (−T)	0	Kurdish (Iranian)
+1: codons 27–28 (+C)	0	Chinese
+1: codon 71 (+T)	0	Chinese
−1: codons 82/83 (−G)	0	Azerbaijani
−1: codon 126 (−T)	+	Italian
−4: codons 128–129, −11: codons 132–135, +5: codon 129	+	Irish
Initiator codon mutants		
ATG→AGG	0	Chinese
ATG→ACG	0	Yugoslavian
RNA Processing Mutants		
Splice junction changes		
IVS-1 position 1 (G→A)	0	Mediterranean
IVS-1 position 1 (G→T)	0	Asian Indian, Chinese
IVS-2 position 1 (G→A)	0	Mediterranean, Tunisian, American black
IVS-1 position 2 (T→G)	0	Tunisian
IVS-1 position 2 (T→C)	0	Black
IVS-1 3′ end (−17 bp)	0	Kuwaiti
IVS-1 3′ end (−25 bp)	0	Asian Indian
IVS-1 3′ end (G→C)	0	Italian
IVS-2 3′ end (A→G)	0	American black
IVS-2 3′ end (A→C)	0	American black
IVS-1 5′ end (−44 bp)	0	Mediterranean

TABLE 4.7. Point Mutations in β-Thalassemia (continued)

Mutant Class	Type*	Origin
IVS-1 3' end (G→A)	0	Egyptian
Consensus changes		
IVS-1 position 5 (G→C)	+	Asian Indian, Chinese, Melanesian
IVS-1 position 5 (G→T)	+	Mediterranean, black
IVS-1 position 5 (G→A)	+	Algerian
IVS-1 position 6 (T→C)	+	Mediterranean
IVS-1 position −1 (G→C) [codon 30]	+	Tunisian, black
IVS-1 position −1 (G→A) [codon 30]	?	Bulgarian
IVS-1 position −3 (C→T) [codon 29]	?	Lebanese
IVS-2 3' end (CAG→AAG)	+	Iranian, Egyptian, black
IVS-1 3' end (TAG→GAG)	+	Saudi Arabian
IVS-2 3' end position −8 (T→G)	+	Algerian
Internal IVS changes		
IVS-1 position 110 (G→A)	+	Mediterranean
IVS-1 position 116 (T→G)	0	Mediterranean
IVS-2 position 705 (T→G)	+	Mediterranean
IVS-2 position 745 (C→G)	+	Mediterranean
IVS-2 position 654 (C→T)	0	Chinese
Coding region substitutions affecting processing		
Codon 26 (G→A)	E	Southeast Asian, European
Codon 24 (T→A)	+	American black
Codon 27 (G→T)	Knossos	Mediterranean
Codon 19 (A→G)	Malay	Malaysian
RNA Cleavage and Polyadenylation Mutants		
AATAAA→AACAAA	+	American black
AATAAA→AATAAG	+	Kurdish
AATAAA→A (−AATAA)	+	Arab
AATAAA→AATGAA	+	Mediterranean
AATAAA→AATAGA	+	Malaysian
Cap Site Mutants		
nt +1 (A→C)	+	Asian Indian
Transcriptional Mutants		
nt −101 (C→T)	+	Turkish
nt −92 (C→T)	+	Mediterranean
nt −88 (C→T)	+	American black, Asian Indian
nt −88 (C→A)	+	Kurdish
nt −87 (C→G)	+	Mediterranean
nt −86 (C→G)	+	Lebanese
nt −31 (A→G)	+	Japanese
nt −30 (T→A)	+	Turkish
nt −30 (T→C)	+	Chinese
nt −29 (A→G)	+	American black, Chinese
nt −28 (A→C)	+	Kurdish, Mexican
nt −28 (A→G)	+	Chinese
Unstable Globins		
$\beta^{\text{Indianapolis}}$ (codon 112; Cys→Arg)	+	European
$\beta^{\text{Showa-Yakushiji}}$ (codon 110; Leu→Pro)	+	Japanese
β^{Houston} (codon 127; Gln→Pro)	+	British
Codons 127–128 (−AGG; Gln, Ala→Pro)	+	Japanese
Codon 60 (Val→Glu)	+	Italian

Source: Kazazian et al. 1991, Ann. N.Y. Acad. Sci.: pp. 3–5.

Note: The total number of point mutations (91) known as of July 1990 is listed. For references, see Kazazian 1990.[60] IVS = intervening sequence.

*0 = β°; + = β⁺; E = βᴱ; Knossos = β^Knossos; Malay = β^Malay; ? = unknown.

TABLE 4.8.   Population-Specific β-Thalassemia Mutations

Population	Mutation
Mediterranean	30 alleles (6 account for 93%)
Chinese/Southeast Asian	15 alleles (4 account for 91%)
Indian	10 alleles (5 account for 90%)
Black	12 alleles
North African/Middle Eastern	13 alleles plus Mediterranean alleles

Source: Phillips and Kazazian 1990, p. 1333.

MCV and MCH are low, the MCHC is relatively normal and the patient is not iron deficient, and the hemoglobin electrophoresis is normal. At birth, hemoglobin Barts may reach 5% in cord blood. The α/β-synthesis ratio is 0.6:0.75, and the genotype in Orientals is usually a single mutation that deletes both α-genes on the same chromosome (Fig. 4.12). A second type of α-thal gene that is dysfunctional but not deleted has been found in Chinese and Cypriots.[54,64] Two percent to 5% of black newborns have mild elevation of hemoglobin Barts (> 2%),[63] and such individuals have been shown to have an α-thalassemia trait phenotype. Restriction endonuclease studies have shown that the α-thalassemia trait phenotype in blacks is usually due to the deletion of a single α-gene on both chromosome 16s (trans, or α-thalassemia$_2$ homozygote) (α-/α-); this contrasts with the usual Oriental genotype (deletion of both α-genes on one chromosome 16 [cis, or α-thalassemia$_1$ heterozygote] [αα/--]).[65]

Silent carriers have α-thalassemia$_2$ genotypes, with the deletion of a single α-gene (αα/α-) in affected Orientals and 28% of blacks.[65] The hematologic findings are normal, because the reduction of α-mRNA is insufficient to produce a significant imbalance in the globin chain (α/β-ratio of 0.8:0.9) (Fig. 4.12). Among Southeast Asians, there is also a second relatively common α-thalassemia$_2$ allele, the α$^{Constant Spring}$ gene; this gene encodes an abnormal α-chain that has 31 additional amino acids at the COOH-terminal end and is synthesized at about 3% of the rate of normal α-chains.[3]

β-THALASSEMIA. In contrast to the α-thalassemia states, in which there are four degrees of severity, the β-thalassemias can be considered to have two. β-Thalassemia major (Cooley anemia) results from two β-thalassemia genes at the β-globin locus; β-thalassemia trait results from a single β-thalassemia gene.

β-Thalassemia major is a severe disease. At birth, affected infants are relatively normal, because the change from γ-chain to β-chain synthesis has not yet occurred (Fig. 4.5). However, by 6 months of age, the infant develops a severely microcytic hemolytic anemia with anisocytosis and poikilocytosis, polychromasia,

and teardrop red cells (Fig. 4.8F).[62] The failure in β-globin production due to absent or greatly decreased β-mRNA leads to an imbalance in α- and β-globin synthesis, and the subsequent precipitation of free α-chains results in inclusion bodies that damage the erythrocyte membrane and lead to the destruction of nucleated red cells in the marrow. The reticulocyte count usually is no greater than 10% because of massive destruction of erythroid precursors in the marrow. To maintain an adequate hemoglobin level, transfusions are usually required every 4 to 8 weeks. Affected children develop hepatosplenomegaly secondary to extramedullary hematopoiesis and a characteristic Oriental facial appearance due to excessive intramedullary hematopoiesis. The bones have expanded marrow cavities, resulting in pathologic fractures and a "hair-on-end" appearance on skull films (Fig. 4.11). Other complications include cholelithiasis, susceptibility to infections, secondary hypersplenism, and delayed growth and maturation.[61,62]

The major causes of mortality are hemochromatosis and overwhelming infections following splenectomy, the former due to excessive iron deposition resulting from blood transfusions and increased gastrointestinal absorption.[66] Excess iron deposited in the heart, pancreas, liver, and other organs damages tissue and leads to cardiac failure, arrhythmias, diabetes mellitus, and liver failure, but given antibiotic and transfusion therapy, many patients survive until their twenties or thirties.[62] Homozygous Greeks and Italians generally follow this course.

Blacks often have a milder disease (β-thalassemia intermedia). Transfusions usually are not required in these patients, even though α/β-synthesis ratios are similar to those observed in homozygous Mediterraneans.[53] β-Thalassemia intermedia also is seen occasionally in other groups, particularly the Portuguese, and is correlated with either a particular mutation in the β-globin gene (which is mild) or the concomitant presence of an α-thalassemia state.

Individuals with β-thalassemia trait (heterozygous β-thalassemia) are usually asymptomatic. They have a mild anemia (10 to 11 g of hemoglobin/100 ml of blood) with decreased MCV (55 to 70) and MCH (16 to 22 pg). Microcytosis, anisocytosis, poikilocytosis, and stippling of the red cells can be seen on the blood smear (Fig. 4.8E),[62] and on physical examination, there is mild to moderate splenomegaly in about half of the cases.

Differential Diagnosis

In the general practice of medicine, many patients present with a mild microcytic anemia; nearly all of

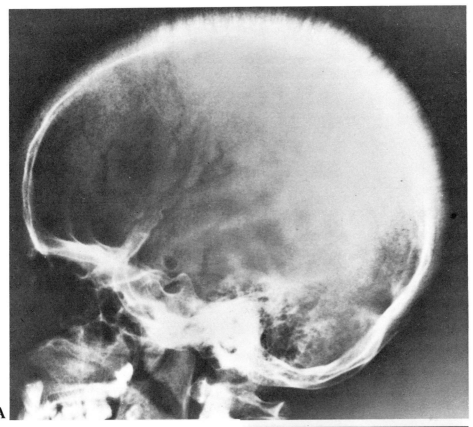

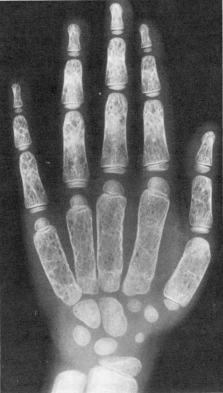

FIGURE 4.11. Radiographic changes in homozygous β-thalassemia. A, Thickened parietal calvaria with outer table destruction and "hair-on-end" appearance. Note the absent pneumatization of the maxillary sinuses and the coincidental epidermoidoma. B, Widened medullary cavities, cortical thinning, and coarse trabeculation secondary to intramedullary hyperplasia. (*Source:* Courtesy of Dr. John Dorst.)

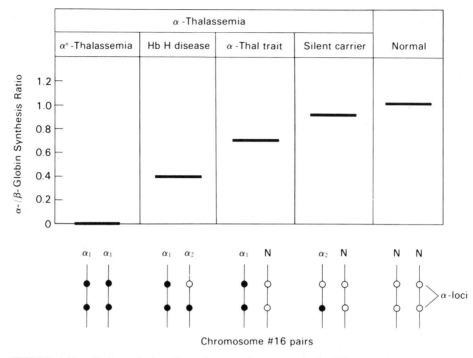

FIGURE 4.12. **Chain synthesis ratios and proposed genotypes in the different α-thalassemia states.** **Genotypes:** *open circle* = **normal,** *N* = **normal,** *closed circle* = **abnormal,** α_1 = **α-thalassemia$_1$,** α_2 = **α-thalassemia$_2$,** α_1N **could also be** α_2-**αs22.** (**Source: Adapted from Nathan 1972. Reprinted by permission of the New England Journal of Medicine.**)

them have iron deficiency anemia or a thalassemia trait. In heterozygous thalassemia, the peripheral smear may be more abnormal than that of iron deficiency and the MCV and MCH decreased, but the MCHC is normal in contrast to the decreased MCHC found in advanced iron deficiency anemia. Also, the MCV in thalassemia traits tends to be lower in relation to the red cell count than the MCV in iron deficiency. This difference is the basis of the Mentzer index (MCV/red cell count [RBC]). MCV/RBC values of less than 11.5 suggest thalassemia trait, while values greater than 13.5 suggest iron deficiency anemia.[67]

A much more definitive approach is to measure hemoglobin A_2 in patients with microcytosis (Fig. 4.13). Patients with microcytosis and normal hemoglobin A_2 should have serum iron or ferritin determinations; a low value suggests iron deficiency anemia, while a normal iron or ferritin value suggests α-thalassemia trait (when documentation obtained in first-degree relatives confirms the diagnosis). When microcytosis and an increased hemoglobin A_2 are found, β-thalassemia trait is the tentative diagnosis,[68] and confirmation is obtained by family studies and chain synthesis ratios. A possible

simple alternative for differentiating iron deficiency from thalassemia trait in patients with low MCVs is to measure the degree of anisocytosis with an electronic red cell counter; anisocytosis is significantly greater in patients with iron deficiency than in those with thalassemia trait.[69]

As seen in Table 4.6, β-thalassemia heterozygotes can have different hemoglobin patterns. The most common is β°-thalassemia or β^+-thalassemia with an increased hemoglobin A_2 (usually 4% to 6%) and a normal or slightly increased hemoglobin F (2% to 5%). In the rare δβ-thalassemia trait, hemoglobin A_2 is normal but hemoglobin F is usually increased. Finally, hemoglobin Lepore trait has 5% to 15% hemoglobin Lepore, which contains a δβ-fusion chain and a slight elevation of hemoglobin F.[52,62] Chain synthesis studies in most β-thalassemia heterozygotes yield α/β ratios of 1.5:2.5.

The term β-*thalassemia intermedia* is sometimes used to describe individuals who are mild homozygotes; blacks homozygous for β^+-thalassemia with a mild clinical course are an example. Homozygous δβ-thalassemia also tends to be clinically mild because, for unknown reasons, the production of hemoglobin F is

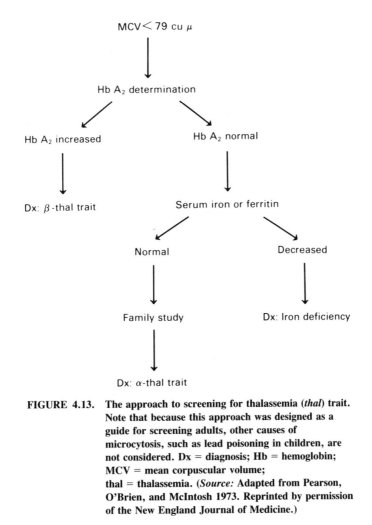

MCV < 79 cu μ

↓

Hb A$_2$ determination

↙ ↘

Hb A$_2$ increased   Hb A$_2$ normal

↓   ↓

Dx: β-thal trait   Serum iron or ferritin

↙ ↘

Normal   Decreased

↓   ↓

Family study   Dx: Iron deficiency

↓

Dx: α-thal trait

FIGURE 4.13. **The approach to screening for thalassemia (*thal*) trait. Note that because this approach was designed as a guide for screening adults, other causes of microcytosis, such as lead poisoning in children, are not considered. Dx = diagnosis; Hb = hemoglobin; MCV = mean corpuscular volume; thal = thalassemia. (*Source:* Adapted from Pearson, O'Brien, and McIntosh 1973. Reprinted by permission of the New England Journal of Medicine.)**

higher in this condition than in other β-thalassemia states and compensates for the absent hemoglobins A and A$_2$. One also can find the combination of α- and β-thalassemia traits in the same individual; this condition is mild because the resulting α/β-synthesis ratio is more normal and there are fewer free α-chains to cause hemolysis.

$\delta\beta$-THALASSEMIA OR F-THALASSEMIA. Homozygous $\delta\beta$-thalassemia usually occurs in Greeks and, as stated earlier, tends to be a mild disorder. The term *F-thalassemia* is used because homozygotes have 100% hemoglobin F and lack hemoglobins A and A$_2$. The mild anemia and hemolysis are due to increased γ-chain synthesis, which makes the imbalance between the synthesis of α- and non-α-chains less than that seen in other β-thalassemias. Patients with heterozygous $\delta\beta$-

thalassemias have mild microcytosis and 5% to 20% hemoglobin F on electrophoresis (Table 4.6).

HEMOGLOBIN LEPORE THALASSEMIA. As previously mentioned, hemoglobin Lepore is a variant of hemoglobin containing a $\delta\beta$-fusion chain. Originally, this chain probably resulted from nonhomologous crossing over between the linked δ- and β-genes during meiosis. Three different Lepore variants are described, which differ in the point at which the $\delta\beta$-fusion occurs. Hemoglobin Lepore has an electrophoretic mobility similar to that of hemoglobin S, and it forms 5% to 15% of the total hemoglobin of heterozygotes (Table 4.6). Decreased hemoglobin Lepore synthesis may be secondary to instability of the $\delta\beta$-mRNA. Heterozygotes are clinically similar to β^0-thalassemia heterozygotes and hemoglobin Lepore homozygotes, and Lepore/β^0-

thalassemia genetic compounds are similar to β^0-thalassemia homozygotes.[62]

γβ-THALASSEMIA. Two full-term newborns with hemolytic, hypochromic anemia and microcytosis have been described. Hemoglobin H and hemoglobin Barts were absent, and globin synthesis studies revealed a deficiency of γ- and β-synthesis in relation to α-synthesis. With time, the peripheral smears and morphology improved and resembled those of the fathers and other relatives with heterozygous β-thalassemia. These cases are probably examples of heterozygous γβ-thalassemia.[70,71] Restriction endonuclease mapping of DNA from one child showed a large deletion that removes all the ε-, ^{G}γ-, ^{A}γ-, and δ-genes from one chromosome 11. Interestingly, the deletion ends 2-kb 5′ to the β-gene, yet that β-gene, while present, is not expressed.[71] In other cases, a deletion has eliminated the entire β-globin cluster.

δ⁰-THALASSEMIA. Heterozygous and homozygous δ⁰-thalassemias have decreased and absent hemoglobin A_2, respectively. However, anemia and changes in peripheral smears are not seen because of the normal low level of δ-chain production (Fig. 4.5).

HEREDITARY PERSISTENCE OF FETAL HEMO-GLOBIN. Hereditary persistence of fetal hemoglobin can occur in many different forms because of different mutations. HPFH heterozygotes differ from thalassemia heterozygotes in that they have no imbalance between the synthesis of α- and non-α-chains (i.e., γ- and β-chains). The HPFH syndromes are characterized by an asymptomatic heterozygous state without microcytosis, and the elevated hemoglobin F ranges from 10% to 15% in the type commonly found in Greeks to 3% to 30% in certain types seen in blacks. The proportion of γ-chain type (^{G}γ vs. ^{A}γ) varies among patients with different HPFHs, and usually, but not always, the hemoglobin F is homogeneously distributed within red cells in contrast to δβ- and other thalassemias.[5] In a few cases, HPFH heterozygotes have two populations of cells: one contains hemoglobin F and the other lacks it. These patients are said to have heterocellular HPFH as opposed to the bulk of patients who have pancellular HPFH.[72]

The β- and δ-genes adjacent to the HPFH gene are often inactive and in fact may be deleted in blacks with two HPFH types, but both are present and active in other HPFH cases involving blacks. In these latter cases, point mutations at −202 and −175 upstream of the ^{G}γ-globin gene have been found. In other ethnic groups, point mutations in the same region 5′ to the ^{A}γ-globin gene have produced nondeletion HPFH. The differences be-

tween HPFH and δβ-thalassemia are subtle, but the clinical picture and blood smears in δβ-thalassemia are somewhat more abnormal and the hemoglobin F has a more heterogeneous cellular distribution. HPFH homozygotes have mild hypochromia, microcytosis, and morphologic changes in the red cells. The hemoglobin is 100% hemoglobin F, and there is no anemia. In some of these cases, α/γ-chain synthesis ratios of 1.5 occur, similar to the α/β-ratios seen in milder β-thalassemia trait. It has been hypothesized that a suppression region for γ-chain synthesis is located between the ^{A}γ- and δ-loci and that HPFH, but not δβ-thalassemia mutations, inhibit its function. However, there appear to be multiple suppression and activation regions in the β-globin gene cluster, and a clear picture has not yet emerged.

The Interaction of Thalassemia with Hemoglobin Variants

Thalassemia and structurally variant hemoglobin genes may or may not interact. An interacting thalassemia gene is one that causes an increased level of the variant hemoglobin chain in the individual who is heterozygous for the variant gene and a thalassemia gene at the same locus. When the presence of both the thalassemia and variant genes does not increase the level of the hemoglobin variant, the thalassemia is noninteracting.

α-THALASSEMIA AND VARIANTS. The genetic compound of α-thalassemia₁ (--) and hemoglobin Q ($α^{47\ Asp\rightarrow His}$) is found mainly in Thailand. The clinical picture is similar to that of hemoglobin H disease, but there is an absence of hemoglobin A synthesis explained by the fact that the $α^Q$-allele occurs on a chromosome from which the second α-gene is deleted ($α^{Q-}$).[73]

Heterozygotes for hemoglobin G Philadelphia ($q^{68\ Asn\rightarrow Lys}$), the most common α-variant in blacks, have been studied, and the amount of the variant seems to be trimodal (22%, 30%, and 41% of the total hemoglobin).[74] Individuals with 30% hemoglobin G have been shown to have chromosomal homologues containing a single $α^G$-gene and two normal $α^A$-genes ($αα/α^{G-}$).[75] Individuals with 22% hemoglobin G have three normal $α^A$-genes in addition to an $α^G$-gene ($αα/α^G α$).

β-THALASSEMIA AND β-VARIANTS. In S/β-thalassemia, the β-thalassemia gene interacts with the $β^S$-gene in the heterozygote to increase the level of hemoglobin S near homozygous sickle cell levels. The S/β-thalassemia heterozygote has a milder clinical course than the sickle cell homozygote, and splenomegaly is a common physical finding. Anemia is present in S/β-thalassemia and is characterized by microcytic red and target cells with occasional sickled forms (Fig. 4.8). Hemoglobin electrophoresis reveals 60% to 90% hemoglobin S, 0% to 30% hemoglobin A, 1% to 20% hemoglobin F, and increased hemoglobin A_2.[62] The percentages of hemoglobins S and A vary depending on whether the β-thalassemia gene is $β^+$ or $β^o$.

β-Thalassemia–hemoglobin C is found among blacks. Splenomegaly and an increased level of hemoglobin C differentiate this genetic compound from that of hemoglobin C heterozygote.

β-Thalassemia–hemoglobin E is a common disorder in Thailand. It results in a clinical picture similar to that of homozygous β-thalassemia.

The Management of Thalassemia

PREVENTION. Table 4.6 outlines matings that can give rise to various types of α- and β-thalassemia. The parents of children homozygous for α- or β-thalassemia are themselves heterozygotes. As such, there is a 25% risk of producing another homozygous child with each pregnancy.

For maximal benefit from genetic counseling, heterozygotes should be identified before they bear affected children. Thalassemia heterozygotes can be diagnosed tentatively by appropriate studies (MCV, hemoglobin electrophoresis, serum iron) (Fig. 4.13), and once the condition is diagnosed, heterozygous individuals should be informed of its presence, inheritance, and the potential for affected children from certain matings so they have an accurate grasp of the risk. In some cases, this would result in the testing of mates who would be identified as noncarriers, and these couples would be at no risk for homozygous offspring. The risk of homozygous offspring when both parents are heterozygous is shown in Table 4.6; other parents also might be at risk for genetic compounds in their offspring.

Prenatal diagnosis may be desired by certain heterozygous couples at risk. The procedure has become widely used, but while it leads to in utero diagnosis, it is merely a preventive measure and not a treatment. From 1975 to 1980, prenatal diagnosis of various thalassemias was done exclusively by analysis of fetal blood. The feasibility of this procedure was based on a number of factors:

1. β-Chains are synthesized by erythroid precursors as early as 5 weeks of fetal age (Fig. 4.5),
2. normal standards of β-chain synthesis at 18 to 20 weeks' gestation are known,

3. fetal cells can be obtained (with a 6% risk of fetal death at present) either by transabdominal placental puncture under ultrasonography or from fetal vessels visualized by fetoscopy,[44] and
4. small numbers of fetal reticulocytes can be separated from maternal red cells by differential agglutination or by preferential lysis of maternal cells.

The fetal blood sample can be incubated with radioactive leucine, and the relative synthesis of α-, β- (or variant β-), and γ-chains can be determined using chromatographic separation.[44] By 1980, approximately 1000 pregnancies had been tested for β-thalassemia in this way.[44] The procedure usually has resulted in adequate fetal blood samples (> 90%) with few technical errors.

In 1978, prenatal diagnosis by restriction endonuclease mapping of DNA came into general use. Fetal amniocytes were obtained for study by amniocentesis, which carries a very low risk of fetal mortality (< 0.5%), and DNA analysis was first carried out on fetuses at risk for α- and δβ-thalassemia in whom deletions could be detected.[76,77] In 1980, polymorphic restriction endonuclease sites in the β-globin gene complex were used for prenatal detection of various β-thalassemias not caused by deletions. Kan et al.[78] first showed that a *Bam* HI site 3′ to the β-globin gene was useful for prenatal diagnosis of a certain $β^o$-thalassemia allele in Sardinian couples at risk. Later, Little et al.[79] demonstrated that other polymorphic sites in the γ-genes could be valuable in prenatal diagnosis in non-Sardinian couples. Using a combination of known DNA polymorphisms and linkage analysis, clinicians could carry out prenatal diagnosis for various β-thalassemia states by amniocentesis alone in 75% of at-risk pregnancies in which the couple had a previous child.[80]

As the various mutations producing β-thalassemia were characterized (Fig. 4.10) and oligonucleotide hybridization techniques were developed for detecting specific nucleotide changes in genomic DNA, prenatal diagnosis by direct mutation detection came into routine use in Sardinia.[81] The development of the polymerase chain reaction technique allowed amplification of the β-globin gene sequences by a millionfold, and this technique can be coupled with oligonucleotide hybridization in dot blots, restriction digestion of amplified product, or direct nucleotide sequencing of the amplified product[82] to allow direct detection of mutations in general prenatal diagnosis of β-thalassemia. At Johns Hopkins in July 1991, the last 225 consecutive prenatal diagnoses of β-thalassemia were carried out in various ethnic groups by direct detection of the mutations involved.

THERAPY. Treatment for severe β-thalassemia is primarily symptomatic. If the anemia is severe enough, transfusions are required to maintain adequate levels of hemoglobin. There are two approaches. First, transfusion may be given when the patient's hemoglobin drops below 8 g/100 ml to avoid symptoms secondary to anemia. Second, hypertransfusion, or repeated transfusions, may be given as frequently as needed to maintain the hemoglobin at a minimum of 10 g/100 ml. This latter approach may require 2 to 3 units every 2 to 4 weeks in adults,[62] and evidence suggests that children maintained on hypertransfusion (hemoglobin greater than 9.5 to 10 g/100 ml) are more active, have fewer infections, and have less frequent complications of cardiac dysfunction, hypersplenism, and bone and dental changes. However, evidence conflicts as to whether this therapy can aid the child in attaining normal growth.[62,83]

Both methods of transfusion increase the iron overload. Iron chelation therapy with deferoxamine has been used to attempt prevention of this side effect of chronic transfusion. The route of administration is important, because 750 mg of deferoxamine intramuscularly (with oral ascorbic acid in patients over 5 years old) resulted in urinary clearance of iron ranging from 2.2 to 44.8 mg/24 hours (before treatment, excretion was 0.1 to 2.5 mg/24 hours). Subcutaneous infusions of 1.5 g deferoxamine over 18 hours further increased iron excretion 2.4-fold, and large doses given intravenously increased clearance over that obtained by subcutaneous infusion.[84,85] The iron excretion attained following intravenous or slow subcutaneous infusion of deferoxamine is far better than excretion when deferoxamine is injected intramuscularly. Other data suggest that while 20 mg of deferoxamine B/kg of body weight given daily by intramuscular injection might reduce the daily iron accumulation somewhat in children, if the deferoxamine is given by overnight infusion, it allows iron balance to be reached even when the child has large transfusion requirements.[83] The relative effectiveness of different doses in thalassemia patients of different ages has been reported.[86] These experimental data suggest that chelation therapy is applicable to clinical practice, and work has intensified on the development of oral iron chelators.

Other side effects of transfusions include hepatitis and cytomegalovirus infections. Also, isoimmunization to minor blood groups may occur, but careful selection of donors may decrease this risk. Using blood with the white cells removed may decrease sensitization to white cell or plasma antigens, and urticaria may be treated with antihistamines as well as epinephrine both before and during transfusion. Febrile reactions may require antipyretics and, if severe, occasionally steroids.[61]

Finally, the increased rate of erythropoiesis can lead to increased folic acid requirements. If folate deficiency occurs, it may cause increased anemia; however, a deficiency is easily avoided by daily oral administration of folic acid.

Splenectomy may be avoided by hypertransfusion therapy, but splenectomy may be necessary to alleviate hypersplenism with worsening of the anemia or pain due to progressive splenomegaly or infarction of the spleen. As mentioned in the discussion on sickle cell disease, splenectomized children, especially those under 6 years of age, are at risk for life-threatening infections. Pneumococcal vaccine as well as prophylactic penicillin should be used in such children, and suspected infections should be treated aggressively.[62,39]

Bone marrow transplantation has been used successfully not only in aplastic anemia and leukemia but also for thalassemia. A large number of affected children have received transplants, with many cures, although there clearly are risks involving graft rejection, morbidity, and death.

Future Treatment

Theoretic approaches to the treatment of thalassemia that may become possible include induction of expression of the deficient globin chain, stabilization of the appropriate mRNA, or activation of nonexpressed γ-genes to reduce the globin chain imbalance. Methods for the insertion of DNA into eukaryotic cells are being developed, but technical as well as ethical problems remain. The application of such techniques to the treatment of thalassemia syndromes, or hemoglobinopathies, should come within the next 3 years.

REFERENCES

1. Bunn HF, Forget BG, Ranney HM. Hemoglobin structure. In: Bunn HF, Forget BG, Ranney HM, eds. Human Hemoglobins. Philadelphia: W. B. Saunders, 1977:4.
2. Baralle EF, Shoulders CC, Proudfoot NJ. The primary structure of the human ε-globin gene. Cell 1980; 21:621.
3. Bunn HF, Forget BG. Human hemoglobin variants. In: Bunn HF, Forget BG, Ranney HM, eds. Human Hemoglobins. Philadelphia: W. B. Saunders, 1986:193.
4. Cooper HA, Hoagland HC. Fetal hemoglobin. Mayo Clin Proc 1972;47:402.
5. Kazazian HH Jr. Regulation of human fetal hemoglobin production. Semin Hematol 1974;11:525.
6. Kazazian HH Jr, Woodhead AP. Hemoglobin A synthesis in the developing fetus. N Engl J Med 1973;289:58.
7. Rieder RF. Human hemoglobin stability and instability: molecular mechanisms and some clinical correlations. Semin Hematol 1974;11:423.
8. Bellingham AJ. Haemoglobins with altered oxygen affinity. Br Med Bull 1976;32:234.
9. Murayama M. In: Nalbandian RM, ed. Molecular Aspects of Sickle Cell Hemoglobin. Springfield, Ill.: Charles C Thomas, 1971.

10. Lawn RM, Fritsch EF, Parker RC, Blake G, Maniatis T. The isolation and characterization of linked δ- and β-globin genes from a cloned library of human DNA. Cell 1978;15:1157.

11. Orkin SH. The duplicated human α globin genes lie close together in cellular DNA. Proc Natl Acad Sci U S A 1978;74:560.

12. Bernards R, Little PFR, Annison G, Williamson R, Flavell RA. Structure of human $^G\gamma$-$^A\gamma$-δ-β globin gene locus. Proc Natl Acad Sci U S A 1979;76:4827.

13. Proudfoot NJ, Baralle F. Molecular cloning of the human ε-globin gene. Proc Natl Acad Sci U S A 1979;76:5435.

14. Lauer J, Schon C-KJ, Maniatis T. The chromosomal arrangement of human α-like globin genes: sequence homology and α-globin gene deletions. Cell 1980;20:119.

15. Fritsch EF, Lawn RM, Maniatis T. Molecular cloning and characterization of the human β-like globin gene cluster. Cell 1980;19:959.

16. Proudfoot NJ, Maniatis T. The structure of a human α-globin pseudogene and its relationship to α-globin gene duplication. Cell 1980;21:537.

17. Slightom JL, Blechl AE, Smithies O. Human fetal $^G\gamma$ and $^A\gamma$ globin genes: complete nucleotide sequences suggest that DNA can be exchanged between these duplicated genes. Cell 1980;21:627.

18. Spritz RA, DeRiel JK, Forget BG, Weissman SM. Complete nucleotide sequence of the human δ-globin gene. Cell 1980;21:639.

19. Lawn RM, Efstradiadis A, O'Connell G, Maniatis T. The nucleotide sequence of the human β-globin gene. Cell 1980;21:647.

20. Efstradiadis A, Posakony JW, Maniatis T, et al. The structure and evolution of the human β-globin gene family. Cell 1980;21:653.

21. Fritsch EF, Lawn RM, Maniatis T. Characterisation of deletions which affect the expression of fetal globin genes in man. Nature 1979;279:598.

22. Grosveld F, van Assendelft GB, Greaves DR, Kollias G. Position independent high level expression of the human β-globin gene in transgenic mice. Cell 1987;51:975.

23. Deisseroth A, Nienhuis A, Turner P, et al. Localization of the human α-globin structural gene to chromosome 16 in somatic cell hybrids by molecular hybridization assay. Cell 1977;12:205.

24. Scott AF, Phillips JA III, Migeon BR. DNA restriction endonuclease analysis for the localization of the human β and δ globin genes on chromosome 11. Proc Natl Acad Sci U S A 1979;76:4563.

25. Gusella J, Varsanyi-Breiner A, Kao F-T, et al. Precise localization of the human β-globin gene complex on chromosome 11. Proc Natl Acad Sci U S A 1979;76:5239.

26. Deisseroth A, Nienhuis A, Lawrence J, Giles R, Turner P, Ruddle FH. Chromosomal localization of human β globin gene on human chromosome 11 in somatic cell hybrids. Proc Natl Acad Sci U S A 1978;75:1456.

27. Tilghman SM, Curtis PJ, Tiemeier DC, Leder P, Weissman C. The intervening sequence of a mouse β-globin gene is transcribed within the 15S β-globin mRNA precursor. Proc Natl Acad Sci U S A 1978;75:1309.

28. Hamer D, Leder P. Splicing and the formation of stable RNA. Cell 1979;18:1299.

29. Kazazian HH Jr, Cho S, Phillips JA III. The mutational basis of the thalassemia syndromes. Prog Med Genet 1977;2:165.

30. Merkel CG, Wood TG, Lingrel JB. Shortening of the poly(A) region of mouse globin messenger RNA. J Biol Chem 1976;251:5512.

31. Seid-Akhavan M, Winter WP, Abramson RK, Rucknagel DL. Hemoglobin Wayne: a frameshift mutation detected in human hemoglobin alpha chains. Proc Natl Acad Sci U S A 1976;73:882.

32. International Hemoglobin Information Center. List of Hemoglobin Variants. Augusta, Ga.: Huisman, T.H.J., 1984.

33. Bunn HF, Forget BG. Hemoglobin: Molecular, Genetic and Clinical Aspects. Philadelphia: W. B. Saunders, 1986.

34. Motulsky AG. Frequency of sickling disorders in US blacks. N Engl J Med 1973;288:31.

35. Nathan DG, Pearson HA. Sickle cell syndromes and hemoglobin C disease. In: Nathan DG, Oski FA, eds. Hematology of Infancy and Childhood. Philadelphia: W. B. Saunders, 1974:419.

36. Barrett-Connor E. Bacterial infection and sickle cell anemia. Medicine 1971;50:97.

37. Dean J, Schechter AN. Sickle cell anemias: molecular and cellular bases of therapeutic approaches. N Engl J Med 1978;299:863.

38. Charache S, Dover GJ, Moyer MA, Moore JW. Hydroxyurea-induced augmentation of fetal hemoglobin production in patients with sickle cell anemia. Blood 1987;69:109.

39. Ammann AJ, Addiego J, Wara DW, Lubin B, Smith WB, Mentzer WC. Polyvalent pneumococcal-polysaccharide immunization of patients with sickle-cell anemia and patients with splenectomy. N Engl J Med 1977;297:897.

40. Akhonkhai VI, Landesman SH, Fikrig SM, et al. Failure of pneumococcal vaccine in children with sickle cell disease. N Engl J Med 1979;301:26.

41. Giebiuk GS, Schillman G, Krivit W, Quie PG. Vaccine type pneumococcal pneumonia: occurrence after vaccination in an asplenic patient. JAMA 1979;241:2736.

42. Hobbins JC, Mahoney MJ. In utero diagnosis of hemoglobinopathies. N Engl J Med 1974;290:1065.

43. Alter BP, Modell CB, Fairweather D, et al. Prenatal diagnosis of hemoglobinopathies. N Engl J Med 1976;295:1437.

44. Alter BP. Prenatal diagnosis of hemoglobinopathies and other hematologic disorders. J Pediatrics 1979;95:501.

45. Kan YW, Dozy AM. Antenatal diagnosis of sickle cell anemia by DNA analysis of amniotic fluid cells. Lancet 1978;ii:910.

46. Phillips JA III, Panny SR, Kazazian HH Jr, et al. Prenatal diagnosis of sickle cell anemia by restriction endonuclease analysis: Hind III polymorphisms in γ-globin genes extend test applicability. Proc Natl Acad Sci U S A 1980;77:2856.

47. Saiki RK, Gelfand DH, Stoffel B, et al. Primer-directed enzymatic amplification of DNA with a thermostable DNA polymerase. Science 1988;239:487.

48. Chehab F, Doherty M, Cai S, Kan YW, Cooper S, Rubin E. Detection of sickle cell anemia and thalassemias. Nature 1987;329:293.

49. Bunn HF, Forget BG, Ranney HM. Unstable hemoglobin variants: congenital Heinz body hemolytic anemia. In: Bunn HF, Forget BG, Ranney HM, eds. Human Hemoglobins. Philadelphia: W. B. Saunders, 1977:282.

50. Nagel RL, Lynfield J, Johnson J, et al. Hemoglobin Beth Israel: a mutant causing clinically apparent cyanosis. N Engl J Med 1976;295:125.

51. Bunn HF. The structure and function of human hemoglobins. In: Nathan DG, Oski FA, eds. Hematology of Infancy and Childhood. Philadelphia: W. B. Saunders, 1974:412.

52. Orkin SH, Nathan DG. Current topics in genetics: the thalassemias. N Engl J Med 1976;295:710.

53. Weatherall DJ. The molecular basis of thalassemia. Johns Hopkins Med J 1976;139:205.

54. Orkin SH, Old JM, Lazarus H, et al. The molecular basis of α-thalassemias: frequent occurrence of dysfunctional α loci among non-Asians with Hb H disease. Cell 1979;17:33.

55. Phillips JA III, Vik TA, Scott AF, et al. Unequal crossing-over: a common basis of single α-globin genes in Asians and American blacks with hemoglobin H disease. Blood 1980;55:1066.

56. Goossens M, Dozy AM, Embury SH, et al. Triplicated α-globin loci in man. Proc Natl Acad Sci U S A 1980;77:518.

57. Embury SH, Miller JA, Dozy AM, Kan YW, Chan V, Todd D.

Two different molecular organizations account for the single α-globin gene of the α-thalassemias-2 genotype. J Clin Invest 1980;66:1319.

58. Pressley L, Higgs DR, Clegg JB, Weatherall DJ. Gene deletions in α-thalassemia prove that the 5′ζ locus is functional. Proc Natl Acad Sci U S A 1980;77:3586.

59. Orkin SH, Kazazian HH Jr. The mutation and polymorphism of the human β-globin gene and its surrounding DNA. Annu Rev Genet 1984;18:131.

60. Kazazian HH Jr. The thalassemia syndromes: molecular basis and prenatal diagnosis in 1990. Semin Hematol 1990;27:209–228.

61. Nathan DG. Thalassemia. N Engl J Med 1972;296:586.

62. Forget BF, Kan YW. Thalassemia and the genetics of hemoglobin. In: Nathan DG, Oski FA, eds. Hematology of Infancy and Childhood. Philadelphia: W. B. Saunders, 1974:450.

63. Wasi D, Na-Nakorn S, Pootrakul S-N. The α thalassemias. Clin Hematol 1974;3:383.

64. Kan YW, Dozy AM, Trecartin R, Todd D. Identification of a non-deletion defect in α thalassemia. N Engl J Med 1977; 297:1081.

65. Dozy AM, Kan YW, Embury SH, et al. α-Globin gene organisation in blacks precludes the severe form of α-thalassemia. Nature 1979;280:605.

66. Bannerman RM, Callender ST, Hardisty RM, Smith RS. Iron absorption in thalassemia. Br J Haematol 1964;10:490.

67. Mentzer WC. Differentiation of iron deficiency from thalassemia trait. Lancet 1973;i:882.

68. Pearson HA, O'Brien RT, McIntosh S. Screening for thalassemia trait by electronic measurement of mean corpuscular volumes. N Engl J Med 1973;288:351.

69. Bessman JD, Feinstein DI. Quantitative anisocytosis as a discriminant between iron deficiency and thalassemia minor. Blood 1979;53:288.

70. Kan YW, Forget BG, Nathan DG. Gamma-beta thalassemia: a cause of hemolytic disease of the newborn. N Engl J Med 1972;286:129.

71. Van der Ploeg LHT, Konings A, Oort M, Roos D, Bernini L, Flavel RA. γ-β-Thalassemia studies showing that deletion of the τ and δ genes influences β-globin gene expression in man. Nature 1980;283:637.

72. Boyer SH, Margolet L, Boyer ML, et al. Inheritance of F cell frequency in heterocellular hereditary persistence of fetal hemoglobin: an example of allelic exclusion. Am J Human Genet 1977;26:256.

73. Lie-Injo LE, Dozy AM, Kan YW, Lopes M, Todd D. The α-globin gene adjacent to the gene for Hb Q-α^{74} $^{Asp \to His}$ is deleted, but not that adjacent to the gene for Hb G α^{30} $^{Glu \to Gin}$: three-fourths of the α-globin genes are deleted in Hb Q-α-thalassemia. Blood 1979;54:1407.

74. Baine RM, Rucknagel, DL, Dublin PA Jr, Adams JG III. Trimodality in the proportion of hemoglobin G Philadelphia in heterozygotes: evidence for heterogeneity in the number of human alpha chain loci. Proc Natl Acad Sci U S A 1976;73:3636.

75. Sancar GB, Tatsis B, Cedeno MM, Rieder RF. Proportion of hemoglobin G Philadelphia (α$_2$^{68} $^{Asn \to Lys}$β$_2$) in heterozygotes determined by α-globin gene deletions. Proc Natl Acad Sci U S A 1980;77:6874.

76. Orkin SH, Alter BP, Altay C, et al. Application of endonuclease mapping to the analysis and prenatal diagnosis of thalassemia caused by globin-gene deletion. N Engl J Med 1978;299:166.

77. Dozy AM, Forman EN, Abuelo DN, et al. Prenatal diagnosis of homozygous α-thalassemia. JAMA 1979;241:1610.

78. Kan YW, Lee KY, Furbetta M, Angius A, Cao A. Polymorphism of DNA sequence in the β-globin gene region. N Engl J Med 1980;302:185.

79. Little PFR, Annison G, Darling S, Williamson R, Camba L, Modell B. Model for antenatal diagnosis of β-thalassemia and other monogenic disorders by molecular analysis of linked DNA polymorphisms. Nature 1980;285:144.

80. Kazazian HH Jr, Phillips JA III, Boehm CD, Vik TA, Mahoney MJ, Ritchey AK. Prenatal diagnosis of β-thalassemia by amniocentesis: linkage analysis of multiple polymorphic restriction endonuclease sites. Blood 1980;56:926.

81. Rosatelli C, Tuveri T, DiTucci A, et al. Prenatal diagnosis of β-thalassemia with the synthetic-oligomer technique. Lancet 1985;i:241.

82. Wong C, Dowling CE, Saiki RK, Higuchi RG, Erlich HA, Kazazian HH Jr. Characterization of β-thalassemia mutations using direct genome sequencing of amplified single copy DNA. Nature 1987;330:384.

83. Weiner M, Karpatkin M, Hart D, et al. Cooley anemia: high transfusion regimen and chelation-therapy, results, and perspective. J Pediatrics 1978;92:653.

84. Propper RD, Cooper B, Rufo RR, et al. Continuous subcutaneous administration of deferoxamine in patients with iron overload. N Engl J Med 1977;297:418.

85. Cohen A, Schwartz E. Iron chelation therapy with deferoxamine in Cooley anemia. J Pediatrics 1978;92:643.

86. Graziano JH, Markenson A, Miller DR, et al. Chelation therapy in β-thalassemia major: I. Intravenous and subcutaneous deferoxamine. J Pediatrics 1978;92:648.

5

Hemolytic Anemia

Thomas S. Kickler, M.D.

A hemolytic disorder occurs when there is premature destruction of circulating red cells; if the rate of destruction exceeds the rate of erythropoiesis, anemia develops. Genetic or acquired abnormalities of the red cell membrane, hemoglobin, or enzymes lead to the intrinsic hemolytic anemias, and the extrinsic hemolytic anemias are acquired disorders caused by interaction of the red cell with environmental, physical, or chemical agents or abnormalities of the vascular system (Table 5.1). A hemolytic disorder may be recognized by reticulocytosis evident as polychromatophilic red cells on examination of the peripheral blood smear. After recognizing the anemia is due to hemolysis, the clinician should determine the specific cause of the condition, and careful and systematic clinical and laboratory investigation is needed to define the cause of the hemolysis.[1]

CLINICAL EVALUATION

Frequently, a thorough clinical history will provide clues to the etiology of the hemolytic anemia (Table 5.2). Anemia since childhood, accompanied by a positive family history, suggests an intrinsic hemolytic anemia; the onset of hemolysis in adulthood without any family history suggests an acquired hemolytic condition. Illnesses such as systemic lupus erythematosus or a lymphoproliferative disorder frequently are associated with immune-mediated hemolysis, and the recent administration of a drug to an individual of Mediterranean or African descent may suggest an intracellular defect (e.g., glucose-6-phosphate dehydrogenase [G6PD] deficiency). Hemolysis may develop in hospitalized patients who have infections, are on drugs, or are undergoing transfusion.

THE INITIAL LABORATORY EVALUATION

Peripheral Smear Morphology

The presence of polychromatophilic macrocytes on a Wright-stained smear suggests hemolysis.[2,3] These blue-orange–staining cells represent early reticulocytes. When the hemolysis is severe, greater marrow stress develops and younger reticulocytes, known as "shift reticulocytes," appear. These cells have fine basophilic stippling. In severe hemolysis, nucleated red cells are readily found, and characteristic morphologic changes of the red cells may suggest a specific disorder (Table 5.3). The absence of polychromatophilia in an anemic patient does not exclude the possibility of shortened red cell survival, because nutritional deficiencies, splenomegaly, or erythroid suppression by drugs may prevent or mask increased erythropoiesis.

In hemolytic anemias, the bone marrow shows erythroid hyperplasia with orderly maturation of erythroid cells. Increased erythroid precursors also may be seen in patients who are bleeding or recovering from marrow suppression. In some cases of hemolytic anemia, reticulocytopenia may develop. Careful examination of the marrow aspirate may indicate whether megaloblastic changes have developed, and this is a clue that folate or vitamin B_{12} deficiency is present, leading to inadequate erythropoiesis. The absence of stainable marrow iron may be seen in chronic intravascular hemolysis; how-

TABLE 5.1.   The Classification of Hemolytic Anemias

Hereditary hemolytic disorders
   Red cell membrane defects
      Hereditary spherocytosis
      Hereditary elliptocytosis
      Hereditary stomatocytosis
      Hereditary pyropoikilocytosis
      Rh-null disease
   Pentose phosphate shunt–glutathione system enzyme deficiencies
      Glucose-6-phosphate dehydrogenase
      Glutathione reductase
      Glutathione synthetase
   Glycolytic enzyme deficiencies
      Pyruvate kinase
      Hexokinase
      Phosphofructokinase
      Triosephosphate isomerase
   Nucleotide enzyme disorders
      Adenylate kinase deficiency
      Pyrimidine 5′ nucleotidase deficiency
   Hemoglobinopathies
      Variant hemoglobins
      Thalassemia
Acquired hemolytic disorders
   Drug induced antibodies
   Alloantibodies
   Transfusion reactions
   Hemolytic disease of the newborn
   Autoantibodies
   Paroxysmal nocturnal hemoglobinuria
   Mechanical hemolysis
      Microangiopathic hemolytic anemia
      Cardiac-valve hemolytic anemia
   Infections
      Viral
      Bacterial
      Malarial
   Chemical agents
   Physical agents
   Liver disease

ever, in most cases of chronic extravascular hemolysis, the iron stores are abundant.

Laboratory Tests

Table 5.4 shows laboratory tests to evaluate hemolysis. The reticulocyte count is the most useful and readily available test to assess the functional capacity of effective erythroid production, but this count must be corrected for the degree of anemia. The degree of reticulocytosis will increase with the severity of the anemia provided adequate iron, folate, and vitamin B_{12} are available and there is no suppression of erythropoiesis as a result of drugs, renal failure, or inflammation. Marrow

TABLE 5.2.   Clues to the Etiology of Hemolytic Anemia

Clinical Setting	Cause of Hemolysis
Childhood onset with familial tendency	Intracellular abnormality
Concomitant illness	
Collagen vascular disease, lymphoproliferative disorders	Immune hemolysis
Malignant hypertension, disseminated intravascular coagulation, prosthetic heart valve, vasculitis, disseminated carcinoma	
Infection	*Clostridia*, malaria, pneumococcus, *Escherichia coli, Bartonella*
Hepatocellular disease	Spur cell anemia
Drug administration	Enzyme deficiency, unstable hemoglobin, immune hemolysis
Recent transfusion	Red cell alloantibody–induced hemolysis

toxins or infection with parvovirus B19 may also lead to an impaired marrow response in patients with a hemolytic anemia.

The most direct measure of red cell survival is isotopically labeling autologous red cells. Chromium-51 is the most widely used isotope for this purpose. To measure the red cell survival, one incubates the patient's anticoagulated red cells with Chromium-51 and reinjects them; the radioactivity of blood samples collected over several days is counted to determine the rate of red cell destruction. Normally, 50% of the injected chromium-51–labeled red cells survive 29 ± 3 days. Because

TABLE 5.3.   Peripheral Smear Morphology in Hemolytic Anemias

Morphologic Abnormality	Disease
Spherocytes	Hereditary spherocytosis
	Immune hemolysis
	Extensive burns
	Clostridial sepsis
	Hb disease
Schistocytes	Red cell fragmentation syndromes
"Blister" cells	G6PD deficiency
Target cells	Hemoglobinopathy
Spiculated cells	Pryuvate kinase deficiency
	Liver disease
Agglutination	Immune hemolysis

Note: G6PD = glucose-6-phosphate dehydrogenase.

TABLE 5.4. Laboratory Evaluation of Hemolysis

Laboratory Test	Result
General tests	
Reticulocyte count	Elevated in hemolysis (also in the presence of hemorrhage or bone marrow recovery from a nutritional deficiency or toxin)
Haptoglobin, hemopexin	Reduced in intra- or extravascular hemolysis
Plasma hemoglobin and urine hemosiderin	Present in intravascular hemolysis
Chromium 51 red cell survival	Reduced
Miscellaneous	
Bilirubin	Elevated unconjugated fraction
Lactic dehydrogenase	Elevated
Carbon monoxide release	Elevated
Specific tests	
Osmotic fragility	Increased with spherocytosis, hereditary or acquired
Direct antiglobulin test	Positive in immune hemolysis
Enzyme assays	Reduced activity
G6PD	
Pyruvate kinase	
Ham or sugar water test	Positive in PNH

Note: G6PD = glucose-6-phosphate dehydrogenase; PNH = paroxysmal nocturnal hemoglobinuria.

the isotope elutes from the red cells, one does not observe the predicted half-life of 60 days (the red cell lifespan is normally 120 days).[4]

In the immune hemolytic anemias, the site of radiolabeled red cell destruction can be quantitated by external counting devices. Although increased sequestration may be seen in the spleen, this does not necessarily predict a response to splenectomy. In patients with severe chronic hemolytic anemia who are transfusion-dependent, survival studies will reflect the storage age of the circulating, transfused red cells. It is best in these cases to use red cells from a freshly collected unit of compatible blood.

The destruction of red cells may occur either intravascularly or extravascularly, and the catabolism of hemoglobin leads to the production of various biochemical products that are useful in substantiating the presence of a hemolytic anemia (Fig. 5.1). If hemolysis is occurring intravascularly, plasma hemoglobin may be increased; this is usually accompanied by hemoglobinuria. With chronic intravascular hemolysis, a Prussian blue stain of the urine sediment will show hemosiderin present in renal tubular cells, and patients with hemolysis caused by a prosthetic heart valve, immune transfusion reactions, or paroxysmal nocturnal hemoglobinuria will have hemosiderinuria, which can lead to iron deficiency.

A variety of chemical determinations are useful in establishing the presence of hemolysis. Bilirubin, an oxidative metabolite of heme, is increased in hemolytic disorders; specifically, the unconjugated or "indirect" form of bilirubin is elevated. The serum level of "direct" or conjugated bilirubin is normal unless hepatic or biliary disease is present.[5] A second indicator of hemolysis is reduced or absent haptoglobin. This α_2-globulin specifically binds free hemoglobin, and the complex is rapidly cleared from the circulation.[6] Thus, patients with significant hemolysis, either intra- or extravascular, have low or absent haptoglobin, and because haptoglobin is an acute phase reactant, hemolysis co-existent with infection or inflammation may not always result in a reduced haptoglobin level. Red cells contain high concentrations of the enzyme lactic dehydrogenase, and serum levels are typically elevated in intravascular hemolysis.

HEMOLYTIC ANEMIAS DUE TO INHERITABLE INTRACELLULAR DEFECTS

Membrane Defects

Viscoelastic properties of the red cell membrane contribute to the deformability of the cell so that it can survive turbulent flow yet be able to pass narrow capillaries. Approximately 15 proteins contributing to the unique structure of red cells can be classified into the integral and the peripheral membrane proteins. The principal components of the peripheral membrane proteins are spectrin, actin, ankyrin, and protein 4.1; these

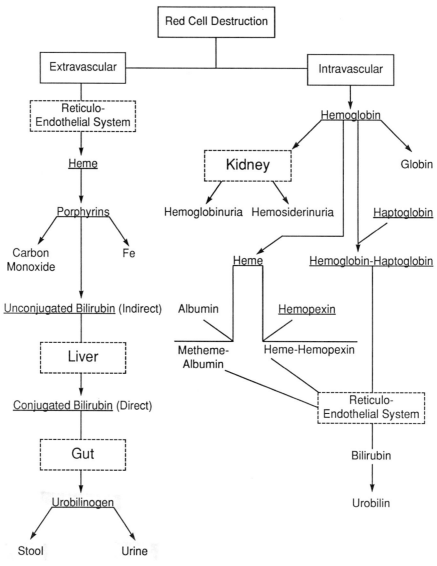

FIGURE 5.1. The catabolism of hemoglobin in red cell destruction.

proteins are confined to the cytoplasmic membrane surface, binding to each other and to sites on the integral membrane proteins. The integral membrane proteins include transport proteins such as protein 3. Qualitative or quantitative defects in the red cell cytoskeletal proteins can lead to a variety of membrane disorders leading to hemolysis, with hereditary spherocytosis the most common.

Hereditary Spherocytosis

The molecular basis of hereditary spherocytosis may involve various red cell membrane proteins. In different kindreds, ankyrin, β- and α-spectrin, and protein 4.2 have been reported as deficient or abnormal.[7] The red cell changes in hereditary spherocytosis lead to a decrease in deformability and splenic sequestration, and once trapped in the spleen, surface area may be further reduced. With an incidence of approximately 1 per 5000, it is one of the most common hereditary hemolytic anemias in the United States.

CLINICAL FEATURES. Hereditary spherocytosis is typically an autosomal dominant inherited defect of the red cell membrane characterized by anemia, spherocytosis, splenomegaly, and increased red cell osmotic fragility. It also may be inherited as a recessive trait, and there is a wide spectrum of severity: some patients are diagnosed incidentally while others have severe hemolytic anemia. The symptoms of hereditary spherocytosis are those characteristic of chronic hemolytic disorders. The disorder frequently is first suspected in the neonatal period because of hyperbilirubinemia, although the disease may be so mild that it goes unrecognized until adulthood. Biliary tract symptoms may be the presenting feature, and by the third decade, cholelithiasis may be seen in more than 40% of patients. Chronic leg ulcers also may complicate the disorder, but inexplicably, this complication may resolve following splenectomy.[8]

The course of the disease may be complicated by episodes of "aplastic crisis" in which erythropoiesis is suppressed yet the hemolytic process continues, leading to profound anemia. As a result, episodes of life-threatening anemia develop. Parvovirus B19 infection of erythroid progenitor cells is a recently described cause for an aplastic crisis,[11,12] and the crisis itself may last from 7 to 14 days. Severe anemia also may develop when the intake of folic acid is inadequate to meet the demands of increased erythropoiesis; consequently, any patient with chronic hemolysis should take folic acid supplements.

LABORATORY FINDINGS. Patients with hereditary spherocytosis will have spherocytes and polychromatophilia on their blood smear. Spherocytes lack central pallor because of the loss of membrane surface area. The mean cell volume is normal, but the mean cell hemoglobin concentration may be elevated (37 to 39 g/dl). The osmotic fragility test is useful in diagnosing the disorder, and because the red cells have a decreased surface-to-volume ratio, they have an increased susceptibility to lysis by hypotonic saline.

In the osmotic fragility test, the lysis of test cells is compared with normal red cells using different concentrations of sodium chloride solution. At higher osmolarities, spherocytic cells are more susceptible to lysis than the control cells. In those patients with only a small population of spherocytic cells, incubating the blood for 24 hours at 37°C will enhance the abnormality. There is no correlation between the degree of anemia and the fragility of the red cells, and it should be noted that in any condition in which spherocytes are present (for example, warm autoimmune hemolytic anemia or ABO incompatibility in the newborn), the osmotic fragility also will be increased.

Spectrin or ankyrin determinations lack specificity and sensitivity as diagnostic tests. Spectrin deficiency may be seen in hereditary pyropoikilocytosis and unstable hemoglobinopathies, and some patients with milder forms of hereditary spherocytosis may have only minimally reduced levels of spectrin, requiring highly sensitive assays whose reliability has not yet been proven.[9,10]

MANAGEMENT. The hemolytic anemia of hereditary spherocytosis may be cured by splenectomy. Transfusions rarely are required unless an aplastic crisis occurs. In any patient who has moderate or severe hereditary spherocytosis, splenectomy should be considered to avert the complications of the disorder, aplastic crisis, cholelithiasis, and chronic leg ulcers. The mortality and morbidity from splenectomy in hereditary spherocytosis are low, and delaying splenectomy to the age of 4 or 5 years may reduce the risk of postsplenectomy sepsis. Before splenectomy, polyvalent pneumococcal vaccine should be given. Prophylactic penicillin also should be given indefinitely to reduce the risk of overwhelming sepsis by encapsulated organisms.[13,14]

Hereditary Elliptocytosis

Hereditary elliptocytosis is characterized by elliptocytic red cells and a variable degree of hemolysis. A variety of abnormalities of the cytoskeletal proteins, involving both α- and β-spectrin and glycophorin C, have been described.[10] Most kindreds exhibit an autosomal dominant inheritance pattern, although hereditary elliptocytosis occasionally is inherited as an autosomal recessive condition. Therapy should be individualized depending on the severity of the anemia, and some patients have required splenectomy.[15]

Hereditary Pyropoikilocytosis

Hereditary pyropoikilocytosis is a subtype of hereditary elliptocytosis characterized by marked poikilocytosis, severe hemolysis, and heat lability of red cells. Inheritance is autosomal recessive, occurring almost exclusively in blacks, and splenectomy may reduce the rate of red cell destruction.[10]

ENZYME DEFECTS

Glucose is the main metabolic substrate for red cells and is metabolized by the Embden-Meyerhof pathway and the hexose monophosphate shunt (Fig. 5.2).[16] Inherited disorders of any enzyme in this pathway may lead to a hemolytic anemia (Table 5.4). The major metabolic product of the Embden-Meyerhof pathway (glycolytic pathway) is ATP, and the pathway also is an important source of NADH, needed to prevent the oxidation of ferrous heme to ferric heme. Phosphoglycerates shunted from the Embden-Meyerhof pathway to the Rapaport-

Lubering shunt result in the formation of high concentrations of 2,3-diphosphoglycerates.

The hexose monophosphate shunt serves to protect the cell (and hemoglobin in particular) from oxidative agents by the generation of glutathione. G6PD is the critical enzyme in the complex enzymatic process that recycles glutathione. G6PD functions to reduce NADP while oxidizing glucose-6-phosphate, thereby providing NADPH, a reducing agent that maintains sulfhydryl groups important in reducing free radicals and peroxides.

Glucose-6-Phosphate Dehydrogenase Deficiency

Glucose-6-phosphate dehydrogenase deficiency is an X-linked hemolytic disorder. Several variants of G6PD have been described[17] at the molecular level, and polymorphisms of the G6PD gene may lead to variants not associated with enzyme deficiency that cause hemolytic anemia only in the presence of chemical or physical stress and others that are sufficiencly impaired functionally to produce a nonspherocytic hemolytic anemia. Males, being hemizygotes, may be markedly deficient in enzyme activity. The majority of heterozygous females show enzyme levels intermediate between the normal and the deficient states. Although a spectrum of enzyme activity may be seen among females, few are as deficient as males with the disorder, and this phenomenon relates to the degree of X-chromosome inactivation in females.

The Mediterranean form of G6PD deficiency is the prototype for the G6PD deficiency states. Although

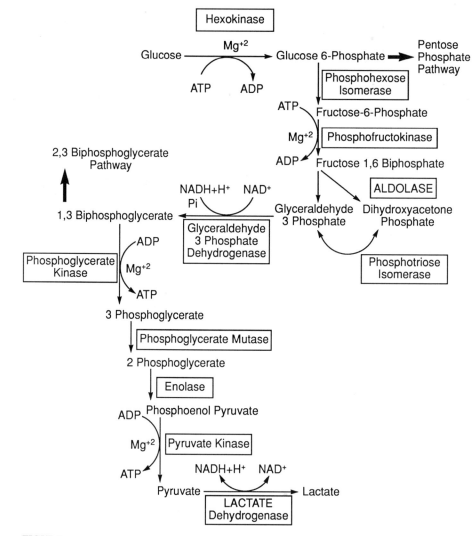

FIGURE 5.2. The glycolytic (Embden-Meyerhof) pathway.

called *Mediterranean,* this form is not limited to individuals from that area. Individuals with G6PD Mediterranean typically have less than 1% enzyme activity, and they are extremely sensitive to oxidant stresses. The fava bean, a common food in the Mediterranean area, may precipitate severe hemolysis.

CLINICAL FEATURES. The typical black individual with G6PD deficiency does not have any evidence of hemolysis unless challenged by oxidant drugs, infection, or noxious agents. These hemolytic episodes are self-limited, and other G6PD variants may have chronic hemolysis punctuated by episodes of accelerated hemolysis. In the acute event, hemolysis occurs intravascularly, and abdominal or back pain may occur in association with hemoglobinuria. In some cases, hemolysis is so severe that acute renal failure may develop; Table 5.5 lists agents implicated in producing hemolysis. A serious effect of G6PD deficiency is neonatal jaundice. Kernicterus may develop unless exchange transfusion therapy is performed.

LABORATORY FINDINGS. The peripheral smear is nondiagnostic. Frequently, cells with displaced hemoglobin, or "blister cells," are evident. A quantitative determination of G6PD establishes the diagnosis; however, because G6PD levels are usually higher in reticulocytes, the enzyme activity is determined at the time of acute hemolysis and reticulocytosis. Normal to low-normal activity may be found, and a low-normal value of G6PD in the presence of reticulocytosis should suggest the disorder. In these cases, the enzyme activity should be measured after the hemolytic episode is over. Quantitative determination of G6PD deficiency in com-

bination with age-related enzymes such as hexokinase also may be helpful.[18,19]

TREATMENT. Individuals with G6PD deficiency should avoid drugs that may induce severe hemolysis. If hemolysis results in severe anemia, transfusions may be life-saving. Splenectomy is not beneficial in hemolytic anemia due to G6PD, and in neonates with severe hemolysis, exchange transfusion may be life-saving.

ENZYMOPATHIES IN THE GLYCOLYTIC PATHWAY

Pyruvate Kinase Deficiency

Pyruvate kinase deficiency is the most common disorder in the glycolytic pathway and is recognized in most ethnic groups.[20] Pyruvate kinase catalyzes the conversion of phosphoenolpyruvate to pyruvate, generating a net gain in ATP production. Without ATP synthesis, there is increased permeability of the red cell to cations. The anemia may vary from mild to severe, and the heterogeneity of phenotypic expression most likely relates to the variability of the molecular lesion. Described abnormalities of the enzyme include reduced specific activity, decreased affinity for the substrate phosphoenolpyruvate, altered stability, and impaired allosteric activation by co-factors.

Morphologically, pyruvate kinase–deficient red cells appear spiculated. The diagnosis is confirmed by specific enzyme assay, and in patients with hemolysis requiring transfusion, splenectomy is usually performed. Postsplenectomy evidence of hemolysis persists, but transfusion requirements may be reduced or eliminated. An acquired form of pyruvate kinase deficiency occurs in patients with myelodysplasia or acute myelogenous leukemia. The severity of the acquired form of pyruvate kinase deficiency varies.

Hexokinase Deficiency

Several kindreds with hexokinase deficiency have been documented in a variety of ethnic groups. The anemia may be mild to severe. There are no diagnostic morphologic changes in the red cells, and the diagnosis is based on enzyme assays. Because hexokinase levels decrease during red cell aging, the level of enzyme activity must be interpreted in relationship to the reticulocyte count.[21–23]

HEMOLYTIC ANEMIAS DUE TO ACQUIRED INTRACELLULAR DEFECTS

Paroxysmal Nocturnal Hemoglobinuria

Paroxysmal nocturnal hemoglobinuria (PNH) is an acquired disorder of hematopoietic stem cells that re-

TABLE 5.5. **Agents Implicated in the Production of Hemolysis in Glucose-6-Phosphate Dehydrogenase Deficiency**

Acetanilid
Doxorubicin
Nalidixic acid
Naphthalene
Niridazole
Nitrofurantoin
Pamaquine
Pentaquine
Phenazopyridine
Primaquine
Sulfacetamide
Sulfamethoxazole
Sulfanilamide
Sulfapyridine

sults in an intrinsic abnormality of red cell, platelet, and granulocyte membranes and also defective cell pro-liferation.[24,25] A susceptibility to complement lysis leads to intravascular hemolysis, and this susceptibility is due to an acquired deficiency of glycosyl-phosphati-dylinositol–anchored membrane proteins, such as de-cay-accelerating factor and homologous restriction fac-tors, that limit the formation of complement attack complexes.[26] The etiology of the stem cell disorder is unknown. Chronic hemolysis dominates the clinical picture.

The most serious complications of PHN are thrombo-sis and marrow aplasia with bleeding or infections. Thrombosis of large intra-abdominal veins, especially hepatic veins, are common.[3] Because the hemolysis is intravascular, iron deficiency may develop in patients[27] with protracted hemolysis, and renal abnormalities may complicate PNH as a result of either thrombosis or chronic hemoglobinuria and hemosiderinuria. Aplas-tic anemia may be the predominant presenting factor in patients with PNH; occasionally, some patients will present with isolated thrombocytopenia. There-fore, in any patient presenting with cytopenias of ob-scure etiology, the diagnosis of PNH should be con-sidered.

The peripheral blood shows no diagnostic features, and the bone marrow characteristically shows erythroid hyperplasia with absent iron stores. When there is pancytopenia, a hypoplastic marrow may be seen. The increased susceptibility to complement lysis forms the basis of the tests used in diagnosing PNH; incubat-ing red cells with sucrose (sugar water test), resulting in hemolysis of red cells with PNH membrane defect, is a sensitive screening test. The acidified-serum lysis test (Ham test) should be done to confirm the diagnosis.

HEMOLYTIC ANEMIAS DUE TO ACQUIRED EXTRACELLULAR DEFECTS

Immune Hemolytic Anemias

Immune hemolytic anemias are caused by antibodies that may be produced as a result of an allo- or autoim-mune response. Drugs also may induce the formation of antibodies to red cells. Table 5.6 classifies the immune hemolytic anemias, and the hallmarks of an immune hemolytic anemia are a positive direct Coombs test and spherocytic red cells.

Warm Autoimmune Hemolytic Anemia

Warm autoimmune hemolytic anemia (AIHA) is the most common type of immune hemolysis, accounting for approximately 70% of cases. Patients of all ages are affected, but there is a higher incidence in females. Neoplasms of the reticuloendothelial system, collagen vascular diseases, inherited and acquired immunodefi-ciency states, and ulcerative colitis frequently are asso-ciated with warm AIHA. The combination of warm AIHA and autoimmune thrombocytopenia is known as Evans syndrome.

PATHOPHYSIOLOGY. IgG antibodies lead to short-ened red cell survival, principally by extravascular destruction in the reticuloendothelial system. The mononuclear phagocytes in these tissues possess Fc receptors for the IgG coating the red cells. If present, complement factors coating the red cells also facilitate phagocytosis by the macrophage. In the process of phagocytosis, small portions of the red cell are ingested by the macrophage, and if the phagocytosis is incom-plete, the released red cell reseals its membrane, loses its typically convex appearance, and seems to be spherical. The principal site of red cell destruction is the spleen, unlike in cold agglutinin disease where the liver plays a predominant role.[28]

PRESENTING SIGNS AND SYMPTOMS. The onset of anemia may be insidious or fulminant. In many patients, symptoms from the associated underlying ill-ness will predominate. Jaundice, hemoglobinuria, and fever are infrequent clinical findings. Splenomegaly is present in about 50% of patients with warm AIHA, and hepatomegaly is present in one third.

TABLE 5.6. **The Classification of Immune Hemolytic Anemias**

Warm autoimmune hemolytic anemia
  Primary warm autoimmune hemolytic anemia
  Secondary warm autoimmune hemolytic anemia
    Collagen vascular disease
    Lymphoproliferative disorders
    Human-immunodeficiency-virus infection
    Ulcerative colitis
Cold autoimmune hemolytic anemia
  Primary cold agglutinin syndrome
  Secondary cold agglutinin syndrome
    Mycoplasmal infections and infectious mononucleosis
    Lymphoproliferative disorders
  Paroxysmal cold hemoglobinuria
Drug-induced immune hemolytic anemias
Alloimmune hemolytic anemias
  Hemolytic transfusion reactions
  Immune hemolytic disease of the newborn

LABORATORY FINDINGS. The hemoglobin concentration is variable, but it is not uncommon to have values less than 7 g/dl. The blood smear shows spherocytes, polychromatophilia, nucleated red cells, and autoagglutination. Bilirubin values are normal in over 50% of patients, and the reticulocyte count typically is elevated. However, reticulocytopenia is not uncommon.[30] In these patients, the marrow does not show erythroid hypoplasia or megaloblastic features suggesting ineffective erythropoiesis.[31] If hemolysis is brisk, persistent reticulocytopenia can lead to life-threatening anemia. Thrombocytopenia and leukopenia also may occur in autoimmune hemolytic anemia.

The hallmark of the disorder is a positive direct antiglobulin test (Coombs test). This test is used to detect increased levels of IgG or complement (specifically C3d) on the surface of the red cell. The test consists of adding goat or rabbit antihuman IgG or C3d, or both, to the patient's red cells to detect in vivo sensitization. Reactivity is determined by the presence of agglutination after incubation and centrifugation. This technique also is used to detect serum antibody by testing the patient's serum against normal red cells (the indirect Coombs test). In rare instances, the direct Coombs test may be negative because of the low sensitivity of the standard direct Coombs test; in this situation, the diagnosis of a Coombs-positive immune hemolytic anemia may be confirmed by more sensitive immunologic techniques such as radioimmunoassay. Some cases of autoimmune hemolytic anemia may be caused by IgA autoantibodies, and special antisera to human IgA are required to diagnose this unusual form of autoimmune hemolytic anemia.

In warm AIHA, IgG is found either alone or in combination with C3. Because IgG and C3 potentiate each other's opsonic function, more severe hemolytic anemia is typical in patients whose red cells demonstrate both IgG and C3. It should be noted, however, that not all patients with positive direct antiglobulin tests have evidence of hemolysis; hypergammaglobulinemia is a common cause of positive direct antiglobulin tests without hemolysis.

THERAPY. The initial therapy for warm AIHA is the administration of corticosteroids. A therapeutic effect, with reduction of hemolysis, is achieved in 80% of patients, and a significant rise in the reticulocyte count frequently precedes this improvement. If this does not occur, other associated conditions, such as iron, folate, or B_{12} deficiency, should be sought. Once the anemia improves, a gradual reduction in the dosage of corticosteroids is warranted; for the patient unable to tolerate long-term steroids or for relapsing anemia after the discontinuation of drug treatment, splenectomy is recommended. Before the introduction of corticosteroid therapy, splenectomy alone was helpful in 50% of patients. Splenectomy should not be undertaken lightly in this disorder, however, because even with skilled surgeons, the morbidity and mortality are significant.

The transfusion of red cells will have shortened survival, paralleling the patient's autologous red cell destruction rate. Nonetheless, if transfusion therapy is considered life-saving, red cells should not be withheld because of the fear of a hemolytic reaction.[31,32] In a patient who has been previously transfused or pregnant, a red cell alloantibody also may be present, and intensive serologic testing may be required to determine that an autoantibody is not masking a clinically important alloantibody.[29]

Cold Agglutinin Disease

In contrast to warm AIHA, cold autoimmune hemolysis involves IgM antibodies. More commonly, the patients are middle-aged or elderly. Accounting for approximately 15% of the immune hemolytic anemias the cold agglutinin syndrome is less frequent than warm AIHA. Cold agglutinin disease may be associated with neoplasms, especially chronic lymphocytic leukemia, Waldenstrom's macroglobulinemia, and lymphoma; in addition, it is associated with mycoplasmal and Epstein-Barr virus infections.

Patients usually have less severe anemia than in warm AIHA. Nonetheless, the most frequent presenting symptoms are related to the anemia. On exposure to cold temperatures, patients may develop hemoglobinuria, and associated with cold exposure and resultant autoagglutination in small capillaries, symptoms of acrocyanosis may occur.

PATHOPHYSIOLOGY. As blood circulates through acral body areas, where ambient temperatures are low, the IgM autoantibodies bind to the patient's red cells and fix complement (C3b) to the red cell membrane. The hemolysis that follows is precipitated by the interaction of the complement-coated red cells with macrophages. Red cell destruction does not go unchecked, however, because a plasma inactivator (factor I) cleaves C3b, converting it to C3d. These C3d cells are resistant to destruction and circulate normally.

LABORATORY FINDINGS. A characteristic finding is autoagglutination of the patient's red cells following phlebotomy. This finding can be observed readily on making a blood smear; other characteristic blood smear findings include mild spherocytosis and polychromatophilia. The characteristic serologic results include a positive direct antiglobulin test with complement sensitization. The presence of IgG on the patient's red cells is not characteristic of cold agglutinin disease, and the responsible IgM antibodies are not detectable as they elute off the red cell at the core body temperature.

Cold-reactive IgM autoagglutinins associated with immune hemolysis usually are present at titers greater than 1000 when tested at 4°C. If the testing is carried out at progressively higher temperatures, the titers decrease. Pathologic IgM autoagglutinins typically react to temperatures of 30°C. In chronic cold agglutinin disease, the IgM antibody usually is a monoclonal protein of the κ-light-chain type. Polyclonal IgM immunoglobulins (with both κ- and λ-light-chain distribution) are found in the form of the disease that is associated with mycoplasmal or Epstein-Barr virus infections.

THERAPY. Therapy is principally preventive in nature. Exposure to cold should be avoided; wearing gloves, hats, and warm clothing when outdoor activities cannot be avoided should be recommended. Steroids and splenectomy are ineffective, and alkylating agents have been tried in patients with severe hemolysis and anemia. However, it is unclear whether this maneuver has provided any long-term benefit. In some cases of cold agglutinin disease associated with lymphoproliferative disorders, interferon-α may be useful in decreasing the titer of the cold agglutinin and in reducing the severity of hemolysis. If transfusions of red cells are required, administration of the blood through a blood warmer is prudent. The cold-reacting antibody may complicate blood typing and compatibility testing, and if the ABO group cannot be determined, group O red cells should be given. Warming the patient's serum during compatibility testing is useful in circumventing the presence of the cold-reacting autoantibody.

Paroxysmal Cold Hemoglobinuria

Paroxysmal cold hemoglobinuria (PCH) is a unique autoimmune hemolytic disorder caused by an IgG autoantibody. The antibody has reactivity against red cell P antigens. The disorder is characterized by an acute onset of fulminant hemolysis associated with fever, chills, and abdominal pain, and hemoglobinuria always occurs. Acute PCH is seen most commonly in children younger than 5 years. PCH frequently develops after a viral illness, and in the past, it was associated with syphilis. The antibody that mediates the disorder is an IgG antibody that binds to the red cell on exposure to the cold. The antibody usually has specificity for the P-blood-group antigen.

The disorder is diagnosed by the Donath-Landsteiner test. This serologic test involves incubating the patient's serum with cells at 4°C, then warming the cells to 37°C to allow the complement activation to proceed. If this type of autoantibody is present, hemolysis of the cells will occur. PCH usually is a self-limited disorder and resolves spontaneously in a few days to weeks. Blood transfusion support, with warmed blood, may be required, and if the antibody has specificity for the P blood group, P-negative blood is necessary. It is unclear whether steroids alter the course of the hemolytic anemia, again because PCH is a self-limited disorder.[30]

Drug-Induced Immune Hemolytic Anemia

Drug administration can lead to immune destruction of red cells by various mechanisms (Table 5.7).[33,34] This type of immune hemolytic anemia accounts for approximately 10% of patients with immune hemolysis, and numerous drugs have been incriminated as inducing immune hemolytic anemia. The usual mode of onset of the anemia is gradual, although with drugs that can induce an immune-complex-type mechanism, the hemolysis may be acute and severe. The direct Coombs test will show IgG and complement sensitization of the red cells, and the administration of methyldopa, unlike any of the other drugs, also frequently will lead to serum antibody (positive indirect Coombs test). Although as many as 20% of patients taking methyldopa will develop a positive direct Coombs test, only a few patients develop hemolysis. The management of drug-induced immune hemolytic anemia is discontinuation of the drug; blood transfusions or steroid therapy are rarely required.

Hemolytic Transfusion Reactions

Red cell alloantibodies may lead to acute hemolytic reactions or delayed hemolytic transfusion reaction. The clinical and serologic aspects of these hemolytic disorders are discussed in the chapter on immunohematology and transfusion practices in this book (Chapter 20).

Fragmentation Syndromes

Physical trauma may be sufficient to cause intravascular hemolysis with hemoglobinuria and hemoglobinemia. The surviving red cells take the form of schistocytes (fragments, helmets, or crescents), which readily

TABLE 5.7. Drugs Associated with Immune Hemolytic Anemia

Immune complex characteristics
  Acetaminophen
  Carbimazole
  Cefotaxime
  Ceftriaxone
  Chlorpromazine
  5-Fluorouracil
  Isoniazid
  Nomifensine
  Phenacetin
  Probenecid
  Quinidine
  Quinine
  Rifampicin
  Stibophen
  Sulphonamides
  Melphalan
  Tolmetin
  Triamterene
  Tetracycline
Autoantibody formation
  Ibuprofen
  Mefanamic acid
  Methyldopa
  Procainamide
  Sulindac
Drug adsorption
  Penicillin
  Semisynthetic penicillins
Undocumented mechanism
  Furosemide
  Hydralazine
  Methadone
  Methysergide
  Streptomycin
  Tolmetin

TABLE 5.8. The Causes of Red Cell Fragmentation

Cardiac abnormality
  Cardiac prothesis
  Unoperated valvular disease
  Valve homografts
  Coarctation of the aorta
Small vessel disease (microangiopathic hemolytic anemia)
  Thrombotic thrombocytopenic purpura
  Vasculitis in collagen vascular diseases
  Hemolytic uremic syndrome
  Malignant hypertension
  Eclampsia
  Disseminated carcinoma
  Giant hemangiomas
  Disseminated intravascular coagulation

distinguish red cell fragmentation disorders from other acquired anemias.

Traumatic Cardiac Hemolysis

Hemolysis may develop following the placement of a prosthetic heart valve or after an ostium primum repair of the atrium with an intracardiac patch; rarely does intrinsic valve disease lead to hemolysis.[35] Aortic prosthetic valves are associated more frequently with hemolysis because of the greater turbulence in flow. The hemolysis accompanying nonsurgically corrected valvular disease is rarely severe. When hemolysis and hemosiderinuria have been prolonged, iron deficiency may develop, and daily iron supplementation should be instituted if significant hemolysis is present. Reoperation may be necessary for some patients with severe hemolysis.

Microangiopathic Hemolytic Anemias

Red cell fragmentation occurring in association with small arterial disease may occur.[36] This type of hemolytic disorder is termed *microangiopathic*. The deposition of fibrin within the microvasculature or severe hypertension provides the conditions for fragmentation, and the diagnosis of a microangiopathic hemolytic anemia is based on the observation of schistocytes and bizarrely misshapen red cells, usually accompanied by reticulocytosis, elevated serum lactate dehydrogenase, and reduced serum haptoglobin. Hemoglobinemia and hemoglobinuria are rarely described.

A variety of clinical syndromes are associated with microangiopathic hemolytic anemia (Table 5.8). One of the most serious disorders is thrombotic thrombocytopenic purpura.

Microangiopathic hemolytic anemia may be a prominent feature of disorders associated with vasculitis. These include polyarteritis and infectious disorders such as in Rocky Mountain spotted fever or Wegener granulomatosis. Also associated with the vasculitis is fibrin disposition, which leads to red cell fragmentation. The peripheral smear of patients with disseminated intravascular coagulation frequently shows red cell fragmentation, and disseminated intravascular coagulation may be the result of a variety of disorders such as sepsis, abruptio placentae, or disseminated carcinoma. In these conditions, the red cell fragmentation is due to fibrin deposition within the microvasculature. The hemolysis is rarely severe, and as the underlying disease is controlled, the fragmentation ceases. Microangiopathic hemolytic anemia in association with thrombocytopenia may complicate massive cutaneous hemangiomas.

MISCELLANEOUS HEMOLYTIC DISORDERS

Hemolysis due to Infection

Several infectious agents can lead to hemolysis. Clostridial sepsis can lead to massive intravascular 10hemolysis as a result of a bacterial lipase that acts on red cell membranes. Malarial infections probably are the most frequent worldwide microbial cause of hemolysis,[37] and the species involved in malaria most frequently associated with severe hemolysis is *Plasmodium falciparum,* which can cause intravascular hemolysis. Babesiosis, bartellonosis, and a variety of bacteria may cause acute or chronic forms of red cell destruction.[38,39]

Hemolysis due to Liver Disease

Anemia of liver disease can have many etiologies, including blood loss, iron deficiency, hypersplenism, folic acid deficiency, and the toxic effects of alcohol on the marrow.[40] In addition, hemolysis may accompany acute or chronic liver disease. Spur cell anemia is a hemolytic anemia found in patients with severe cirrhosis, and the peripheral smear shows a predominance of acanthocytes, polychromatophilia, and nucleated red cells. Spur cell membranes contain high levels of cholesterol with normal phosphatidylcholine content, and the membranes are rigid, leading to splenic entrapment and eventual extravascular lysis.

REFERENCES

1. Ballas SK. The pathophysiology of hemolytic anemia. Transfusion Med Rev 1990;4:236–56.
2. Deiss A, Kurth D. Circulating reticulocytes in normal adults as determined by the new methylene blue method. Am J Clin Pathol 1970;53:481.
3. Hillman RS. Characteristics of marrow production and reticulocyte maturation in normal man in response to anemia. J Clin Invest 1969;48:443.
4. Najean Y, Cacchione R, Dresch C, Rain JD. Methods of evaluating the sequestration site of red cells labeled with [51]Cr: a review of 96 cases. Br J Haematol 1975;29:495.
5. Berlin NI, Berk PD. Quantitative aspects of bilirubin metabolism for hematologists. Blood 1981;57:983.
6. Nyman M. Serum haptoglobin: methodological and clinical studies. Scand J Clin Lab Invest 1959;(suppl 39):11.
7. Palek J, Lux SE. Red cell membrane skeletal defects in hereditary and acquired hemolytic anemias. Semin Hematol 1983;20:189.
8. Weed RI. Hereditary spherocytosis. Arch Intern Med 1975;135:1316.
9. Agre P, Aismos A, Casella JF, et al. Inheritance pattern and clinical response to splenectomy as a reflection of erythrocyte spectrin deficiency in hereditary spherocytosis. N Engl J Med 1983;315:1579.
10. Lux SE. Disorders of the red cell membrane. In: Nathan DG, Oski FA, eds. Hematology of Infancy and Childhood. Third Edition. Philadelphia: W. B. Saunders, 1987.
11. Young N. Hematologic and hematopoietic consequences of B19 parvovirus infection. Semin Hematol 1988;25:159.
12. Saarinen UM, Chorba TL, Tattersall P, et al. Human parvovirus B19 induced epidemic acute red cell aplasia in patients with hereditary hemolytic anemia. Blood 1986;67:1411–17.
13. Rutkow IM. Twenty years of splenectomy for hereditary spherocytosis. Arch Surg 1981;116:306–16.
14. Schwartz SI, Bernard RP, Adams JT, et al. Splenectomy for hematologic disorders. Arch Surg 1970;101:338.
15. Palek J. Hereditary elliptocytosis and related disorders. Clin Hematol 1985;14:45–87.
16. Murray RK, Granner DK, Mayes PA, eds. Harper's Biochemistry. Englewood Cliffs, N.J.: Appleton and Lange, 1990.
17. Beutler E. Glucose-6-phosphate dehydrogenase deficiency and non-sphereocytic hemolytic anemia. Semin Hematol 1985;2:91.
18. Hirono A, Beutler E. Enzymatic diagnosis in nonspherocytic hemolytic anemia. Medicine 1988;67:110–6.
19. Luzzatto L, Battistuzzi G. Glucose 6 phosphate dehydrogenase. Adv Human Genet 1985;14:217–329.
20. Tanka KR, Valentine WN, Miva S. Pyruvate kinase deficiency hereditary nonspherocytic hemolytic anemia. Blood 1962;19:267.
21. Valentine WN, Tanaka KJ, Paglia DE. Pyruvate kinase and other enzyme disorders of the erythrocyte. In: Scriver CR, et al., eds. The Metabolic Basis of Inherited Disease. Sixth Edition. New York: McGraw Hill, 1989:2341.
22. Valentine WN. Hemolytic anemia and inborn errors of metabolism. Blood 1979;54:549.
23. Valentine WN, Tanaka KR, Paglia DE. Hemolytic anemias and erythrocyte enzymopathies. Ann Intern Med 1985;103:245–57.
24. Hartman RC, Jenkins DE. The sugar water test for paroxysmal nocturnal hemoglobinuria. N Engl J Med 1966;275:155.
25. Hartman RC, Jenkins DE, McKee LC et al. Paroxysmal nocturnal hemoglobinuria: clinical and laboratory studies relating to iron metabolism and therapy with androgen and iron. Medicine 1966;45:331.
26. Rosse W. Phosphatidyl linked proteins and paroxysmal nocturnal hemoglobinuria. Blood 1990;75:1595–601.
27. Hartman RC, Luther AB, Jenkins DE et al. Fulminant hepatic venous thrombosis in paroxysmal nocturnal hemoglobinuria: definition of a medical emergency. Johns Hopkins Med J 1980;146:247.
28. Frank MM, Schreiber AD, Atkinson JP. Pathophysiology of immune hemolytic anemias. Ann Intern Med 1977;87:210.
29. Petz LD, Garraty G. Acquired Immune Hemolytic Anemias. New York: Churchill Livingstone, 1980.
30. Liseveld JL, Rowe JM, Lichtman MA. Variability of the erythropoietic response in autoimmune hemolytic anemia: analysis of 109 cases. Blood 1987;69:820.
31. Conley CL, Lippman SM, Ness PM. Autoimmune hemolytic anemia with reticulocytopenia: a medical emergency. JAMA 1980;244:1688–90.
32. Rosenfield RE, Jagathambal. Transfusion therapy for autoimmune hemolytic anemia. Semin Hematol 1976;13:1311.
33. Petz LD, Branch DR. Drug induced immune hemolytic anemia. In: Chaplin H, ed. Methods in Hematology. Immune Hemolytic Anemias, Volume 4. New York: Churchill Livingstone, 1985:47–94.

34. Garratty G, Petz LD. Drug induced immune hemolytic anemia. Am J Med 1975;48:398.

35. McClung JA, Stein JH, Ambrose JA, Herman MV, Reed GE. Prosthetic heart valves: a review. Prog Cardiovasc Dis 1983; 26:237–70.

36. Brain MC. Microangiopathic hemolytic anemia: the possible role of vascular lesions in pathogenesis. Br J Haematol 1962;8:358.

37. Miller LH. Malaria. In: Warren KW, Mahmoud AAF, eds. Tropical and Geographical Medicine. New York: McGraw Hill, 1983.

38. Rosner F, Zarrali MH, Benach JL, et al. Babesiosis in splenectomized adults. Am J Med 1984;76:696.

39. Dooley JR. Haemotropic bacteria in man. Lancet 1980;ii:1237.

40. Cooper RA. Hemolytic syndromes and red cell membrane abnormalities in liver disease. Semin Hematol 1980;17:103.

6

Normocytic Anemia

Jeanette Mladenovic, M.D., and G. David Roodman, M.D., Ph.D.

In 1930, Wintrobe described a method for classification of anemias based on the size and hemoglobin content of the red blood cell. These erythrocyte indices have come to form a basis for the clinical evaluation of patients with decreased hemoglobin.[1] While such a classification may not always allow for the easy correlation of disease states with the newest concepts of pathogenetic mechanisms, it continues to prove useful to the clinician faced with the initial evaluation of the anemic patient.

Anemia accompanied by normal-sized cells (normocytic) is the most frequently encountered type, and it encompasses a diverse group of diseases. This chapter presents the differential diagnoses of normocytic anemias and concentrates on those specific entities unique to this category of anemia and not covered elsewhere in this textbook.

CLINICAL SIGNS AND SYMPTOMS

In most instances, the patient who presents with a normocytic anemia will be asymptomatic from the anemia itself. A fall in hemoglobin to 9 to 11 g/dl, often over a prolonged time period, physiologically should not compromise the normal individual. However, in patients who have underlying cardiac or pulmonary disease, even a modest reduction in oxygen-carrying capacity may exacerbate their symptoms. A more rapid fall to lower levels of hemoglobin may result in typical signs and symptoms of decreased oxygen-carrying capacity: fatigue, dyspnea on exertion, palpitations, pallor, and tachycardia.

Often, however, normocytic anemia simply presents as a laboratory abnormality accompanying a systemic disease, with symptoms of that disease being the primary clinical manifestation. The patient with laboratory anemia alone presents a particular challenge, because this abnormality may be the first early clue to a new illness.

INITIAL LABORATORY EVALUATION

The initial characterization of anemia is returned to the physician with the standard complete blood count. Modern Coulter counters have replaced the older, manual methods and directly measure the hemoglobin, number of red cells, and their size or mean corpuscular volume (MCV). These values result in calculated values of the hematocrit and other characteristics of the red cell: the hemoglobin content per cell (MCH) and the hemoglobin concentration per cell (MCHC). Table 6.1 shows the normal range of values for these measurements. While all the red cell indices are reported, practically speaking, only the MCV is required for a useful pathophysiologic classification of anemias.[2] A simplified version of this classification is presented in Table 6.2. However, there may be exceptions to this classification in some diseases.

The normal MCV range is 80 to 96 fl/red cell. However, this value represents an average cell volume for the entire cell population; thus, it may not detect abnormalities of mixed cell populations. Also, simple reliance on the electronic MCV would miss patients whose cells are dimorphic (such as in sideroblastic

TABLE 6.1. Normal Red Cell Values

	Men	Women
Hemoglobin, *g/dl*	14.0 to 17.5	12.3 to 15.3
Hematocrit, *ratio*	0.42 to 0.50	0.36 to 0.45
Red cell count, $\times 10^{12}/L$ *blood*	4.52 to 5.90	4.10 to 5.10
Mean corpuscular volume, *fl/red cell*	80.0 to 96.1	
Mean corpuscular hemoglobin, *pg/red cell*	27.5 to 33.2	
Mean corpuscular hemoglobin concentration, *g/dl red blood cells*	33.4 to 35.5	
Red cell distribution width, %	11.5 to 14.5	

Source: Williams WJ, Nelson DA, Morris MW. Examination of the blood, in Williams WJ, Beutler E, Erslev AJ, Lichtman MA, eds., *Hematology,* 4th ed., New York: McGraw-Hill, 1990:10.

anemia) but whose MCV is in the normocytic range. Therefore, evaluation of the peripheral blood smear remains an important exercise, especially when the Coulter counter shows evidence of variation in cell size as measured by an increased red cell distribution width (RDW).

With the finding of anemia, a determination of the marrow response to the anemia must be made. Evaluation of the leukocyte and platelet counts may yield some initial information about marrow function; however, the adequacy of the erythroid response to anemia is best evaluated by the reticulocyte count. The reticulocyte is a newly made red blood cell released from the marrow with some RNA still present in its cytoplasm. This RNA, which will degrade over the next 1 to 2 days, is manifested by a blue hue on peripheral smear of these cells (polychromatophilia) or can be seen with a special reticulin stain. The number of reticulocytes serves as a measure of marrow red cell production, normally approximately 1% of the red cells per day; because the reticulocyte count often is given as a percentage of the total red cells, its value must be corrected downward in the presence of anemia to provide a more accurate measure of daily production (corrected reticulocyte count).

In response to a fall in hemoglobin, the marrow is able to more than triple its capacity to produce red blood

cells. For this to occur, the marrow must have adequate stem and progenitor cells; adequate supplies of nutrients; and adequate production of erythropoietin, the major hormone governing erythropoiesis and released by the kidney during hypoxic stress. Therefore, the reticulocyte count serves as a measure of the total marrow response to anemia, and it represents an additional useful test in the classification of normocytic anemias.

After the complete blood count is obtained, the initial laboratory evaluation of the anemic patient always includes the reticulocyte count. It also includes evaluation of the peripheral blood smear to detect mixed cell populations or to find clues in the red or other cell lines as to the underlying diagnosis.

DIFFERENTIAL DIAGNOSIS

Table 6.3 shows differential diagnosis of normocytic anemia. Anemia is defined as a decrease in the red cell mass and not simply a decrease in hematocrit or hemoglobin concentration. Thus, a decreased hemoglobin or hematocrit concentration may be the result of a fall in the red cell mass or an increase in plasma volume. Decreases in hematocrit due to increased plasma volume rather than decreased red cell mass are termed *spurious anemias,* and although it is possible to measure the

TABLE 6.3. The Differential Diagnosis of Normocytic Anemias

Spurious anemias
  Pregnancy
  Volume-overload states
Absolute anemias
  Increased production (reticulocytes > 2%)
    Blood loss
    Hemolysis
  Hypoproliferative (reticulocytes < 2%, usually < 1%)
    Primary marrow disorder
      Stem cell failure
        Aplastic anemia
        Preleukemia (myelodysplastic syndromes)
        Myeloid metaplasia
      Pure red cell aplasia
      Myelophthisic diseases
      Sideroblastic anemias
    Secondary to systemic conditions
      Chronic renal failure
      Endocrine diseases
      Protein deficiency
    Combined defects
      Anemia of chronic diseases
      Early iron deficiency
      Mixed deficiencies

TABLE 6.2. The Classification of Anemia Based on Cell Size

Microcytic (Low MCV)	Normocytic (Normal MCV)	Macrocytic (High MCV)
Iron deficiency	All others	Vitamin B_{12} deficiency
Thalassemias		Folate deficiency

Note: MCV = mean corpuscular volume.

plasma volume, the diagnosis of spurious anemia is best made by the clinical situation. Spurious anemias usually are mild in degree and are accompanied by a normal reticulocyte count for the degree of anemia. Anemias that characteristically have expanded plasma volumes as a significant pathophysiologic mechanism are included in this category. Anemia attributed to dilutional causes in congestive heart failure or other volume-overload states should occur only in the obvious clinical setting, when other contributory factors (e.g., occult gastrointestinal bleeding, or shortened survival on a cardiac valve) are ruled out, and when improvement in the volume status leads to correction of the anemia.

Patients with *absolute anemia* are further categorized by the reticulocyte count. Although many anemic states represent a combination of decreased production and shortened red cell survival (e.g., those of chronic disease, or chronic renal failure), the reticulocyte count will define the major pathophysiologic abnormality underlying the anemia. Patients with acute blood loss or increased red cell destruction (hemolysis) with an intact marrow response manifest an increased reticulocyte count, and an overwhelming reticulocytosis in response to hemolysis may even result in a falsely high MCV because of the high percentage of young reticulocytes (large cells with a high MCV) in circulation. The diagnosis of hemolytic anemia may be supported further by findings on the peripheral blood smear and evidence of the products of red cell breakdown. (Chapter 5 provides further discussion of these points.)

Most normocytic anemias, however, are not accompanied by an appropriate reticulocyte response and are hypoproliferative in nature. Termed *Hypoproliferative anemias,* these may be divided into groups based on the primary reason their marrow does not respond appropriately, such as an intrinsically impaired bone marrow (primary bone marrow disorder), lack of responsiveness in otherwise healthy bone marrow (anemia due to nutritional deficiencies or other systemic conditions), or a result of multiple or unknown defects.

Those anemias accompanying primary stem cell failure, and the primary defects of iron deficiency and vitamin B_{12} or folate deficiency, are discussed in detail in other chapters. In the case of primary stem cell failure, abnormalities of the white cells and platelets are particularly helpful in suggesting this etiology. Patients with folate or vitamin B_{12} deficiency classically have a macrocytic anemia, and those with iron deficiency classically have a microcytic anemia. However, it has become clear that these classical presentations may be less frequent both because of complicating illnesses, especially in hospitalized patients, and the earlier clinical presentation of these patients to the physician.

With an increasing number of older patients, anemia of the elderly is a concern in the evaluation of a normocytic anemia. While it is true that marrow reserves may decrease with age, it also is likely that many of the diseases that cause anemia increase in frequency with age.[3] Appropriate evaluation of the elderly patient with anemia should proceed as usual; however, should no overt cause for a mild anemia be found, invasive procedures are not likely to uncover any surprising, underlying pathophysiology in the absence of other clinical or laboratory abnormalities.

SPURIOUS ANEMIA

During pregnancy, physiologic changes occur that decrease the hematocrit from its normal range (0.36 to 0.45) to 0.30 or less. This "physiologic anemia of pregnancy" arises from an increase in plasma volume which is greater than the increase in red cell mass that normally occurs during pregnancy. The red cell mass only increases by approximately 300 ml during pregnancy, while the total plasma volume increases by up to 1000 ml. This increased plasma volume most probably results from an increased need to maintain circulatory volume and to ensure perfusion of the placenta during pregnancy.[4] The plasma volume increases most dramatically during the second trimester and then reaches a plateau; the red cell mass increases slowly during the entire 9 months of pregnancy. During the third trimester, the hematocrit remains relatively stable.

The increased red cell mass during pregnancy is due to increased erythropoietin production. Erythropoietin production is thought to be stimulated by increased prolactin, progesterone, and placental gonadotropin levels in pregnant patients. The red blood cells are normocytic and, occasionally, may show a slight increase in their MCV. During pregnancy, the white blood cell count may increase to levels of 9 to 15×10^9 cells/L, but the platelet count usually remains normal. The serum iron is decreased modestly while the total iron-binding capacity is increased. The serum ferritin is in the normal range. Table 6.4 summarizes the hematologic parameters in pregnancy.

If the pregnant patient has a hematocrit less than 0.3, then causes for the decreased hematocrit other than hemodilution should be sought. The most common causes of anemia in pregnancy are iron and folate deficiency. If patients are both iron and folate deficient, they can present with a normocytic anemia that may resemble the "physiologic anemia of pregnancy." Iron deficiency anemia is the most common cause of anemia in pregnancy, occurring in 70% to 80% of patients who do not receive iron supplementation; folate deficiency,

TABLE 6.4. Hematologic Values in Pregnancy

	Normal	Iron Deficient
Hematocrit, *ratio*	0.36 to 0.45	< 0.30
Hemoglobin, *g/d*	10 to 13	< 10
Mean corpuscular volume, *fl/red cell*	90 ± 10	70 to 80
White cell count, ×*10⁹/L blood*	9 to 15	9 to 15
Platelets, ×*10⁹/L blood*	140 to 440	140 to 440
Serum iron, *μg/dl*	30 to 100	< 30
Total iron-binding capacity, *μg/dl*	200 to 350	> 400
Saturation, *%*	15 to 30	< 10
Ferritin, *ng/ml*	> 35	< 10

due to the increased demand for folic acid by the developing fetus, is usually mild and causes only modest decreases in the hematocrit.

Laboratory evaluation of the pregnant patient with "physiologic anemia of pregnancy" shows a modestly increased white blood cell count, a normal platelet count, a normal to mildly elevated MCV, and a normal serum ferritin. Tests required to make the diagnosis include measuring the serum iron, total iron-binding capacity, and red cell folate levels to exclude folate or iron deficiency as a cause. No treatment is required for the "physiologic anemia of pregnancy."

ANEMIA ACCOMPANIED BY INCREASED RED CELL PRODUCTION

Rapid loss of large amounts of blood induces a compensatory increase in plasma volume and a progressive decrease in hematocrit over a 3-day period. The red blood cells are normocytic, and iron stores are normal. If blood loss becomes chronic, iron stores become depleted, the serum iron falls, the total iron-binding capacity increases, and the serum ferritin decreases. Eventually, such patients develop the microcytic anemia of iron deficiency.

Healthy young subjects can tolerate up to 15% loss of their blood volume with few, if any, symptoms. With rapid blood loss of 20% to 30% of the total volume, patients will develop hypotension, tachycardia, and orthostasis. There is a normocytic anemia and perhaps a mild increase in the platelet count on laboratory examination. The erythropoietin level increases within 6 hours after an acute bleed, and polychromatophilia from the reticulocytosis may be seen on the peripheral blood smear. The hematocrit and hemoglobin levels may not equilibrate following an acute bleed for up to 72 hours, so measurements during the first 24 to 48 hours may not accurately reflect the degree of blood loss.

It is imperative that a search for the site of the bleeding be undertaken. Blood loss can occur from the gastrointestinal tract, retroperitoneally, or from gynecologic sources. In the hospitalized patient, extensive phlebotomy for laboratory testing may be a source of blood loss and a common cause of acquired anemia. Treatment of these patients includes transfusions of packed red blood cells and intravenous fluids to correct hypovolemia. Once the bleeding site is identified and the bleeding is under control, no further therapy is necessary, but if the blood loss is severe and has not been replaced by transfusion, iron therapy should be instituted, especially if the blood loss was chronic.

ANEMIA ACCOMPANIED BY DECREASED RED CELL PRODUCTION

Primary Marrow Failure

PURE RED CELL APLASIA.Pure red cell aplasia is a rare disorder that occurs in both children and adults. This disease is characterized by severe anemia accompanied by a marked decrease or absence of red cell precursors in the bone marrow. Other myeloid and megakaryocytic elements are normal in the marrow and in the peripheral blood.

Pure red cell aplasia can be either acquired or congenital. The acquired type is seen in about 5% of patients with thymoma and can be corrected by thymectomy; the disease also occurs in the absence of thymoma. IgG antibodies that are directed against red cell precursors have been demonstrated in serum from patients with acquired pure red cell aplasia. In some patients, a T-cell–mediated immunity that suppresses the growth of red cell precursors may be found;[5] thus, acquired pure red cell aplasia is often an autoimmune disease. It also has been associated with lymphoproliferative diseases such as chronic lymphocytic leukemia and lymphoma and importantly with parvovirus B19 infection.[6] In most patients with pure red cell aplasia, erythropoietin levels are markedly elevated; however, the antibody directed against erythroid precursors either destroys these cells or prevents them from responding to erythropoietin.

On laboratory presentation, patients have a profound anemia associated with an absolute reticulocytopenia. Examination of the bone marrow shows an absence of red cell precursors but normal numbers of myeloid precursors and megakaryocytes. In a significant proportion of these patients, bone marrow culture studies reveal an antibody directed against red cell precursors. Other laboratory features include an elevated serum iron with an iron saturation of almost 100%, because no red cell precursors are being made to utilize the iron. When present, thymic enlargement usually is detected on chest radiography, but computed tomography or magnetic resonance imaging may be needed to demonstrate the tumor.

Treatment of patients with pure red cell aplasia may require aggressive transfusion therapy to maintain the hematocrit in the 20% to 30% range. If a thymic mass is present, a thymectomy should be performed. Otherwise, glucocorticoids should be instituted to alleviate the transfusion requirement. If the patient does not respond to glucocorticoids, other immunosuppressive agents such as azathioprine or cyclophosphamide have been used with success. Approximately 25% of patients with pure red cell aplasia either with or without thymoma will have a remission in response to immunosuppressive therapy.[7] However, most patients will require transfusions and glucocorticoid therapy, and approximately 50% of those patients will enter a remission, with a median survival of more than 10 years.

MYELOPHTHISIC ANEMIA. Marrow infiltration by cells that are capable of altering the marrow microenvironment results in a myelophthisic anemia. The anemia itself may vary in severity and have minimal to marked variations in cell size and shape on the peripheral blood smear. Leukopenia and thrombocytopenia may accompany the anemia; however, leukocytosis and even thrombocytosis are also possible. Characteristically, some nucleated red blood cells and immature granulocytes circulate in the blood, a finding referred to as *leukoerythroblastosis*.[8]

The pathogenesis of these abnormalities results from extramedullary hematopoiesis or a disruption in the normal egress of marrow elements into the peripheral blood. Mature blood elements are thought to migrate from their site of origin through small pores in the endothelial cells to reach the circulation. Infiltration with abnormal cells disrupts the marrow architecture so that immature cells, whose cell membrane is such that they otherwise would not be able to use this route, gain entrance into the circulation; erythrocyte deformities may result from membrane loss and disruption during movement of cells through the injured marrow. Abnormal peripheral blood cell counts are not correlated directly with the amount of infiltration seen in the marrow, and may be related to release of inhibitory, fibroblastoid, or stimulatory factors produced by the infiltrating or reactive marrow cells. Other factors also may contribute to the severity of the myelophthisic anemia in some patients with malignant infiltration. Splenic sequestration or destruction and disseminated intravascular coagulation can lead to a shortened red blood cell survival, and nutritional deficiency and che-

motherapy administration can further compromise marrow function in patients with malignant diseases.

The most common etiology of myelophthisic anemia is metastatic carcinoma.[9] While all cancers may metastasize to the bone marrow, carcinomas of the lung (especially small-cell carcinoma), breast, and prostate most commonly do so at presentation and during the courses of their disease. The development of myelophthisic anemia with leukoerythroblastosis signals metastases, but metastatic foci of these tumors frequently are found in the absence of any findings on the peripheral blood smear. Hematologic malignancies also are capable of causing a myelophthisic anemia; however, the lymphoid malignancies seem less likely to cause the structural injury that results in the typical findings of leukoerythroblastosis and a myelophthisic smear.

Myelofibrosis, a proliferation of fibrous tissue in the marrow, results from either a primary stem cell disorder (myeloid metaplasia) or a secondary reactive process during marrow infiltration.[10,11] In the primary myelofibrosis of myeloid metaplasia, extensive replacement of the marrow with fibrous tissue is accompanied by prominent extramedullary hematopoiesis in the liver and spleen.

Although less common overall, nonmalignant disorders also are capable of damaging the marrow and resulting in myelophthisic anemia. These disorders include miliary tuberculosis, disseminated fungal infections, and granulomatous and lipid storage diseases.

Clinical manifestations of myelophthisic anemia usually relate to the underlying disease process. In advanced cases of marrow infiltration, bone pain and palpation tenderness may be present. Peripheral blood counts may vary, and examination of the peripheral smear shows evidence of leukoerythroblastic changes with a spectrum of cells at all levels of maturity possible. Thus, myelocytes, nucleated red cells, and polychromatophilic cells all may be present, and the finding of red cells in teardrop shapes is particularly suggestive of marrow infiltration even in the absence of obvious leukoerythroblastosis.

The diagnosis of marrow infiltration is made by bone marrow biopsy, especially in areas of bony tenderness. Marrow aspiration may not be successful ("dry tap") or easily interpretable in patients with myelofibrosis. Even if an initial biopsy is negative for infiltrating cells, a repeat biopsy is warranted to increase the diagnostic yield for those diseases known to frequent the marrow.

Treatment is aimed at the management of the primary disease and blood-product support as needed for life-threatening cytopenias. Overall, marrow infiltration remains a poor prognostic sign for most patients with malignancy. However, in patients with tumor present in the marrow and an otherwise treatable malignancy, chemotherapy should not be withheld because of marrow infiltration; if a response to chemotherapy is obtained, improvement in blood counts and marrow fibrosis may ensue. Also, if severe hypersplenism significantly contributes to pancytopenia, temporary improvement in peripheral blood counts may be anticipated with splenectomy in selected patients.

SIDEROBLASTIC ANEMIA. The sideroblastic anemias comprise a group of disorders characterized by an abnormality of heme incorporation.[12] They are included in the group of normocytic anemias because anemia may present with normal MCV by electronic evaluation. However, if the peripheral smear is evaluated, a mixed population of large and small cells with variable hemoglobin concentrations (dimorphic population) classically is found. Alternatively, an increased or decreased MCV is also consistent with the diagnosis of sideroblastic anemia.

Sideroblastic anemias may be classified as either acquired or congenital, with the acquired types being further divided into primary or secondary sideroblastic anemias. Several biochemical defects have been described, all likely related to abnormalities early in the heme synthetic pathways at the level of δ-aminolevulinic acid (ALA) synthesis. This blockade allows iron to accumulate in the mitochondria of red cell precursors rather than being incorporated into heme; the net result is that marrow proliferation of cells continues but is ineffective (i.e., cells are destroyed in the marrow prior to being released into the circulation).

Primary acquired sideroblastic anemia is considered a clonal abnormality of the myeloid stem cell, and it falls into a preleukemic category of disease.[13] Secondary acquired sideroblastic anemia results from drugs that interfere with pyridoxal phosphate metabolism, a co-vitamin required for the synthesis of ALA.[14] Alcohol and antituberculous agents (isonicotinoylhydrazine, cycloserine, and pyrazinamide) can cause sideroblastic anemia by this mechanism, and chronic lead intoxication also results in sideroblastic anemia through the interference of several heme synthetic enzymes.

Clinically, asymptomatic anemia may be detected while the patient is undergoing evaluation for other reasons. Alternatively, the disease may be detected during treatment for alcoholism or evaluation for symptoms or circumstances suggesting lead intoxication. The anemia may be mild initially, with normal leukocyte and platelet counts, so the peripheral smear is particularly important in encouraging the clinician to pursue the workup. The smear characteristically shows basophilic stippled red cells, with small and normal or large cells present and accompanied by mild variations in shape. Nucleated red cells may be present, but the reticulocyte

count is inappropriate for the degree of anemia. Examination of the bone marrow establishes the diagnosis of sideroblastic anemia; it shows increased cellularity consistent with ineffective erythropoiesis, iron-laden macrophages, and characteristic ringed sideroblasts. These cells are red cell precursors that have accumulated large amounts of iron in their mitochondria which, on iron stain, form a coarse granular ring surrounding the nucleus. If serum iron studies are obtained, high levels of ferritin and iron saturation are seen and are consistent with the diagnosis. In primary acquired sideroblastic anemia, chromosomal studies are abnormal in approximately 50% of the reported patients. Lead intoxication should be evaluated by measuring levels in the blood or urine when the appropriate clinical history or situation dictates.

The treatment of patients with a trial of high-dose pyridoxine is warranted, but the likelihood of response in acquired sideroblastic anemias is small. Discontinuation of any known offending drugs should also occur. Transfusional support should be used judiciously because of the possibility of iron overload (hemosiderosis) in patients with ineffective erythropoiesis.

Secondary to Systemic Conditions

CHRONIC RENAL FAILURE. Anemia virtually always accompanies chronic renal failure when the creatinine exceeds 5 mg%. Although the etiology of this anemia is multifactorial, lack of the hormone erythropoietin is considered the major cause. As destruction of renal parenchyma occurs, less erythropoietin is produced to respond to the hypoxic stress of anemia, resulting in low circulating levels of the hormone. Because several other factors contribute to the anemia in chronic renal failure, this erythropoietic response is not adequate to maintain normal levels of hemoglobin.[15,16]

Other factors known to contribute to anemia in chronic renal failure include gastrointestinal or other blood loss exacerbated by the platelet dysfunction found in uremia, a mild shortening of the red cell lifespan that is seen during uremia, and the possibility that undefined retained uremic toxins might inhibit erythropoiesis. During the treatment of patients for their chronic renal failure, additional factors also aggravate the anemia. Dialyzer blood loss, aluminum overload (from the utilization of phosphate binders), and secondary hyperparathyroidism with osteitis fibrosa may further compromise erythropoiesis.

The anemia of chronic renal failure is characteristically hypoproliferative, with a normal MCV, a reticulocyte count that is low for the degree of anemia and a bone marrow that has a decreased ratio of erythroid to myeloid cells. The diagnosis of anemia due to erythropoietin deficiency requires the presence of an elevated creatinine for a prolonged period (months) and the exclusion of known complicating factors. The iron status of patients should be ascertained utilizing the serum ferritin and the iron saturation, and a review of the peripheral blood smear also may help to determine the extent of the workup for other complicating factors or diseases. Folic acid deficiency and aluminum overload should be considered if the peripheral smear or clinical situation dictates. While folic acid is lost in dialysis and may be maintained poorly in nutritionally deficient patients, most patients receive folic acid supplements; aluminum overload is decreasing in incidence and is usually recognized by a low MCV.

Treatment of the anemia of chronic renal failure has changed dramatically with the availability of recombinant erythropoietin.[17,18] Erythropoietin has replaced the use of androgens or transfusion therapy, and avoids the associated risk of iron overload. For the patient with hematocrit of less than 0.3, erythropoietin therapy should be considered.[19] Virtually all patients respond to treatment with an increase in hematocrit and a dramatic increase in their well-being. Manageable complications of erythropoietin therapy include exacerbated hypertension in one third of patients and iron deficiency in up to one half of the patients during treatment. Blood pressure should be carefully monitored, especially during the rise in hematocrit, and treated as necessary; iron deficiency should be treated with supplementation, which often may require intravenous iron dextran. While a ferritin level of 100 ng/ml and an iron saturation of 20% at the onset of therapy is sufficient for initial responsiveness to the hormone, erythropoietin therapy results in such rapid iron utilization that a relative iron-deficient state (as manifested by a low iron saturation with normal ferritin levels) results. In addition to iron deficiency, inflammatory states (or even surgery or viral infections), osteitis fibrosa, and aluminum overload may blunt the response to erythropoietin.

ENDOCRINE DISEASES. Several types of endocrine dysfunction can result in a mild to moderate anemia.[20] This may be seen in pituitary, thyroid, adrenal, and testes deficiency states. An unexplained normocytic anemia also has been reported in patients with hyperparathyroidism.

The pathophysiology underlying the anemia associated with endocrine disorders is not well-characterized. In vivo selective ablation of the anterior pituitary, thyroid gland, adrenal glands, or testes in animals causes a decrease in the rate of red cell production that is correctable with replacement hormones. In vitro, thyroid, gonadal, and growth hormones; some steroid congeners; and insulin can enhance erythropoietin-dependent red cell formation.[21] Both androgen and thyroid hormones can also directly stimulate erythropoietin secretion.

In patients with panhypopituitarism, a normocytic anemia develops and is corrected with hormonal replacement that includes thyroid hormone. In Addison disease, there is both a decrease in red cell mass and plasma volume, and because the decrease in plasma volume is much greater than the decrease in the red cell mass, it partially masks the severity of the anemia. A mild normocytic anemia occurs in many patients with uncomplicated hypothyroidism and is corrected by the increased cellular metabolism occurring with thyroid replacement therapy.[22] The anemia, however, also may be complicated by iron deficiency from the menorrhagia seen in many women with myxedema. Also, vitamin B_{12} deficiency has been associated with thyroid and adrenal deficiencies and is due to an autoimmune process.

On presentation, patients usually have a normocytic anemia, a low reticulocyte count, and an unremarkable peripheral smear; they may have a microcytic anemia if they have hypothyroidism complicated by iron deficiency. Patients usually have normal white blood cell and platelet counts, but a finding of eosinophilia may suggest Addison disease. Correction of the anemia is centered on treatment of the endocrine disorder.

PROTEIN DEFICIENCY. Mild normocytic anemia develops after 6 months of semistarvation and after 3 months of severe starvation. This anemia is due in part to a relative increase in plasma volume compared with the decrease in body weight and red cell mass. In chronic protein deficiency, decreased red cell production accompanies the reduced metabolic demand, and protein deficiency also decreases production of erythropoietin, an observation that formed the basis for an early animal assay to measure erythropoietin levels from clinical samples.[23] Amino acid supplementation during protein deficiency results in enhanced erythropoietin production, and other nutritional deficiencies and blood loss are seen frequently in patients with protein and calorie malnutrition. Thus, these patients must be evaluated for nutritional deficiencies and blood loss as part of the evaluation of the anemia. With severe malnutrition, white blood counts will also fall.

On laboratory presentation, the patients have a normocytic anemia and may have a modestly decreased white blood cell count if protein and calorie malnutrition are severe and prolonged. In children, the hemoglobin may decrease to as low as 8 g/dl, but the folate and iron status must be evaluated. A gradual improvement in the anemia occurs over 1 to 2 months following refeeding if the anemia is due to protein and calorie malnutrition.

Combined Defects

ANEMIA OF CHRONIC DISEASE. Anemia is a common finding in patients with malignancies, chronic inflammatory diseases such as rheumatoid arthritis, and long-standing infections. This anemia is seen without any evidence of bone marrow involvement by the malignant or infectious process, and it is characterized by a mild or moderate nonprogressive hypoproliferative anemia, decreased serum iron and total iron-binding capacity, and normal or increased reticuloendothelial iron stores.

Many studies have attempted to determine the etiology of the anemia of chronic disease. This anemia probably results from a combination of causes that include shortened red cell survival, decreased intrinsic red cell production, and inadequate production of erythropoietin in response to the anemia.

The red cell lifespan is reduced by about 20% to 30% in patients with the anemia of chronic disease. This decreased red cell survival is not due to a defect intrinsic to the red cell, because cells from patients with the anemia of chronic disease have normal survival when transfused into normal recipients. It is possible that the activation of macrophages by the chronic disease processes results in increased red blood cell destruction from increased activity of the reticuloendothelial system. However, the modest decrease in red cell lifespan seen in chronic disease is insufficient to explain the anemia seen in these patients, because the normal bone marrow easily should be capable of compensating for this level of decreased survival. Therefore, the major problem in patients with the anemia of chronic disease is suppressed red blood cell production.

The most characteristic features of this type of anemia are a low serum iron, low total iron-binding capacity, and an elevated serum ferritin. These findings show that iron present in the macrophages is not readily available for use in red blood cell production. However, despite the low iron and total iron-binding capacity, the anemia of chronic disease does not resemble iron deficiency anemia, nor does it respond to oral or parental iron therapy. Thus, factors other than absolute iron deficiency are likely to play a role in the decreased red cell production. The erythropoietin response for the degree of anemia in patients with solid tumors is much less than that seen in patients with a similar degree of iron deficiency anemia alone,[24] and this blunted erythropoietin response, also reported in patients with rheumatoid arthritis,[25] could be responsible in part for the anemia

seen in these patients. In addition, factors produced by activated macrophages, such as tumor necrosis factor–α and interleukin-1, can suppress erythropoiesis both in vitro and in vivo.[26,27] These macrophage products may play a role in decreased red cell production either directly or by affecting the availability of iron for red cell precursors. Most likely, combinations of these defects result in the decreased red blood cell production seen.

The anemia of chronic disease is a diagnosis of exclusion, because patients with chronic illnesses can have multiple causes for their anemia, including blood loss, hemolysis, and marrow suppression from various therapeutic modalities (e.g., chemotherapy, radiation therapy). The evaluation includes determining the iron status of these patients, searching for evidence of occult blood loss in the stool and urine, and examination of the peripheral blood smear for signs of hemolysis. The peripheral smear usually shows a normocytic anemia, but it may show a mild microcytosis. The reticulocyte count is low, consistent with a hypoproliferative anemia. The percentage of iron saturation (ratio of the serum iron to the total iron-binding capacity) usually is less than 20%, but when this is less than 10%, it is consistent with relative iron deficiency and suggests that a more aggressive evaluation for iron deficiency should be undertaken. The serum ferritin also may help in the differential diagnosis of iron deficiency and the anemia of chronic disease. The bone marrow can be examined for iron stores, but this usually is not required to make the diagnosis. Table 6.5 contrasts the laboratory findings of the anemia of chronic disease with those of iron deficiency.

Treatment of the anemia of chronic disease requires treatment of the underlying disease process. Erythropoietin may also prove to be a useful treatment, as it was recently demonstrated that patients with malignancies[28] and rheumatoid arthritis can respond to infusions of recombinant erythropoietin.[29] However, because most patients with chronic disease have a mild anemia, it is unclear whether increasing the hematocrit will significantly improve their quality of life.

Anemia in acquired immunodeficiency syndrome may represent a somewhat different situation from that

TABLE 6.5.   Hematologic Values in Patients with Iron Deficiency or the Anemia of Chronic Disease

	Iron Deficiency	Anemia of Chronic Disease	Normal
Serum iron, $\mu g/ml$	<60	<60	60 to 100
Transferrin saturation, %	<15	<20	20 to 60
Ferritin, ng/ml	<20	>100	20 to 30

found in patients with other chronic diseases.[30] Anemia is a prominent feature in 20% to 30% of patients who harbor asymptomatic human-immunodeficiency-virus (HIV) infection and is a severe problematic finding in up to 90% of patients during the course of their disease and treatment. This anemia is initially normocytic and fulfills all criteria for the anemia of chronic disease. A high incidence of positive antiglobulin tests is found, but significant red cell destruction is not. Accompanying iron deficiency anemia also may be found, and the incidence of thrombocytopenia and neutropenia is also high and erythropoietin production is suppressed.[31] Bone marrow examination reveals normal or increased cellularity in most patients, with variable abnormalities present in red cells, white cells, and megakaryocytes.[29,32] This anemia is further aggravated by treatment of HIV and its consequential infections, at which time the anemia may become macrocytic in character. Erythropoietin therapy appears to be beneficial in improving the hematocrit during primary therapy with current drugs for HIV infection.[33]

EARLY IRON DEFICIENCY. Early iron deficiency presents as a normocytic anemia in up to 30% of patients. These patients present with a mild anemia, normal white blood cell counts, and usually normal or modestly elevated platelet counts. Evaluation of the peripheral blood smear is unremarkable. The serum iron is decreased, the total iron-binding capacity is increased, and the serum ferritin is less than 20 ng/L. Because the temporal sequence for development of iron deficiency first results in depleted iron stores, a bone marrow examination shows absent iron; after severe and prolonged iron deficiency, patients develop a more pronounced peripheral smear with microcytosis and variation in the size of the red cells. Iron deficiency and its treatment are discussed in Chapter 2.

TWO ABNORMALITIES. A normal MCV may result from combined defects of hematopoiesis that involve abnormalities affecting both nuclear maturation and cytoplasmic heme synthesis. In this situation, the megaloblastosis of folate or vitamin B_{12} deficiency may be masked by iron deficiency, chronic disease, or even thalassemia minor.[34] Examination of the peripheral blood smear should help in the differential diagnoses by showing evidence of large and small cells as well as hypersegmented granulocytes as evidence of megaloblastosis. Serum iron studies obtained in the presence of folate or vitamin B_{12} deficiency may not reflect iron deficiency, because the ineffective erythropoiesis results in underutilization of the iron available from intramedullary red cell breakdown. Bone marrow examination may not reveal as pronounced a picture of

megaloblastosis in the red cells, but the white cell abnormalities remain diagnostic. A combined abnormality also should be considered when a patient shows an incomplete response to replacement therapy with the presumed deficient hematinic. In these cases, typical megaloblastosis may emerge with iron treatment, or iron deficiency will be diagnosed easily by repeat serum studies as the response to folate or vitamin B_{12} stops short of correcting the anemia.

REFERENCES

1. Wintrobe MM. Anemia: classification and treatment on the basis of differences in the average volume and hemoglobin content of the red corpuscles. Arch Intern Med 1934;54:256.
2. Seward SJ, Safra C, Marton KI, Robinson SH. Does the mean corpuscular volume help physicians evaluate hospitalized patients with anemia? J Gen Intern Med 1990;5:198.
3. Lipschitz DA. Nutrition, aging, and the immunohematopoietic system. Clin Geriatr Med 1987;3:319.
4. Chesley LC. Plasma and red cell volumes during pregnancy. Am J Obstet Gynecol 1972;112:440.
5. Hoffman R, Zanjani ED, Vila J, Zalusky R, Lutton JD, Wasserman LR. Diamond-Blackfan syndrome: lymphocyte-mediated suppression of erythropoiesis. Science 1976;193:899.
6. Harris JW. Parvovirus B19 for the hematologist. Am J Hematol 1992;39:119.
7. Clark DA, Dessypris EN, Krantz SB. Studies on pure red cell aplasia. XI. Results of immunosuppressive treatment of 37 patients. Blood 1984;63:277.
8. Weick JK, Hagedorn AB, Linman JW. Leukoerythroblastosis: diagnostic and prognostic significance. Mayo Clin Proc 1974;49:111.
9. Delsol G, Guiu-Godfrin B, Guiu M, et al. Leukoerythroblastosis and cancer frequency, prognosis, and physiologic significance. Cancer 1979;44:1009.
10. Ward HP, Block MH. The natural history of agnogenic myeloid metaplasia and a critical evaluation of its relation with the myeloproliferative syndrome. Medicine 1971;50:357.
11. Varki A, Lottenberg R, Griffith R, et al. The syndrome of idiopathic myelofibrosis. Medicine 1983;62:353.
12. Bottomley SS, Muller-Eberhard U. Pathophysiology of heme synthesis. Semin Hematol 1988;256:282.
13. Gattermann N, Aul C, Schneider W. Two types of acquired sideroblastic anemia (AISA). Br J Haematol 1990;74:45.
14. Cazzola M, Barosi G, Govvi PG, Invernizzi R, Riccardi A, Ascari E. Natural history of idiopathic refractory sideroblastic anemia. Blood 1988;71:305.
15. Eschbach JW, Adamson JW. Anemia of end-stage renal disease (ESRD). Kidney Int 1985;28:1.
16. Paganini EP. Overview of anemia associated with chronic renal disease: primary and secondary mechanisms. Semin Nephrol 1989;1:3.
17. Eschbach JW, Egrie JC, Downing MR, Browne JK, Adamson JW. Correction of the anemia of end-stage renal disease with recombinant human erythropoietin. N Engl J Med 1987;316:73.
18. Adamson JW. Treatment of the anemia of chronic renal disease with recombinant erythropoietin. Annu Rev Med 1990;41:349.
19. Eschbach JW, Adamson JW. Guidelines for recombinant human erythropoietin therapy. Am J Kidney Dis 1989;14:2.
20. Orwoll FS, Orwoll JL. Hematologic abnormalities in patients with endocrine and metabolic disorders. Hematol Oncol Clin North Am 1987;1:261.

21. Adamson JW, Popvic WJ, Brown JE. Hormonal control of erythropoiesis. In: Golde DW, Cline MJ, Metcalf D, eds. Hematologic Cell Differentiation. New York: Academic Press, 1978:53.

22. Green ST, Ng JP. Hypothyroidism and anaemia. Biomed Pharm 1986;40:326.

23. Caro J, Silver R, Erslev AJ, Miller OP, Birgegard G. Erythropoietin production in fasted rats. J Lab Clin Med 1981;98:860.

24. Miller CB, Jones RJ, Piantadosi S, Abeloff MD, Spivak JL. Decreased erythropoietin response in patients with the anemia of cancer. N Engl J Med 1990;322:1689–1692.

25. Baer AN, Dessypris EN, Goldwasser E, Krantz SB. Blunted erythropoietin response to anaemia in rheumatoid arthritis. Br J Haematol 1987;66:559.

26. Johnson RA, Waddelow TA, Caro J, Oliff A, Roodman GD. Chronic exposure to tumor necrosis factor in vivo preferentially inhibits erythropoiesis in nude mice. Blood 1989;74:130.

27. Schooley JC, Kullgren B, Allison AC. Inhibition by interleukin-1 of the action of erythropoietin on erythroid precursors and its possible role in the pathogenesis of hypoplastic anaemias. Br J Haematol 1987;67:11.

28. Ludwig H, Fritz E, Kotzmann H, Hocker P, Gisslinger H, Barnas U. Erythropoietin treatment of anemia associated with multiple myeloma. N Engl J Med 1990;322:1693.

29. Pincus T, Olsen NJ, Russell IJ, Wolfe F, Harris ER, Schnitzer TJ, Boccagno JA, Krantz SB. Multicenter study of recombinant human erythropoietin in correction of anemia in rheumatoid arthritis. Am J Med 1990;89:161–168.

30. Spivak JL, Bender BS, Quinn TC. Hematologic abnormalities in the acquired immunodeficiency syndrome. Am J Med 1984; 77:224.

31. Spivak JL, Barnes CD, Fuchs E, Quinn TC. Serum immunoreactive erythropoietin in HIV-infected patients. JAMA 1989; 261:3104.

32. Treacy M, Lai L, Costello C, Clark A. Peripheral blood and bone marrow abnormalities in patients with HIV-related disease. Br J Haematol 1987;65:289.

33. Fischl M, Galpin JE, Levine JD, et al. Recombinant human erythropoietin for patients with AIDS treated with zidovudine. N Engl J Med 1990;322:1488.

34. Spivak JL. Masked megaloblastic anemia. Arch Intern Med 1982;142:2111.

7

Porphyrias, Lead Poisoning, and Sideroblastic Anemias

Sylvia S. Bottomley, M.D.

Heme (iron-protoporphyrin IX) plays a central role in the function of all cells. It is formed in every nucleated cell to provide the prosthetic moiety of cytochromes in the mitochondrial respiratory chain for the generation of cellular energy. Heme is required for the function of many other hemoproteins, and some tissues have a much greater demand for heme than others. Most of the total heme in the body is synthesized by erythroid cells for assembly into hemoglobin, but substantial amounts also are produced by the liver for various hemoproteins, particularly the microsomal P-450 proteins for the biosynthesis of steroid hormones and bile acids, the processing of certain cell mediators, and the metabolism of most drugs and environmental agents. Other hemoproteins provide for the storage of oxygen (myoglobin), methemoglobin reduction (cytochrome b_5 in erythrocytes), and fatty-acid synthesis (microsomal cytochrome b_5 in the liver). Because of these many roles for heme in normal cell physiology, it may be predicted that disturbances of heme production would involve multiple tissues and biochemical processes. Differences in the mechanisms that regulate heme biosynthesis are being revealed between tissues (e.g., in hepatocytes vs. erythroid cells) and help clarify the pathophysiology of the diverse disorders of heme synthesis.

Inherited defects of enzymes of the heme synthetic pathway account for the various porphyrias and are now well-characterized. The DNA sequences for most of these enzymes have been cloned, and specific mutations causing the defects have been identified. However, the physiologic mechanisms of the clinical manifestations in the porphyrias are only partly understood. Chronic lead intoxication mimics certain porphyrias clinically, and among its adverse biochemical effects, lead also interferes with heme biosynthesis. The sideroblastic anemias represent a third category of disorders, in which production of heme is impaired only in the erythroid cell.

THE BIOSYNTHESIS OF HEME AND ITS REGULATION

The formation of heme proceeds through a complex pathway of eight enzymatic steps that are compartmentalized between the mitochondrion and the cytosol of the cell (Fig. 7.1). The enzymes catalyzing the mitochondrial steps (four) also are encoded by nuclear DNA, and after being produced on cytoplasmic ribosomes, they must be imported into mitochondria. 5-Aminolevulinate (ALA) synthase catalyzes the first step, forming ALA from succinyl CoA and glycine within the mitochondrion, and requires pyridoxal phosphate as a coenzyme. On exit from the mitochondrion, two molecules of ALA are condensed by the cytosolic enzyme ALA dehydratase to the pyrrole porphobilinogen (PBG). In the cytosol, PBG deaminase polymerizes four molecules of PBG to the unstable intermediate hydroxymethylbilane (HMB), a linear tetrapyrrole that is rapidly closed to the macrocycle of uroporphyrinogen (URO′gen) III by URO′gen III synthase. In the absence of this enzyme,

101

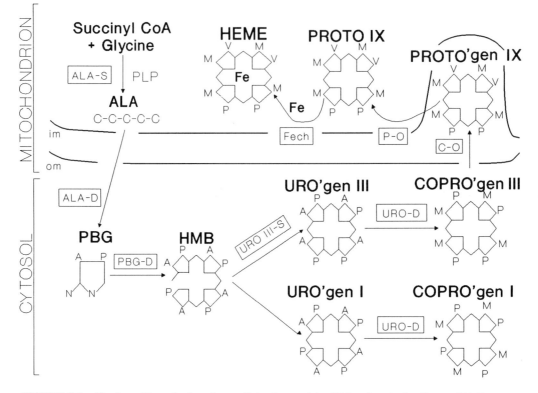

FIGURE 7.1. **The heme biosynthesis pathway.** *Note:* **A** = acetate; **ALA** = 5-aminolevulinate, **ALA-D** = 5-aminolevulinate dehydratase; **ALA-S** = 5-aminolevulinate synthase; **C-O** = coproporphyrinogen oxidase; **CoA** = coenzyme A; **COPRO'gen** = coproporphyrinogen; **Fech** = ferrochelatase; **HMB** = hydroxymethylbilane; **im** = inner membrane; **om** = outer membrane; **M** = methyl; **P** = propionate; **PBG** = porphobilinogen; **PBG-D** = porphobilinogen deaminase; **PLP** = pyridoxal phosphate; **P-O** = protoporphyrinogen oxidase; **PROTO** = protoporphyrin; **PROTO'gen** = protoporphyrinogen; **URO III-S** = uroporphyrinogen III synthase; **URO-D** = uroporphyrinogen decarboxylase; **URO'gen** = uroporphyrinogen; **V** = vinyl.

the unstable HMB cyclizes nonenzymatically to URO'gen I. The last cytosolic enzyme in the pathway, URO'gen decarboxylase, sequentially removes carboxyl groups from the acetyl side chains on the four pyrrole rings of URO'gen III to form coproporphyrinogen (COPRO'gen) III. It also decarboxylates URO'gen I to COPRO'gen I, but this isomer cannot be used further in the pathway. Decarboxylation/oxidation of COPRO'gen III by COPRO'gen oxidase in the intermembrane space of the mitochondrion yields protoporphyrinogen IX, which is then oxidized by protoporphyrinogen oxidase on the inner mitochondrial membrane to protoporphyrin IX. Ferrochelatase, likewise located on the inner membrane, inserts iron into protoporphyrin to form heme.

The sequence of these enzymatic reactions proceeds with little accumulation of respective intermediates, because their maximum activity is not utilized. However, two enzymes, ALA synthase and PBG deaminase, have much lower relative activities and thus serve regulatory functions; defects of these enzymes compromise heme production much more readily than defects of the remaining enzymes in the pathway.[1] In addition, the expression and regulation of these two enzymes is distinct in erythroid cells and all other tissues. Two isoforms of PBG deaminase, one ubiquitous in all tissues and the other found solely in erythroid cells, are encoded by one gene, but separate promoters control expression of the two mRNAs.[2] The necessity for the two forms probably relates to the programming of heme biosynthesis in the developing erythroid cell, where the enzyme activity appears to be less rate-limiting than in the liver. In the case of ALA synthase, two separate genes encode two distinct enzymes: a ubiquitous or housekeeping ALA synthase, and an erythroid-specific ALA synthase.[3] These genes are also located on separate chromosomes, the housekeeping gene on chromosome 3 and the erythroid on the X chromosome.[4,5] Production of the housekeeping enzyme is adapted for a rapid response to prevailing cellular needs for heme, and heme levels tightly regulate transcription of its mRNA in a "feedback" manner (Fig. 7.2). The erythroid gene is activated and transcribed in concert with other events of erythroid differentiation, and production of the enzyme protein is controlled further at the level of translation.[3,6,7] This translational regulation is most likely by available iron through an iron-responsive element present in its mRNA, analogous to the regulation of apoferritin synthesis by iron (Fig. 7.2). Additional control over at least the housekeeping form of ALA synthase occurs by heme, which retards its transport into mitochondria.[6]

As the erythroid cell matures and its hemoglobin content increases, there is progressive loss of the heme synthetic enzymes. However, sufficient ribosomal and mitochondrial elements with their enzymes remain in the reticulocyte for continued heme (as for globin) synthesis to still manufacture as much as the last 30% of the erythrocyte's complement of hemoglobin. The cytosolic enzymes of the heme synthetic pathway persist throughout the lifespan of the red cell. Thus, all of the enzymes can be assessed in peripheral red blood cells for study and for diagnosis.

Substrate intermediates of impaired heme synthetic enzymes, as discussed later, accumulate above the normal trace amounts when enzyme activities are 50% or lower, are released from cells into plasma and bile, and are excreted in urine or feces according to their water solubility; the porphyrin precursors ALA and PBG are lost exclusively in the urine. The water solubility of porphyrins (their colorless, nonfluorescent native substrate forms [the porphyrinogens] already variably oxidized to the porphyrins in tissues) is determined by the number of carboxyl groups on the molecule. With eight carboxyls, uroporphyrin is excreted mainly in urine, protoporphyrin only in feces, and coproporphyrin through both routes. Excretion profiles of excess porphyrins and their precursors characteristically reflect the position of an enzymatic defect in the heme synthetic pathway, and their analysis is the standard method for establishing the diagnosis of the porphyrias. All of the intermediates can be detected also in plasma, but in smaller amounts; plasma measurements are not used routinely.

THE PORPHYRIAS

In clinical practice, the porphyrias are relatively rare disorders. They are characterized by a unique and

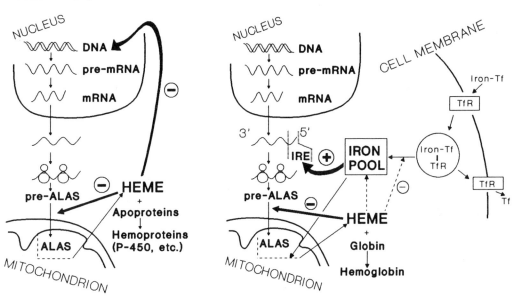

HEPATOCYTE **DIFFERENTIATING ERYTHROID CELL**

FIGURE 7.2. The postulated regulation of the hepatic (housekeeping) and the erythroid 5-aminolevulinate synthase (*bold arrows*). *Note:* ⊖ = inhibition; ⊕ = stimulation; ALAS = 5-aminolevulinate synthase; IRE = iron-responsive element; Tf = transferrin; TfR = transferrin receptor.

long-known spectrum of neural and dermatologic features, the reasons for which have been discovered in enzymic abnormalities in the heme biosynthesis pathway. All seven human porphyrias represent discrete, inherited partial deficiencies of each of the seven enzymes beyond the first and rate-limiting ALA synthase step of the pathway (Table 7.1). While the abnormal porphyrinogenesis resulting from these enzyme defects appears to be largely confined to the liver and bone marrow (the sites where the vast majority of heme is made), the clinical and pathologic phenotype of each porphyria is dictated by the defective enzyme and the mode of inheritance. Variability of the clinical picture within each type of porphyria may be attributed to genetic heterogeneity (i.e., the specific molecular lesions of the enzyme proteins), and particularly to certain metabolic and environmental factors. Three kinds of general metabolic derangements result from the various enzymatic defects (Table 7.1):

1. apparent marginal production of heme that intermittently compromises the function of neural tissues,
2. accumulation of porphyrin substrates that elicit only cutaneous photosensitivity, and
3. both an apparent heme deficit and an accumulation of skin-damaging porphyrin intermediates.

It is worth noting that, except for a few rare homozygous forms, the defects in all seven porphyrias do not sufficiently compromise erythroid heme synthesis to produce a significant anemia.

Acute Porphyrias

INCIDENCE, GENETICS, AND THE METABOLIC ABNORMALITIES. Defects of four different enzymes underlie the acute porphyrias (Table 7.2).[8] The acute intermittent porphyria (AIP) defect is the most common, affecting 1 per 10,000 in the United States and Europe. This dominant trait usually is expressed in half-normal activity of PBG deaminase and is detectable in all tissues examined to date. With molecular studies, marked genetic heterogeneity of the defect is being found.[9] Various mutations in one PBG deaminase allele result in no expression of the enzyme protein, while others encode an abnormal protein that is inactive.[9,10] The partial deficiency of the enzyme causes accumulation of its substrate, PBG, and to a lesser degree ALA, and a consequent relative deficit of cellular heme induces ALA synthase, accentuating the accumulation of these porphyrin precursors.

Coproporphyria (CP) is uncommon. Heterozygotes have half-normal COPRO′gen oxidase activity, homozygotes have 2% residual activity of the enzyme, and its substrate, coproporphyrin, accumulates. Variegate porphyria (VP) is most prevalent in South Africans of Dutch ancestry (1 per 300) but occurs worldwide. Heterozygotes have half-normal and homozygotes 10% of normal PROTO′gen oxidase activity, and the oxidized substrate protoporphyrin accumulates. In CP and VP, PBG and ALA also accumulate, but usually only during clinical attacks when heme requirements exceed the capacity of the restricted pathway, ALA synthase is induced, and PBG deaminase becomes rate-limiting. In addition, the accumulated coproporphyrin and protoporphyrin inhibit the PBG deaminase.

Acute porphyria due to ALA dehydratase deficiency (plumboporphyria), the last porphyria to be discovered and so far observed in four reported patients, is manifested only in homozygotes in whom residual enzyme activity is reduced to 1% to 2% of normal.[8,11] In the cases characterized at the molecular level distinct point mutations were found in each dehydratase allele.[12,13] The enzyme becomes rate-limiting in the production of heme, and the accumulated substrate is ALA.

TABLE 7.1.   Genetic and Clinical Characteristics of the Porphyrias

Disorder	Inheritance	Defective Enzyme	Enzyme Activity, %* Heterozygote	Enzyme Activity, %* Homozygote	Clinical Manifestations
ALA dehydratase deficiency	AR	ALA-D	36	1 to 2	Neurovisceral
Acute intermittent porphyria	AD	PBG-D	50	15	Neurovisceral
Congenital erythropoietic porphyria	AR	URO III-S	50	20	Cutaneous
Porphyria cutanea tarda	AD	URO-D	50	3 to 27	Cutaneous
Coproporphyria	AD	C-O	50	2	Neurovisceral and cutaneous
Variegate porphyria	AD	P-O	50	10	Neurovisceral and cutaneous
Protoporphyria	AD	Fech	20	6.5	Cutaneous (liver disease)

Note: AR = autosomal recessive; AD = autosomal dominant; ALA-D = 5-aminolevulinate dehydratase; PBG-D = porphobilinogen deaminase; URO III-S = uroporphyrinogen III synthase; URO-D = uroporphyrinogen decarboxylase; C-O = coproporphyrinogen oxidase; P-O = protoporphyrinogen oxidase; Fech = ferrochelatase.
   *Percentage of normal.

TABLE 7.2.   Intermediates Accumulated and Excreted in Excess in the Acute Porphyrias

Disorder	ALA	PBG	URO	COPRO	PROTO
ALA dehydratase deficiency	+	−	−	+	(+)
Acute intermittent porphyria	+	+	+	+/−	−
Coproporphyria	+	+	+/−	+	−
Variegate porphyria	+	+	+/−	+	+

Note: ALA = 5-aminolevulinate; PBG = porphobilinogen; URO = uroporphyrin; COPRO = coproporphyrin; PROTO = protoporphyrin.

THE CLINICAL PICTURE. The acute porphyrias have in common acute attacks of neuropsychiatric illness whose clinical manifestations are not distinguishable among the four types.[8,14–16] Symptoms and signs may be protean and vary greatly, but represent neurovisceral and psychiatric deficits. Most often, the acute attack is an autonomic neuropathy manifest in colicky abdominal pain, vomiting, constipation, without rigidity or rebound tenderness, and abdominal radiographs showing segmental intestinal dilatation and spasm. Other common findings are tachycardia and labile hypertension or paradoxical hypotension, or urinary retention. Less frequently, and with prolonged attacks, peripheral nerve deficits, potential life-threatening bulbar and respiratory muscle paralysis or anxiety with emotional lability that can progress to confusion and frank psychosis occur. Grand mal seizures can be attributed to hyponatremia from inappropriate ADH secretion, reflecting hypothalamic dysfunction. If peripheral nerve deficits develop, they may clear slowly, over months or even years. Pathologic studies show patchy demyelination and axonal degeneration of nerves.[17] Chronic or intermittent symptoms also occur, and they tend to be nonspecific and are often difficult to evaluate, especially in carriers of a trait who have not had documented acute attacks.

How to link these clinical manifestations to the well-characterized biochemical abnormalities remains a major problem. Three mechanisms have been postulated (Fig. 7.3). The first is that the porphyrin precursor ALA, produced in excess in all the acute porphyrias, causes neurotoxicity. Some studies in animals indicate that it can alter neural structure and function, perhaps by acting as a γ-aminobutyric acid agonist.[18] Urine levels of ALA and PBG correlate poorly with symptoms and signs, although ALA and PBA excretion tends to increase during attacks. A second postulated mechanism is that episodic depletion of cellular heme from marginal to critical levels deprives enzymatic oxidations and energy-producing reactions involving hemoproteins in neural tissue. Thirdly, experimental work in animals indicates that depletion of heme impairs catabolism of L-tryptophan by the heme-dependent hepatic tryptophan pyrrolase and results in accumulation to neurotoxic levels of tryptophan and serotonin.[19,20] The relevance of this mechanism in patients with porphyria also remains to be determined. The well-documented effectiveness of intravenously administered hematin in often reversing the clinical manifestations of acute attacks as well as in reducing ALA and PBG levels is consistent with all these postulates.

The clinical expression of the acute porphyria defects not only is episodic and variable, even between affected siblings, but is overall infrequent, and there are many more latent carriers than symptomatic individuals. Contributory factors (e.g., genetic, metabolic, and environmental) are important for clinical expression.[8] Gonadal hormones, especially the 5β-steroids and ovarian hormones or their metabolites, play a role, and while certain cytochrome hemoproteins are necessary for their synthesis, they can induce ALA synthase and thus stress a defective heme synthesis pathway. In one study, the additional deficiency of hepatic steroid 5α-reductase, and a presumed consequent excess of 5β-steroid metabolites, correlated with clinical expression of AIP.[21] Clinical attacks of acute porphyria occur rarely if ever before puberty and are more common in women, and in women susceptible to attacks during the luteal phase (high progesterone) of the menstrual cycle, the benefit of the luteinizing hormone releasing hormone analog peptides can be attributed to induction of pituitary refractoriness to luteinizing hormone releasing hormone to suppress production of progesterone and its 5β metabolites.[22] Yet, paradoxes abound in that oral contraceptives aggravate porphyria in some women but relieve premenstrual symptoms in others; pregnancy may be complicated by porphyric symptoms, may be benign, or may even reduce manifestations. The prevailing view is that pregnancy should not be interdicted in patients who have porphyria. Countless drugs, with barbiturates and sulfonamides heading the list, can precipitate porphyric attacks and usually do so by inducing hepatic apocytochrome P-450 for their metabolism via microsomal hydroxylation, thereby increasing the need for hepatocellular heme. Again, the response of patients is highly variable. Furthermore, an intercurrent illness and decreased caloric intake may precede acute attacks. As shown in experimental settings as well, carbohydrate administration can block the associated induction of ALA synthase, tip heme biosynthesis toward the normal, and improve symptoms.[14,23,24]

Cutaneous photosensitivity is absent in AIP and ALA dehydratase deficiency, because porphyrins proper do not accumulate. It occurs in 20% to 30% of patients with CP and in up to 80% of those with VP, because

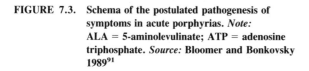

Block in heme synthesis

↑ALA Synthase

↑ALA

Critical heme deficiency

[↑Tryptophan from liver ?]   [↑Neuronal ATP production ?]

Neuronal dysfunction

Neurovisceral symptoms

FIGURE 7.3. Schema of the postulated pathogenesis of symptoms in acute porphyrias. *Note:* ALA = 5-aminolevulinate; ATP = adenosine triphosphate. *Source:* Bloomer and Bonkovsky 1989[91]

porphyrin substrates of the defective enzymes do accumulate.[8] The photocutaneous manifestations occur independently of acute neurovisceral attacks and resemble those found in porphyria cutanea tarda.

DIAGNOSIS. The diagnosis is firmly established by quantifying excreted porphyrin precursors and porphyrins for the distinctive pattern of each form of porphyria. During a symptomatic phase, urinary excretion of the respective substances, as listed in Table 7.2, is always raised; an increased urinary PBG is the biochemical hallmark of AIP. During acute attacks, the PBG is sufficiently elevated (at least 5 to 10 mg/L) to usually yield a positive qualitative or Watson-Schwartz test. When performing the test, false-positive results from urobilinogen, drugs, and drug metabolites must be eliminated using appropriate extraction steps with chloroform and n-butanol.[25] However, the test is unsuitable for screening asymptomatic patients or possible carriers who may have mild or no increases of urinary PBG. In all situations, specific quantitation of PBG in a 24-hour urine collection must be carried out to establish the diagnosis or, occasionally, a carrier state. Excess urine uroporphyrin is also found in AIP but represents either extracellular conversion of PBG or porphobilin, a polymer of PBG that forms with time in the urine and more rapidly in sunlight. CP and VP are distinguished from AIP by finding a very high urinary level of coproporphyrin during attacks. CP and VP are differentiated by finding excess fecal or bile[26] coproporphyrin in the

former and mainly excess protoporphyrin in the latter. Profiles of fecal porphyrins also detect the defects in patients with CP and VP between attacks, when the urine is more likely to be normal than in AIP, as well as in asymptomatic carriers. In ALA dehydratase deficiency, urine ALA is increased but PBG is normal. It should be emphasized that the so-called "urine porphyrin screen" commonly carried out is nonspecific; it merely detects and does not quantitate an increased level of urine coproporphyrin, which can be associated with a variety of illnesses.

In AIP, a diminished erythrocyte PBG deaminase activity is another useful measurement for diagnosis and the detection of relatives with the latent defect. However, even if combined with pedigree analysis, the erythrocyte value may be indeterminate or normal in less than 10% of cases due to genetic heterogeneity of the mutations and not involving the erythroid isoform of the enzyme.[9,27,28] The approach of linkage analysis using intragenic restriction fragment length polymorphisms in amplified DNA of PBG deaminase has been used to identify haplotypes for more definitive detection of presymptomatic carriers of the genetic defect within AIP families.[29] Assay of erythrocyte ALA dehydratase activity detects the rare deficiency of this enzyme and the low enzyme activity is differentiated from that caused by lead poisoning in that it is not reversed by sulfhydryl reagent. The assays of COPRO'gen oxidase and PROTO'gen oxidase are complex and remain research procedures.

MANAGEMENT. Prevention of symptoms is the cornerstone of managing the acute porphyrias and includes identification of carriers among relatives of patients with the disorders. Preventive measures for affected individuals consist of avoiding most drugs and fasting, and a caloric intake sufficient to maintain a normal body weight should be practiced.

The acute porphyric attack is managed by removal of any precipitating factor or factors; control of pain with analgesics and narcotics; treatment of fluid, electrolyte, and caloric deficits; and maintenance of morale and alleviation of fear. Vigorous carbohydrate administration (e.g., 500 g of dextrose/day through a central catheter) alone can modify or remit the attack.[14] Propranolol has been effective in reducing the tachycardia and hypertension, but it must be used cautiously in patients with hypovolemia. Intravenous hematin (solubilized crystalline heme chloride) is effective therapy in the acute porphyrias but should be used only in very ill patients and in those who have progressive neurologic manifestations.[30–32] Because of the instability of hematin in solution, phlebitis, coagulopathy, and renal failure can occur from its degradation products.[33] These problems largely have been circumvented with the more stable Finnish preparation heme-arginate, but at present, it is not available in the United States.[34] For the special circumstances of seizures and surgical anesthesia, non-barbiturate agents must be used. The better understanding of the pathogenesis of these illnesses, the advent of hematin, and modern intensive care methods have reduced sharply the morbidity and mortality from acute porphyric attacks.

Porphyria Cutanea Tarda

This most commonly encountered porphyria results from defects of uroporphyrinogen decarboxylase (URO-D), causing accumulation of uroporphyrins in hepatocytes and their eventual release into plasma and excretion in urine.[8] Clinical manifestations are limited to the skin in the form of a photosensitivity dermatosis, a consequence of the circulating uroporphyrins. Neurovisceral symptoms never occur in this porphyria; moreover, the usual, heterozygous enzyme defect is manifested clinically only in the presence of certain hepatotoxins and is silent in many persons. The skin disorder occurs spontaneously and early in life in those rare individuals who inherit homozygous defects of the URO-D enzyme (also called hepatoerythropoietic porphyria).

GENETICS. Two general forms of porphyria cutanea tarda (PCT) are distinguished, one called *sporadic* (type I) and the other *familial* (type II). The sporadic form is considered more common and was believed previously to be an acquired defect. The enzyme deficiency is detectable only in liver tissue and so far is characterized by decreased enzyme activity without a decrease of enzyme protein.[35] After treatment and remission of symptoms, the low enzyme activity reverts to normal. Recent findings indicate that this form of PCT can also be inherited, suggesting either a novel tissue-specific genetic control of the enzyme or some other heritable factor that affects the normal enzyme.[36]

Familial PCT (type II) follows dominant inheritance. In heterozygous individuals, half-normal URO-D activity is demonstrable in all tissues and results from various mutations in one of the URO-D alleles. To date, point mutations in the coding regions of the URO-D gene, but most often a splice-site mutation, have been discovered and produce an unstable or inactive enzyme protein.[37,38] In the rare homozygous individuals, residual enzyme activity has ranged from 3% to 27% of normal.[1]

CLINICAL FEATURES. The damaging effects of the excess uroporphyrin are targeted on the sun-exposed areas of the skin, such as the face and the distal extremities. Usually, there is no discomfort with sun exposure per se, and blue (visible) light only triggers an insidious cutaneous damage. Like all porphyrins, the uroporphyrin absorbs light at 400 to 410 nm (Soret band); in this excited state it not only yields its energy as fluorescence but also generates reactive oxygen species in the aerobic environment of tissues. Irradiation of uroporphyrin activates complement which promotes the release of proteases from dermal mast cells.[39] The dermal–epidermal junction becomes disrupted and leads to skin fragility and the formation of vesicles and bullae that easily rupture, and sclerodermoid changes of the skin occur due to a light–independent effect of the uroporphyrin on collagen synthesis by skin fibroblasts. The pathogenesis of the mottled hyper- and hypopigmentation and the periorbital hypertrichosis, also common in PCT, is not understood.

In most individuals with a heterozygous URO-D defect, the factors that correlate with development of the dermatosis include alcoholism with or without liver disease, and less often other forms of hepatocellular disease or estrogen ingestion.[40,41] Generous liver iron stores are another prerequisite for the clinical expression, and at least in patients with sporadic PCT, HLA-linked hemochromatosis alleles have been shown to be commonly present.[42] Occasionally, concomitant inheritance of hereditary hemochromatosis alone, after sufficient iron has been assimilated, precipitates symptoms in persons who have a URO-D defect.[43] Iron somehow plays an important part in impairing the residual enzyme activity in the hepatocytes, either through possible direct oxidant effects on the enzyme or via oxidation of uroporphyrinogen to uroporphyrin.[1,8,36] This key role of iron is shown by the uniformly successful clearance of symptoms and uroporphyrinuria with phlebotomy treatment to a de-ironed state as initiated by Ippen in 1961.[44] Patients with renal disease on hemodialysis may in time manifest the PCT clinically because of a transfusional iron overload and or because dialysis does not remove the protein-bound porphyrins from the plasma.[41]

Patients with PCT are reported to have a 100- to 200-fold risk for the development of hepatocellular carcinoma.[45,46] This may be compounded by associated cirrhosis or hepatitis. Unusual cases of benign and malignant hepatic tumors which produced uroporphyrin with typical photodermatosis that was reversed when the tumor was removable also are on record.[47] Thus, it seems prudent to perform a liver scan at the initial evaluation of patients with PCT.

DIAGNOSIS. Clinical diagnosis is confirmed by demonstrating the characteristic large excretion of uroporphyrin in urine. Usually, some excess coproporphyrin is also found, and fecal excretion of isocoproporphyrin, a by-product of the impaired URO′gen III decarboxylation, is pathognomonic of PCT.[8] It rarely is necessary to perform fecal porphyrin analysis to distinguish PCT from variegate porphyria or coproporphyria. In anuric patients, plasma porphyrin analysis confirms the diagnosis. Dermatologists also favor performance of skin biopsy to demonstrate "diagnostic" immunoglobulin and complement deposits around dermal vessels and at the dermal–epidermal junction.

TREATMENT. Removal of factors that contribute to the clinical expression of the disease (i.e., alcohol, estrogen, iron supplements) is advised, but phlebotomies of 500 ml at 1- to 2-week intervals constitute the definitive treatment. Initial serum transferrin iron saturation and ferritin values are obtained to define the iron burden present. With regular monitoring of the hemogram before bleedings, a de-ironed state is heralded by a low normal mean corpuscular volume (e.g., 80 fl), and usually 5 to 10 phlebotomies are necessary. Although further overproduction of uroporphyrin is halted thereafter the chronically accumulated hydrophilic porphyrins are released slowly from the liver. Hence, formation of new skin lesions ceases gradually, and full recovery often extends over several months to a year or more. After the de-ironing a relapse is unlikely and even indefinite in the usual patient.

Administration of chloroquine in low doses is an effective alternative treatment when phlebotomy is contraindicated. This drug forms water-soluble complexes with the porphyrins in hepatocytes, thereby aiding their removal and urinary excretion.[41] Its action also involves hepatocyte destruction. For the anemic patient with end-stage renal disease in whom the skin disorder may be particularly severe, use of recombinant erythropoietin followed by phlebotomies as necessary is preferable to the alternative, the iron chelator deferoxamine.[48]

Protoporphyria (Erythropoietic Protoporphyria)

Deficiency of the mitochondrial enzyme ferrochelatase causes the relatively common protoporphyria, and it appears to be inherited in an autosomal dominant manner.[8] Mutations of one or both alleles are being discovered[49,50] and their effects on the functional form of the enzyme as a dimer[51] may account for the enzyme activity of only 20% of normal in affected individuals. Although low enzyme activity is detectable in all tissues, protoporphyrin, the substrate of the enzyme, mainly if not exclusively accumulates in erythroid cells and does so during their last stages of maturation, when the enzyme normally becomes rate-limiting for heme production. Erythroid heme synthesis is compromised minimally in some individuals (< 30%) who carry a marginal hypochromic-microcytic anemia,[52,53] and unlike zinc protoporphyrin, which accounts as the raised red cell protoporphyrin in iron-deficiency states because ferrochelatase is not defective, the excess porphyrin here is unchelated. It is loosely bound to globin chains and diffuses out of new erythrocytes in a few days so that only the youngest circulating cells fluoresce.[54] Because of its low water solubility, the protoporphyrin is excreted exclusively through the biliary tract.

The liver appears to play a variable role in the accumulation of the porphyrin, and its contribution is not well-defined. The porphyrin deposits observed in the liver and in commonly occurring protoporphyrin gall stones may be attributed to an erythroid source alone. Hepatic heme synthesis is not known to be compromised by the enzyme defect, perhaps because the normal relative activity of hepatic ferrochelatase is the highest of all the heme synthetic enzymes.[1] Why at times, and unpredictably, an unrelenting and fatal liver disease develops in some patients by mid-life is also not understood. The erythrocyte and fecal porphyrin levels are the highest in such cases, possibly because of impaired biliary excretion of the protoporphyrin.[55,56]

The variable clinical expression of the defect is presumably in part due to heterogeneity of mutations.[49] It is unclear why obligate carriers usually show some elevations of erythrocyte, fecal protoporphyrin, or both but often no symptoms. Symptoms generally correlate with the plasma and red cell concentration of protoporphyrin, and the typical picture is an acute solar photosensitivity that nearly always begins in childhood. In contrast to the cutaneous manifestations in the other porphyrias, this patient experiences an immediate, painful burning of the skin after a short exposure to the sun as well as to unshielded fluorescent lighting. Hours later, erythema, urticaria, and edema ensue. Photoexcitation of the protoporphyrin generates reactive oxygen species that enhance hydrogen peroxide and lipid peroxide formation and thus damage cell membranes, and an inflammatory response is elicited by activation of complement and release of mediators from mast cells.[39] Fibroblast proliferation also is stimulated by the activated porphyrin and accounts for a characteristic waxy thickening of the skin.

Diagnosis is established by demonstrating high free erythrocyte and fecal protoporphyrin levels. Sunscreens and administration of the singlet oxygen scavenger β-carotene constitute the major symptomatic treatment available; the progressive liver disease has been interrupted by liver transplantation.[57]

Congenital Erythropoietic Porphyria (Gunther Disease)

Congenital erythropoietic porphyria is a very rare disorder and is inherited as an autosomal recessive trait.[8] The defect resides in the enzyme URO'gen III synthase, and several point mutations in the gene have been identified recently.[58,59] Heterozygotes have half-normal enzyme activity and no symptoms or metabolic abnormalities. A residual enzyme activity of 20% in homozygous individuals results in marked overproduction of uroporphyrin I from HMB, the substrate of the enzyme (Fig. 7.1), and is expressed visibly only in the erythron. Erythroid hyperplasia in response to associated anemia accentuates this porphyrin overproduction, and a variably severe anemia is due to an apparent dyserythropoiesis and sometimes a peripheral hemolysis. Strangely, the porphyrin is found mainly in the nuclei of developing erythroblasts and is thought to affect their maturation. The mechanism for the hemolysis has not been worked out.

The very large amounts of uroporphyrin formed and released are not only excreted but also have a predilection for bones and teeth, producing a characteristic brown staining of these tissues that fluoresce under ultraviolet light. The principal symptomatology and morbidity is from severe photodermatosis, with friability and blistering of the skin over light-exposed body regions, especially the hands and face. Constant phototoxic injury by the uroporphyrin from infancy with associated repetitive infections leads to extensive scarring, epidermal atrophy, and deformity due to mutilating resorption of acral structures such as the nose, eyelids, ear lobes, and digits. Milder phenotypes have been observed, with onset in later life, and are likely due to genetic heterogeneity of the defect although URO'gen III synthase activity is as low in these cases as in those more severe.[10]

The diagnosis is confirmed easiest by demonstrating markedly raised levels of uroporphyrin in the blood and urine. Specific assays of URO'gen III synthase activity in erythrocytes and cultured lymphocytes, fibroblasts, and amniotic fluid cells also have been developed.[8] Supportive treatment is aimed at measures to shield the skin from light and trauma, but in most cases, this is only minimally successful. Occasionally, splenectomy may be beneficial in attenuating the overproduction of porphyrin by reducing the erythroid proliferation if the hemolytic component of the disease or a hypersplenism is significant. Hypertransfusion to suppress the defec-

tive erythroid cell line is effective, and together with iron chelation, it can be proposed as the optimal current management even though it is costly and not without risk.[60] The most definitive treatment can be expected to be a normal marrow graft and, in the future, perhaps transfer of the normal gene into hematopoietic stem cells.

LEAD POISONING

An increased body lead burden mimics the porphyrias both biochemically and clinically, and cases of plumbism have been mistaken for porphyria when the source of the lead was not immediately evident. The toxic effects of lead include impairment of many, and potentially all, of the enzymes of heme biosynthesis and a neurologic syndrome of autonomic neuropathy (abdominal pain and ileus) and motor neuropathy. Only rarely has photosensitivity been reported. Evidence of renal dysfunction (lead nephropathy) also may prompt the diagnosis.

A wide and interesting array of materials has been found to be the source of inorganic lead intoxication, ranging from lodged bullets to inhaled particles of the metal in a firing range, its fumes in industries, ingested contaminated herbs and food supplements, or beverages containing lead solubilized from glazes of utensils and linings of stills.[61] Organic lead is acquired by absorption through the skin or by gasoline sniffers. Individuals heterozygous for hereditary ALA dehydratase deficiency are said to be susceptible to lower levels of lead exposure as are persons with one or both genes for the less common allele ($ALAD_2$) of the enzyme.[1] However, the clinical encounter of lead toxicity appears to be reduced as this metal is being eliminated from consumer products and occupational exposure is better monitored.

Lead is known to inhibit a variety of enzymes by displacing an essential metal or reacting with active-site thiol groups, and in high concentrations, it can denature proteins. Blockade of the enzymatic steps of heme biosynthesis by lead in vivo is evident in the accumulation and excretion of various substrate intermediates in the pathway (Table 7.3) as in the porphyrias, and these quantitatively correlate with the levels of lead present. ALA dehydratase is most sensitive to lead both in vitro and in vivo; such is the sensitivity of the dehydratase that its activity in erythrocytes as well as urinary excretion of ALA was used effectively to monitor blood lead levels in human lead poisoning before lead determinations could be easily performed. The other readily susceptible enzymatic steps are catalyzed by ferrochelatase and COPRO'gen oxidase, so increased erythrocyte protoporphyrin and urine coproporphyrin levels are found regularly in persons with chronic lead intoxication.

The lead effects on the production of heme also are interrelated with iron metabolism.[62] A reciprocal relationship exists between the intestinal absorption of iron and lead. In erythroid cells, lead limits the intracellular delivery of iron, and the surrogate metal zinc is inserted into protoporphyrin by ferrochelatase, as it is in iron deficiency. Consequently, access of the mitochondrial ferrochelatase to iron rather than the activity of the enzyme limits heme formation. These features are consistent with observations, contrary to past statements, that mitochondrial iron deposits and ring sideroblasts are uncommon in lead poisoning, if they occur at all. The ultimate manifestations in the erythron are modified by yet other effects of lead: red cell membrane ATPase is inhibited and leads to cellular loss of K^+, pyrimidine 5'-nucleotidase activity is reduced and promotes hemolysis, globin synthesis is inhibited, and erythroid hypoplasia may occur.[62]

Despite these multiple effects on erythroid cells, they cause relatively little harm in the clinical setting as anemia is usually mild.[61] It is more severe in children because of a commonly associated iron deficiency. Peripheral blood findings of lead poisoning, when present, are only suggestive abnormalities and include mild hypochromia, basophilic stippling, and nonspecific size and shape alterations. The diagnosis can be accurately surmised by measuring erythrocyte ALA dehydratase and the heme synthesis intermediates, but it is appropriately established by blood and/or urine lead determinations (Table 7.3). Occasionally, the urinary lead excretion that is enhanced by a standardized ethylenediaminetetraacetic acid infusion must be measured to fully assess a toxic lead burden. Treatment is removal of the lead source and administration of courses of intravenous calcium ethylenediaminetetraacetic acid.

TABLE 7.3. Laboratory Abnormalities in Chronic Lead Intoxication

Erythrocyte	
5-Aminolevulinate dehydratase activity	
−DTT	Low
+DTT	Normal
Protoporphyrin	High
Lead concentration (whole blood)	> 40 μg/dl
Urine	
5-Aminolevulinic acid	High
Porphobilinogen	Normal*
Uroporphyrin	Trace
Coproporphyrin	High
Lead	> 150 μg/24 h
after EDTA infusion	> 500 μg/24 h

Note: DTT = 1,4-dithiothreitol; EDTA = ethylenediaminetetraacetic acid.

  *Occasionally high.

SIDEROBLASTIC ANEMIAS

Sideroblastic anemias constitute a heterogeneous group in which the biosynthesis of heme in the developing erythroid cell is disrupted from diverse causes. As in other erythropoietic disorders of cytoplasmic or nuclear maturation (e.g., thalassemias, megaloblastic erythropoiesis), defective precursor cells are destroyed in the marrow environment (intramedullary hemolysis), and the characteristic picture of ineffective erythropoiesis, with marrow erythroid hyperplasia and peripheral reticulocytopenia, is observed. Varying proportions of defective, hypochromic, and microcytic erythrocytes are released into the circulation and there provide the initial clue to the diagnosis (Fig. 7.4A,B). The diagnostic hallmark is the ring sideroblast in the Prussian blue–stained marrow aspirate, representing an erythroblast with a perinuclear collar of iron-laden mitochondria (Fig. 7.4C,D). These siderotic mitochondria may be retained in circulating erythrocytes that denote the nearly pathognomonic siderocytes in the peripheral blood smear. On rare occasions, these diagnostic features can be masked almost completely by an associated iron deficiency from any cause (e.g., chronic blood loss), and the disorder declares itself after iron therapy.[63]

Several exogenous factors and genetic lesions of the erythroid cell line underlie both the reversible and irreversible forms of sideroblastic anemia, respectively (Table 7.4). A defective heme biosynthesis is implied in these disorders, as the pathways for globin synthesis and for iron delivery are intact. What causes this aberration is understood least in the irreversible forms; in vitro biosynthetic studies and enzyme assays of the abnormal erythroid cells, a striking erythropoietic response in some patients to pyridoxine in doses above normal daily requirements, as well as the production of characteristic sideroblastic anemia in experimental models of vitamin B_6 deprivation, all point to ALA synthase as one vulnerable site in the pathogenesis.[62,63] Alternative mechanisms may involve mitochondrial defects, because mutations in the mitochondrial genome also have been noted in the ring sideroblastic abnormality.[64] Presently, the specific types of sideroblastic anemia are defined by detailed clinical and laboratory studies.

Inherited Types

GENETICS. Hereditary sideroblastic anemia is uncommon and follows X-linked inheritance in most kindreds. Minimal expression of hematologic abnormalities is frequent in female carriers and consistent with X inactivation affecting the mutant locus of the disorder. However, in some kindreds, prominent anemia has occurred only in females, suggesting that the defect may be lethal in males during fetal development or that it is not an X-linked disorder.[65,66] In several kindreds where another known X-linked disorder also was present, the defect segregated with the anemia,[67,68] while in another with factor IX deficiency, there was discordance.[69] In a few families, the trait appeared to be transmitted in an autosomal manner.[70,71]

Together with the occurrence of isolated congenital forms of sideroblastic anemia, these varied inheritance patterns suggest a considerable spectrum of fundamental defects. Defects in erythroid-specific ALA synthase are being defined in some cases of the X-linked type and are consistent with the gene for this enzyme mapped to the X chromosome.[5] Moreover, in cases that respond to pyridoxine, activity of the bone marrow ALA synthase is consistently low,[72,73] which could imply a mutation affecting the active site or the stability of the enzyme. However, alternative defects must be proposed in the other inherited forms.

CLINICAL ASPECTS. Severity of anemia varies widely between families. A mild anemia may be discovered fortuitously, or it sometimes curiously worsens and first comes to medical attention in adulthood. The red cell indices are invariably small, and marrow erythro-

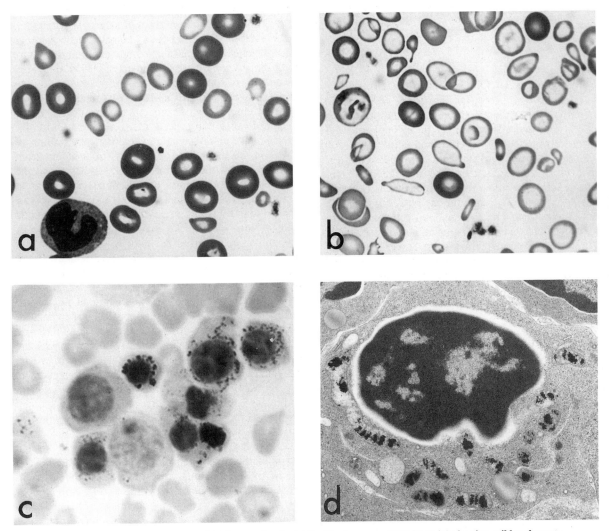

FIGURE 7.4.   The morphology in sideroblastic anemia. A and B, Blood smears (Wright stain) showing mild and severe hypochromic red cell morphology, respectively. C, A Bone marrow smear (Prussian blue stain) showing ring sideroblasts. D, Electronmicrograph of an erythroblast with iron-laden mitochondria.

TABLE 7.4.   The Classification of Sideroblastic Anemias

Hereditary
  X-linked*
  Autosomal, dominant or recessive*
  Congenital
    Isolated, inheritance undetermined*
    Associated with mitochondrial cytopathy (Pearson's
      syndrome)
Acquired
  Reversible
    Alcoholism
    Certain drugs (isoniazid, chloramphenicol)
    Copper deficiency (nutritional, zinc toxicity)
    Hypothermia
    Vitamin B_6 deprivation (in animals)
  Idiopathic acquired*
  Associated with myelodysplasia, myeloproliferative disorders,
    hematologic malignancies

*Some of these respond to pyridoxine.

blasts have poor hemoglobinization, with the ring sideroblast feature dominating the late forms of erythroid maturation. Most patients exhibit manifestations of iron overload at diagnosis; such may be evident in a hepatosplenomegaly and is documented with a high iron saturation of serum transferrin and a raised serum ferritin level. In some kindreds and some isolated congenital cases, the anemia is very responsive to variable doses of vitamin B_6, and the hemoglobin is often restored to normal. The abnormal red cell morphology usually is attenuated following such a response, but it never becomes normal. In unresponsive cases with severe anemia, transfusion therapy is necessary and predictably accelerates any prior iron overload.

Acquired Types

REVERSIBLE SIDEROBLASTIC ANEMIA. Several diverse factors are recognized that can usher in a sideroblastic anemia that is fully reversible when the cause is removed (Table 7.4). In chronic alcoholism with advanced nutritional deficits, and folate depletion in particular, a transient ring sideroblast defect is one of several features reflecting disrupted erythropoiesis (and hematopoiesis).[74,75] However, a number of studies have not provided a clear explanation for a defective heme synthesis in this setting. Isoniazid interferes with pyridoxine metabolism and impairs ALA synthase by depleting its cofactor pyridoxal phosphate; the uncommon occurrence of anemia with the use of this drug suggests an additional predisposition.[63] The reversible toxicity of chloramphenicol is associated with a ring sideroblast defect because of mitochondrial injury,[76] and this drug

preferentially inhibits mitochondrial protein synthesis in the erythroid cell line and probably secondarily also impairs ALA synthase and ferrochelatase. Copper deficiency from dietary lack[77] or inhibited absorption following megadose zinc ingestion[78] can result in severe sideroblastic anemia and is regularly accompanied by neutropenia. Copper deficiency reduces iron release from storage sites, but it also impairs iron utilization for heme synthesis in mitochondria by an unknown mechanism.[79] Interestingly, individuals with the episodic hypothermia syndrome during clinical attacks develop the ring sideroblast defect as well as thrombocytopenia;[80] these reverse after recovery, suggesting thermo-sensitive steps in the formation of heme.

IDIOPATHIC ACQUIRED SIDEROBLASTIC ANEMIA. This most-common form of sideroblastic anemia occurs later in life. It is a clonal hematopoietic disorder where a genetic change in a precursor cell imparts to its erythroid progeny a defect (or defects) that somehow selectively disrupts heme synthesis.[81] A nonrandom cytogenetic abnormality has not been found, but among a host of reported cytogenetic alterations, defects in the X chromosome have been observed.[82] In those instances, one could postulate potential aberrations of erythroid ALA synthase. However, information from crude assays of the enzyme are inconclusive, and the response of this category of sideroblastic anemias to vitamin B_6 is very unusual. A defect in iron delivery or intracellular transport in erythroblasts is not evident from in vitro studies.[83] It may be that perturbation of iron utilization occurs at the mitochondrial level, where mutations of mitochondrial DNA could produce a loss of intrinsic proteins that interferes with heme synthesis or iron pathways.[84]

The typical peripheral blood finding in this clonal disorder is a dual erythrocyte population of hypochromic-microcytic and normal or macrocytic cells. The size of the small cell population roughly correlates with the severity of anemia, but the percentage of marrow ring sideroblasts correlates poorly. The erythropoietin drive, in response to the anemia, may accelerate development and release of cells from the normal clone and account for the macrocytic cell population and attendant macrocytic red cell indices that frequently are seen. Associated dyserythropoiesis or, occasionally, a folate deficit would be alternative reasons for the macrocytosis. The extent of intramedullary destruction of the aberrant clone and the size of the persisting normal clone probably determine the severity of anemia. Over time, often years, the defective clone tends to predominate or erythroid hypoplasia may develop, and the patient becomes dependent on transfusions.[85] That the stem cell from which the sideroblastic erythropoiesis emanates is more susceptible to additional genetic change can be postulated, because a subset of patients (10%) unpredictably develops acute leukemia.[63] Other patients exhibit myeloproliferative features, and others have associated leukopenia or thrombocytopenia, with or without dysplastic features of the granulocytic and megakaryocytic cell lines, that greatly increase the risk of leukemic transformation.[86] This clinical spectrum of the disorder also provides the basis for its inclusion among the myelodysplastic syndromes.

Iron Overload in Sideroblastic Anemia

Some iron overload is usually evident at diagnosis in all the irreversible sideroblastic anemias, but more consistently so in the inherited types. The chronic or lifelong ineffective erythropoiesis alone may be sufficient to increase intestinal iron absorption and, in time, produce parenchymal iron deposition indistinguishable from hereditary hemochromatosis. Because an iron overload is not constant in all cases, either inherited or acquired, the presence of at least one allele for hereditary hemochromatosis may be another determinant. Alternatively, it has been proposed that one hemochromatosis allele may be required for the pathogenesis of some sideroblastic anemias.[87] Inappropriate ingestion of medicinal iron and necessary blood transfusions greatly accelerate the iron overload.

The iron status is initially surveyed with serum iron, serum transferrin and serum ferritin measurements. Evident iron overload should be assessed further with liver histology and liver iron quantitation for long-term management and prognosis. Evaluation of cardiac and endocrine function also is appropriate.[88]

The inevitable consequences of multiple organ damage due to the iron burden (i.e., liver cirrhosis, cardiac myopathy, endocrinopathies, and others) must be prevented by iron-removal maneuvers. If already established, they can be variably reversed.[88] Graded phlebotomies are well-tolerated and preferred in persons with mild or moderate anemia and in the absence of certain contraindications, such as heart disease or advanced age. When anemia is more severe or transfusions are given, the iron chelating agent deferoxamine must be administered; its effectiveness, long-term benefits, and safety outweigh the attendant concerns of inconvenience, cost, minimal discomfort, and minor risks until an oral iron-chelating agent becomes available.[89,90] Occasionally, anemia improves with de-ironing, although the reason for this is not understood.

REFERENCES

1. Bottomley SS, Muller-Eberhard U. Pathophysiology of heme synthesis. Semin Hematol 1988;25:282.

2. Chretien S, Dubart A, Beaupain D, et al. Alternative transcription and splicing of the human porphobilinogen deaminase gene result either in tissue-specific or in housekeeping expression. Proc Natl Acad Sci U S A 1988;85:6.

3. May BK, Bhasker CR, Bawden MJ, et al. Molecular regulation of 5-aminolevulinate synthase: diseases related to heme biosynthesis. Mol Biol Med 1990;7:405.

4. Sutherland GR, Baker E, Callen DF, et al. 5-Aminolevulinate synthase is at 3p21 and thus not the primary defect in X-linked sideroblastic anemia. Am J Hum Genet 1988;43:331.

5. Cox TC, Bawden MJ, Abraham NG, et al. Erythroid 5-aminolevulinate synthase is located on the X chromosome. Am J Hum Genet 1990;46:107.

6. Dierks P. Molecular biology of eukaryotic 5-aminolevulinate synthase. In: Dailey HA, ed. Biosynthesis of Heme and Chlorophyll. New York: McGraw-Hill, 1990:201.

7. Cox TC, Bawden MJ, Martin A, et al. Human erythroid 5-aminolevulinate synthase: promoter analysis and identification of an iron-responsive element in the mRNA. EMBO J 1991;10:1891.

8. Kappas A, Sassa S, Galbraith RA, et al. The porphyrias. In: Scriver CR, Beaudet AL, Sly WS, Valle D, eds. The Metabolic Basis of Inherited Disease. New York: McGraw-Hill, 1989:1305.

9. Nordman Y, deVerneuil H, Deyback J-C, et al. Molecular genetics of porphyrias. Ann Med 1990;22:387.

10. Delfau MH, Picat C, De Rooij F, et al. Molecular heterogeneity of acute intermittent porphyria: identification of four additional mutations resulting in the crim-negative subtype of the disease. Am Hum Genet 1991;49:421.

11. Mercelis R, Hassoun A, Verstraeten L, et al. Porphyric neuropathy and hereditary δ-aminolevulinic acid dehydratase deficiency in an adult. J Neurol Sci 1990;95:39.

12. Plewinska M, Thunnel S, Holmberg L, et al: δ-Aminolevulinate dehydratase deficient porphyria: identification of the molecular lesions in a severely affected homozygote. Am J Hum Genet 1991;49:167.

13. Ishida N, Fujita H, Fukuda Y, et al. Cloning and expression of the defective genes from a patient with δ-aminolevulinate dehydratase porphyria. J Clin Invest 1992;89:1431.

14. Stein JA, Tschudy DP. Acute intermittent porphyria: a clinical and biochemical study of 46 patients. Medicine 1970;49:1.

15. Goldberg A, Rimington C, Lochhead AC. Hereditary coproporphyria. Lancet 1967;i:632.

16. Eales M. Porphyria as seen in Cape Town: a survey of 250 patients and some recent studies. S Afr J Lab Clin Med 1963;9:151.

17. Ten Eyck FW, Martin WJ, Kernohan JW. Acute porphyria: necropsy studies in nine cases. Proc Staff Meet Mayo Clin 1961;36:409.

18. Brennan MJW, Cantwell RC. δ-Aminolevulinic acid is a potent agonist for GABA autoreceptors. Nature 1979;280:514.

19. Litman DA, Correia MA. Tryptophan: a common denominator of biochemical and neurological events of acute porphyria? Science 1983;22:1031.

20. Litman D, Correia MA. Elevated brain tryptophan and enhanced 5-hydroxytryptamine turnover in acute hepatic heme deficiency: clinical implications. J Pharm Exp Ther 1985;232:337.

21. Anderson KE, Bradlow HL, Sassa S, et al. Studies in porphyria. VII. Relationship of the 5α-reductase metabolism of steroid hormones to clinical expression of the genetic defect in acute intermittent porphyria. Am J Med 1979;66:644.

22. Anderson KE, Spitz IM, Bardin W, et al. A gonadotropin releasing hormone analogue prevents cyclical attacks of porphyria. Arch Intern Med 1990;150:1469.

23. Welland FH, Hellman ES, Gaddis EM, et al. Factors affecting the excretion of porphyrin precursors by patients with acute intermittent porphyria. I. The effect of diet. Metabolism 1964;13:232.

24. Bonkowsky HL, Magnussen CR, Collins AR, et al. Comparative effects of glycerol and dextrose on porphyrin precursor excretion in acute intermittent porphyria. Metabolism 1976;25:405.

25. Watson CJ, Bossenmaier I, Cardinal R. Acute intermittent porphyria: urinary porphobilinogen and other Ehrlich reactors in the diagnosis. JAMA 1961;175:1087.

26. Logan GM, Weimer MK, Ellefson M, et al. Bile porphyrin analysis in the evaluation of variegate porphyria. N Engl J Med 1991;324:1408.

27. Lamon JM, Frykholm BC, Tschudy DP. Family evaluations in acute intermittent porphyria using red cell uroporphyrinogan I synthase. J Med Genet 1979;16:134.

28. Bottomley SS, Bonkowsky HL, Kreimer-Birnbaum M. The diagnosis of acute intermittent porphyria. Usefulness and limitations of the erythrocyte uroporphyrinogen I synthase assay. Am J Clin Pathol 1981;76:133.

29. Lee JS, Lindsten J, Anvret M. Haplotyping of the human porphobilinogen deaminase gene in acute intermittent porphyria by polymerase chain reaction. Hum Genet 1990;84:241.

30. Dhar GJ, Bossenmaier BA, Petryka Z, et al. Effects of hematin in hepatic porphyria. Ann Intern Med 1975;83:20.

31. Watson CJ, Pierach CA, Bossenmaier I, et al. Postulated deficiency of hepatic heme and repair by hematin infusions in the "inducible" hepatic porphyrias. Proc Natl Acad Sci U S A 1977;74:2118.

32. Lamon JM, Frykholm BC, Hess RA, et al. Hematin therapy for acute porphyria. Medicine 1979;58:252.

33. Goetsch CA, Bissell DM. Instability of hematin used in the treatment of acute hepatic porphyria. N Engl J Med 1986;315:235.

34. Mustajoki P. Heme in the treatment of porphyrias and hematological disorders. Semin Hematol 1989;26:1.

35. Elder GH, DeSalamanca RE, Urquhart AJ, et al. Immunoreactive uroporphyrinogen decarboxylase in the liver in porphyria cutanea tarda. Lancet 1985;ii:229.

36. Elder GH, Roberts AG, DeSalamanca RE. Genetics and pathogenesis of human uroporphyrinogen decarboxylase defects. Clin Biochem 1989;22:163.

37. Garey JR, Hanson JL, Harrison LM, et al. A point mutation in the coding region of uroporphyrinogen decarboxylase associated with familial porphyria cutanea tarda. Blood 1989;73:892.

38. Garey JR, Harrison LM, Franklin KF, et al. Uroporphyrinogen decarboxylase: a splice site point mutation causes the deletion of exon 6 in multiple families with familial porphyria cutanea tarda. J Clin Invest 1990;86:1416.

39. Lim HW. Pathophysiology of cutaneous lesions in porphyrias. Semin Hematol 1989;26:114.

40. Grossman ME, Bickers DR, Poh-Fitzpatrick MB, et al. Porphyria cutanea tarda. Clinical features and laboratory findings in 40 patients. Am J Med 1979;67:277.

41. Pimstone NR. Porphyria cutanea tarda. Semin Liver Dis 1982;2:132.

42. Edwards CQ, Griffen LM, Goldgar DE, et al. HLA-linked hemochromatosis alleles in sporadic porphyria cutanea tarda. Gastroenterology 1989;97:972.

43. Bottomley SS. Porphyria cutanea tarda and hereditary hemochromatosis. Bollet Instit Dermatol S Gallic 1986–87;13:237.

44. Ippen VH. Allgemeinsymptome der Spaten Hautporphyrie (porphyria cutanea tarda) als Himweise fur deren Behandlung. Dtsch Med Wochenschr 1961;86:127.

45. Kordac V. Frequency of occurrence of hepatocellular carcinoma in patients with porphyria cutanea tarda in long-term follow up. Neoplasma 1972;19:135.

46. Solis JA, Betancor P, Campos R, et al. Association of porphyria cutanea tarda and primary liver cancer. J Dermatol 1982;9:131.

47. Grossman ME, Bickers DR. Porphyria cutanea tarda: a rare cutaneous manifestation of hepatic tumors. Cutis 1978;21:782.

48. Anderson KE, Goeger DE, Carson RW, et al. Erythropoietin for the treatment of porphyria cutanea tarda in a patient on long-term hemodialysis. N Engl J Med 1990;322:315.

49. Lamorie J, Boulechfar S, de Verneuil H, et al. Human erythropoietic protoporphyria: two point mutations in the ferrochelatase gene. Biochem Biophys Res Commun 1991;181:594.

50. Nakahashi Y, Fujita H, Taketani S, et al. The molecular defect of ferrochelatase in a patient with erythropoietic protoporphyria. Proc Natl Acad Sci (U S A) 1992;89:281.

51. Straka JG, Bloomer JR, Kempner ES. The functional size of ferrochelatase determined *in situ* by radiation inactivation. J Biol Chem 1991;266:24637.

52. Bottomley SS, Tanaka M, Everett MA. Diminished erythroid ferrochelatase activity in protoporphyria. J Lab Clin Med 1975;86:126.

53. Mathews-Roth MM. Anemia in erythropoietic protoporphyria. JAMA 1974;230:824.

54. Piomelli S, Lamola AA, Poh-Fitzpatrick MB, et al. Erythropoietic protoporphyria and lead intoxication. The molecular basis for differences in cutaneous photosensitivity. J Clin Invest 1975;56:1519.

55. Bloomer JR. The liver in protoporphyria. Hepatology 1988;8:402.

56. Morton KO, Schneider F, Weimer MK, et al. Hepatic and bile porphyrins in patients with protoporphyria and liver failure. Gastroenterology 1988;94:1488.

57. Bloomer JR, Weimer MK, Bossenmaier IC, et al. Liver transplantation in a patient with protoporphyria. Gastroenterology 1989;97:188.

58. Deybach J-C, deVerneuil H, Boulechfar S, et al. Point mutations in the uroporphyrinogen III synthase gene in congenital erythropoietic porphyria (Gunther's disease). Blood 1990;75:1763.

59. Warner CA, Yoo H-W, Roberts AG, et al. Congenital erythropoietic porphyria: Identification and expression of exonic mutations in the uroporphyrinogen III synthase gene. J Clin Invest 1992;89:693.

60. Piomelli S, Poh-Fitzpatrick MB, Seaman C, et al. Complete suppression of the symptoms of congenital erythropoietic porphyria by long term treatment with high level transfusions. N Engl J Med 1986;314:1029.

61. Cullen MR, Robins JM, Eskanzi B. Adult inorganic lead intoxication: presentation of 31 new cases and a review of recent advances in the literature. Medicine 1983;62:221.

62. Bottomley SS. Sideroblastic anaemia. In: Jacobs A, Worwood M, eds. Iron in Biochemistry and Medicine II. London: Academic Press, 1980:363.

63. Bottomley SS. Sideroblastic anaemia. Clin Haematol 1982;11:389.

64. Rötig A, Cormier V, Blanche S, et al. Pearson's marrow-pancreas syndrome. A multi-system mitochondrial disorder of infancy. J Clin Invest 1990;86:1601.

65. Lee GR, MacDiarmid WD, Cartwright GE, et al. Hereditary, X-linked sideroachrestic anemia. The isolation of two erythrocyte populations differing in Xg^a blood type and porphyrin content. Blood 1968;32:59.

66. Weatherall DJ, Pembrey ME, Hall EG, et al. Familial sideroblastic anaemia: problem of Xg and X chromosome inactivation. Lancet 1970;ii:744.

67. Prasad AS, Tranchida L, Konno ET, et al. Hereditary sideroblastic anemia and glucose-6-phosphate dehydrogenase deficiency in a Negro family. J Clin Invest 1968;47:1415.

68. Pagon RA, Bird TD, Detter JC, et al. Hereditary sideroblastic anaemia and ataxia: an X-linked recessive disorder. J Med Genet 1985;22:267.

69. Hast R, Miale T, Westin J, et al. Hereditary ring sideroblastic anaemia and Christmas disease in a Swedish family. Scand J Haematol 1983;30:444.

70. Kasturi J, Basha HM, Smeda SH, et al. Hereditary sideroblastic anaemia in 4 siblings of a Libyan family: autosomal inheritance. Acta Haematol 1982;68:321.

71. Van Waveren Hogervorst GD, von Roermund HCP, Snijders PJ. Hereditary sideroblastic anaemia and autosomal inheritance of erythrocyte dimorphism in a Dutch family. Eur J Haematol 1987;38:405.

72. Aoki Y, Maranaka S, Nakabayashi K, et al. 5-Aminolevulinic acid synthetase in erythroblasts of patients with pyridoxine-responsive anemia. J Clin Invest 1979;64:1196.

73. Bottomley SS, Healy HM, Brandenburg MA, et al. 5-Aminolevulinate synthase in sideroblastic anemias: mRNA and enzyme activity levels in bone marrow cells. Am J Hematol 1992;41:76.

74. Eichner ER, Hillman RS. The evolution of anemia in alcoholic patients. Am J Med 1971;50:218.

75. Pierce HI, McGuffin RG, Hillman RS. Clinical studies of alcoholic sideroblastosis. Arch Intern Med 1976;136:283.

76. Yunis AA. Chloramphenicol toxicity: 25 years of research. Am J Med 1989;87(3N):44.

77. Zidar BL, Shadduck RK, Zeigler Z, et al. Observations on the anemia and neutropenia of human copper deficiency. Am J Hematol 1977;3:177.

78. Broun ER, Greist A, Tricot G, et al. Excessive zinc ingestion. A reversible cause of sideroblastic anemia and bone marrow depression. JAMA 1990;264:1441.

79. Williams DM, Loukopoulos D, Lee GR, et al. Role of copper in mitochondrial iron metabolism. Blood 1976;48:77.

80. O'Brien H, Amess JAL, Mollin DL. Recurrent thrombocytopenia, erythroid hypoplasia and sideroblastic anaemia associated with hypothermia. Br J Haematol 1982;51:451.

81. Prchal JT, Throckmorton DW, Carroll AJ, et al. A common progenitor for human myeloid and lymphoid cells. Nature 1978;274:590.

82. DeWald GW, Brecher M, Travis LB, et al. Twenty-six patients with hematologic disorders and X chromosome abnormalities: frequent (X)(q13) chromosomes and Xq13 anomalies associated with pathologic ring sideroblasts. Cancer Genet Cytogenet 1989;42:173.

83. Bottomley SS. The spectrum and role of iron overload in sideroblastic anemia. Ann N Y Acad Sci 1988;526:331.

84. Linnane AW, Ozawa T, Marzuki S, et al. Mitochondrial DNA mutations as an important contributor to ageing and degenerative diseases. Lancet 1989;ii:642.

85. Cazzola M, Barosi G, Gobbi PG, et al. Natural history of idiopathic refractory sideroblastic anemia. Blood 1988;71:305.

86. Gattermann N, Aul C, Schneider W. Two types of acquired sideroblastic anaemia (AISA). Br J Haematol 1990;74:45.

87. Cartwright GE, Edwards CQ, Skolnick MH, et al. Association of HLA-linked hemochromatosis with idiopathic sideroblastic anemia. J Clin Invest 1980;65:989.

88. Schafer AI, Rabinowe S, LeBoff MS, et al. Long-term efficacy of desferrioxamine iron chelation therapy in adults with acquired transfusional iron overload. Arch Intern Med 1985;145:1217.

89. Hoffbrand AV, Wonke B. Results of long-term subcutaneous desferrioxamine therapy. Bailliere's Clin Haematol 1989;2:345.

90. Brittenham GM. Iron chelating agents. In: Brain MC, Carbone PP, eds. Current Therapy in Hematology-Oncology-3. Toronto: B. C. Decker, 1988:149.

91. Bloomer JR, Bonkovsky HL. The porphyrias. Dis Mon 1989;35:1.

8

Erythrocytosis and Polycythemia

Maura J. McGuire, M.D., and Jerry L. Spivak, M.D.

Under normal circumstances, the red cell mass is maintained within narrow limits (28 ± 3 ml/kg for men and 25 ±3 ml/kg for women) and is relatively constant. The production of red cells is regulated by erythropoietin, a 30,400-d glycoprotein hormone produced mainly by the kidneys in adults. The production of erythropoietin appears to be mediated primarily by the tissue oxygen demand, although because of its important regulatory functions, erythropoietin is never absent from plasma, even in the anephric state or with extreme erythrocytosis. While the usual serum level of this hormone is 4 to 26 mU/ml, this level increases substantially in the setting of hypoxia.

Erythrocytosis may occur either as a primary disorder, as in polycythemia vera (where an increased red cell mass develops independently of erythropoietin), or as a secondary event due to increased erythropoietin production, as in hypoxic states. Secondary erythrocytosis also can occur because of inappropriate production of erythropoietin by certain tumors. In all of these situations, if the red cell mass exceeds a certain limit, systemic oxygen transport actually declines owing to increased blood viscosity (Fig. 8.1). An elevated blood viscosity also can occur in certain "stress" states in which the hematocrit is elevated due to a reduction in plasma volume rather than to an absolute increase in red cell mass. The pathophysiology, diagnosis, and management of these conditions are the subjects of this chapter.

OXYGEN TRANSPORT AND ERYTHROCYTE PHYSIOLOGY

The principle function of blood is to deliver oxygen from the lungs to the tissues. Because body oxygen stores are only 20 ml/kg while basal metabolic processes consume 4 ml/kg/min of oxygen, adequate and continuous oxygen transport is vital. Oxygen transport is dependent on the red cell mass and the oxygen affinity of hemoglobin as well as on cardiopulmonary factors, regional blood flow, and ambient tissue oxygen tension. Transient changes in oxygen demand can be effected by changes in minute ventilation, cardiac output, and blood-flow redistribution, as well as by changes in hemoglobin-oxygen affinity within the internal milieu of the erythrocyte.[1–3]

The oxygen affinity of normal hemoglobin is affected by pH in the range of 6.0 to 8.5, such that increased acidity reduces oxygen affinity; this results in increased oxygen delivery in tissues where elevated P_{CO_2} produces an acid environment. Hemoglobin-oxygen affinity is also regulated by 2,3-diphosphoglycerate (2,3-DPG), which is present in red cells in an amount equimolar to hemoglobin.[4] When 2,3-DPG binds to hemoglobin, its oxygen affinity is reduced and tissue oxygen delivery enhanced. Synthesis of 2,3-DPG is enhanced in states of respiratory alkalosis, making this an important adaptive mechanism inhypoxic states where hyperventilation is usually the rule.

Figure 8.2 shows the relationship of the red cell mass to arterial oxygen saturation, and the relationship of red cell mass to arterial oxygen tension is shown in Figure 8.3. While the red cell mass varies directly with the arterial oxygen saturation, the oxygen tension (P_{O_2}) must fall below 67 mm Hg before an elevation in the red cell mass occurs.[5] Arterial oxygen saturation thus is a better measure of tissue hypoxia in assessing the appropriateness of an elevated red cell mass; an arterial

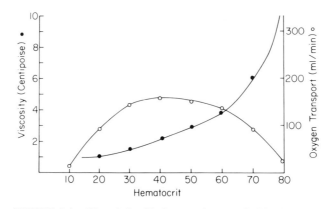

FIGURE 8.1. The relationship between hematocrit, blood viscosity, and oxygen transport. *Source:* Pirofsky 1953[111] and Murray 1965[6]

oxygen saturation of greater than 92% in the setting of an elevated red cell mass suggests erythrocytosis is inappropriate.[6] With standard blood gas analysis, the arterial oxygen tension (Pao_2) and pH are measured directly, and the arterial oxygen saturation is calculated from a standard oxygen-hemoglobin dissociation curve (Fig. 8.4). However, the calculated oxygen saturation may be inaccurate in the settings of a high oxygen-affinity hemoglobin, severe hypoxia, or carbon monoxide intoxication. Because carbon monoxide binds hemoglobin with 230 times the avidity of oxygen, a Pco of only 0.4 mm Hg will cause half the blood hemoglobin to be saturated with carbon monoxide instead of oxygen.[7] Thus, arterial oxygen saturation (Sao_2) should be measured directly by oximetry when evaluating erythrocytosis.

Oxygen transport also is affected by blood viscosity, as shown in Figure 8.1. Oxygen transport declines at hematocrits above 45% to 50%, and it declines rapidly as the hematocrit exceeds 60%. A reduction in hematocrit in men with polycythemia to a level of 45%, or 42% in women, generally will enhance oxygen delivery, particularly to the brain.[8]

THE PHYSIOLOGY OF ERYTHROPOIETIN

Erythropoietin is the principle hormone regulating the production of red blood cells. The gene for human erythropoietin has been localized to human chromosome 7 (7q11–22)[9] and consists of a single copy with five exons encoding a 193–amino acid peptide; a 27–amino acid N-terminal leader sequence is cleaved, leaving an active peptide with 166 amino acids and a predicted MW of 18,400 d.[10] Erythropoietin is heavily glycosylated. Purified human urinary erythropoietin, and a recombinant form produced in Chinese hamster ovary cells, has an observed MW of 30,400 d in the sodium dodecyl sulfate-polyacrylamide gel electrophoresis technique corresponding to a carbohydrate content of 30% to 40%.[11–13] The carbohydrate content is essential for secretion from the cell, survival in the circulation, and biological activity. Desialated recombinant erythropoietin is rapidly cleared from the circulation and metabolized in liver,[14] while incompletely glycosylated erythropoietin is retained intracellularly or has reduced bioactivity.[15]

Approximately 90% of circulating erythropoietin is produced in the kidneys, and smaller amounts are

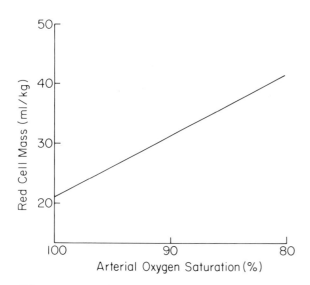

FIGURE 8.2. The relationship between red cell mass and arterial oxygen saturation. *Source:* Weil et al. 1968[5]

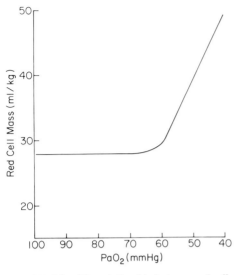

FIGURE 8.3. **The relationship between red cell mass and arterial oxygen tension.** *Source:* **Weil et al. 1968[5]**

appear to affect the rate of hormone production in the cells that produce it constitutively.[23] Erythropoietin production in the liver occurs primarily in hepatocytes but also in a population of as yet undefined interstitial cells. Hepatic erythropoietin production appears to require a greater degree of hypoxia for its initiation and, in contrast to kidney production, does not occur in an all-or-none fashion.[24] Rather, the hepatocytes around central veins appear to regulate their erythropoietin production according to the level of tissue hypoxia.

Erythropoietin only interacts with cells that have receptors for it. Such receptors in humans have been identified only on committed erythroid progenitor cells, but erythropoietin is not the only growth factor that interacts with erythroid progenitor cells. Early erythroid progenitor cells are affected by granulocyte-macrophage colony-stimulating factors, interleukin-3, and interleukin-9,[25–27] but for late erythroid progenitor cells, only erythropoietin appears to be obligatory for maturation. As they mature, these cells lose their erythropoietin receptors so that mature red cells are not influenced by the hormone.

When the supply of oxygen exceeds the demand, as in autonomous erythrocytosis, the production of erythropoietin is reduced, the rate of red cell production falls, and the red cell mass decreases. If, however, oxygen demand exceeds supply and the deficit cannot be corrected by circulatory, respiratory, or red cell metabolic changes, there is an increase in erythropoietin production, followed by increased erythropoiesis and an increased red cell mass.

synthesized in liver.[16–18] Under normal circumstances, erythropoietin is produced constitutively by peritubular interstitial cells in the inner cortex of the kidney[19–21] which appear to contain the renal oxygen sensor as well. The oxygen sensor seems to be a heme protein that controls the expression of erythropoietin mRNA in an unknown fashion.[22] Anemia or hypoxia recruit additional cells to synthesize erythropoietin, but they do not

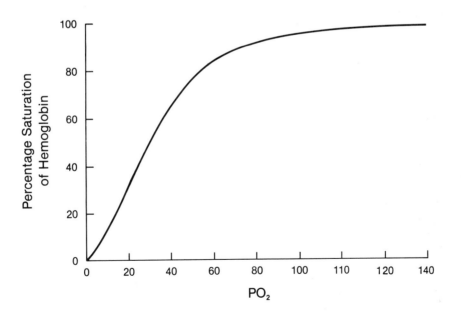

FIGURE 8.4. **The oxygen-hemoglobin dissociation curve.**

Exposure to hypobaric hypoxia results in a detectable increase in circulating erythropoietin within 2 hours,[28] but the increased production is not sustained unless the hypoxia is severe.[29–31] However, an elevation in the red cell mass can occur and be maintained after erythropoietin levels have fallen into the normal range.[29] Because hypoxia also leads to changes in minute ventilation, heart rate, tissue blood flow, and reduces hemoglobin-oxygen affinity by increasing production of 2,3-DPG, thus enhancing tissue oxygen delivery, tissue oxygen demands may be met by immediate adaptive mechanisms without triggering sustained erythropoietin elevation. It is worth noting also that nonsustained periodic episodes of hypoxia can cause an increase in the red cell mass, as seen in patients with the sleep apnea syndrome[32] or the supine hypoventilation syndrome.[33]

If other mechanisms of compensating for hypoxia are ineffective, elevation of erythropoietin production will be sustained, leading first to an increase in the total erythroid progenitor cell pool and ultimately to an increase in the red cell mass. If the elevation in the red cell mass corrects the tissue hypoxia, erythropoietin production will decline and the plasma erythropoietin level fall into the normal range, though it will probably remain slightly higher than the basal rate for that particular patient. This slight increase in production will be sufficient to maintain the elevated red cell mass. The ability of the kidneys to produce erythropoietin in response to tissue hypoxia also will be greater than expected.[34]

THE CAUSES OF A HIGH HEMATOCRIT

Spurious Erythrocytosis

Table 8.1 shows the various causes of an elevated hematocrit. This can result either from an increased red cell mass or from a reduction in plasma volume; spurious erythrocytosis, also known as relative or benign erythrocytosis, or Geisbock syndrome, is characterized by a chronically elevated hematocrit in the presence of an elevated or normal red cell mass and a reduced plasma volume. It is associated most commonly with cigarette smoking,[35,36] although it also may be induced by hypertension, alcohol, diuretic use, or hypoaldosteronism.[37–39] Spurious erythrocytosis is the diagnosis in the majority of patients who present for evaluation of an elevated hematocrit.[40]

At least in the setting of tobacco abuse, spurious erythrocytosis appears to result from chronic carbon monoxide intoxication. Carbon monoxide avidly occupies oxygen-binding sites on hemoglobin, reducing the amount of oxygen that can be bound, shifting the oxygen-hemoglobin dissociation curve to the left, and

TABLE 8.1. The Causes of a High Hematocrit

Relative or spurious erythrocytosis
  Hemoconcentration secondary to dehydration (diarrhea, diaphoresis, diuretics, deprivation of water, emesis, ethanol), hypertension, pre-eclampsia, pheochromocytoma, carbon monoxide intoxication
Absolute erythrocytosis: hypoxia
  Carbon monoxide intoxication
  High oxygen-affinity hemoglobin
  High altitude
  Pulmonary disease
  Supine hypoventilation syndrome
  Sleep apnea syndrome
  Right-to-left cardiac shunts
  Neurologic defects (respiratory center dysfunction)
Renal disease
  Cysts, hydronephrosis
  Renal artery stenosis
  Focal glomerulonephritis
  Renal transplantation
Tumors
  Hypernephroma, Wilms tumor
  Hepatoma
  Cerebellar hemangioblastoma
  Uterine fibromyoma
  Adrenal tumors
  Pheochromocytoma
Androgen therapy
Bartter syndrome
Familial erythrocytosis (with normal hemoglobin function)
Polycythemia vera

reducing oxygen unloading in the tissues. It also suppresses 2,3-DPG production[41] and causes, for unknown reasons, a diminution in plasma volume.[32] In addition, there usually is an elevation in red cell mass if the hypoxia due to carbon monoxide intoxication is severe.[36]

Although the term *benign polycythemia* has been used to describe this condition, there is an increased incidence of thromboembolic events,[35,42] and in one series, a mortality rate 6 times greater than expected for unaffected individuals of the same age was observed.[42] Although efforts in the treatment of this condition should be directed at correcting any underlying disorder and smoking cessation, phlebotomy of symptomatic patients will correct the abnormalities of plasma volume and red cell mass, reduce blood viscosity, and improve the delivery of oxygen to the tissues.

Hypoxic Erythrocytosis

Hypoxic erythrocytosis encompasses a variety of conditions in which erythropoietin is appropriately produced in response to impaired tissue oxygenation, resulting in an elevated red cell mass.

Hypobaric Hypoxia

Exposure to high altitudes produces acute changes in minute ventilation, heart rate, and hemoglobin-oxygen affinity as described earlier. It also causes a transient elevation in serum erythropoietin. Erythropoietin eventually falls to normal levels unless hypoxia is extreme,[31] but the red cell mass and hematocrit will increase because of expansion of the erythroid progenitor pool as a consequence of the initial erythropoietin elevation. It appears that normal levels of the hormone can sustain this pool once it has been expanded by the initial elevation in erythropoietin production.

Concomitant with these changes, there is a reduction in plasma volume.[43] Other adaptive changes that occur with sustained altitude exposure include an increased lung volume and capillary density.[3] For unknown reasons, a blunted respiratory response to hypoxia develops in some patients[44,45] that results in chronic mountain sickness, a state of symptomatic hyperviscosity in which the red cell mass far exceeds that expected for the degree of hypobaric hypoxia.[46]

Chronic Pulmonary Disease

Hypoxia occurring during chronic lung disease represents a less-homogenous picture than hypobaric hypoxia, because the erythrocytosis expected for the degree of hypoxia is not always present. In part, this is because patients often present with complicating illnesses that can impair erythropoiesis. In general, however, patients with impaired pulmonary function and elevated hematocrit demonstrate the expected correlation between red cell mass and arterial oxygen saturation. Two special situations in which hypoxic erythrocytosis can develop without evidence of overt pulmonary disease are the sleep apnea syndrome and supine hypoventilation; both cause only intermittent hypoxia but result in red cell mass elevation.[32,33,47] These two conditions should be considered in the differential diagnosis of erythrocytosis, because routine measurements of pulmonary function may not reveal their presence.

Cyanotic Congenital Heart Disease

Congenital heart disease with right-to-left shunting and poor blood oxygenation is a predictable cause of erythrocytosis. Because erythrocytosis usually compensates for arterial oxygen desaturation, serum erythropoietin is normal in these patients.[48] Phlebotomy, however, will result in a marked increase in erythropoietin. These patients frequently have hemostatic abnormalities with low fibrinogen and platelet counts,[49–51] but strokes appear to be uncommon.[52] Hematologic management of these patients can be complicated,[53] but phlebotomy often produces symptomatic improvement, probably because of improved cerebral blood flow.[54,55]

High Oxygen-Affinity Hemoglobin

High oxygen-affinity hemoglobins that are unable to unload oxygen to the tissues at venous oxygen tension are an uncommon but interesting cause of erythrocytosis. The first high-affinity hemoglobin, hemoglobin Chesapeake, was identified in an 81-year-old man being evaluated for angina pectoris.[56] Since then, more than 40 of these variants have been described. Affected patients are heterozygous individuals with approximately 40% abnormal hemoglobin.[57]

A high oxygen-affinity hemoglobin should be suspected in patients with elevated red cell mass and a family history of erythrocytosis or thrombosis.[58] Because these hemoglobins often have a normal electrophoretic mobility due to the internal location of the amino acid substitution, a hemoglobin P-50 determination is required to establish this diagnosis; Po_2 and calculated oxygen saturation will, of course, be normal and do not reflect the tissue hypoxia that is present.

Inappropriate Erythropoietin Secretion

RENAL DISEASE. Because the kidneys are the major site of erythropoietin production, renal disease may cause erythrocytosis as well as anemia. A number of renal conditions, including cystic renal disease,[59] renal transplantation,[60] focal glomerulonephritis,[61,62] and renal artery stenosis,[63] have been documented to cause erythrocytosis.

Although it seems that an interruption of renal blood flow should result in tissue hypoxia and stimulate the production of erythropoietin, experimental constriction of the renal artery in animals does not stimulate erythropoietin production to the same extent as induced anemia.[64] While it has been suggested that erythrocytosis in the setting of hypertension may be a clue to the presence of renal artery stenosis,[65] primary hypertension may result in relative erythrocytosis because of a reduction in plasma volume, and renal artery stenosis accounts for erythrocytosis in only a few patients.

Patients with polycystic renal disease maintain higher hematocrits than patients with other forms of renal disease,[59,66–68] and acquired renal cysts in patients undergoing hemodialysis are associated with erythrocytosis.[69] In autosomal dominant polycystic kidney disease, interstitial cells external to the cysts appear to be the site of erythropoietin production.[59] Hydronephrosis is associated with erythrocytosis, possibly because of tissue hypoxia resulting from increased pressure in the kidney.[70] Focal glomerulonephritis, with or without nephrotic syndrome, may be complicated by erythrocytosis,[61,62] although anemia frequently develops as the disease progresses. Also, Bartter syndrome is an unusual cause of erythrocytosis.[71,72]

While successful renal transplantation is associated with restoration of renal function and amelioration of anemia, 9% to 17% of patients develop erythrocytosis for unclear reasons.[60,73,74] The onset varies from 3 to 90 months after transplantation, with a peak at 12 months, and may be transient or persistent. The posttransplant kidney appears to respond to the usual stimuli regulating erythropoietin production. A biphasic change in plasma erythropoietin levels appears to occur in uncomplicated renal transplantation, with an initial transient rise in the postoperative period and a smaller but more sustained increase that is associated with recovery of graft function.[73] While erythropoietin levels return to normal as the hematocrit rises above 32%, a persistent elevation of serum erythropoietin was noted in patients who developed erythrocytosis or were iron deficient. Acute graft rejection appears to be associated with falling erythropoietin levels,[60,74,75] although in chronic graft rejection, elevated levels are often observed.[75] An elevated erythropoietin level, however, is not an unequivocal indicator of graft rejection; more likely it is a sign of a healthy graft unless erythrocytosis is present.

A review of risk factors in 53 patients with post–renal transplantation erythrocytosis implicated smoking, diabetes mellitus, and a rejection-free course but not rejection, renal artery stenosis, or obstruction.[60] Another study implicated diuretic therapy as a cause of apparent erythrocytosis.[76] It has been postulated that the native kidneys may resume normal endocrine function, which may result in erythrocytosis with correction of uremia,[77,78] but the physiologic basis of the erythrocytosis that develops in some patients remains unclear. The type of transplant, whether cadaveric or living donor, does not appear to be a factor.

ECTOPIC PRODUCTION OF ERYTHROPOIETIN.

A number of tumors secrete erythropoietin, causing an elevation in the red cell mass and symptomatic erythrocytosis.[79] Table 8.2 lists the tumors most commonly associated with erythropoietin production and prominently includes tumors of the kidneys and liver, the organs where erythropoietin is produced. In renal cell

TABLE 8.2. Tumors Associated with Inappropriate Production of Erythropoietin

Tumor	Characteristics
Hypernephroma	More common in men. Erythrocyte sedimentation rate is often elevated. Associated with von Hippel-Lindau disease.
Wilms tumor	
Renal adenoma	
Undifferentiated renal carcinoma	
Hepatoma	More common in men. Increase in plasma volume may obscure the elevated red cell mass.
Liver hamartoma	
Cerebellar hemangioblastoma	More common in men. Metastases can be confused with those of a hypernephroma. Associated with von Hippel-Lindau disease.
Uterine fibromyoma	Tumor extracts (only from very large tumors) contain erythropoietic activity.
Pheochromocytoma	Rare. Spurious elevation of the hematocrit can occur because of decreased plasma volume. Associated with von Hippel-Lindau disease.
Adrenal adenoma or hemangioblastoma	Associated with von Hippel-Lindau disease.
Paraganglioma	

Source: Thorling 1972[79]

carcinoma, the tumor has been demonstrated to be the site of erythropoietin production,[80] but because only a few studies of presumed ectopic production of erythropoietin have used sensitive and specific assays, the consistency of its elevation in these conditions is unknown. An elevated serum erythropoietin level in the absence of hypoxia should prompt evaluation for an ectopic source of hormone production.

FAMILIAL ERYTHROCYTOSIS. Several cases of familial erythrocytosis presumed due to defects in erythropoietin regulation have been reported.[58,81,82] Some studies suggest there may be a defect in erythropoietin production in certain families; in others, there may be a defect at the level of the erythroid progenitor cell.[83,84] Other family cohorts with erythrocytosis have red cell enzyme abnormalities.[85]

POLYCYTHEMIA VERA

Polycythemia vera is a clonal disorder of a pluripotent hematopoietic stem cell, marked by an increase in the production of phenotypically normal red cells, white cells, and platelets. It is an uncommon disorder of middle-aged and elderly people, with an incidence of 0.6 to 1.8 per 100,000. There is a slight predominance of males, and the mean age of onset is 60 years. Familial forms of polycythemia vera have been identified.[86,87] The cause of polycythemia vera is unknown, but the increase in blood cell production appears to be autonomous.[88]

In women with polycythemia vera and glucose-6-phosphate dehydrogenase deficiency, it has been possible to study the behavior of the abnormal clone. Early in the illness, hematopoietic progenitor cells from normal and abnormal clones co-exist; however, within the circulation, only progeny from the abnormal clone are found.[89] This suggests that proliferation of normal cells is inhibited relative to that of the mutant line.[90]

The symptoms of patients with polycythemia are similar to those seen with other forms of erythrocytosis (with the exception of pruritus), especially after a warm bath or shower, and the symptoms associated with splenomegaly, which occurs in 75% of patients. The symptoms of polycythemia also include those of secondary gout, which develops in about 10 percent of patients. Other findings on physical examination include hepatomegaly in about 30% of patients, plethora, ruddy cyanosis, fundal vein engorgement, and systolic hypertension.

Along with an elevated hematocrit, leukocytosis (which can be substantial) with an orderly shift to the left is found in 40% of patients, thrombocytosis in 60%, reticulocytosis in 50%, elevation of leukocyte alkaline phosphatase in 70%, histaminemia in 90%, and an elevated vitamin B_{12} level in 30%.[91] Hyperuricemia is seen in about 40% of patients.[92] Red cell morphology is normal unless hemorrhage or phlebotomy have caused iron deficiency, but morphologically bizarre platelets may be seen. Blood basophil levels are often increased,[91] and bone marrow aspiration is not required to make the diagnosis and is normal except for hypercellularity and absence of stainable iron. Bone marrow scanning reveals extension of active marrow into long bones.[93]

The diagnosis of polycythemia vera is based on criteria adopted in 1968 by the Polycythemia Vera Study Group,[91] which are listed in Table 8.3. Diagnosis is made if all three category A parameters are met or if any two category B parameters are met in conjunction with elevated red cell mass and arterial oxygen saturation above 92%. Because peptic ulcer disease is common in patients with polycythemia vera, iron deficiency anemia may initially mask the diagnosis. While the diagnosis of polycythemia vera may be a relatively simple matter in patients with elevated red cell mass who present with leukocytosis, thrombocytosis, and organomegaly, there is no specific diagnostic test for this disorder; in many cases, the diagnosis may not be obvious early in the course of the illness.

TABLE 8.3. Criteria for the Diagnosis of Polycythemia Vera

Category A
1) Total red cell mass
   Male $\geq$ 36 ml/kg
   Female $\geq$ 32 ml/kg
2) Arterial oxygen saturation $\geq$ 92%
3) Splenomegaly

Category B
1) Thrombocytosis (platelets $> 400 \times 10^3$ μl)
2) Leukocytosis (white blood cells $> 12 \times 10^3$/μl)
3) Increased leukocyte alkaline phosphatase score
4) Serum vitamin $B_{12} > 900$ pg/ml or vitamin B_{12}–binding capacity > 2200 pg/ml

Source: Berlin 1975[91]
Note: Polycythemia vera is diagnosed when the parameters A1, A2, and A3, or A1 and A2 and any two from category B are met. However, it must be understood that polycythemia vera is a clonal disorder and the criteria listed above are only phenotypic.

Polycythemia vera is associated with decreased life expectancy because of complications and the natural history of the illness. The major complication of polycythemia vera is hyperviscosity due to the elevated red blood cell mass, and this may result in thrombophlebitis; pulmonary or myocardial infarction; stroke; or splenic, portal, or hepatic vein thrombosis. Paradoxically, hemorrhage can also occur as well, and it is estimated that almost 50% of deaths from polycythemia vera result from thrombosis or bleeding. The risk of surgical bleeding or thrombosis appears to be less once the red cell mass has been normalized,[94] but unfortunately, many physicians do not appreciate that a hematocrit of 50% may be associated with a substantial increase in red cell mass in patients with polycythemia vera.[91] As a consequence, thrombotic events are all too common in this disease.

In some patients, the disease enters a "spent" phase, characterized by increasing anemia and often the development of myelofibrosis and myeloid metaplasia,[95] and in these patients, the need to transfuse replaces the need for phlebotomy. A small number of untreated patients develop acute leukemia, but leukemia actually is uncommon unless the patient has been treated with alkylating agents or radioactive phosphorus.[96,97]

The initial treatment of polycythemia vera is phlebotomy to reduce the hematocrit to a level below 45% in men (hemoglobin 15 g%) and 42% in women (hemoglobin 12 g%), thus reducing the source of hyperviscosity and its complications. After reducing the red cell mass, the goal of long-term treatment is to retard autonomous red cell proliferation so that the state of erythrocytosis and hyperviscosity does not recur. This is most safely accomplished by using phlebotomy to a state of iron deficiency, thus reducing the capacity for red cell proliferation; once a state of iron deficiency has been attained, phlebotomies may be required only every 3 or 4 months. It is never the case that the erythrocytosis of polycythemia cannot be controlled by phlebotomy.

The excess thrombotic morbidity noted by the Polycythemia Vera Study Group in patients treated with phlebotomy alone was due to the target hematocrit of 52% used in the initial study. This is higher than the recommended level of 42% to 45% that is felt to minimize hyperviscosity; thus, the thrombotic tendency in these patients was not maximally treated.

Pharmacologic therapies, mainly phosphorus 32 and myelosuppressive agents, have been used in treatment of the disease, but a study undertaken by the Polycythemia Vera Study Group showed these agents to be leukemogenic.[97] Between 1967 and 1985, 431 patients were assigned randomly to receive phlebotomy versus treatment with phosphorus 32 or chlorambucil.[97] The median survival of the phlebotomized group was 13.9 years, compared with 11.8 years for the group receiving phosphorus 32 and 8.9 years for the chlorambucil group. However, these differences were not statistically significant. Leukemia developed in 10.3% of the phosphorus 32 group, 13.5% of the chlorambucil group, but only 1.5% of the phlebotomy group. Thus, alkylating agents are not indicated to control the red cell mass in polycythemia vera.

Hydroxyurea may be useful to control splenomegaly, pruritus, or erythrocytosis when phlebotomy is technically unfeasible.[98] There has been much speculation concerning the theoretic risk of thrombosis due to the elevated platelet count seen in polycythemia vera, but no controlled study has ever documented any adverse consequences of thrombocytosis in these patients.[99,100] In fact, thrombocytosis appears to be a risk factor for bleeding and not for thrombosis, and it is well-documented that aspirin may enhance the risk of bleeding in patients with polycythemia vera.[101] Indeed, the only indication for aspirin in these patients is the presence of erythromelalgia.[102] Until a more effective and less hazardous therapy is found, phlebotomy remains the treatment of choice to control the red cell mass in polycythemia vera; thrombocytosis in the asymptomatic patient requires no therapy.[103] Also, it is a myth that the induction of iron deficiency by phlebotomy to control erythrocytosis either increases blood viscosity[104] or impairs functional aerobic performance.[105]

THE DIAGNOSIS AND TREATMENT OF ERYTHROCYTOSIS

Clinical Evaluation

Symptoms commonly encountered with erythrocytosis include headaches, dizziness, weakness, tinnitus, and visual disturbances. Pruritus is distinctly suggestive of polycythemia vera, and a history of smoking, drug, alcohol, or medication use (including over-the-counter agents) should be obtained. A family history may suggest an inherited hemoglobin abnormality or familial renal disease, and physical examination may reveal plethora, venous engorgement, or hypertension. Marked obesity, lung disease, heart murmurs, renal bruits, organomegaly, and neurologic findings may focus the evaluation further. Routine laboratory evaluation should include a complete blood count, electrolytes including blood urea nitrogen and creatinine, and urinalysis. Evaluation of a peripheral blood smear always should be done.

Laboratory and Diagnostic Tests

In this era of automated chemistry and hematologic profiles, most elevated hematocrits are detected in asymptomatic patients and, as stated previously, most will have a normal red cell mass. Figure 8.5 shows a decision-tree analysis of an approach to the diagnosis of erythrocytosis, and Table 8.4 shows the costs of the various tests and procedures used to evaluate erythrocytosis.

In an asymptomatic patient with mildly elevated hematocrit (< 54%) and no other hematologic or chemical abnormalities, the likelihood of erythrocytosis is low, and evaluation for common causes of spurious erythrocytosis is indicated.[40] If these are found, the patient should be counseled about smoking and ethanol use, and diuretics should be stopped if possible. If the hematocrit remains elevated despite these maneuvers, a red cell mass should be performed. A normal red cell mass suggests a diagnosis of spurious erythrocytosis, and if the red cell mass indicates true erythrocytosis, a serum erythropoietin level and arterial oxygen saturation should be determined. An elevated erythropoietin level with a normal oxygen saturation requires evaluation for ectopic hormone production, and if the oxygen saturation is reduced, primary pulmonary disease should be considered.

Polycythemia vera is diagnosed based on the criteria shown in Table 8.3. Even after a thorough evaluation, the etiology of erythrocytosis in many cases may remain unclear. Phlebotomy should be considered in every patient with an elevated red cell mass, even if the cause is uncertain.

RED CELL MASS. Red cell mass is determined by isotope dilution. An aliquot of the patient's red cells is tagged with chromium 51 and allowed to equilibrate with the patients cells. Plasma volume can be measured similarly with radiolabelled albumin. Because an elevated red cell mass can be associated with hyperviscos-

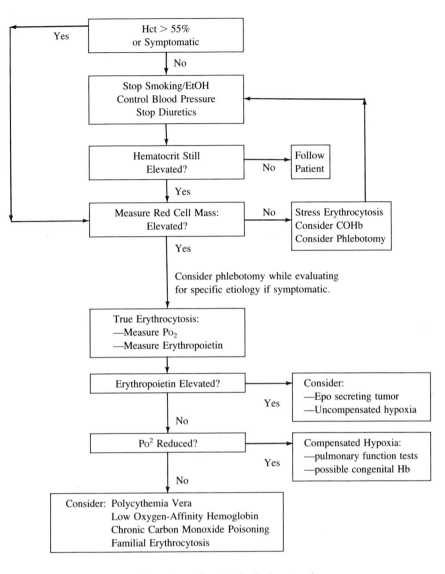

FIGURE 8.5. **Evaluation of persistent elevation in the hematocrit.**

ity, particularly if splenomegaly is present, adequate time for mixing of the labelled cells with the blood pool should be allowed.

THE MEASUREMENT OF ERYTHROPOIETIN. Sensitive and specific radioimmunoassays for serum erythropoietin levels are available and allow precise measurement of this hormone. Low to normal levels may be seen in polycythemia vera, but levels are normal in most patients with erythrocytosis. Because erythrocytosis suppresses erythropoietin production unless tissue hypoxia is severe, a normal or even low erythropoietin level does not exclude hypoxia as a cause for erythrocy-

tosis. Clinically, this test is most useful in suggesting which patients require evaluation for ectopic hormone production; with secondary erythrocytosis, hormone levels can vary substantially in the same patient on different occasions.[106]

ARTERIAL OXYGEN SATURATION. Arterial oxygen saturation (Sao_2) is a measure of the actual oxygen content of hemoglobin compared to its maximum potential oxygen-carrying capacity. This can be measured directly using a blood oximeter, which spectrophotometrically determines saturation.

TABLE 8.4. The Costs of Tests Commonly Used in the Evaluation of Erythrocytosis

Test	Approximate Cost, US$
Complete blood count with differential	6 to 10
Electrolytes, blood urea nitrogen, creatinine	7 to 20
SMA-12 (LFTs and uric acid)	17 to 42
Vitamin B_{12}	17 to 42
Arterial blood gas	20 to 25
Erythropoietin	40 to 45
Urinalysis	7 to 10
Hemoglobin electrophoresis	40 to 50
Red cell volume	132
Plasma volume	141
Abdominal CT scan	380
Head CT scan with contrast	380

Note: All costs are as of 1991. CT = computed tomography.

Treatment

Phlebotomy will provide symptomatic improvement in patients with erythrocytosis and is the treatment of choice in polycythemia vera and in erythrocytosis without a correctable cause. Volumes of 500 ml of blood may be removed at weekly or biweekly intervals until a hematocrit level of 45% is reached; smaller volumes should be removed in elderly patients or patients with heart disease. More frequent phlebotomy will be required initially in patients with polycythemia vera. Maintenance can be achieved with phlebotomy every 1 to 3 months, and because 200 mg of iron is removed with each unit of blood, iron deficiency will limit erythropoiesis. As mentioned previously, iron deficiency does not cause hyperviscosity[104] or impair cardiovascular performance.[105]

The decision to phlebotomize patients with hypoxic erythrocytosis because of congenital heart disease or pulmonary disease may be difficult; symptoms of hypoxia may mimic symptoms of hyperviscosity. In these patients, a trial of phlebotomy may indicate whether a patient is likely to benefit from a reduction in hematocrit,[54,55,107–109] and symptomatic response and serum erythropoietin levels, as a reflection of tissue hypoxia, can be used to gauge the extent of phlebotomy.

Patients with relative or spurious erythrocytosis also are likely to benefit from phlebotomy, because cerebral blood flow and oxygenation are limited by hyperviscosity due to the elevated hematocrit.[110] In patients with a low plasma volume, phlebotomy will stimulate an increase in plasma volume.

REFERENCES

1. Torrance JD, Lenfant C, Cruz J, et al. Oxygen transport mechanisms in residents at high altitude. Respir Physiol 1970;11:1.
2. Heistad DD, Abboud FM. Circulatory adjustments to hypoxia. Circulation 1980;61:463.
3. Frisancho AR. Functional adaptation to high altitude hypoxia. Science 1975;187:313.
4. Benesch R, Benesch RE. Intracellular organic phosphates as regulators of oxygen release by haemoglobin. Nature 1969;221:618.
5. Weil JV, Jamieson G, Brown DW, et al. The red cell mass-arterial oxygen relationship in normal man. J Clin Invest 1968;47:1627.
6. Murray JF. Arterial studies in primary and secondary polycythemic disorders. Am Rev Respir Dis 1965;92:435.
7. Hlastala MP, McKenna HP, Franada RL, et al. Influence of carbon monoxide on hemoglobin-oxygen binding. J Appl Physiol 1976;41:893.
8. Thomas DJ, Marshall J, Russell R, et al. Cerebral blood-flow in polycythaemia. Lancet 1977;ii:161.
9. Law ML, Cai GY, Lin FK, et al. Chromosomal assignment of the human erythropoietin gene and its DNA polymorphism. Proc Natl Acad Sci U S A 1986;82:6920.
10. Lai PH, Everett R, Wang FF, et al. Structural characterization of human erythropoietin. J Biol Chem 1986;261:3116.
11. Davis JM, Arakawa T, Strickland TW, Yphantis DA. Characterization of recombinant human erythropoietin produced in Chinese hamster ovary cells. Biochemistry 1987;26:2633.
12. Miyake T, Kung CKH, Goldwasser E. Purification of human erythropoietin. J Biol Chem 1977;252:5558.
13. Sasaki H, Bothner B, Dell A, Fakuda M. Carbohydrate structure of erythropoietin expressed in Chinese hamster ovary cells by a human erythropoietin cDNA. J Biol Chem 1987;262:12059.
14. Spivak JL, Hogans BB. The in vivo metabolism of recombinant human erythropoietin in the rat. Blood 1989;73:90.
15. Dube S, et al. Glycosylation at specific sites of erythropoietin is essential for biosynthesis, secretion, and biological function. J Biol Chem 1988;263:17516.
16. Jacobson LO, Goldwasser E, Fried W, Plzak L. Role of the kidney in erythropoiesis. Nature 1957;179:633.
17. Fried W. The liver as a source of extrarenal erythropoietin. Blood 1972;40:671.
18. Bondurant MC, Koury MJ. Anemia induces accumulation of erythropoietin mRNA in the kidney and liver. Mol Cell Biol 1986;6:2731.
19. Lacombe C, Da Silova JL, Bruneval P. Peritubular cells are the site of erythropoietin synthesis in the murine hypoxic kidney. J Clin Invest 1988;81:620.
20. Koury ST, Bondurant MC, Koury MJ. Localization of erythropoietin synthesizing cells in murine kidneys by in situ hybridization. Blood 1988;71:524.
21. Caro J, Erslev AJ. Biologic and immunologic erythropoietin in extracts from hypoxic whole rat kidneys and in their glomerular and tubular fractions. J Lab Clin Med 1984;103:922.
22. Goldberg MA, Dunning SP, Bunn HF. Regulation of the erythropoietin gene: evidence that the oxygen sensor is a heme protein. Science 1988;242:1412.
23. Koury ST, Koury MJ, Bondurant MC, et al. Quantitation of erythropoietin-producing cells in kidneys of mice by in situ hybridization: correlation with hematocrit, renal erythropoietin mRNA, and serum erythropoietin concentration. Blood 1989;74:645.
24. Koury ST, Bondurant MC, Koury MJ, Semenza GL. Localiza-

tion of cells producing erythropoietin in murine liver by in situ hybridization. Blood 1991;77:2497.

25. Goldwasser E, et al. The effect of interluekin-3 on hemopoietic precursor cells. In: Golde DW, Marks PA, eds. Normal and Neoplastic Hematopoiesis. New York: Alan R. Liss, 1983:301.

26. Donahue RE, et al. Demonstration of burst-promoting activity of recombinant human GM-CSF on circulating erythroid progenitors using an assay involving the delayed addition of erythropoietin. Blood 1985;66:1479.

27. Donahue RE, et al. Human P40 T-cell growth factor (Interleukin 9) supports erythroid colony formation. Blood 1990;75:2271.

28. Schuster SJ, Badiavas EV, Costa-Giomi P, et al. Stimulation of erythropoietin gene transcription during hypoxia and cobalt exposure. Blood 1989;73:13.

29. Abbrecht PH, Littell JK. Plasma erythropoietin in men and mice during acclimatization to different altitudes. J Appl Physiol 1972;32:54.

30. Fried W, Johnson C, Heller P. Observations on the regulation of erythropoiesis during prolonged periods of hypoxia. Blood 1970;36:607.

31. Milledge JS, Cotes PM. Serum erythropoietin in humans at high altitude and its relation to plasma renin. J Appl Physiol 1985;59:360.

32. Zwillich CW, Sutton FD, Pierson DJ, et al. Decreased hypoxic ventilatory drive in the obesity-hypoventilation syndrome. Am J Med 1975;59:343.

33. Ward HP, Bigelow DB, Petty TL. Postural hypoxemia and erythrocytosis. Am J Med 1968;45:880.

34. Adamson JW. Oxygen delivery by abnormal hemoglobins: effects on erythropoietin production. In: Stohlman F Jr, ed. Hemopoietic Cellular Proliferation. New York: Grune & Stratton, 1970:112.

35. Russell RP, Conley CL. Benign polycythemia: Gaisbock's syndrome. Arch Intern Med 1964;114:734.

36. Smith JR, Landaw SA. Smoker's polycythemia. N Engl J Med 1978;298:6.

37. Chrysant SG, Frohlich ED, Adamopoulous PN, et al. Pathophysiologic significance of "stress" or relative polycythemia in essential hypertension. Am J Cardiol 1976;37:1069.

38. Weintreb NJ, Shih CF. Spurious polycythemia. Semin Hematol 1975;12:397.

39. Leth A. Changes in plasma and extracellular fluid volumes in patients with essential hypertension during long-term treatment with hydrochlorothiazide. Circulation 1970;42:479.

40. Lederle FA. Relative erythrocytosis: an approach to the patient. J Gen Intern Med 1987;2:128.

41. Astrup P. Intraerythrocytic 2,3-diphosphoglycerate and carbon monoxide exposure. Ann N Y Acad Sci 1970;174:252.

42. Burge PS, Johnson WS, Prankerd TAJ. Morbidity and mortality in psuedopolycythaemia. Lancet 1975;i:1266.

43. Sanchez C, Merino C, Figallo M. Simultaneous measurement of plasma volume and cell mass in polycythemia of high altitude. J Appl Physiol 1970;28:775.

44. Kryger M. Breathing at high altitude: lessons learned and application to hypoxemia at sea level. Adv Cardiol 1980;27:11.

45. Kryger M, McCullough R, Doekel R, et al. Excessive polycythemia of high altitude: role of ventilatory drive and lung disease. Am Rev Respir Dis 1978;118:659.

46. Monge CC, Whittembury J. Chronic mountain sickness. Johns Hopkins Med J 1976;139:87.

47. Moore-Gillon JC, Treacher DF, Gaminara EJ, et al. Intermittent hypoxia in patients with unexplained polycythaemia. BMJ 1986;293:588.

48. Haga P, Cotes PM, Till JA, et al. Serum immunoreactive erythropoietin in children with cyanotic and acyanotic congenital heart disease. Blood 1987;70:822.

49. Henriksson P, Varendh G, Lundstrom NR. Haemostatic defects in cyanotic congenital heart disease. Br Heart J 1979;41:23.

50. Ekert H, Gilchrist GS, Stanton R, et al. Hemostasis in cyanotic congenital heart disease. J Pediatr 1970;76:221.

51. Jackson DP. Hemorrhagic diathesis in patients with cyanotic congenital heart disease: preoperative management. Ann N Y Acad Sci 1964;115:235.

52. Rosove MH, Hocking WG, Canobbio MM, et al. Chronic hypoxaemia and decompensated erythrocytosis in cyanotic congenital heart disease. Lancet 1986;ii:313.

53. Perloff JK, Rosove MH, Child JS, Wright GB. Adults with cyanotic congenital heart disease: hematologic management. Ann Intern Med 1988;109:406.

54. Rosenthal A, Nathan DG, Marty AT, et al. Acute hemodynamic effects of red cell volume reduction in polycythemia of cyanotic congenital heart disease. Circulation 1970;42:297.

55. Oldershaw PJ, Sutton MG. Haemodynamic effects of haematocrit reduction in patients with polycythaemia secondary to cyanotic congenital heart disease. Br Heart J 1980;44:584.

56. Charache S, Weatherall DJ, Clegg JB. Polycythemia associated with a hemoglobinopathy. J Clin Invest 1966;45:813.

57. Bunn HF, Forget BG. Hemoglobin: Molecular, Genetic, and Clinical Aspects. Philadelphia: W. B. Saunders, 1986.

58. Adamson JW. Familial polycythemia. Semin Hematol 1975;12:383.

59. Eckardt K-U, Mollmann M, Neumann R, et al. Erythropoietin in polycystic kidneys. J Clin Invest 1989;84:1160.

60. Wickre CG, Norman DJ, Bennison A, et al. Post renal transplant erythrocytosis: a review of 53 patients. Kidney Int 1983;23:731.

61. Basu TK, Stein RM. Erythrocytosis associated with chronic renal disease. Arch Intern Med 1974;133:442.

62. Sonneborn R, Perez G, Epstein M, et al. Erythrocytosis associated with the nephrotic syndrome. Arch Intern Med 1977;137:1068.

63. Bacon BR, Rothman SA, Ricanati ES, et al. Renal artery stenosis with erythrocytosis after renal transplantation. Arch Intern Med 1980;140:1026.

64. Pagel H, Jelkmann W, Weiss C. A comparison of the effects of renal artery constriction and anemia on the production of erythropoietin. Pflugers Arch 1988;413:62.

65. Tarazi RC, Frohlich ED, Dustan HP, et al. Hypertension and high hematocrit. Another clue to renal artery disease. Am J Cardiol 1955;18:855.

66. McGonigle RJS, Husserl F, Wallin JD, et al. Hemodialysis and continuous peritoneal dialysis effects on erythropoiesis in renal failure. Kidney Int 1984;25:430.

67. Chandra M, Miller ME, Garcia JF, et al. Serum immunoreactive erythropoietin levels in patients with polycystic kidney disease as compared with other hemodialysis patients. Nephron 1985;39:26.

68. Pavlovi'c-Kentera V, Clemons GK, Djukanovi'c L, et al. Erythropoietin and anemia in chronic renal failure. Exp Hematol 1987;15:785.

69. Shalhoub RJ, Rajan UMA, Goldwasser E. Erythrocytosis in patients on long-term hemodialysis. Ann Intern Med 1982;97:686.

70. Toyama L, Mitus WJ. Experimental renal erythrocytosis. III. Relationship between the degree of hydronephrotic pressure and production of erythrocytosis. J Lab Clin Med 1966;68:740.

71. Montagnac R, Manceaux M Cl, Boffa G, et al. Syndrome de Bartter et erythrocytose. Semin Hosp Paris 1985;21:1513.

72. Erkelens DW, Statius van Eps LW. Bartter's syndrome and erythrocytosis. Am J Med 1973;55:711.

73. Sun CH, Ward JH, Paul WL, et al. Serum erythropoietin levels after renal transplantation. N Engl J Med 1989;321:151.

74. Besarab A, Caro J, Jarrell BE. Dynamics of erythropoiesis following renal transplantation. Kidney Int 1987;32:526.

75. Rejman ASM, Grimes AJ, Cotes PM, et al. Correction of anaemia following renal transplantation: serial changes in serum immunoreactive erythropoietin, absolute reticulocyte count and red cell creatinine levels. Br J Haematol 1985;61:421.

76. Pollak R, Maddux MS, Cohan J, et al. Erythrocythemia following renal transplantation: influence of diuretic therapy. Clin Nephrol 1988;29:119.

77. Dagher FJ, Ramos E, Erslev AJ, et al. Are the native kidneys responsible for erythrocytosis in renal allorecipients? Transplantation 1979;28:496.

78. Dagher FJ, Ramos E, Erslev A, et al. Erythrocytosis after renal allotransplantation: treatment by removal of the native kidneys. South Med J 1980;73:940.

79. Thorling EB. Paraneoplastic erythrocytosis and inappropriate erythropoietin production. Scand J Haematol 1972;17:13.

80. Da Silva JL, Lacombe C, Bruneval P, et al. Tumor cells are the site of erythropoietin synthesis in human renal cancers associated with polycythemia. Blood 1990;75:577.

81. Yonemitsu H, Yamaguchi K, Shigeta H, et al. Two cases of familial erythrocytosis with increased erythropoietin activity in plasma and urine. Blood 1973;42:793.

82. Adamson JW, Stamatoyannopoulos G, Kontras S, et al. Recessive familial erythrocytosis: aspects of marrow regulation in two families. Blood 1973;41:641.

83. Greenberg BR, Golde DW. Erythropoiesis in familial erythrocytosis. N Engl J Med 1977;296:1080.

84. Daniak N, Hoffman R, Lebowitz AL, et al. Erythropoietin-dependent primary pure erythrocytosis. Blood 1979;53:1076.

85. Rosa R, Prehu M-O, Breuzard Y, et al. The first case of a complete deficiency of diphosphoglycerate mutase in human erythrocytes. J Clin Invest 1978;62:907.

86. Miller RL, Purvis JD, Weick JK. Familial polycythemia vera. Cleve Clin J Med 1989;56:813.

87. Ratnoff WD, Gress RD. The familial occurrence of polycythemia vera: report of a father and son, with consideration of the possible etiologic role of exposure to organic solvents, including tetrachloroethylene. Blood 1980;56:233.

88. Spivak JL, Cooke CR. Polycythemia vera in an anephric man. Am J Med Sci 1976;272:339.

89. Adamson JW, Fialkow PJ, Murphy S, et al. Polycythemia vera: stem-cell and probable clonal origin of the disease. N Engl J Med 1976;295:913.

90. Adamson JW, Singer JW, Catalano P, et al. Polycythemia vera: further in vitro studies of hematopoietic regulation. J Clin Invest 1980;66:1363.

91. Berlin NI. Diagnosis and classification of the polycythemias. Semin Hematol 1975;12:339.

92. Yu TF. Secondary gout associated with myeloproliferative diseases. Arthritis Rheum 1965;8:765.

93. Van Dyke D, Anger HO. Patterns of marrow hypertrophy and atrophy in man. J Nucl Med 1965;6:109.

94. Wasserman LR, Gilbert HS. Surgical bleeding in polycythemia vera. Ann N Y Acad Sci 1964;115:122.

95. Silverstein MN. Postpolycythemic myeloid metaplasia. Arch Intern Med 1974;134:113.

96. Landaw SA. Acute leukemia in polycythemia vera. Semin Hematol 1986;23:156.

97. Berk PD, Goldberg JD, Silverstein MN, et al. Increased incidence of acute leukemia in polycythemia vera associated with chlorambucil therapy. N Engl J Med 1981;304:441.

98. Kaplan ME, Mack K, Goldberg JD, et al. Long-term management of polycythemia vera with hydroxyurea: a progress report. Semin Hematol 1986;23:167.

99. Kessler CM, Klein HG. Untreated thrombocythemia in chronic myeloproliferative disorders. Br J Haematol 1982;50:157.

100. Pearson TC, Wetherly-Mein G. Vascular occlusive episodes and venous haematocrit in primary proliferative polycythaemia. Lancet 1978;ii:1219.

101. Tartaglia AP, Goldberg JD, Berk PD, Wasserman LR. Adverse effects of antiaggregating platelet therapy in the treatment of polycythemia vera. Semin Hematol 1986;23:172.

102. Michiels JJ, Abels J, Steketee J, Van Vliet HHDM, Vuzevski VD. Erythromelalgia caused by platelet-mediated arteriolar inflammation and thrombosis in thrombocythemia. Ann Intern Med 1985;102:466.

103. Schafer AI. Bleeding and thrombosis in the myeloproliferative disorders. Blood 1984;64:1.

104. Birgegard G, Carlsson M, Sandhagen B, et al. Does iron deficiency in treated polycythemia vera affect whole blood viscosity? Acta Med Scand 1984;216:165.

105. Rector WG Jr, Fortuin NJ, Conley CL. Non-hematologic effects of chronic iron deficiency: a study of patients with polycythemia vera treated solely with venesections. Medicine 1982;61:382.

106. Cotes PM, Dore CJ, Yin JAL, et al. Determination of serum immunoreactive erythropoietin in the investigation of erythrocytosis. N Engl J Med 1986;315:283.

107. Dayton LM, McCullough RE, Scheinhorn DJ, et al. Symptomatic and pulmonary response to acute phlebotomy in secondary polycythemia. Chest 1975;68:785.

108. York EL, Jones RL, Menon D, et al. Effects of secondary polycythemia on cerebral blood flow in chronic obstructive pulmonary disease. Am Rev Respir Dis 1980;121:813.

109. Wallis PJW, Skehan JD, Newland AC, et al. Effects of erythrapheresis on pulmonary haemodynamics and oxygen transport in patients with secondary polycythaemia and cor pulmonale. Clin Sci 1986;70:91.

110. Humphrey PRD, Marshall J, Russell RWR, et al. Cerebral blood-flow and viscosity in relative polycythaemia. Lancet 1979;ii:873.

111. Pirofsky B. The determination of blood viscosity in man by a method based on Poiseuille's law. J Clin Invest 1953;32:292.

9

Neutrophils

William P. Hammond, M.D.

In a classic paper in 1880, Paul Ehrlich described the differential staining of blood leukocytes and introduced the terms *neutrophil, basophil,* and *acidophil* (later replaced by *eosinophil*) for the polymorphonuclear leukocytes in blood.[1] In 1883, Elie Metchnikov described studies of the phagocytic capacity of the "ameboid cells" of blood, introducing this direct function of the neutrophil for the first time. These observations, for which Ehrlich and Metchnikov shared the 1909 Nobel Prize, laid the foundations for our understanding of the "neutrophil." Strictly speaking, the terms *polymorphonuclear neutrophil,* referring to *polymorphonuclear,* and *granulocyte,* including basophils and eosinophils as well as neutrophils, are less specific. Here, we refer to neutrophils as the neutrophilic polymorphonuclear leukocytes originally described by Ehrlich.

The function of the neutrophil as a component of a complex host defense mechanism is primarily the ingestion and killing of invading microorganisms. Recent studies suggest that secretion of its cellular constituents or of various cytokines may contribute to its function in vivo, and these will be discussed later. Our understanding of the normal physiology of the neutrophil has been built on discoveries of specific pathophysiologic defects in neutrophil production and function in both inherited and acquired disease states. The neutrophil plays a major role in defense against bacterial pathogens, and it may contribute to defense against fungal infections as well. Interestingly, the century-old debate as to the relative importance of phagocytic and immune components of the host defense system begun by Metchnikov still persists today. While humoral and cellular immune responses by B and T lymphocytes appear critical to the prevention of numerous viral diseases, the contribution of neutrophils to defense against these pathogens remains unclear. Virchow recognized the neutrophil as a component of pus in the mid-1850s and inferred a role in wound healing from his early observations; in addition, it is clear that the neutrophil plays a major role in inflammatory states due to many causes, including certain pathologic states where its effects may be deleterious. In this chapter, we review the morphology and development of neutrophils, their function, and several pathologic disorders of neutrophil number and function, and we discuss clinical management, including differential diagnosis of neutrophil disorders and newer biologic therapies.

MORPHOLOGY AND DEVELOPMENT

Neutrophils are formed in the bone marrow from morphologically unrecognizable precursor cells called *stem cells.* Stem cells are characterized by capacities for extensive self-renewal and for the production of multiple differentiated cell types. To produce neutrophils, the stem cell commits its progeny to differentiation into cells of the granulocytic and/or macrophage lineages, and subsequent generations ultimately lose the capacity for differentiation into any cell lineage other than neutrophils. These "committed" neutrophilic precursor cells then begin a process of differentiation leading to morphologically identifiable cells within the marrow, namely, myeloblasts, promyelocytes, and meylocytes, all of which retain the capacity for mitosis (the "mitotic" neutrophilic compartment). Beyond the myelocyte

MARROW

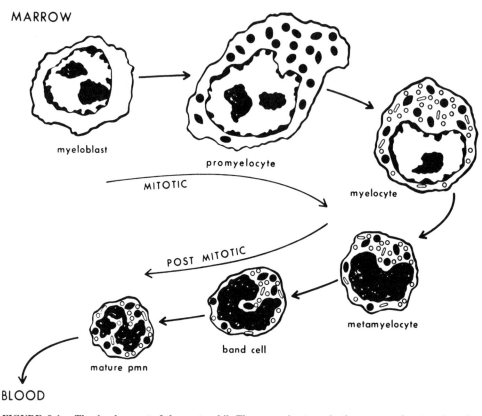

myeloblast

promyelocyte

MITOTIC

myelocyte

POST MITOTIC

metamyelocyte

band cell

mature pmn

BLOOD

FIGURE 9.1.   **The development of the neutrophil. There are six stages in the process of maturation of the cell from the first recognizable component of the mitotic pool to the fully mature, segmented neutrophil. The maturation process is divided into the mitotic and postmitotic phases, reflecting the loss of capacity for cell division after the myelocyte stage.** *Note:* **pmn = polymorphonuclear.** *Source:* **Bainton 1971 Reproduced by copyright permission of the Rockefeller University Press.**

stage, these precursors lose the capacity for mitosis and undergo a process of maturation with identifiable stages referred to as the *metamyelocyte, band,* and *segmented neutrophils*. These stages are often referred to as the "postmitotic" compartment of the marrow neutrophilic precursors (Figs. 9.1, 9.2, and 9.3).

As stated, the mitotic compartment contains three morphologic identifiable cell types. The myeloblast is the earliest morphologically recognizable precursor of the neutrophil; it has fine nuclear chromatin, prominent nucleoli, and no cytoplasmic granules. The promyelocyte is the precursor in which primary or "azurophilic" granule formation begins; it has a prominent Golgi apparatus and often two to five nucleoli. The last neutrophil precursor capable of cell division is the myelocyte, and it is identified by the onset of secondary (or "specific") granule formation. Primary granule formation ceases at this point.

The postmitotic compartment also contains three identifiable stages. The metamyelocyte is the earliest cell in this "maturational" phase, and its nucleus becomes indented or horsehoe shaped, beginning the process of nuclear condensation. Secondary granules far outnumber primary granules by this stage in development. The nuclear chromatin is further condensed in the band neutrophils, or second stage; there are no segments to the nuclear chromatin here. Finally, the mature bone marrow neutrophil is identical to the blood neutrophil, with a fully segmented, condensed nucleus.

The process of development from myeloblast through meylocyte in the mitotic compartment is believed to take 3 or 4 days, while the maturation process appears to take between 6 and 8 days.[2] The time for complete maturation of the cells and release into the peripheral blood is also referred to as the *marrow transit time,* and it appears to be regulated in part by an intrinsic program of

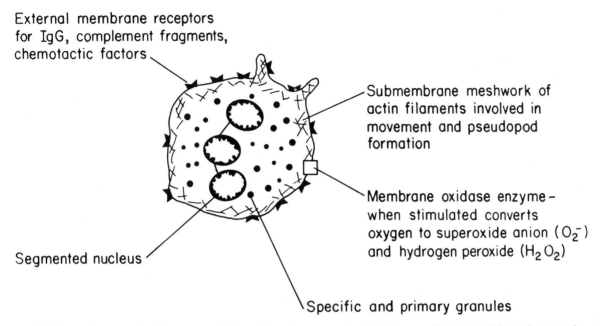

External membrane receptors
for IgG, complement fragments,
chemotactic factors

Submembrane meshwork of
actin filaments involved in
movement and pseudopod
formation

Membrane oxidase enzyme—
when stimulated converts
oxygen to superoxide anion (O_2^-)
and hydrogen peroxide (H_2O_2)

Segmented nucleus

Specific and primary granules

FIGURE 9.2. **The anatomy of the neutrophil. Five different components of the structure of the neutrophil are shown; each contributes to the normal function of the cell.** *Source:* **Babior and Stossel 1990[4]**

differentiation and in part by exogenous stimuli from the bone marrow microenvironment and beyond.

The anatomy of the mature neutrophil can be viewed as consisting of five major components, with functional implications somewhat unique to this cell (Fig. 9.2).[3] First, there are external membrane receptors on its surface that direct its responses: receptors for IgG (Fc receptors), complement fragments and chemotactic factors (e.g., f-*met-leu-phe*), as well as leukocyte adhesion molecules that mediate and regulate its interactions with other cells in the body. These signal a variety of responses for the cell and are discussed later. Second, there is a submembranous cytoskeleton of actin filaments interacting with myosin and other proteins which subserves directed ameboid motion and phagosome creation. Third, numerous primary and secondary granules contain constituents for killing and digesting invading organisms (Table 9.1). Fourth, there exists a pool of oxidase enzymes that are "stored" in the resting state but capable of movement to and activation into the phagocytic vacuolar membrane with appropriate stimulation. Finally, the neutrophil's nucleus is condensed and segmented in a unique fashion, presumably related in some manner to the cell's need for extraordinary mobility and deformability in carrying out its function.[4]

Once fully matured, the neutrophil spends a period of time within the marrow space in a storage pool of cells called the *marrow neutrophil reserves*. This population of cells is roughly 10 times the size of the total quantity

TABLE 9.1. **Constituents of Azurophilic and Specific Granules from Human Neutrophils**

Azurophilic	Secondary
Myeloperoxidase	Collagenase
Lysozyme	Lysozyme
Elastase	Lactoferrin
Cathepsins G, B, D	Vitamin B_{12}–binding protein
Proteinase 3	Plasminogen activator
β-glucuronidase	Histaminase
L-mannosidase	Laminin
Defensins	Cytochrome *b*

Source: Williams et al. 1990[2]

in the circulation, and it serves both as the source of continuing resupply of blood neutrophils and as the reactive reserve under conditions of increased demand. The mechanisms regulating egress of marrow neutrophils into the blood are not precisely known, but they are believed to involve alterations of both the neutrophils' surface leukocyte adhesion molecules and the bone marrow vascular endothelial cell lining. Within the blood stream, approximately 50% of the neutrophils circulate freely in the central axial stream of the blood, while the remainder become loosely adherent to endothelial cell surfaces throughout the body. These two populations, called *circulating* and *marginated* blood neutrophil pools, respectively, are in a dynamic equilibrium. Individual cells flow in the blood, then adhere to a surface for a while, then release and flow again. The cells must adhere more firmly as the first step to leaving the blood and entering tissues where their primary function is carried out, a process requiring alteration of surface ligands on both the neutrophils and endothelial cells. Studies employing radioactively tagged neutrophils demonstrate that egress from blood to the tissues follows first-order kinetics, with a half-life of approximately 6 hours. This first-order kinetic behavior demonstrates that neutrophils leave the circulation randomly, not as a function of age, and thus are most likely do so in relation to local tissue needs and not any intrinsic property of the cell itself.

FUNCTION

The primary function of neutrophils is to ingest and kill microorganisms. To carry out these functions, the neutrophil must be motile, with a functional intracellular contractile system and appropriate energy sources (ATP), and must be capable of directed motion in response to chemical signals in its environment, a process termed *chemotaxis*. To reach its target site, the neutrophil also must be capable of adherence, first to the surfaces of endothelial cells to allow egress from the blood into the tissue, a process termed *adhesion,* followed by a capacity to adhere to and ingest the organism, a process termed *phagocytosis*. During phagocytosis, an abrupt increase in oxygen consumption occurs with production of toxic oxygen species, a process referred to as the *metabolic burst,* followed by fusion of primary and secondary granules with the phagosome, termed *degranulation,* and finally, killing and digestion of the microorganism occurs.[5]

The first processes, cell motility and chemotaxis, are dependent on a cytoskeletal filamentous system. This system works via a process of pseudopod formation and an ATP-dependent interaction of actin with myosin and other proteins that pulls the cell body toward the sites of attachment much like a crawling, tank-tread mechanism.[4] Calcium ionic fluxes appear to play an important role in this process. Chemotaxis, or the directed movement of cells toward foreign substances, is stimulated by the release of molecules from sites of inflammation to which the neutrophil responds in a concentration-dependent fashion; among the in vivo chemotactic factors are fragments of complement (C5a), bacterial oligopeptides, fibrinopeptide B, and leukotriene B_4. In vitro, the small peptide f-*met-leu-phe* is used as a convenient test for chemotaxis. This directed motility may be distinguished from a generalized activation of cell motility that occurs with certain stimuli.

Having arrived in the vicinity of the invading microorganism, the neutrophil must recognize that microorganism as foreign. Microbes are rendered recognizable by a process of coating with plasma proteins called *opsonization*. The major plasma opsonins are IgG and complement fragments C3b and C3bi, for which specific receptors exist on the neutrophil surface. The adherence of the neutrophils to the opsonized organism triggers a series of events including pseudopod formation around and engulfing the microbe, invagination of membrane to create space around it called the *phagocytic vacuole* or *phagosome,* beginning the release of secondary and then primary granule contents into the phagosome (creating a "phagolysosome"), and activation of the "metabolic burst." The phagosome localizes the invading foreign agent and provides an environment in which lysis can occur. Secondary granules, followed by primary granules, empty their contents into the phagosome by a process of organelle membrane fusion that brings together the multiple components of the killing system.

The metabolic burst involves a set of reactions that begin as the neutrophil initiates phagocytosis. Flux of calcium ions, alteration of lipid metabolism (including phosphoinositide breakdown), and movement of various glycoprotein molecules and enzymes to the surface and to phagosomal membranes occur with a burst of oxygen consumption. The oxygen consumption provides energy for these reactions, and it also generates activated oxygen forms that directly participate in the microbicidal process. There is increased glycolysis; increased hexose monophosphate shunt activity; decreased pH within the phagocytic vacuole; and increased production of superoxide, H_2O_2, and hydroxyl radical.

The mechanisms whereby microorganisms are killed are multiple. Both oxygen-independent and -dependent systems are brought to bear within the phagosomes, including multiple proteases and the myeloperoxidase-hydrogen peroxide-halide system. The specific mechanism whereby hydrogen peroxide and halide contribute to the killing appears to involve the formation of toxic oxygen radicals (OH^- and O_2^-) and then hypochlorous acid; the contribution of myeloperoxidase is crucial to this system.[5] The precise role and mechanism of the antimicrobial activity of lactoferrin and the neutral proteases remains to be elucidated.

PATHOPHYSIOLOGY

Pathophysiologic abnormalities of neutrophils can be considered in three categories: abnormalities in the number of neutrophils, neutrophil dysfunction, and the contributions of neutrophils to tissue damage in inflam-

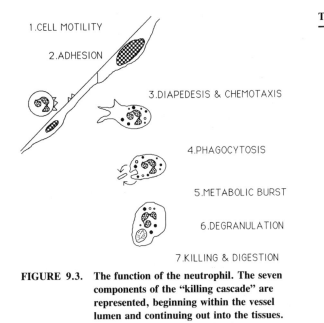

FIGURE 9.3. The function of the neutrophil. The seven components of the "killing cascade" are represented, beginning within the vessel lumen and continuing out into the tissues.

1.CELL MOTILITY
2.ADHESION
3.DIAPEDESIS & CHEMOTAXIS
4.PHAGOCYTOSIS
5.METABOLIC BURST
6.DEGRANULATION
7.KILLING & DIGESTION

TABLE 9.2. The Classification of Neutrophilia

Demargination
   Exercise
   Seizures
   Epinephrine
   Corticosteroids
   Asplenia
Blocked egress
   Corticosteroids
   Leukocyte adhesion deficiency syndrome
Increased marrow release
   Endotoxin
   Etiocholanolone
   Corticosteroid (including Cushing syndrome)
   Colony-stimulating factors (G-CSF, GM-CSF)
   Thyroid storm
Increased production
   Malignancy
   Colony-stimulating factors (G-CSF, GM-CSF)
   Myeloproliferative disorders
   Chronic inflammation
   Chronic myelogenous leukemia
   Lithium
   Idiopathic

Note: G-CSF = granulocyte colony-stimulating factor; GM-CSF = granulocyte-macrophage colony-stimulating factor.

matory states. Abnormal increases in neutrophil counts other than those caused by malignant disorders frequently herald infections, but these may represent a major presenting feature of noninfectious inflammatory disorders. Multiple causes of neutropenia exist and require a careful differential diagnosis, and neutrophil dysfunction may be either congenital or acquired and be caused by factors either extrinsic or intrinsic to the neutrophil itself. Congenital disorders of neutrophil function have provided insights into the normal physiology of neutrophil function, as predicted from Garrod's work many years ago.[6] Recent work on the mechanisms of neutrophil function have allowed experimental studies to examine the role of neutrophils in inflammatory states, including the postreperfusion syndromes, and suggest a major role for the neutrophil in the pathophysiology of tissue damage following ischemia.[7]

Neutrophilia

Neutrophilia is defined as an increase in the neutrophil count above the upper limit of the normal range (1800 to 7500 cells/μl), but increases in the neutrophil count above 10,000/μl generally are considered significant. The increase is limited to segmented neutrophils, bands, and rare metamyelocytes; appearance of more immature neutrophilic cells in the blood suggests more abnormality and may represent leukemia or a leukemoid reaction (discussed later). The importance of neutrophilia lies in its identification of an underlying abnor-

mality in the host. In general, marked increases in the neutrophil count are tolerated by the body without deleterious effects up to at least 50,000/μl.

The mechanisms of neutrophilia include two in which the delivery to tissues appear as not to be increased and two in which delivery probably is increased (Table 9.2). The first two are *demargination* and *decreased egress.* Demargination is movement of cells from the marginated neutrophil pool into the circulating pool, resulting in an increase in the count of blood neutrophils without any increase of immature cell forms seen in the blood. This typically occurs with exercise and has been demonstrated experimentally to follow epinephrine administration; it usually appears within a few minutes and disappears within 30 minutes. Decreased egress increases the count due to less movement from the vascular space out into tissues; the decrease in egress has been documented with corticosteroid treatment and certainly contributes to the increased cell count during steroid treatment. The rare inherited lack of leukocyte adhesion molecules (discussed later) is typically associated with neutrophilia due to this mechanism.

Two mechanisms of neutrophilia also probably increase delivery of neutrophils to tissues. First is release of cells from the bone marrow neutrophil reserve, also increasing the neutrophil count. The bone marrow neutrophil reserve contains approximately 10 times as many neutrophils as are normally present in the total blood neutrophil pool (the sum of the "circulating" and "marginated" pools). Release of these cells from the marrow may occur with infection but also may occur directly in response to glucocorticosteroids and the colony-stimulating factors.

Increased production of neutrophils driven by the stimuli of infection or inflammatory mediators can be massive and is the fourth mechanism of neutrophilia. This occurs through the action of the hematopoietic growth factors, including granulocyte-macrophage colony-stimulating factor (GM-CSF) and granulocyte colony-stimulating factor (G-CSF). Increases in blood neutrophil counts, with an associated increased number of immature forms ("left shift"), may reach 10- to 20-fold. Recent studies with recombinant human hematopoietic growth factors such as GM-CSF and G-CSF have shown that these increased numbers of cells are also activated, with associated increases in cell volume, granularity, and retained RNA (identifiable as Döhle bodies) in the case of G-CSF treatment. Drugs, including lithium and prednisone, regularly produce increased neutrophil counts.

In the absence of treatment with growth factors, the degree of increase depends on the duration and severity of the inflammatory stimulus. The marked though short-term stimulation of a delayed hemolytic transfusion reaction, for example, can produce extreme increases in blood neutrophil counts with less shift, a pattern indistinguishable from chronic myelogenous leukemia or one of the myeloproliferative disorders and hence called a *leukemoid reaction*. Chronic stimulation also can produce massive increases in neutrophil count, including chronic infection such as bacterial abscesses and certain malignancies that appear to increase production by synthesizing hematopoietic growth factors in an unregulated manner. I define an increase in neutrophil count in adults to more than 25,000/μl as a leukemoid reaction, with chronic granulomatous diseases, a persisting undrained abscess, and solid tumors (especially breast and lung cancers) being the most common causes. It should be noted, however, that children typically mount a more exuberant neutrophil-count response to infection and thus require a count in excess of 50,000/μl to be called a leukemoid reaction.

Neutropenia

Neutropenia is defined as a decrease in neutrophil count below the lower limit of the normal range ($<$ 1800/μl). It may occur as an isolated decrease in neutrophils, such as agranulocytosis or chronic idiopathic neutropenia, or as one component of a broader hematologic abnormality such as aplastic anemia or leukemia. To qualify as chronic neutropenia, a duration in excess of 6 months must be documented; to be considered severe, the neutrophil count must be under 500/μl. If neutrophil function is otherwise normal, risk of infection (bacterial and possibly fungal) clearly rises below 500/μl, with further increases in risk at less than 200/μl and less than 100/μl. Thus, both the duration and severity of neutropenia contribute to the risk of developing infection.

The mechanisms of neutropenia parallel those for neutrophilia. In the first, an increased margination may occur, with a corresponding decrease in the circulating cell count. This typically occurs with splenomegaly and has led to the terms *sequestration neutropenia* and *pseudoneutropenia,* examples of which are the neutropenia seen in chronic malaria and dialysis neutropenia.[8,9] The second is an accelerated egress of neutrophils from the blood into the tissue. Acute endotoxemia is the classic cause of sudden falls in the blood neutrophil count; if a patient is seen before the marrow has had sufficient time to proliferate in response to the infection and thus increase production to meet demand, neutropenia may be the consequence. This is presumed to be the cause of neutropenia associated with overwhelming bacterial infections.[3] A third mechanism causing neutropenia is an accelerated removal of cells from the circulation, usually due to antibody-mediated destruction or the so-called "immune neutropenia," the best-documented form of which is neonatal isoimmune neutropenia.[10] Immunologically mediated neutropenias have been identified by the presence of excess IgG on the surface of neutrophils in patients with systemic lupus erythematosus, Felty syndrome, and in some with rheumatoid arthritis without splenomegaly.[11,12] Finally, neutropenia may be caused by decreased production of cells by the marrow, either because of true hypoproliferative marrow states or ineffective neutrophil production by the marrow. A host of causes for hypoproliferation exist: radiation therapy, alkylating agents, idiosyncratic drug reactions, aplastic anemia, certain viral infections, and several inherited diseases cause this type of neutropenia; ineffective production is a state of the marrow in which neutrophilic precursor proliferation has occurred but final maturation and release into the blood have not taken place. The classic causes of this type of relatively mild neutropenia are folate and vitamin B_{12} deficiencies, with the most common cause being the folate antagonist trimethoprim, given for urinary tract infections. In at least some patients with the myelodysplastic syndromes (preleukemia), ineffective production contributes to the neutropenia.

To facilitate differential diagnosis (discussed later), it usually is helpful to classify neutropenic disorders beginning with the clinical characterization of the patient. Patients with an acute onset (occurring within less than 1 month) appear to have a different spectrum of disease (Table 9.3) than those with chronic or congenital neutropenia (Table 9.4). The presence or absence of splenomegaly, lymphadenopathy, bone tenderness, or features suggesting prior or ongoing infection may help to identify generalized disorders of hematopoiesis, which then can be confirmed by platelet count, hematocrit and/or hemoglobin concentration, and blood smear analysis. The presence of autoimmune disorders, recent or even remote exposure to radiation or drugs, or serious viral illness could suggest a cause for the neutropenia.

In patients with chronic or congenital neutropenia (Table 9.4), additional disorders also must be considered. Infectious causes are more likely to be chronic mycobacterial infections or parasitic diseases, and immunologic causes are less likely to be drug-induced and more likely to be autoimmune disease–related. Some of the disorders of myeloid or lymphoid cell origin that may present as acute neutropenia also may present with a more gradual onset, especially hairy-cell leukemia and the syndrome of large granular lymphocytosis with neutropenia. Among the congenital disorders, onset of neutropenia with recurrent and/or severe infections in the first 6 months of life suggests Kostmann syndrome or reticular dysgenesis. Findings associated with particular inherited disorders, such as pancreatic exocrine deficiency in Shwachman-Diamond syndrome or oculocutaneous albinism in Chédiak-Higashi syndrome (discussed later), are helpful in identifying these congenital diseases. The presence of ineffective granulocytopoiesis in patients with long-standing neutropenia should suggest one of the rarer forms of congenital neutropenia, such as myelokathexis, or an acquired myelodysplastic syndrome in adults.

Neutrophil Function Disorders

Neutrophil function disorders have taught us a great deal about the normal physiology of the neutrophil. Humoral factors clearly play an important role by affecting cellular function either directly (such as ethanol or aspirin ingestion, hyperglycemia, and hypercortisolism) or indirectly via opsonization and the generation of chemotactic peptides (Table 9.5). Complement deficiencies, particularly autosomal recessive C3 deficiency and C3b inactivator deficiency, are associated with severe, recurrent pyogenic infections, particularly those caused by virulent encapsulated organisms (e.g., *Haemophilus influenzae* and *Streptococcus pneumoniae*). Hypogammaglobulinemia likewise is associated with similar pyogenic infections, and deficient serum chemo-

TABLE 9.3. The Classification of Acute and Acquired Neutropenias

Increased margination
  Dialysis neutropenia–complement activation
  Endotoxemia
  Typhoid fever
Accelerated egress
  Endotoxemia, acute and severe
  Overwhelming bacterial infection (sepsis)
Accelerated removal
  Alloimmune neonatal neutropenia
  Autoimmune neutropenia
    Idiopathic
    Pure white cell aplasia
    Drug-induced
      Aminopyrine
      Semisynthetic penicillins
      Diphenylhydantoin (possibly)
  Neutropenia with autoimmune diseases
    Felty syndrome
    Systemic lupus erythematosus
    Rheumatoid arthritis without splenomegaly
    Large granular lymphocytosis
Decreased production
  Hypoproliferation
    Radiation exposure, alkylating agents
    Primary stem cell diseases–leukemia, aplastic anemia
    Lymphoproliferative diseases
      Hairy-cell leukemia
      Chronic lymphocytic leukemia
      Large granular lymphocytosis with neutropenia
    Drug-induced
      Phenothiazines
      Antithyroid medications
      Chloramphenicol, sulfonamides, penicillins
      Penicillamine, captopril
    Viral diseases
      Infectious mononucleosis (Epstein-Barr virus, possibly cytomegalovirus)
      Hepatitis A
      Human-immunodeficiency-virus infection (ineffective production?)
      Rubeola
  Ineffective production
    Folate deficiency
      Dietary
      Drug-induced (trimethoprim, methotrexate, diphenylhydantoin)
    Vitamin B_{12} deficiency
      Pernicious anemia
      Malabsorption
      Transcobalamin II deficiency
    Myelodysplastic syndrome (preleukemia)

Note: This category of neutropenias includes those with a history of less than 1 month.

TABLE 9.4. The Classification of Chronic and Congenital Neutropenias

Increased margination
  Infections, usually with splenomegaly
    Tuberculosis, other mycobacterial infections
    Brucellosis
    Malaria
    Kala-azar
Accelerated removal
  Autoimmune neutropenia
    Idiopathic
    Pure white cell aplasia
    Drug-induced
      Diphenylhydantoin (possibly)
      Semisynthetic penicillins
  Neutropenia with autoimmune disorders
    Felty syndrome
    Systemic lupus erythematosus
    Rheumatoid arthritis without splenomegaly
    Large granular lymphocytosis with neutropenia
Decreased production
  Hypoproliferation
    With generalized marrow damage*
    Lymphoproliferative diseases*
    Congenital disorders
      Kostmann syndrome (infantile genetic agranulocytosis)
      Reticular dysgenesis
      Shwachman-Diamond syndrome
      Neutropenia with hypogammaglobulinemia
      Cartilage-hair hypoplasia syndrome
      Idiopathic neutropenia
      Chédiak-Higashi syndrome
      Cyclic neutropenia
    Acquired disorders
      Chronic idiopathic neutropenia
      Cyclic neutropenia
      Copper deficiency (with anemia)
  Ineffective production
    Myelodysplastic syndrome(s)
    Myelokathexis
    Lazy leukocyte syndrome
    Transcobalamin II deficiency
    Neutropenia with dysgranulopoiesis

Note: This category of neutropenias includes those with a history longer than 6 months.
*See Table 9.2 for more information.

TABLE 9.5. The Classification of Neutrophil Function Disorders

Defective motility
  Congenital
    Lazy leukocyte syndrome
    Neutrophil action dysfunction
Defective adherence
  Congenital
    CD116/CD18 deficiency (C3bi receptor deficiency)
    Neutrophil action dysfunction
  Acquired
    Treatment with monoclonal antibody to CD116/CD18
    Alcohol, glucocorticoid, aspirin
Defective chemotaxis and/or phagocytosis
  Congenital
    Complement protein deficiencies (especially C3)
    Immunoglobulin deficiency
    Neutrophil action dysfunction
    Hyperimmunoglobulin syndrome
    Neonatal developmental immaturity
    Chédiak-Higashi syndrome
    Plasminogen proactivator (Fletcher factor) deficiency
  Acquired
    Ethanol ingestion (usually chronic)
    Glucocorticoid excess, hyperglycemia
    Hypophosphatemia due to hyperalimentation
    Immune complex diseases (rheumatoid arthritis, systemic lupus erythematosus, cirrhosis)
Defective metabolic burst
  Chronic granulomatous disease, X-linked
  Chronic granulomatous disease variants, autosomal recessive
  Glucose-6-phosphate dehydrogenase deficiency, severe (with hemolytic anemia)
Granule function deficiency and organelle abnormalities
  Chédiak-Higashi syndrome
  Specific granule deficiency
  May-Hegglin anomaly
  Alder-Reilly anomaly
  Fechtner syndrome
  Pelger-Huët anomaly
Defective microbial activity
  Chronic granulomatous disease and its variants
  Glucose-6-phosphate dehydrogenase deficiency
  Myeloperoxidase deficiency

tactic or opsonic activity has been associated with autoimmune disorders including rheumatoid arthritis, systemic lupus erythematosus, and immune complex disease as well as cirrhosis, sickle cell anemia, sarcoidosis, and other inflammatory states.

Defects in neutrophil function inherent to the neutrophil include the apparent motility disorder of the "lazy leukocyte" syndrome and the neutrophil actin dysfunction syndrome; in the latter, defective adherence also is seen. The recent elucidation of CD11b/CD18 deficiency in patients with recurrent bacterial infection and an inability to generate pus has provoked a great deal of interest.[13] This heterodimeric (α- and β-subunits) surface glycoprotein is a member of the integrin family of leukocyte adhesion molecules found on multiple different leukocytes. It serves to hold the neutrophil onto endothelial cell surfaces (as well as possibly being involved in attachment to opsonized microorganisms), and its expression is normally upregulated by certain inflammatory mediators and activators of degranulation. The defective gene for the β_2-subunit (CD18) on chromosome 21 results in decreased expression of the heterodimer on the cell surface and a markedly reduced expression on stimulation. Thus, neutrophils egress from the blood stream poorly and, in the presence of infection, accumulate within the circulation, producing massive neutrophilia as described previously, sometimes exceeding 100,000/μl. Severe deficiency of the protein is correlated with severe recurrent infections and high mortality.

Defective chemotaxis and phagocytosis occur with the generalized motility disorder of the actin dysfunction syndrome and in neonates with developmentally immature neutrophils. In Chédiak-Higashi syndrome, the granule dysfunction (discussed later) is associated with neutropenia as well as a generalized defect in membrane activation and chemotactic responsiveness. Hypophosphatemia because of hyperalimentation (without adequate phosphate replacement) was reported to cause defective chemotaxis and phagocytosis, but with closer monitoring of plasma phosphate during such therapy, now this is rarely observed.

An abnormal metabolic burst and defective microbicidal activity against catalase-producing bacteria were identified in patients characterized by recurrent microabscesses and granuloma formation and called *chronic granulomatous disease of childhood*.[2,14] The original cases were X-linked, but subsequent studies demonstrated about 30% of cases to have an autosomal recessive form of inheritance. The normal membrane oxidase cytochrome *b* is absent in the majority of patients with the X-linked disease, whereas a cytosolic factor required for normal function of the heterodimeric oxidase is lacking in most patients with the autosomal recessive disease.[15] Additional variants have been reported, which imply a complex of factors involved in the normal assembly, transport, and function of this membrane oxidase. The pathogenesis of infection in these patients is due to the failure to generate sufficient H_2O_2 to exceed the capacity of bacterially produced catalase to neutralize the microbicidal activity of H_2O_2 and its metabolites. Some organisms, such as streptococci, produce some H_2O_2 without catalase, hence providing an endogenous source of the co-factor of the myeloperoxidase-H_2O_2-halide system to kill them. Other organisms, such as staphylococci, gram-negative enteric rods, *Candida albicans,* and *Aspergillus* species, produce catalase and cannot be eliminated by chronic granulomatous disease cells, thus leading to chronic infections with these organisms.[16]

Abnormalities of organelles within the cytosol, mostly granules and their precursors, are readily identified morphologically on Wright- and Giemsa-stained blood smears. In the Chédiak-Higashi syndrome, giant granules are readily identified by light microscopy. The defect in this disease appears to be a generalized defect in granule membrane function, because these neutrophil granules are unable to empty their contents into the phagocytic vacuole in a normal fashion and other granules, such as those in platelets and melanocytes, are also abnormal. Thus, various forms of albinism and a propensity to abnormal bleeding also are features of this disorder.[5]

Among the other structural abnormalities, the Pelger-Huët anomaly is probably the most common. In this entity, the nucleus of the neutrophil fails to segment normally (termed *hyposegmentation*), and neutrophils are bilobed or even appear mononuclear. Pelger-Huët cells are seen in an inherited form and in acquired disorders, particularly the myelodysplastic syndromes.

Neutrophils in Inflammation and Injury

On occasion, the neutrophil may contribute to injury instead of host defense. Examples include rheumatoid arthritis in which neutrophilic exudates within the joint space are believed to contribute to injury by release of toxic oxygen species and/or various destructive proteins (e.g., collagenase) from their granules,[5] and penicillamine may ameliorate symptomatic rheumatoid arthritis by inhibition of the action of hydrogen peroxide within the joint space. Similarly, neutrophils may contribute to the pathophysiology of emphysema via their production of elastase in the lung. Proof of the role of neutrophils in the pathophysiology of the "postreperfusion injury" syndrome is probably the strongest, however; in a number of different animal model systems, inhibition of neutrophil function mediated by exogenously administered antibody to leukocyte adhesion molecules has markedly reduced or even eliminated the expected postischemia injury.[7] Recent studies have shown marked reduction in the multiorgan failure syndrome by antibody treatment following shock in a primate model, suggesting an extremely important contribution to clinical care may derive from basic studies of the pathophysiologic role of the neutrophil in ischemic injury.[17]

CLINICAL MANAGEMENT

Differential Diagnosis

The differential diagnosis of neutrophil disorders begins with the clinical history and physical examination. The prior exposure to various medications or toxins, particularly chemotherapeutic agents, is a very important part of the history. Symptoms or signs of clinical infection will often explain abnormal neutrophil counts; it is important to remember that, in general, disorders of neutrophils are indicators of the presence of disease rather than primary causes in and of themselves. Usually, we begin the differential diagnosis by determining whether there are abnormalities in the number or function of neutrophils by the combination of clinical evaluation and the neutrophil count. Functional disorders can be inferred only by a clinical history of recurrent infections without lowered counts to explain them, but occasionally, they also may be suspected based on morphologic examination of the peripheral blood smear. Automated differential counting techniques that specifically stain cells for myeloperoxidase can demonstrate myeloperoxidase deficiency.

After determining that the number of neutrophils is abnormal, the most important next step is to determine whether other cell lines also are involved. For example, decreases in neutrophils also associated with decreases in other cell types should suggest a more generalized marrow disorder. Similarly, in patients with elevated neutrophil counts, elevations of other cell counts, such as red cells or platelets (and particularly basophils), should suggest a primary myeloproliferative disorder. When isolated neutrophilia is present, the number of possibilities actually is relatively small; infections, drugs (steroids, lithium, or one of the colony-stimulating factors), chronic myelogenous leukemia, or a leukemoid reaction because of a chronic inflammatory disorder or malignancy should be considered. When isolated neutropenia is present, drugs and infections, particularly viral infections, are the most common causes numerically, and because these are reversible, simple observation usually is sufficient as a starting point. When isolated neutropenia is known to have been present for some time, or when the degree of neutropenia is extreme ($<200/\mu l$), the workup must include bone marrow examination to rule out several of the causes which can be determined only by marrow examination. The particular syndrome causing the neutropenia often can be identified with a careful personal and family history as well as the physical examination. Blood counts and the peripheral blood smear, along with a bone marrow examination including cytochemistry, cytogenetics, and cell surface markers, will then complete the diagnostic evaluation of the patient.

Treatment

Until recently, there has been no specific treatment for neutrophil count disorders per se, save for the occasional patient with apparently immunologic neutro-

penia responsive to steroids or splenectomy. Neutrophilia does not require treatment itself; its identification points the clinician toward an underlying disease process or a primary myeloproliferative disorder. Testosterone and lithium therapy have been reported to increase neutrophil counts in scattered cases of patients with neutropenia, but they have not been generally effective. In situations where neutropenia is caused by a known factor, it is often reversible by elimination of the specific cause, such as overwhelming bacterial infection or drug-induced neutropenia.

The mainstray of supportive therapy for neutropenic disorders has been the management of acute infection. Antibiotics have been shown to help in the management of acute neutropenia when fever is present, even when a specific cause of the infection is not readily identified. Neutrophil transfusion was employed in the treatment of patients undergoing chemotherapy who had become neutropenic and were apparently refractory to empiric antibiotic regimens; however, because the research evidence to support the efficacy of neutrophil transfusion was limited to certain defined situations, and the number of neutrophils available for transfusion represent a small fraction of the normal daily endogenous production, neutrophil transfusion has been used considerably less frequently in recent years. One situation in which neutrophil transfusions continue to be indicated is in the management of patients with severe forms of neutrophil dysfunction. For example, patients with severe leukocyte adhesion molecule deficiency can benefit significantly from transfusion of normally functioning neutrophils, even with the relatively small numbers available by present collection methods.

Various antibiotics have been used as prophylactic therapy in neutropenic patients as well. Prophylactic penicillin and ampicillin regimens have been tried, but as resistant organisms increased in frequency, this method of prophylactic therapy was found to be of limited use. Prophylactic trimethoprim-sulfamethoxazole combination therapy has been thought to be beneficial in certain patient groups. Also, patients with severe chronic neutropenia, particularly children with congenital neutropenias, frequently have been maintained on long-term prophylactic antibiotics, although clear-cut proof of the benefits from this approach are unavailable in the literature.

The recent introduction of the recombinant human colony-stimulating factors, G-CSF and GM-CSF, promises to alter significantly the management of this group of patient problems. Early clinical trial data demonstrate that both G-CSF and GM-CSF can decrease the severity and duration of neutropenia caused by chemotherapy for various malignant diseases.[18,19] In addition, both factors appear capable of shortening the period of severe neutropenia following autologous bone marrow transplantation for lymphoma or solid tumors.[20,21] The availability of these hematopoietic growth factors to increase the peripheral blood neutrophil count certainly will change the spectrum of problems occurring in patients during various forms of cancer chemotherapy, and developmental issues will appear around the appropriate use of these factors to increase the dose of chemotherapy to be administered and raise questions about whether prophylactic treatment or therapeutic intervention after the development of neutropenia is the most appropriate approach. The specific indications for each factor will evolve over the next few years, and additional clinical experience will be required to determine their relative merits and proper place in our armamentarium.

In the case of neutropenic syndromes unassociated with cancer chemotherapy, there is a developing body of literature that suggests the efficacy of recombinant human G-CSF for neutropenic disorders. G-CSF has been shown both to increase counts and decrease infectious complication rates in several varieties of severe chronic neutropenia,[22–24] and comparative trials in the syndrome of infantile genetic agranulocytosis (Kostmann syndrome) suggest that G-CSF may be superior to GM-CSF for this entity.[25] Further studies will be required to identify the precise indications for these factors in nonmalignant causes of neutropenia.

Because these recombinant CSFs have been demonstrated to affect the function of cells as well as their production, trials have been initiated to determine their effects in some of the rarer neutrophil function disorders. The data are insufficient to reach conclusions at this time, but further work continues. In chronic granulomatous disease of childhood, studies suggest the efficacy of interferon-γ in improving cell function and diminishing infectious complication rates.[26] The role of other biologic factors in altering neutrophil function and potentially benefitting this group of patients has only begun to be examined.

Given the significant role of neutrophils in inflammatory responses, and particularly the contribution of neutrophils to the "postreperfusion injury" syndromes, the prospect for management of neutrophil-induced diseases is beginning to be appreciated. Initial preclinical investigations have demonstrated that inhibiting neutrophil function can provide protection from this severe injury. Infarct size in a dog model of myocardial infarction, reperfusion injury following reattachment of severed ears in rabbits, and shock in primates have improved dramatically with administration of murine monoclonal antibodies that inhibit leukocyte adhesion molecule function.[7] Experimental studies in humans using this novel approach have just begun.

The advent of newer biologic agents capable of increasing the numbers and function of neutrophils have allowed a new approach to patients with neutrophil disorders. This advance in therapeutics will compel physicians toward an increasingly more precise differential diagnosis of neutrophil disorders. The identification of particular syndromes of neutropenia and neutrophil function disorders that will respond to these newer therapies has just begun. In the past, neutrophil disorders were identified largely as markers for other diseases, mostly infections and primary marrow disorders that reduced their number; today, neutrophil disorders also include a number of primary processes amenable to modification that offer an opportunity to improve the care of patients.

REFERENCES

1. Craddock CG. Defenses of the body: the initiators of defense, the ready reserves, and the scavengers. In: Wintrobe MM, ed. Blood, Pure and Eloquent. New York: McGraw-Hill, 1980:417–54.
2. Williams WJ, Beutler E, Erslev AJ, Lichtman MA, eds. Hematology, Fourth Edition. New York: McGraw-Hill, 1990:761–834.
3. Zucker-Franklin D, Greaves MF, Grossi CE, Marmont A. Atlas of Blood Cells: Function and Pathology. Philadelphia: Lea & Febiger, 1981.
4. Babior BM, Stossel TP. Hematology: A Pathophysiological Approach, 2nd ed. New York: Churchill Livingstone, 1990:265–89.
5. Klebanoff SJ, Clark RA. The Neutrophil: Function and Clinical Disorders. New York: North Holland, 1978.
6. Garrod AE. Inborn errors of metabolism. Lancet 1908;ii: 1,73,142,214.
7. Harlan JM, Vedder NB, Winn RK, Rice CL. Mechanisms and consequences of leukocyte-endothelial interaction. West J Med 1991;155:365–9.
8. Dale DC, Wolff SM. Studies of the neutropenia of acute malaria. Blood 1973;41:197–205.
9. Skubitz KM, Craddock PR. Reversal of hemodialysis granulocytopenia and pulmonary leukostasis. J Clin Invest 1981;67:1383.
10. Price TH, Dale DC. The selective neutropenias. Clin Haematol 1978;7:501–21.
11. Starkebaum G, Price TH, Lee MY, Arend WP. Autoimmune neutropenia in systemic lupus erythematosus. Arthritis Rheum 1978;21:504.
12. Starkebaum G, Singer JW, Arend WP. Humoral and cellular immune mechanisms of neutropenia in patients with Felty's syndrome. Clin Exp Immunol 1980;39:307.
13. Anderson DC, Springer TA. Leukocyte adhesion deficiency: an inherited defect in the Mac-1, LFA-1, and p150,95 glycoproteins. Annu Rev Med 1987;38:175.
14. Dinauer MC, Orkin SH, Brown R, et al. The glycoprotein encoded by the X-linked chronic granulomatous disease locus in a component of the neutrophil cytochrome b complex. Nature 1987;327:717.
15. Curnutte JT, Berkow RL, Roberts RL, et al. Chronic granulomatous disease due to a defect in the cytosolic factor required for nicotinamide adenine nucleotide phosphate oxidase activation. J Clin Invest 1988;81:606.
16. Babior BM, Crowley CA. Chronic granulomatous disease and

other disorders of oxidative killing by phagocytes. In: Stanbury JB, Wyngaarden JB, Frederickson DS, eds. Metabolic Basis of Inherited Disease. New York: McGraw-Hill, 1983:1956–85.

17. Mileski WJ, Winn RK, Vedder NB, Pohlman TH, Harlan JM, Rice CL. Inhibition of CD18-dependent neutrophil adherence reduces organ injury after hemorrhagic shock in primates. Surgery 1990;108:206–12.

18. Antman KS, Griffin JD, Elias A, et al. Effect of recombinant human granulocyte-macrophage colony-stimulating factor on chemotherapy-induced myelosuppression. N Engl J Med 1988;319:593–8.

19. Crawford J, Ozer H, Stoller R, et al. Reduction by granulocyte colony-stimulating factor or fever and neutropenia induced by chemotherapy in patients with small-cell lung cancer. N Engl J Med 1991;315:164–70.

20. Nemunaitis J, Rabinowe SN, Singer JW, et al. Recombinant granulocyte-macrophage colony-stimulating factor after autologous bone marrow transplantation for lymphoid cancer. N Engl J Med 1991;324:1773–8.

21. Sheridan WP, Morstyn G, Wolf M, et al. Granulocyte colony-stimulating factor and neutrophil recovery after high-dose chemotherapy and autologous bone marrow transplantation. Lancet 1989;ii:891–5.

22. Hammond WP, Price TH, Souza LM, Dale DC. Treatment of cyclic neutropenia with granulocyte colony-stimulating factor. N Engl J Med 1989;320:1306–11.

23. Jakubowski AA, Souza L, Kelly F, et al. Effects of human granulocyte colony-stimulating factor in a patient with idiopathic neutropenia. N Engl J Med 1989;320:38–42.

24. Bonilla MA, Gillio AP, Ruggeiro M, et al. Effects of recombinant human granulocyte colony-stimulating factor on neutropenia in patients with congenital agranulocytosis. N Engl J Med 1989;320:1574–80.

25. Welte K, Zeidler C, Reiter A, et al. Differential effects of granulocyte-macrophage colony-stimulating factor and granulocyte colony-stimulating factor in children with severe congenital neutropenia. Blood 1990;75:1056–63.

26. Ezekowitz RAB, Orkin SH, Newburger PE. Recombinant interferon gamma augments phagocyte superoxide production and X-chronic granulomatous disease gene expression in X-linked variant chronic granulomatous disease. J Clin Invest 1987;80:1009.

10

Monocytes and Macrophages

David S. Newcombe, M.D.

The monocyte–macrophage system and polymorphonuclear leukocytes, as professional phagocytes, represent the major cellular elements of the innate immune system and the primary host defense against infectious agents.[1-3] Monocytes and macrophages also are key components of the lymphocyte-mediated adaptive immune system, because these cells process antigens and present partially degraded antigen on their surface where it is recognized by lymphocytes, with the subsequent generation of antibodies.[4]

Cells of the monocyte–macrophage system consist of monoblasts and promonocytes arising from stem cells in the bone marrow and residing there until maturation is complete, when the mature monocyte is released into the blood stream as a circulating cell.[5-9] Circulating monocytes migrate to various tissues, where they undergo further maturation into free or fixed tissue macrophages. Both blood monocytes and free tissue macrophages are mobile cells that can migrate to sites of chronic inflammation, where their phagocytic properties and secretory products are utilized to attack invading organisms or tumor cells and to participate in tissue repair and remodeling processes.[10,11] In acute inflammatory reactions, monocytes also may assist neutrophils, especially with infectious agents that parasitize macrophages and undergo intracellular replication.[12,13]

Monocytes and macrophages also assist in the regulation of erythropoiesis and granulopoiesis through secretion of the colony-stimulating factor (CSF) for human colony-forming unit–granulocyte macrophage as well as a factor essential for the growth of erythroid burst-forming units.[14,15] Furthermore, macrophages residing in the spleen ingest senescent erythrocytes, and the catabolism of hemoglobin from these erythrocytes releases iron for transfer to developing erythroblasts.[16]

Tissue macrophages are widely distributed in the body, and these cells undergo adaptations to function effectively in their local environments.[17-24] In many instances, evaluations of free macrophages recovered from body sites such as the bronchoalveolar spaces, peritoneal cavity, pleural cavity, and bone marrow may be useful as adjuncts to the diagnosis and management of specific disease processes. Furthermore, analyses of fixed macrophages in biopsy specimens have illustrated clearly the morphologic and functional heterogeneity that exists in peripheral blood monocytes and tissue macrophage populations.[24-29] Subsets of monocytes and macrophages have been recognized by differences in size and cell density as well as by differences in their membrane receptors, secretory products, and responses to stimuli (Table 10.1).[30-33] Some variations have been studied most extensively in the peripheral blood monocyte and pulmonary macrophages recovered by lung lavage. The challenge to the clinician is to relate such cellular variations to physiologic and pathologic states.

Similar to disorders of other cells of the hematopoietic system, disorders of monocyte and macrophage function give rise to pathologic processes, and changes in monocyte and macrophage cell numbers sometimes are associated with specific diseases. Such pathologic processes include malignant disorders of monocytes and macrophages,[34-38] abnormalities in the processing of phagocytosed materials (storage disorders),[39] genetic defects in monocyte and macrophage secretory components and membrane receptors,[40,41] defective migration,[42-47] and impaired phagocytosis and chronic gran-

TABLE 10.1. The Heterogeneity of Monocyte Subsets

Surface Antigen/Function	Large Monocyte	Small Monocyte
Ia	+	+
Leu M3	+	+
Nonspecific esterase	+	+
Leu 10 (B cells; monocytes)	50%	−
Phagocytosis	Increased	N
Superoxide production	Increased	N
Myeloperoxidase activity	Increased	N
Antigen presentation	+ +	+ + + +
Prostaglandin E$_2$ production	+ + +	+ +
Activated function	Immunosuppression	Immunostimulation

Source: Esa et al. 1986[33]; Gonwa et al. 1983[285]; Yasaka et al. 1981[286]; Norris et al. 1979[287]

Note: N = normal; − = absent; + = present.

ulomatous processes including both reactive hyperplasia and destructive neoplastic processes such as Wegener granulomatosis.[48–52]

Understanding monocytes and macrophages in both health and disease provides the hematology student with the biochemical basis of cell differentiation, emigration and chemotaxis, transmembrane signaling and cell secretion, phagocytosis and cytotoxic mechanisms, and the regulation of both host defense systems and inflammatory processes by recombinant products and other molecules. Such a plenary comprehension is essential as the new age of immunotherapy with recombinant products emerges.

MONOCYTOPOIESIS

In fetal life, the yolk sac, liver, and spleen serve as the site of hematopoiesis until the seventh intrauterine month, at which time the bone marrow becomes the primary site of hematopoiesis, including monocytopoiesis.[53–55] Monocytes and their precursor cells are difficult to identify in bone marrow preparations, because they constitute less than 1% of the approximately 10^{12} hematopoietic progenitor cells. The bone marrow is tightly regulated to permit only the generation and differentiation of sufficient numbers of monocytes to perform their normal physiologic functions and to respond to certain pathophysiologic needs. Alterations in such regulatory mechanisms may contribute to abnormal states of bone marrow production such as in leukemias.

The maturation of bone marrow precursor cells to mature blood and tissue macrophages requires stimula-

tion by specific growth factors,[56] and these growth factors have certain common properties. They are all extracellular proteins heavily glycosylated to protect them from proteolysis in inflammatory settings and to increase their stability and solubility,[57] but such glycosylation has little effect on their functional properties. The genes for the growth factors involved in monocyte production (interleukin [IL]-3), granulocyte-macrophage colony-stimulating factor (GM-CSF), macrophage colony-stimulating factor (M-CSF), and the cell receptor for M-CSF all reside on the long arm of human chromosome 5 (5q), where other growth factors (endothelial cell growth factor and platelet-derived growth factor) are also found.[58] All growth factors act on cells a short distance from where they are generated and are therefore termed *paracrine* factors. Their action usually is not restricted to a single progenitor cell type, which may have significance regarding the differential regulation of proliferation and differentiation observed with some growth factors. These growth factors also alter the functions of terminally differentiated cells; for example, IL-3 enhances the cell division and phagocytosis of differentiated macrophages, and GM-CSF increases macrophage phagocytic activity and intracellular killing.[59–61]

The most immature progenitor cell for monocytes is the pluripotent stem cell (colony-forming unit [CFU]-blasts), which also serves as a progenitor cell for erythrocytes, basophils, neutrophils, eosinophils, and platelets.[62] Relatively small numbers of these cells (10^6 to 10^7) exist in human marrow, but such stem cells have an enormous capacity for self-renewal.[63,64] In fact, less than 5% of the total marrow stem-cell population is required for the regeneration of bone marrow after transplantation, and both IL-3 (multi-CSF) and GM-CSF trigger the proliferation of puripotent stem cells. IL-3 is produced primarily by antigen or IL-1–stimulated T cells.[57] Human IL-3 is a species-specific molecule (20 to 26 kd) that binds to a 72.4-kd receptor on human peripheral blood monocytes and bone marrow cells with an affinity constant in the range of 10^{-10} M.[57,65] Human GM-CSF is also species specific, with a molecular mass of 14 to 35 kd, and binds to neutrophils, macrophages, and bone marrow cells with an affinity constant of about 4×10^{-9} M.[57] Both IL-3 and GM-CSF are essential for the generation of monocytes from bone marrow progenitor cells and have the capacity to stimulate the following monocyte precursors: CFU-blast, colony-forming unit–granulocyte-erythroid-macrophage-megakaryocyte, and CFU–granulocyte macrophage. The complete molecular mechanism for the modes of action of these growth factors on progenitor cells remains to be resolved, but it is known that IL-3 translocates protein kinase C from cytoplasm to membrane without an accompanying change in phospho-inositide metabolism.[66,67]

Macrophage colony-stimulating factor (or CSF-1) is a 26-kd protein released from activated monocytes, endothelial cells, and fibroblasts that triggers the maturation of macrophage progenitor cells to monoblasts and peripheral blood monocytes.[57,65] It also enhances phagocytic activity in monocytes. This growth factor is macrophage-specific and binds to a 16.5-kd receptor on monocytes and macrophages; the M-CSF receptor has tyrosine kinase activity and is identical to the c-*fms* proto-oncogene product.[68–70] In murine systems, this receptor negatively regulates the production of M-CSF by lowering M-CSF concentrations in the blood. In the steady state, the concentration of M-CSF is related inversely to the number of macrophages[71]; when the number of macrophages increases, there is more receptor-mediated endocytosis and lysosomal degradation of M-CSF as well as a lower concentration of CSF in the blood. Thus, fewer progenitor cells in the marrow are triggered to differentiate into monocytes and macrophages. Based on a generation time of 48 hours per progenitor cell, it has been estimated that it takes approximately 6 days to differentiate from primitive precursor to circulating monocyte.[72] However, because additional progenitor cells have been defined, the transit time may be somewhat longer than had been initially postulated. Both monoblasts and promonocytes can be differentiated from fully matured monocytes by their morphology and the presence of azurophilic granules. Also, there is little or no bone marrow pool of monocytes, such as exists for neutrophils, because the monocytes are released soon after they attain maturity (1 to 2 days). The average generation time for monocytes is believed to be 13 hours.

THE MORPHOLOGY OF MONOCYTES AND MONOCYTE-DERIVED CELLS

Monocytes viewed in fresh peripheral blood smears stained with Wright stain usually are easy to differentiate from other cells.[73] However, monocytes may be difficult to distinguish from large lymphocytes, and in this setting, histochemical stains have been used to characterize specific markers of the monocyte and macrophage series. Peripheral blood monocytes give weakly positive reactions both with the periodic acid–Schiff reaction for carbohydrates and with the Sudan black B reaction for lipids, but the membrane-localized nonspecific esterase reaction represents an enzyme marker reasonably specific for cells of the monocyte and macrophage series.[74] The monocyte–macrophage nonspecific esterase activity can be differentiated from the esterase activity of granulocytes by sodium fluoride, which inhibits monocyte esterases but not the granulocyte enzyme. Monocyte esterase has now been purified to homogeneity, and its kinetic parameters are well defined.[75]

The monocyte itself is about 12 to 15 μm in diameter, with a reniform nucleus comprising almost 50% of the cell's total area. Nuclear chromatin is aggregated along the internal surface of the nuclear membrane, and nucleoli usually are present. The nuclear chromatin with its small strands gives a "raked" appearance, and with Wright stain, the cytoplasm of the monocyte has a characteristic bluish-gray color containing fine pinkish-purple as well as large azurophilic granules and clear cytoplasmic vacuoles.[73] By phase microscopy, the eccentric nucleus of the monocyte can be seen to have a central depression that contains a centrosome, and the most striking appearance of the monocyte by both phase and transmission electron microscopy is the undulating and ruffled cell margin with its numerous microprojections. The monocyte and macrophage both have well-developed Golgi complexes associated with mitochondria.

By electron microscopic histochemistry, the monocyte is observed to have two populations of cytoplasmic granules. Such granule populations either are analogous to the azurophilic granules of the granulocyte and contain acid phosphatase, arylsulfatase, and peroxidase or represent granules without defined cytochemical reactivity. Lysosomal granules contain digestive enzymes and can be characterized by their lysosomal enzymes.

The population of monocytic granules is similar to the azurophilic granules of granulocytes, and its chemical reactivity is heterogenous. Such granules represent modified primary lysosomes. The peroxidase-positive granules of the monocyte are small and less numerous than those of the neutrophil.

The macrophage represents a much more mature cell than the monocyte, and its cytochemical and histologic features reflect both its geographic location and its function at that site. Macrophages usually have a diameter of 25 to 50 μm, two to three times that of their precursor, the monocyte. Their nuclear shape is either reniform or fusiform, with one or two nucleoli. The nucleus is eccentric, and the chromatin is localized along the nuclear membrane or in clumps in the interior of the nucleus. As might be expected for a phagocytic cell, the plasma membrane is intensely ruffled, permitting adherence and migration through the function of these lamellipodia. There usually also are numerous cytoplasmic vacuoles at the periphery of the cell indicative of the cell's pinocytotic activity.

The most characteristic feature of the macrophage is its membrane-bound lysosomes, which often can be seen fusing with phagosomes to form phagolysosomes containing microbial structures or particulates. Phagolysosomes are secondary lysosomes that digest and dispose of phagocytosed materials. Macrophages also have a well-developed Golgi complex (because it performs secretory functions) and generous mitochondria to provide the energy for endocytosis. Splenic and liver macrophages (Kupffer cells) are characterized by the appearance of ingested erythrocytes and aggregated ferritin in their cytoplasm; bone marrow, splenic, and hepatic macrophages also have a central role in the storage and transfer of iron. Macrophages from the pleural and peritoneal cavities contain the structural elements necessary for endocytosis, and histochemical analyses of macrophages easily identify heterogeneity in this population. This is especially true when lysosomes are stained for specific enzymatic activity.[76]

Monoblasts and promonocytes are the immediate precursors of the monocyte, and the monoblast, the most primitive cell of the macrophage series, is indistinguishable from the granulocyte precursor, the myeloblast. This cell has a very large nucleus occupying most of the cell except for a small cytoplasmic rim. The nucleus contains multiple nucleoli, and peroxidase-positive reactions are identified in the rough endoplasmic reticulum, the cysternae of the Golgi complex, and the occasional developing azurophilic granules. The promonocyte, the immediate precursor of the peripheral blood monocyte, also is difficult to distinguish from the progranulocyte (promyelocyte). It has an indented nucleus and visible nucleoli, and cytochemical studies show its characteristic nonspecific esterase activity, which identifies it as a cell of the monocyte–macrophage series. The cytoplasm of this monocyte precursor has a well-developed Golgi complex and contains bundled or single filaments; such filaments and deeply indented nuclei with an irregular shape are said to distinguish these cells from progranulocytes. Peroxidase-positive reactions are visualized throughout the cell structures participating in cell secretion (which includes the rough endoplasmic reticulum), cysternae of the Golgi and perinuclear area, and in immature and mature granules. Such peroxidase-positive granules distinguish exudate macrophages that have recently migrated from the bone marrow and blood from resident macrophages that have lost their peroxidase reactivity.[77] The same secretory apparatus also gives positive reactions for acid phosphatase and arylsulfatase.

DISTRIBUTION

Monocytes are produced in humans at a rate of 7×10^6 cells/hour/kg body weight under homeostatic condi-

tions; this rate may increase fourfold in inflammatory states.[78] The pool size of blood monocytes has been determined to be in the range of 3×10^5 cells/ml of blood, or an average circulating pool of 1.8×10^7 cells/kg body weight. These cells remain in the blood for 1 to 3 days, with an average daily turnover rate of 1.9×10^9 cells/kg and a half-life in blood of between 8 and 71 hours. The heterogeneity of circulating monocytes has been clearly established with respect to size, density, morphology, surface antigens, and perhaps function.[29] Small peripheral blood monocytes manifest more immunogenic activity, whereas large monocytes appear to be more immunosuppressive.[33] However, despite the isolation and characterization of both monocyte and macrophage subsets, the origin of such heterogeneity remains in question. The prevailing evidence seems to suggest that such heterogeneity develops after migration from the bone marrow, but some evidence still remains from animal systems that such variation may arise from different progenitor subtypes in the marrow. Because adherence-promoting glycoproteins result in the attachment of monocytes to endothelial cells, a marginating pool of monocytes probably exists in the capillaries, but conclusive proof of such a pool in humans remains to be established.[79,80] However, recent citations indicate that the circulating monocyte pool consists of a marginating and a circulating pool, with the marginating pool being three times the size of the circulating. Such data have been derived in part from epinephrine studies that examined the marginating pool of neutrophils,[81] and such studies receive additional support from the knowledge that leukocyte adherence proteins exist in the monocyte.

Monocytes migrate from the circulating pool to the extravascular pool on a random basis, and there they undergo transformation into tissue macrophages. Little is known about the regulation of monocyte maturation into tissue macrophages, but the process appears to be under the control of local factors. Once monocytes migrate to tissue sites, they do not return to the circulating pool of cells, and certain generalizations can be made about tissue macrophages. Heterogeneity exists in both the size and the density of free-macrophage populations. The lifespan of tissue macrophages is much longer than the life span of the precursor cells, and studies of patients who underwent bone marrow ablation demonstrate that host macrophages are replaced by donor cells approximately 3 months after transplantation. Proof that human macrophages have a hematopoietic origin has been clearly shown for alveolar macrophages and Kupffer cells, because these macrophages from bone marrow transplant recipients express the sex karyotype of the donor marrow.[82,83] Nonetheless, there also is evidence that tissue macrophages can expand their population by local proliferation.[20,82] This evidence favors the predominance of hematopoietic sources for tissue macrophages over local replication. The lifespan of tissue macrophages is more than likely variable, depending on the tissue site and function, but such cells clearly remain viable for months. In the case of skin macrophages that have ingested tattoo dye and no longer retain their functional properties, the lifespan is measured in years.

In acute inflammation, both the rate of monocyte distribution to tissue sites and their metabolic activity are altered. Similar changes also occur in chronic inflammatory states. In the chronic states, the terminal stage of monocyte development gives rise to two new cell types: multinucleated giant cells and epithelioid cells. Furthermore, suppressive drugs used in the management of such pathologic states also alter the kinetics and metabolism of monocytes.

The numbers of circulating monocytes usually increase during acute or chronic infection, and the degree of this numeric change is related to the biologic characteristics of the inflammatory vector. The numbers of monocytes and macrophages also increase in those tissue sites involved in an infectious process. In part, such increases are secondary to influxes of cells from the bone marrow and circulating blood, but increments in cell numbers also occur as a result of local proliferation. Macrophages found at the site of infection are exudate macrophages, which can be differentiated from resident macrophages by their increased peroxidatic activity and monoclonal antibodies with specificity for such cells. Exudate macrophages appear to follow the arrival of monocytes from the circulation and originate primarily from blood monocytes rather than resident macrophages. Studies of acute inflammatory responses in both mice and rats have shown that total monocyte production increases more than 60% and that the half-life of circulating monocytes shortens significantly.[20] Furthermore, a substance isolated from mouse and rabbit serum or plasma during acute infections, called *factor-increasing monocytopoiesis*, has been characterized.[84] This factor is different from IL-1 and CSF-1 and has the capacity to reduce the cell-cycle time of promonocytes, increase the rate of monoblast division, and increase the number of promonocytes. Factor-increasing monocytopoiesis is synthesized and secreted by macrophages at the site of inflammation,[85] and during the late phases of an inflammatory responses, serum also contains a factor that inhibits monocytopoiesis.[86] These substances, however, have not yet been isolated from human sources.

In chronic inflammation, the cellular changes observed are dependent on the stimulus, because agents that are not easily degraded cause the production of granulomas whereas substances that can be disposed of easily cause the production of monocytes in a manner similar to that seen in acute processes. There are two fundamental types of granuloma: immune and nonimmune.[87–90] Immune granulomas are discussed in the section titled granulomas and macrophages. Nonimmune granulomas usually are characterized by foreign-body multinucleated giant cells derived for the most part by the fusion of young, recently populating monocytes with aging monocytes, the absence of epithelioid cells and lymphocytes, and the rapid turnover of immune granuloma cells in contrast to the slow turnover of cells comprising a foreign-body granuloma.[87] Epithelioid cells in those granulomas have a typical histologic appearance and are less phagocytic than their precursor cells, the monocyte and macrophage, and the lifespan of such cells is relatively short (1 to 4 weeks). Thus, monocyte–macrophage cell lineages play a significant role in both acute and chronic inflammatory processes and are especially prominent effector cells in chronic inflammatory reactions.

It should not be surprising to find that pharmacologic modulators of the immune system such as corticosteroids and purine analogues alter the kinetics and functions of monocytes and macrophages. Glucocorticoids administered to humans in pharmacologic dosages cause a reduction in the absolute and relative numbers of peripheral blood monocytes.[92–94] Two hours after a 3-day course of prednisone (50 mg) every 12 hours for six doses, a profound monocytopenia is observed.[95] Absolute numbers of monocytes as low as 50 monocytes/mm^3 have been documented after steroids, and recoveries of monocyte numbers to greater than normal levels were observed within 12 hours after the cessation of steroid treatment. The mechanism for this glucocorticoid-induced monocytopenia remains unknown, but it may have to do with changes in monocyte traffic. Independent of these alterations in cell numbers, glucocorticoids also induce functional changes in the monocyte and macrophage that will be discussed later. The purine analogues, 6-mercaptopurine and azathioprine, also reduce monocyte numbers, but kinetic studies have been characterized only for animals. Also, because the sensitivity to these agents varies among species, such data cannot be extrapolated directly to humans.[96,97] Low dosages of methotrexate (amethopterin), a folic acid analogue, also appear to reduce the number of peripheral blood monocytes in humans.[98] In animals, low dosages of this antimetabolite also reduces macrophage IL-1 synthesis and Ia antigen expression.[99]

MONOCYTE EMIGRATION

As effectors of inflammatory reactions and cell-mediated immune responses, mononuclear phagocytes must emigrate from the blood stream to sites where their regulatory capacities are required. Both leukocyte adhesion proteins and chemotaxis are essential for monocytes to emigrate.[100–102] The chemotactic substances, N-formylmethionyl peptides (FMLP) and the C5a complement fragment, bind with high affinity to specific receptors on monocytes and granulocytes,[103] and as a consequence of this receptor binding of chemoattractants, the surface expression of a family of adhesive glycoproteins, Mac-1 (complement receptor [CR]3) and p150,95, is rapidly increased.[101] The recent discovery of patients deficient in Mac-1, lymphocyte function-associated antigen 1 (LFA-1), and p150,95 glycoproteins has enhanced the understanding of the functions and molecular biology of these adhesive glycoproteins.[101] These patients express a deficiency in a subunit of the glycoproteins that includes the α-subunits of Mac-1, LFA-1, and p150,05 and a common β 95-kd subunit. This leukocyte adhesion protein deficiency is inherited as an autosomal recessive mutation with a variable phenotypic expression. When less than 0.2% of these adhesive substances are expressed, it is a severe type; when only 5% are found, it is a moderate deficiency. The defective protein has been identified as an abnormal β-chain, which is essential for processing and transporting the various 150- to 190-kd α-subunits bound noncovalently to the β-unit to the cellular pool and cell surface when required for adhesion. A deficiency in these glycoproteins results in recurrent soft tissue infections, because neither granulocytes nor monocytes can migrate to inflammatory sites. Chemotactic responses of granulocytes and monocytes are suppressed, and chemotaxis-induced cell orientation also is deficient. Such glycoprotein-deficient monocytes are unable to adhere to endothelial cells during diapedesis and migration to inflammatory sites. Blood monocytes express more CR3 than p150,95, whereas the expression of these two components in tissue macrophages is reversed. The p150,95 protein is the key component for monocyte adhesion and chemotaxis, whereas the Mac-1 appears to be more important for neutrophil migration. The genes encoding the α- and β-subunits of these leukocyte adhesion proteins are located on chromosomes 16 and 21, respectively.

A variety of substances have been characterized as chemoattractants for monocytes and macrophages (Table 10.2); some have specificity for only these cell types, whereas others have broader specificity. The most potent monocyte chemotaxin appears to be transforming growth factor-beta, because under certain conditions, monocytes can respond to femtomolar concentrations of this lymphokine or platelet-derived product.[104,105] The chemoattractants with the most relevance to pathologic processes involving monocyte- and macrophage-dependent processes are: lymphocyte-derived chemotactic

TABLE 10.2.   Monocyte Chemotactic Factors

Activated T-lymphocyte product (LDCF)
Activated B-lymphocyte chemotactic products
Bacterial products
    N-formylated oligopeptides
Complement-derived components
    C5a
Connective tissue products
    Elastin peptides
    Desmosine
    Collagen
    Collagenase-digested collagen (collagen peptides)
    Fibronectin fragments
Denatured albumin and hemoglobin
Neuropeptides
    Opiate peptides (β-endorphin and dynorphin)
    Bombesin
    Substance P
    Benzodiazepines (Valium)
Platelet-derived growth factor
Prekallikrein-derived chemotactic factor
Thrombin
Transforming growth factor-β
Tumor cell–derived chemotactic factors

Note: LDCF = lymphocyte-derived chemotactic factor.

factor, C5a, elastin-derived peptides, collagen-derived peptides, platelet-derived growth factor, and TGF-β.[105–111] Chemotaxis is dependent on the reaction of the chemotactic ligand with a specific cell surface receptor; monocyte and macrophage receptors central to chemotactic responses usually express a high affinity for the chemotactic ligand. Such interactions of chemotactic ligand with cell receptors are concentration-dependent, and at the levels that induce directional movement (chemotaxis), these substances also increase random motility (chemokinesis), cell-to-substrate adherence, and cell–cell aggregation. Higher concentrations of chemotaxins may induce the release of lysosomal enzymes, the production of reactive oxygen species, and IL-1. The initial event in chemotaxis is monocyte membrane hyperpolization, which leads to an activation of an N protein by guanosine triphosphate.[100,102,113] Activated N protein stimulates phospholipase C, which hydrolyzes phosphatidylinositol 4,5-biphosphate into two intracellular messengers, 1,2-diacylglycerol and inositol triphosphate. These second messengers activate protein kinase C and release ionic calcium from intracellular stores. The increment in intracellular calcium mediates protein phosphorylation either by protein kinase C or by calcium and calmodulin-dependent kinases, and such phosphorylated proteins like gelsolin permit actin-filament assembly and cell propulsion. Retractive movements are regulated by calcium-dependent myosin activity, and the chemotactic response is terminated by elevated levels of cyclic adenosine monophosphate and the cessation of phosphatidylinositol 4,5-biphosphate hydrolysis by inactivation of the N protein via protein kinase C activity. While these mechanisms of cell chemotaxis are best characterized for human neutrophils, these findings serve as models for monocyte chemotaxis.[100,102,103]

PINOCYTOSIS AND PHAGOCYTOSIS

Once monocytes have emigrated to the sites of inflammation or their normal tissue locale (sinusoids of the liver and spleen, pulmonary alveoli, pleural and peritoneal serous cavities, brain as microglial cells, skin, and connective tissues as well as the synovial membrane of joints), they usually participate in tissue remodeling and repair or respond to infection and inflammation by the ingestion of cellular debris and/or microorganisms. Pinocytosis is a receptor-mediated endocytic system for the ingestion of fluid and small molecules that has several differences from the more traditional phagocytic system.[114] Many cells can pinocytose, but the attachment and ingestion of particles by phagocytosis is restricted to "professional phagocytes." Particles ingested by receptor-mediated pinocytosis are less than 1 μm in diameter and use clathrin-coated vesicles for this process. Cytochalasins alter phagocytosis by inhibiting the formation of actin filaments but do not impede pinocytosis, which occurs at lower temperatures (18°C) than phagocytosis. Therefore, pinocytosis is not a function specific to monocytes whereas phagocytosis is.

Mononuclear phagocytes contain a variety of plasma membrane receptors essential for phagocytosis. These include immunoglobulin Fc receptors (FcRI, FcRII, and FcRIII), complement receptors (CR1 [C3b], CR3 [C3bi]), and CR4 [C3d,g]), glycoprotein receptors (mannosyl-, fucosyl-, and N-acetylglucosaminyl glycoproteins), fibronectin receptors, and acetylated low-density lipoprotein receptors.[115–120] Particles opsonized by immunoglobulin, complement, or fibronectin are ingested via specific Fc, CR, and fibronectin receptors, whereas mannose- or fucose-terminal glycoprotein or acetylated receptors bind substances directly. The Fc receptors also have specificity in that FcRI binds monomers of IgG with high affinity and with preference for IgG_1, then IgG_3, then IgG_4, and with much less preference for IgG_2, with a K_a of 1 to 3×10^8 M^{-1}.[121] FcRII is present on tissue macrophages and binds immune complexes with low avidity, with preference for IgG_1 and IgG_3 over IgG_2 and IgG_4, and FcRIII binds aggregates of IgG_1 and IgG_3. The expression of FcRI on monocytes is enhanced by interferon-γ, and binding to

this receptor increases the generation of superoxide radicals.[122,123] Antibody-dependent cellular cytotoxicity also is mediated via this receptor,[124] but the absence of FcRI receptors on human monocytes does not appear to result in abnormal pathology.[125]

Complement receptors also mediate the binding and ingestion of complement-coated particles. CR1 contains two complement recognition sites, one for C3b and one for C4b, whereas CR3 binds iC3b with a requirement for a divalent cation, magnesium, or calcium.[117,126] CR1 requires no cations for its binding, and its affinity for dimeric C3b is 5×10^7 M^{-1}. The CR3 receptor also recognizes coagulation factor X, fibrinogen, and a membrane protein of *Leishmania* parasites as well as molecular components of *Salmonella typhimurium* and *Histoplasma capsulatum*.[127–129] Other microbes that grow inside monocytes and macrophages, such as *Mycobacterium tuberculosis, Mycobacterium leprae,* and *Legionella pneumophilia,* also are presumed to bind to the CR3 receptor.[130–133] Unlike the Fc receptor, ligand binding to complement receptors does not induce any other cellular responses, which perhaps accounts for the absence of oxidant-induced damage to the microorganisms ingested by such receptors. Yeasts are ingested by mannose glycoprotein receptors, and unopsinized gram-negative bacteria bind to CR3, LFA-1 and p150,95 receptors.[127,134] CR3 receptors increase in number as monocytes become macrophages, and individuals with a deficiency of CR3 receptors are susceptible to recurrent microbial infections. Interferon-γ treatment of monocytes and macrophages significantly reduces the binding of C3b and iC3b to CR1 and CR3 receptors in contrast to the up-regulation of Fc receptors by this lymphokine;[135] this reduction in binding appears to result from a conformational change in the receptor molecules. Such changes in binding activity can be enhanced by interactions with fibronectin, serum amyloid P component, and laminin bound to extracellular matrices,[136–138] and these proteins are all present in basal lamina attached to elastin fibers. In addition, soluble fibronectin, which in its unbound form does not activate C3 complement receptors, binds to thrombi, denatured collagen, and microbes. Fibronectin in this bound form serves to enhance macrophage phagocytosis via activated C3 complement receptors.[121] In animals, lymphokines also can activate C3 complement receptors, but a human counterpart has yet to be described. The mechanism of activation is incompletely understood, but it may occur via protein phosphorylation and subsequent clustering of receptors. Protein synthesis is not a requirement for the activation of complement receptors.

Both Fc and CR receptors regulate phagocytosis and can act either independently or cooperatively to ingest particles.[126,139] It is essential to understand the differences and commonalities between the functions of these receptors. The binding of C3bi to CR3 receptors is a temperature-dependent process, whereas the binding to Fc receptors is not. Clustering of immunoglobulins or complement fragments on particles enhances attachment to their respective receptors, and Fc receptors behave in a constitutive fashion, with attachment followed by ingestion, whereas complement receptors require activation to ingest particles. Furthermore, Fc-mediated phagocytosis is accompanied by the production of superoxide radicals, the synthesis and release of arachidonic acid metabolites, and protein phosphorylation; phagocytosis via activated CR receptors does not generate these synthetic products. Phagocytosis requires energy, which comes from glycolysis and the large glycogen stores in macrophages,[140] and macrophages also utilize energy derived from creatine phosphate stores.[141] In Fc-mediated phagocytosis, the oxygen uptake is increased, and the reduction of this oxygen to superoxide results in the release of this free radical that is active in microbial killing. However, the respiratory burst of oxygen uptake associated with phagocytosis is not an essential component of this process.[142] The engulfment of Fc or complement-coated particles occurs by a similar mechanism which has received the eponym "the zipper hypothesis."[143] After the ligand and receptor make initial contact, continuing contact is made between pseudopods formed by the assembly and cross-linking of actin filaments in the cytoplasm beneath the receptors, such that ligand-receptor interaction occurs in the fashion of a "zipper" as the particle is surrounded by a protein-tight seal. As the pseudopods from either side of the engulfed particle approach, membrane fusion occurs and forms a phagosome inside the cell. The phagocytosis of multiple particles can result in the internalization of large quantities of plasma membrane, but the large stores of plasma membrane within the cell as well as the efficient recycling of phagosomes permit these cells to maintain more than sufficient surface area to continue phagocytosis.

As might be expected, a variety of signal transduction mechanisms have been postulated to account for the process of phagocytosis, but none has led to a complete understanding of this process.[144] Inhibitors of monocyte metabolism (deoxyglucose or fluoride) and actin assembly (cytochalasins) block the ingestion of phagocytes, and monovalent cation fluxes and altered calcium concentrations may alter accessory functions associated with phagocytosis but appear not to affect phagocytosis directly. Pertussis toxin has been shown to diminish Fc-mediated phagocytosis by human monocytes, and such data suggest that pertussis toxin–sensitive G proteins may be involved in particle ingestion by this receptor. In addition, macrophage protein phosphoryla-

tion has been associated with Fc- and complement-mediated phagocytosis.[121,127,145] Further work is necessary to characterize the signals essential for phagocytosis, but it is clear that the assembly and disassembly of the macrophage cytoskeleton are essential for the phagocytic process. However, the process is even more complex, because one ligand can interact with more than one receptor and one receptor is able to transmit more than one transductive signal.

TISSUE MACROPHAGES: THE RESPONSE TO INJURY AND INFECTION

Monocytes that have emigrated to a site of inflammation are stimulated by a variety of molecules associated with the inflammatory process that alter both the structure and function of these cells during their differentiation to macrophages.[88,146,147] Furthermore, the vast array of secretory products of the monocyte and macrophage attest to the essential role of this cell type in tissue remodeling and the regulation of inflammation (Table 10.3). Stimulated or inflammatory macrophages contain more protein per cell than resident macrophages, which accounts for their increased size, and a significant increase in plasma membrane ruffling accounts for the increased capacity of inflammatory macrophages both to adhere to artificial surfaces (plastic and glass) and to ingest fluid and particulates. Both the endocytic and migratory capacities of these inflammatory macrophages also are increased, as are the biochemical functions associated with those activities.[88,146,147] Such biochemical changes include increases in lysosomal enzyme activity, number of lysosomes and lysosomal fusion vacuoles, secreted enzymes capable of tissue-matrix breakdown, number of mitochondria, enzymes essential for glycolysis, and Fc receptors.[148] One might assume that such plump endocytic inflammatory macrophages would be sufficient to respond to any challenge, but these cells cannot destroy certain infectious agents or neoplastic growths despite their capacity to invade inflammatory and neoplastic lesions.[149–151] The activation of macrophages is required for these processes.

Unlike the maturation process from resident macrophage or migratory monocyte to inflammatory macrophage, the activation of macrophages requires a cell-mediated immune process to generate macrophages with both antitumor cytotoxicity and the capacity to destroy intracellular parasites.[152–154] This activation process occurs in a stepwise fashion and has immunologic specificity through its antigen-driven, sensitized-T-lymphocyte activation to produce macrophage "activating" lymphokines; the effector functions of the activated

TABLE 10.3. Monocyte and Macrophage Secretory Products

Coagulation factors
  Factors V, VII, IX, X
  Fibrinolysis inhibitor
  Prothrombin
  Protein kinase
  Thrombospondin
  Thromboplastin
Complement components
  C1, C4, C2, C3, C5
  C3b inactivator
  Factors B and D
  B1H
  Properdin
Enzymes
  Acid glycosidases
  Acid lipases
  Acid nucleases
  Acid phosphatases
  Acid proteases
  Acid sulfatases
  Arginase
  Collagenase
  Cytolytic proteinase
  Elastase
  Lipoprotein lipase
  Lysozyme
  Phospholipase A_2
Enzyme inhibitors
  α_2-Macroglobulin
  α_1-Antiprotease
  α_1-Antichymotrypsin
Hematologic and immunoregulatory proteins
  Colony stimulating factors
  Erythropoietin
  Fibronectin
  Haptoglobin
  Interferon-α and -β
  Interleukin-1
  Platelet-derived growth factor
  Transferrin
  Transcobalamin II
  Thymosin B_4
  Transforming growth factor-β
Lipid mediators
  Prostaglandins (E_2, F_2, and I_2)
  Thromboxane A_2
  Leukotrienes B, C, D, and E
  Monohydroxyeicosatetraenoic acids
  Platelet-activating factor
Reactive oxygen intermediates
  Hydrogen peroxide
  Hydroxyl radical (OH·)
  Hypohalous acid
  Superoxide (O_2^-)
Other metabolites
  Glutathione
  Purines
  Pyrimidines

macrophage express nonspecific cytotoxicity. Inflammation still plays a central role in macrophage activation, because sensitized T cells from lymph nodes draining an inflamed area migrate to such sites. There, the sensitized T cells are more than likely to make contact with sensitizing antigens and be triggered by them to proliferate and produce lymphokines. Furthermore, inflammatory macrophages are converted more easily to activated than resting macrophages, and such activated cells are cytotoxic toward antigen-inducing lymphokine production by the T lymphocyte. Thus, macrophages primed by factors from an inflammatory process are easily activated to become cytotoxic macrophages, which regulate the cytotoxic response by eliminating the antigen responsible for the production of the activating lymphokine similar to a negative feedback loop.

Macrophage activation factor remained elusive for a long time, until interferon-γ and macrophage activation factor were found to be functionally identical. Subsequently, GM-CSF and IL-4 (B-cell stimulatory factor 1) also were shown to be capable of inducing macrophage cytotoxicity for tumors and microbes.[155,156] The complex pattern of interferon-γ receptors on monocytes and macrophages may provide clues to the reasons for this redundancy in cytokines capable of inducing the activation of macrophages. Mature human macrophages express two classes of interferon-γ receptors, one set with a kD_1 of $(4.3 \pm 0.3) \times 10^{-10}$ M and the other with a kD_2 of $(6.4 \pm 1.1) \times 10^{-9}$ M.[157] Monocytes express only one receptor for interferon-γ with a kD_2 of 1×10^{-9} M; the high-affinity interferon-γ macrophage receptor has a greater affinity for the interferon-γ antagonists, interferon-β and interferon-α. Low-affinity interferon-γ receptors are not subject to this antagonism by noninterferon-γ molecules. It has been postulated that such a complex regulatory system for interferon-γ relates to the need to suppress macrophage activation at sites distant from inflammatory reactions where interferon-α and -β can prevent interferon-γ from activating macrophages and inducing tissue damage, whereas at the site of the inflammation, interferon-γ is present in sufficient concentrations to bind to the low-affinity macrophage receptors and overcome the inhibition of binding by noninterferon-γ molecules and activation of the high-affinity receptors.

Interferon-γ in the process of activation induces a number of changes in macrophages.[157] Some of these are associated directly with macrophage cytotoxicity, whereas the relationship of other changes to cytotoxicity remains to be determined. Interferon-γ increases the expression of HLA-DR, Fc receptors, lipopolysaccharide binding sites, and LFA-1, whereas this lymphokine decreases mannosyl-fucosyl glycoproteins, CR1, and transferrin receptors. Binding to the CR3 receptor is decreased by interferon-γ but is reversible with fibronectin; interferon-γ also induces the expression of IL-2 receptors on monocytes. The biologic rationale for these changes in receptor density defies a sound explanation at present, because some of these changes are not easily reconciled with the biology of macrophage activation.

The mechanism of macrophage cytotoxicity has centered on the effects of reactive oxygen intermediates. This is despite the fact that activated macrophages either are induced or show an enhanced capacity to secrete a variety of other molecules toxic to cells and microbes.[158] In addition to reactive oxygen intermediates, such toxic substances include bioactive lipids such as the arachidonic metabolites, enzymes such as hydrolases and proteases, lysozyme, IL-1α, IL-1β, TGF-β, tumor necrosis factor (TNF), interferon-γ, and reactive nitrogen intermediates.[157,159] This array of toxic agents clearly indicates that processes other than reactive oxygen intermediates likely play a role in macrophage cytotoxicity, but the products of oxygen metabolism remain the most well-characterized antibacterial defense mechanisms. Secretion of the reactive oxygen intermediates (superoxide anion and hydrogen peroxide) is triggered in the activated macrophage by phagocytosis or binding of immunoglobulins or complement fragments (C5a) to their receptors, which then give rise to an increased uptake of oxygen that has been termed *the respiratory burst*. Through an incompletely characterized reaction sequence, a plasma-membrane-resident NADPH- and flavoprotein-dependent oxidase in association with a cytochrome *b* cofactor and umbiquinone reduces oxygen to the superoxide anion, which subsequently is converted to hydrogen peroxide by superoxide dismutase. Blood monocytes also contain a peroxidase in their cytoplasmic granules identical to the myeloperoxidase in neutrophils, but the myeloperoxidase concentration in monocytes is roughly one third that observed in neutrophils. Thus, monocytes generate an antimicrobial system against bacteria and fungi through the reaction of hydrogen peroxide, ferrous ions, and iodide to form a toxic iodide species.[158] In addition, monocytes can synthesize a chlorinating substance through reactions between myeloperoxidase, hydrogen peroxide, and halides.[158] The killing of *Toxoplasma gondii, Candida albicans,* and *Aspergillus fumigatus* is in part myeloperoxidase-dependent, but nonoxidative killing mechanisms also may contribute to these cytocidal effects.[160–162] As monocytes differentiate into macrophages, they lose their granule-associated peroxidase; this change is accompanied by a decrease in the magnitude of the respiratory burst. Activated macrophages, however, have a greater respiratory burst than

resident macrophages, but such changes are unrelated to myeloperoxidase activity, which is deficient, and results instead from changes in the affinity of NADPH oxidase for NADPH.[163,164] Thus, the K_m for the NADPH oxidase substrate, NADPH, is higher (low affinity) in resident than in activated macrophages.

Another monokine with cytotoxic activity specifically toward tumors is TNF, which causes hemorrhagic necrosis and regression of TNF-sensitive tumors.[165,166] Interferon-γ, GM-CSF, CSF-1, and TNF itself can induce the synthesis and release of TNF from activated macrophages. IL-1 enhances the release of TNF from monocytes, and Sendai virus triggers the production of TNF by macrophages. Receptors for TNF have been identified on human cells, and interferon-γ increases the number of TNF receptors. The mechanisms for the cytotoxic effects of TNF are incompletely understood, but in vitro effects of TNF require the presence of TNF receptors on the target cell. Also, the inhibition of protein synthesis markedly enhances the capacity of TNF to destroy tumors. In vivo, TNF may cause cytotoxicity by somewhat different mechanisms, because it can stimulate the production of superoxide radicals by neutrophils, the degranulation and release of proteases from neutrophils, and the generation of procoagulant activity by endothelial cells with vessel thrombosis. Such effects may cause tumor cytotoxicity by impairing the vascular supply to the tumor as well as inducing the generation of tissue-damaging oxidants.

Tumor necrosis factor also is relevant to inflammatory responses, because it has many properties similar to IL-1. These include the induction of fever and acute phase reactants (such as α_1-acid glycoprotein, C3, factor B, haptoglobin, serum amyloid A, and serum amyloid P), the release of collagenase by synovial cells, the resorption of proteoglycan, the inhibition of proteoglycan synthesis, the proliferation of fibroblasts and wound repair, and the activation of osteoclasts to resorb bone.[166] In addition to these effects on the inflammatory response, TNF also has immunoregulatory properties that are especially important with respect to T-cell activation. In this way, TNF may amplify certain events related to the activation of macrophages, because it enhances the proliferation of activated T cells to antigen; increases IL-2 receptor expression and, as a result, the response to IL-2; and induces interferon-γ production, a key mediator of macrophage activation.[166] Human TNF also increases the number of antibody-forming cells to T-dependent antigens in a mouse model, and it may stimulate the proliferation of B cells. It also has the capacity to increase the expression of major histocompatibility complex (MHC) class I and class II antigens under very defined conditions, as well as to induce the expression of intercellular adhesion molecule 1, which is essential for the binding of T cells to antigen-presenting cells.[167] Such activity emphasizes the role that TNF may play in another key monocyte-dependent process, antigen presentation, which suggests that TNF may participate in protecting the host from reinfection through its facilitation of monocyte–T cell interactions.

The destruction of tumor cells by macrophages occurs through several different mechanisms: mediator-regulated suppression of cell proliferation, mediator-dependent cytostasis, antibody-independent tumor cytolysis, and antibody-dependent cellular cytotoxicity.[168] Mediator-regulated suppression of cell proliferation usually is related to the capacity of small numbers of macrophages to release mediators that inhibit lymphocyte proliferation in response to antigens or polyclonal mitogens; such suppressive activity is believed to be mediated by prostaglandin E_2 (PGE_2) and related compounds.[169] Mediator-dependent cytostasis is a poorly characterized process that requires large numbers of macrophage. It is not specific for tumor cells, because normal cells also have their entry into the S phase of cell division and DNA replication inhibited by such cytostatic macrophages. This effect occurs rapidly (within hours) in the absence of apparent contact between cytostatic macrophages and target cells, and for these reasons, mediators such as prostaglandin, thymidine, arginase, IL-1, and TNF have been postulated as the mediators of this cytostatic reaction. Cytostasis requires activated macrophages, and it is not restricted to the MHC.

Macrophage-mediated tumor cytolysis is a very specific process that requires the binding of activated macrophages to tumor cells and is independent of any antibody requirement. This process occurs over 24 to 48 hours and in two stages: the binding of macrophage to tumor cell, and the release of toxic substances.[150,151,170] Macrophage binding to tumor cells has high specificity for a variety of malignant cells of syngeneic, allogeneic, or xenogeneic origin,[171] and such macrophages are highly selective in their binding and select tumor cells from normal cells without error. The initial binding is weak and easily disrupted; early binding becomes stronger over time (1 hour at 37°C) and requires an intact microtubular and microfilamentous system. There is some suggestion that such binding occurs through a macrophage-specific receptor, the identity of which remains unknown at present. Binding to tumors can be disrupted completely by pre-incubating macrophages with proteases, which suggests that a specific protein or proteins are required for binding; the release of substances toxic to tumor cells appears to be dependent on a serine protease and TNF. The activity of the serine protease secreted by macrophages is blocked by serum antiproteases, and its activity as a cytotoxin may be required directly for cytotoxicity or, more likely, may

represent a requirement for the activity of other cytotoxic substances. TNF and reactive oxygen intermediates have known cytotoxic activities, but the activity of TNF is restricted to a very few sensitive targets. Thus, the active cytotoxic substance or substances required for macrophage-mediated tumor cytolysis remain to be characterized more completely.

Antibody-dependent cellular cytotoxicity is a well-characterized mechanism by which leukocytes, including macrophages, destroy antibody-coated cells.[150,151,171,172] This process has received prominence recently, because monoclonal antibodies have been prepared against surface molecules on tumor cells. Such antibodies recognize tumor cells through an interaction between the Fab portion of the antibody and tumor cell surface antigens; the Fc portion of the antibody serves as the link between the antibody and the macrophage Fc receptors. Antibody-coated cells make contact through the Fc receptor specific for IgG_1, IgG_{2a}, IgG_{2b}, or IgG_3 isotypes, but IgG_{2a} antibodies are much more efficient in their binding capacity than the other isotypes. The primary mechanism of cell cytotoxicity is through the release of toxic oxygen metabolites, and there appear to be two different rates of cell destruction by the antibody-dependent cellular cytotoxicity mechanism, one rapid (5 to 6 hours) and one slow (24 to 48 hours). The rapid lytic response requires a fully activated macrophage and tumor cell targets sensitive to small quantities of hydrogen peroxide; the slow mechanism is mediated by macrophages incompletely activated that require 24 to 48 hours to lyse their target cells. Additional cytotoxic substances may be released during the course of antibody-dependent cellular cytotoxicity, but they remain incompletely characterized at this time.

In conclusion, certain generalizations can be drawn regarding the activation of macrophages. First, macrophage membrane structures play a key role in the activation process whether viewed from the perspective of the receptors necessary for the induction of activation, the generation of toxic reactive oxygen intermediates, or the capacity of activated macrophages to bind to antigenically different tumor cells. Furthermore, as will be shown later, the chronic expression of activation can lead to tissue damage, and in most instances, the activated state is short-lived precisely to avoid such destructive responses. Down-regulation of the activated state is controlled by autocrine factors like prostaglandins, TNF, IL-1, interferon-γ, and CSF-1 secreted by macrophages and lymphocytes. In addition, further differentiation of activated macrophages results in the inability of the cell to respond to lymphokines and to express its cytotoxic capacities. Thus, macrophage plasma membranes play a critical role in the induction and deactivation of macrophage cytotoxicity. Second, there is significant variation in the susceptibility of microorganisms and tumors to the effects of cytotoxic macrophages and their products. Close correlations exist between the generation and release of hydrogen peroxide and macrophage cytotoxicity toward *Candida, Leishmania, Mycobacterium, Toxoplasma,* and *Trypanosoma* species, but there also are significant differences, even within the same species, in the dosage of toxicant necessary to kill.[159] Indeed, organisms at different stages of development may vary in their susceptibility to cytotoxic molecules; for example, *Leishmania* promastigotes are more sensitive to hydrogen peroxide than *Leishmania* mastigotes.[173] Furthermore, oxygen-independent mechanisms likely participate in some killing responses, because cells from patients with chronic granulomatous disease and impaired NADPH oxidase activity can mediate partially the killing of some organisms.[51]

Monocytes and macrophages ingest and destroy bacteria, but their rate of ingestion, capacity to kill, and total dependence on oxygen-requiring metabolic pathways for phagocytosis separate them from neutrophils. Neutrophils have a more efficient process for ingesting and killing bacteria and utilize oxygen-independent pathways, in part, for phagocytosis. In the transition from monocyte to macrophage, less myeloperoxidase is present, and there is a decrease in the capacity of these cells to generate superoxide radical and hydrogen peroxide. The macrophage may compensate for these changes by using catalase in the myeloperoxidase, hydrogen peroxide, and halide microbial killing system; lipid peroxidation and the generation of malonyldialdehyde, a substance with antibacterial activity, also may contribute to the killing of bacteria.

In the intracellular environment, phagocytosed microbes may be killed and catabolized, killed and incompletely degraded, or sequestered as dormant microorganisms.[159] *M. tuberculosis, L. pneumophilia,* and *M. leprae* have all developed mechanisms to avoid destruction by macrophages. In the absence of immune serum, *M. tuberculosis* is ingested, but phagosomes and lysosomes do not fuse because of the presence of a microbial anionic trehalose glycolipid.[174] Tissue-resident organisms of this class are totally resistant to monocyte and macrophage lysosomal enzymes discharged into the extracellular milieu, and *M. leprae* and certain rickettsia also are equipped to avoid destruction by phagolysosomal enzymes.[10,175] These same rickettsial species thrive and multiply in the cytoplasm of macrophages in the absence of specific antibody. *L. pneumophilia* also are able to circumvent destruction by preventing the migration of lysosomes to phagosomes as well as their ultimate fusion.

Both cell-mediated and humoral immunity are effective in preventing toxoplasmosis. Trophozoites are killed effectively by macrophages in the presence of antibody and/or complement; in their absence, these organisms multiply within macrophages until the cell bursts and the parasite is released. Delayed hypersensitivity assists in the destruction of *Toxoplasma* species through the production of migration inhibition factor and interferon-γ, preventing macrophage migration and activating macrophages to kill the parasite. Delayed hypersensitivity also plays a role in establishing immunity and the destruction of parasites in other disorders such as leishmaniasis, trypanosomiasis, and trichinosis. Cell-mediated immunity is suppressed when amebic abscesses exist, but delayed hypersensitivity is reacquired after such liver abscesses are cured. With the facility of travel in the modern world, such seemingly rare parasitic diseases for those residing in the United States are becoming more common.

GRANULOMAS AND MACROPHAGES

In the face of persistent irritants it is unable to digest, the host develops a chronic inflammatory reaction consisting primarily of macrophages, which is termed a *granuloma*. Such granulomatous inflammation is not tissue specific and can be observed in the liver, lung, blood vessel, bowel, and other organs in such disorders as primary biliary cirrhosis, berylliosis, giant cell arteritis, and Crohn disease of the bowel.[87–90] Irritants that lack antigenic properties give rise to foreign-body granulomas consisting primarily of macrophages, epithelioid cells, and giant cells such as one might see in response to talc, suture material, or a uric acid tophus; irritants that evoke an immune response, such as *Mycobacterium tuberculosis* or beryllium, give rise to an immune granuloma. Immune granulomas have been termed *hypersensitivity-type granulomas* and are comprised of T and B lymphocytes, activated macrophages, epithelioid cells, giant cells, and fibroblasts. The immunopathogenesis of pulmonary hypersensitivity responses has recently been reviewed and provides a detailed discussion of these reactions.[91]

The monocyte is the centerpiece of both foreign-body and hypersensitivity granulomas, and it is both the incapacity of these cells to digest irritants efficiently as well as the capacity to synthesize autocrine and paracrine mediators that cause the formation and maintenance of a granuloma. The inability to digest an irritant may occur because the chemical composition resists macrophage mechanisms to degrade it, the chemical continues to complex with tissue antigenic proteins in a nonspecific fashion (such as beryllium oxide does), or the irritant is too large to be ingested and digested as is the case with some parasites. In foreign-body granulomas, the persistent irritant is nonimmunogenic, whereas in hypersensitivity granulomas, the irritant is immunogenic and elicits an immune reaction. Bacteria, fungi, chlamydia, and protozoa that form granulomas usually are degraded slowly, creating a persistent irritant, or contain an undegradable molecule that persists as an irritant.

In hypersensitivity granulomas, the earliest cell types attracted are small mononuclear cells that eventually aggregate and mature into macrophages with ruffled membranes and cytoplasmic organelles. In many cases, such macrophages develop further, under a variety of stimuli, to form epithelioid cells that often align in a pallisading pattern. Epithelioid cells represent a heterogenous population of macrophage-derived cells either with granular endoplasmic reticulum and mitochondria or with cytoplasmic vacuoles containing pale fibrillar material. The functions of these epithelioid cells are understood incompletely, but they express microbicidal activity with less phagocytic activity than macrophages. They also have the machinery to secrete their contents, and a number of digestive and metabolizing enzymes have been detected in their cytoplasm. Immune granulomas also contain another macrophage-derived cell called the *Langhans giant cell;* these giant cells develop either as fusion products of macrophages or epithelioid cells under the influence of lymphokines or as attempts to ingest large structures. Giant cells have a characteristic appearance, with their nuclei arranged in a ring just beneath the peripheral cell membrane. Their function is unknown, but they are not phagocytic cells. It sometimes is difficult to separate foreign-body and immune granulomas on a structural basis, because some foreign-body granulomas, like the lesions induced by silica or asbestos, are active and destructive. Nonetheless, immune granulomas are amplified from the simple foreign-body granuloma to a more complex structure by lymphokines provided by sensitized lymphocytes and by monokines generated by activated macrophages. Sensitized lymphocytes are induced to proliferate and produce monocyte chemotaxins as well as blastogenic and other lymphokines, which cause the activation of macrophages (macrophage activation factor) and inhibit their migration (migration inhibition factor).

Such monokines and other monocyte products perform a variety of regulatory functions that have a key role in the expression and regression of granulomas.[176] IL-1 and prostaglandin (PG)E_2 both serve as regulators of lymphocyte activation and proliferation; IL-1 also induces monocyte chemotactic protein 1 mRNA in human fibroblasts as well as the expression of neutrophil-activating protein-1 or IL-8 and monocyte chemotactic protein 1 in other immune and nonimmune cells. Monocyte chemotactic protein 1 and monocyte-derived neutrophil chemotactic factor represent novel cytokines of a supergene family functioning as inflammatory mediators and regulators of immune function. The monokine TNF appears to be more significant in the maintenance of granulomas, whereas IL-1 has an important role in the induction of such lesions. Studies using granuloma models have identified large quantities of lipid mediators such as hydroxyeicosatetraenoic acid and leukotrienes in the cell recruitment phase of granuloma development, whereas the cyclooxygenase product and immunoregulatory substance, PGE_2, seems to be the predominant lipid mediator during the maintenance of the granuloma. The monokine IL-1 has been determined to be one of the key mediators of granuloma formation, because elevated levels of this regulatory substance have been measured in the culture media derived from monocytes recovered from patients with clinical granulomatous disorders such as leprosy and tuberculosis as well as from monocytes obtained from experimental granulomas in animals. The IL-1 species recovered has been determined to be predominantly IL-1β (60%), as compared with a lesser quantity of IL-1α (20%). It was also determined that IL-1α and IL-1β were cell-associated in foreign-body granulomas, whereas IL-1β was secreted by the giant cells in delayed-type hypersensitivity reactions. Furthermore, stimulated macrophages from foreign-body granulomas produce far less TNF (one fifth) than hypersensitivity granulomas, and both IL-1 and TNF levels are reduced in resolving granulomas.

Prostaglandin E_2 is known to suppress the production of TNF by lipopolysaccharide (LPS)–stimulated macrophages but has no effect on the production of IL-1α or IL-1β, triggers for the synthesis and release of arachidonic acid metabolites.[177] PGE_2 also can increase the production of the B-lymphocyte differentiating factor, IL-6. Thus, PGE_2 and IL-1 together appear to regulate the proliferation and regulation of B cells. In addition to these regulatory routes, both IL-1 and TNF can induce the production of additional IL-1 by monocytes. Transforming growth factor-beta also can suppress the production of TNF but not IL-1. From these data, it appears that macrophage TNF production is more susceptible to regulation than is IL-1, but the rationale for these differences in regulation remains unknown. TNF is a potent mediator of fibroblast proliferation, and perhaps such tight regulation serves to prevent excessive organ and tissue fibrosis.

It has been demonstrated clearly that macrophage-derived mediators also influence the production of mediators by nonimmune cells such as fibroblasts, endothelium, and epithelium. Thus, not only is the generation of granulomatous reactions a macrophage-dependent process, but mediators from these cells clearly influence other cell types known to be associated with the formation and maintenance of granulomas.

The usual structure of an immune granuloma contains a central area of macrophages surrounded by aggregated epithelioid cells that are rimmed by T-helper and -suppressor lymphocytes and fibroblasts.[87] Granulomatous lesions may resorb over time, shrink under the influence of suppressive factors such as those generated by T-suppressor cells, or persist in association with tissue damage and fibrosis. Structural integrity is altered by such space-occupying lesions exerting pressure on nearby tissues, by the release of reactive oxygen intermediates from activated macrophages, by the release of lysosomal enzymes during frustrated phagocytosis (inability to completely engulf particulates, with associated loss of phagolysosomal contents to the exterior), or by the secretion of hydrolytic enzymes as well as other toxic substances. As might be expected, macrophages in a hypersensitivity granuloma have a rapid turnover, whereas these same cells have a slow turnover in foreign-body granulomas.

In animal models, bacillus Calmette-Guérin, the antigens evoking extrinsic allergic alveolitis such as extracts of pigeon droppings and *Micropolyspora faeni* antigen, the Schistosome egg granuloma, and bentonite antigen-coated particles induce an immune granuloma. The human counterparts to these granulomas include silicosis, berylliosis, hard metal disease, hypersensitivity pneumonitis, and a variety of granulomatous reactions associated with bacterial (tuberculosis, leprosy, salmonellosis, brucellosis, listeriosis, syphilis, Q fever), viral (cat scratch fever), helminthic (schistosomiasis, trichiniasis, filariasis, capillariasis), fungal (histoplasmosis, blastomycosis, paracoccidioidomycosis, cryptococcosis, coccidioidomycosis), and chlamydial (lymphogranuloma venereum) infections. There also are a number of granulomas of unknown cause (sarcoidosis, primary biliary cirrhosis, granulomatous ileitis and colitis, and certain vasculitides); in fact, sarcoidosis has been a primary contributor to knowledge about immune granulomas. Chronic granulomatous reactions of the skin also may be observed with exposure to zirconium, nickel, or chromium.

Although granulomatous hypersensitivity is the most significant form of delayed hypersensitivity, skin reactions observed with contact- and tuberculin-type antigens that involve a bone marrow–derived macrophage cell expressing Fc, CR1, and HLA-DR surface receptors are important lymphocyte–macrophage integrated reactions of significance to the clinical physician.[178,179] Delayed-type skin hypersensitivity is an antigen-specific, T cell–dependent reaction requiring lymphocytic memory cells and dendritic Langerhans cells that are bone marrow–derived cells related to mononuclear

phagocytes accounting for 2% to 5% of the epidermal cell population.[180,181] These latter cells reside in the epidermis between the basal cell layer and the keratinized epithelium; such cells contain a well-developed endoplasmic reticulum and mitochondrial systems but have limited, if any, capacity for phagocytosis. They express significant quantities of ATPase activity and class II MHC receptors on their membrane and contain a characteristic ultrastructural morphologic marker, the "tennis racquet"–shaped Birbeck granule. Such cells react with an F4/80 monoclonal antibody that also recognizes a macrophage protein and an antibody against the cortical thymocyte antigen, CD1. The term *Langerhans-dendritic cell* arose from the fact that these cells have a number of thin membranous projections (dendrites) that are considered to give these cells the appearance of being "veiled." The significance of these cells is that they serve to present antigen to sensitized lymphocytes.

Contact hypersensitivity results when haptens such as nickel, chromium, poison oak, or poison ivy come in contact with skin and react with tissue proteins to form neoantigens. These neoantigens create a population of sensitized cells, so a second contact with hapten triggers a hypersensitivity reaction. Langerhans cells, which can act as antigen-presenting cells instead of macrophages, migrate from the epidermis and lymphocytes from the dermal vessels, and within 48 hours, lymphocytes and macrophages infiltrate the epidermis. Within 72 hours, the epidermis is edematous. Contact hypersensitivity reaches a peak in 72 hours, and the pathology is expressed primarily in the epidermis. The Langerhans cell is the principal cell presenting antigen in contact sensitization. Ultraviolet light blocks the induction of contact sensitivity at the irradiated site, which results form the destruction of HLA-DR$^+$ Langerhans cells by ultraviolet–radiation and the induction of antigen-specific CD8$^+$ suppressor cells. These latter cells suppress the CD4$^+$ lymphocytes participating in the skin pathology, and the destruction of Langerhans cells blocks antigen presentation to CD4$^+$ cells.

Tuberculin-type hypersensitivity is predominantly a dermal reaction. This reaction tests the previous exposure of individuals to organisms like *M. tuberculosis, M. leprae,* and *L. tropica,* because 48 to 72 hours after the intradermal administration of the microorganism's antigen, red induration of the skin is apparent in sensitive hosts. The pathology of this lesion in its earliest stage shows dermal infiltration with CD4$^+$ and CD8$^+$ cells, in a 2:1 ratio, as well as macrophages in the first 12 hours.[178,179] Between 24 and 48 hours, Langerhans cells begin to migrate from the epidermis and appear in the dermis. Infiltrating lymphocytes and macrophages are likely to express HLA-DR antigens, as are some keratinocytes. The appearance of HLA-DR$^+$ keratinocytes both in tuberculin-type and contact hypersensitivity remain a functional enigma in these reactions. Both macrophages and CD1$^+$ Langerhans cells are the antigen-presenting cells in this reaction and account for cellular traffic from the dermis to the regional lymph nodes and back to the lesion. The anergy to tuberculin skin reactivity observed in sarcoidosis results from the activity of CD8$^+$ T cells and not a defect in antigen presentation.

THE IMMUNOREGULATION OF HUMORAL AND CELL-MEDIATED IMMUNITY BY MACROPHAGES

As alluded to in the preceding discussions, macrophages have the unique capacity to process and present antigens to T lymphocytes, and through this mechanism, these cells play a central role in the regulation of both cell-mediated and humoral immunity.[180–184] At present, antigen processing by macrophages is understood reasonably well, and the components of this process include an understanding of class II MHC molecules on macrophages, the internalization and biochemical processing of antigens by macrophages, and the accessory molecules essential for the presentation of antigen. Accessory cells such as macrophages are cells that cooperate with lymphocytes and assist in the recognition and elimination of antigens; antigen presentation represents a key function of accessory cells.

The central role for class II MHC molecules in antigen processing was identified initially through the use of antibodies to class II MHC molecules; antigen-presenting cells are unable to initiate T-cell proliferation in response to appropriate immunogens in the presence of such antibodies. Animal experiments also determined that T cells only respond to accessory cells bearing syngeneic MHC molecules. Such responses of T lymphocytes to accessory cells are restricted to CD4 T cells, which have been termed *helper* or *inducer T lymphocytes* because of their role in the proliferation of such T cells as well as the secretion of lymphokines such as IL-2 and interferon-γ that enhance both the growth and differentiation of other lymphocytes.[185] Although this is the usual circumstance, there are times when CD4 T cells can be cytolytic to cells bearing class II MHC molecules or when CD8 T cells can behave like helper lymphocytes, releasing the lymphokine IL-2. These latter reactions remain to be characterized further.

Protein antigens require internalization by processing cells, and specific intracellular biochemical reactions are essential for the preparation of antigen for representation on the macrophage surface and its ultimate recognition by T lymphocytes. Peptide fragments of 10 to 12 amino acids do not require internalization, and such peptides are insensitive to agents that inhibit antigen presentation by interrupting intracellular biochemical processes.[186] Once internalized, protein antigens are digested in vesicles at an acid pH; in fact, chemical agents like the lysosomotropic amines, chloroquine and ammonium chloride, inhibit antigen processing by neutralizing the acidic digestion of antigens.[187] It takes approximately 30 to 60 minutes from the initial antigen exposure for processing to membrane antigen expression. More than one protein antigenic epitope may be present in each protein molecule, and therefore, more than one antigen can be presented by macrophages. Despite this capacity for heterogeneity in the antigen presented by a single protein, there usually is a dominant antigen peptide presented to which most of the T cells respond. Nonetheless, T-cell clones may have subtle alterations in their specificity for a single antigen on the macrophage membrane. Class II MHC molecules bind antigens with affinities in the range of 10^{-6} M, and such bound molecules can also dissociate from these MHC sites. However, the rates of dissociation are slower than those for association. In animals, the affinity of antigen for class II MHC molecules is related directly to their immunogenicity. Because peptides bind to these MHC molecules, present dogma states that the MHC molecules have a key role in the intracellular transport of peptide antigens;[180,181] it also follows that peptides may compete for binding to class II MHC molecules and that protein structures exist in such MHC molecules as binding sites. Recent experiments also have demonstrated that single amino acid changes in a peptide can alter its affinity for binding to MHC molecules. Peptides bound in a particular configuration to MHC molecules are what the T lymphocyte recognizes, and variable binding by the class II MHC molecules is likely to account for the allelic variations in antigen presentation. It is of some interest to note that trypsin, a proteolytic enzyme, does not disrupt antigen presentation, suggesting that immunogenic peptides are resistant to proteolysis. Despite the focus on antigen presentation by macrophages in this discussion, it is clear that many other cells also have the capacity to present antigens when endowed with class II MHC molecules, and such cells include vascular endothelia, cells purported to be related to macrophages phylogenetically, fibroblasts, and epithelial cells.

In addition to the class II MHC molecules and intracellular processing, there are accessory substances that assist antigen presentation either by enhancing contact between macrophages and CD4$^+$ T cells or by triggering proliferation of T cells. Substances that increase cell-to-cell adherence have been discussed previously, and the only additional facet that merits comment is that antibodies against LFA-1 can block antigen presentation.[188] However, such inhibition does not prevent antigen presentation in all cases. It has been suggested that the density of LFA-1 molecules may play a role in the interaction between macrophages and $CD4^+$ T cells, and IL-1, a product of many cells (including macrophages), has a multiplicity of effects, some of which relate to antigen presentation. This monokine is produced primarily by macrophages and keratinocytes in vivo, and it needs a stimulus to initiate gene transcription and monokine release. The contact of T cell and macrophage through an antigen-dependent, MHC-restricted process can trigger IL-1 production, and a number of microbial products such as endo- and exotoxins also can stimulate its release. The data at hand would suggest that IL-1 may play a central role in the immunoregulation of antigen presentation, because it may induce both positive and negative regulators of macrophage and T-lymphocyte activity. The presentation of tetanus toxoid to fresh T cells requires IL-1–producing macrophages. IL-1 also may be necessary for some T cells to respond and produce IL-2, but there is ample evidence that T cells themselves may produce IL-1 and use it to regulate their own proliferation. IL-1 also enhances the capacity of dendritic cells to present antigen, and negative regulators induced by IL-1 include prostaglandins, especially PGE_2, released by macrophages triggered by IL-1 and the production of corticotropin-releasing factor, which triggers the release of adrenocorticotropic hormone from the pituitary and the subsequent release of immunosuppressive glucocorticoids from the adrenal glands. Furthermore, IL-1 induces the release of TNFs, CSFs, and IL-1 itself. These costimulators of antigen presentation, as well as the whole process of antigen presentation itself, is only partially understood; further studies are likely to clarify mechanisms of T cell and macrophage interaction in processing antigen.

It is essentially the sensitized T cell that seeks out antigen peptides of the same type to which the T cells have become sensitized on the B-cell membrane. Such sensitized T cells signal B cells to become activated, and they also release lymphokines that bind to B-cell receptors and trigger such B cells to proliferate into antibody-producing cells. In addition, sensitized T cells enter the circulation of the host and seek cells with membrane expression of the antigens to which the T cell is sensitized. Recognition of such antigens may lead to cytolysis of the target cell by the sensitized T cells or other reactions such as delayed type-hypersensitivity depending on what T-cell subset is involved. Thus, the ablation of antigen presentation by macrophages will block the generation of sensitized T cells and lead to suppression of both cell-mediated and humoral immunity. Mono-

cytes and macrophages play a central role in the host defense systems against microorganisms and tumors through their participation in acute and chronic inflammation; regulation of immune responses; secretion of complement, fibronectin, IL-1, and other immunoregulatory and inflammatory effector substances; as well as their release of cytostatic molecules. Furthermore, these cells have a major role in wound repair and tissue remodeling with their innate capacity to regulate coagulation, fibrinolysis, neovascularization, and scavenging of dead cells and inhaled particulates. As monocyte-derived osteoclasts, they also function as regulators of bone deposition and resorption; such cells also participate directly in lipid metabolism and the development of atherosclerotic plaques. As producers of CSFs and erythropoietin, monocytes and macrophages also regulate hematopoiesis.

On the basis of such a broad spectrum of functional activities, it should not be surprising to find that these cells secrete a wide variety of products (Table 10.3) and express many different receptors on their cell surface (Table 10.4). It is likely that additional roles for these multifunctional cells will be found, and their roles in the metabolism and detoxification of xenobiotic compounds will continue to be documented further, such that the term *wandering hepatocyte* may become more justified to describe these circulating biochemical factories. Excellent reviews of granulomatous inflammation and antigen presentation are available in recent publications, and these monographs should be consulted for additional details of these physiologic and pathologic processes.[168,169,189]

ABNORMALITIES OF MONOCYTES AND MACROPHAGES

Abnormalities of monocytes and macrophages are recognized as either increases or decreases in cell numbers, changes in cell morphology, or functional disorders. Peripheral blood monocytes represent only a small percentage (1% to 6%) of the total peripheral blood leukocytes. Macrophages are tissue resident cells and usually are expressed as the percentage of the total cell numbers in specific body cavities such as the alveolar spaces of the lung. In the case of the lung, pulmonary macrophages represent approximately 90% to 95% of the total cells recovered by lung lavage from normal, healthy, nonsmoking volunteers.

Tables 10.5 and 10.6 show the common causes of blood monocytosis and monocytopenia. In adults, the mean peripheral blood monocyte count is 4×10^5 monocytes/ml of peripheral blood; when this number exceeds 8×10^5 monocytes/ml or 500 monocytes/mm^3,

TABLE 10.4. Mononuclear Phagocyte Receptors

Cytokine receptors
  Colony-stimulating factors (CSF-1, GM-CSF)
  Interferons (α, β, and γ)
  Interleukins (1α, 1β, 2, 3, and 4)
  Tumor necrosis factor
  Transforming growth factor-β
Complement and immunoglobulin receptors
  C1q
  C3a, C5a
  CR1 (C3b), CR3 (C3bi), CR4 (C3d,g)
  Factor H (B1H)
  IgG (Fc), aggregated IgG, IgE
Local and systemic hormone receptors
  Arginine vasopressin
  β-adrenergic
  Calcitonin
  Cyclic adenosine monophosphate
  Glucagon
  Histamine
  Insulin
  Leukotrienes and prostaglandins
  Neuropeptides (enkephalins, endorphins, and so on)
  Parathormone
  Serotonin
  Somatostatin
  Thyrotropin
  Vitamin D
Inflammatory and blood product receptors
  α_2-Macroglobulin-protease complexes
  Factors VII and VIIa
  Fibrin
  Fibronectin
  Lactoferrin
  Mannosyl-, fucosyl-, and N-acetylglucosaminyl
Terminal glycoproteins
Bacterial product receptors
  N-formyl peptides
  Endotoxic lipopolysaccharides
Lipoprotein receptors
  Acetylated low-density lipoproteins
  Apolipoproteins B and E

Note: GM-CSF = granulocyte-macrophage colony-stimulating factor.

TABLE 10.5. Common Causes of Blood Monocytosis

Disorders of unknown cause
  Sarcoidosis
  Weber-Christian disease
  Langerhans cell histiocytosis
    Hand-Schüller-Christian syndrome
    Eosinophilic granuloma
    Letterer-Siwe disease
    Pure cutaneous histiocytosis
    Langerhans cell granulomatosis
    Type II histiocytosis
    Hashimoto syndrome
    Nonlipid reticuloendotheliosis
Environmental disorders
  Tetrachlorethane poisoning
Gastrointestinal diseases
  Inflammatory bowel diseases
  Sprue
Hematologic disorders (nonneoplastic)
  Postsplenectomy
  Agranulocytic and neutropenic syndromes
    Chronic hypoplastic neutropenia
    Chronic granulocytopenia
    Cyclic neutropenia
    Familial benign chronic neutropenia
    Infantile genetic agranulocytosis
    Recovering drug-induced agranulocytosis
Infectious diseases
  Cytomegalovirus virus infection
  Histoplasmosis
  Salmonellosis
  Subacute bacterial endocarditis
  Syphilis
  Toxoplasmosis
  Tuberculosis
Malignant disorders
  Acute monocytic leukemia
  Chronic myelomonocytic leukemia
  Histiocytic medullary reticulosis
  Lymphomas
  Multiple myeloma/Waldenström macroglobulinemia
  Nonhematologic malignancy
Parturition

monocytosis is said to exist. No carefully documented monocyte studies have been done to define when monocytopenia exists, but in general, less than 1×10^5 monocytes/ml constitutes monocytopenia. Common causes include the premalignant phase of specific leukemias, aplastic anemia, and infection with the human immunodeficiency virus.[189–191] Radiotherapy and severe thermal injuries also can result in monocytopenia, and these conditions usually are obvious to the clinician.[192] Preleukemic phases of myelogenous leukemias can be first observed either as hypoplastic hemopoiesis with aplastic anemia and pancytopenia, or as ineffective hemopoiesis and chronic monocytosis, and this latter feature may exist for years before the complete clinical expression of the leukemia. Obviously, drug-induced marrow aplasia also will be associated with monocytopenia when pancytopenia exists. Approximately 30% of patients infected with human immunodeficiency virus will be monocytopenic, and in addition to an absolute decrease in the number of peripheral blood monocytes in acquired immunodeficiency syndrome, there are associated monocyte functional abnormalities. Such functional defects include decreased chemotaxis to C5a,

TABLE 10.6.   Common Causes of Blood Monocytopenia

Acute myelogenous leukemia
Aplastic anemia
Glucocorticoid therapy
Hairy-cell leukemia
Human-immunodeficiency-virus infection
Preleukemic states
Thermal injuries

FLMP, lymphocyte-derived chemotactic factor, diminished expression of class II MHC molecules, production of an IL-1 inhibitor, increased release of TNF, and diminished clearance of IgG- and C3-opsonized erythrocytes. It is thought that such changes diminish the capacity of the host to present antigen to helper lymphocytes and to suppress cell-mediated immunity, contribute to the weight loss and cachexia of HIV-infected hosts through the activity of TNF, and cause the dissemination of virus-infected cells to a variety of organ systems including the central nervous system.

Hairy-cell leukemia is a rare lymphoproliferative malignancy that is observed in patients with generalized weakness, weight loss, and splenomegaly. Approximately 80% of patients have monocytopenia,[190,194] and the diagnosis is based on the clinical features and typical appearance of the bone marrow with the characteristic fried-egg appearance of hairy cells in marrow infiltrates.

The most common cause of monocytopenia is the transient decrease in blood monocytes observed between 4 and 8 hours after the administration of glucocorticoids.[195] Such a decrease is short term (24 hours), and a reactive monocytosis may occur subsequently. Long-term glucocorticoid therapy also causes functional monocyte abnormalities; there is a decrease in the expression of IgG, C3, mannose and low-density lipoprotein receptors on monocytes and macrophages; a diminished release of IL-1, plasminogen activator, prostaglandins and leukotrienes, lysosomal enzymes; and a suppression of the recruitment of monocytes and macrophages to inflammatory lesions.[92,195] In addition, glucocorticoids decrease monocyte bactericidal and fungicidal activities, and cutaneous delayed hypersensitivity is decreased so that skin tests with tuberculin and other antigens may give false-negative results.[196–198]

A variety of different disorders may be observed with monocytosis of the peripheral blood, but the primary clinical problems expressing this change are those associated with chronic or subchronic infections,[199–207] neutropenias,[208–212] and malignant disorders.[34,35,213–224] Chronic monocytosis may precede acute leukemia by months, and monocytosis associated with drug-induced agranulocytosis usually heralds recovery. Hodgkin disease has an associated monocytosis in 25% of cases, and

20% of patients with subacute bacterial endocarditis (SBE) have elevated peripheral blood monocyte counts. Occasionally, monocytosis follows the resolution of an acute infectious process; unexplained monocytosis should trigger an investigation for an underlying infection and also should exclude the possibility of an undetected malignancy. Autoimmune disorders such as rheumatoid arthritis, systemic lupus erythematosus, giant cell arteritis, polymyositis, and polyarteritis nodosa often are listed as causes of monocytosis.[49,225–227] Certainly, monocytosis has been documented in such disorders, but it is much less useful as a marker than the thrombocytopenia and leukopenia of systemic lupus erythematosus, the thrombocytosis of rheumatoid arthritis, and the tissue changes observed by biopsy in the others. Obviously, monocytosis is not an absolute finding in any of these disorders, and its absence in association with such disorders has little significance.

In terms of the disorders associated with changes in macrophage number and dysfunction, the numbers of macrophages may increase in a variety of conditions associated with pathology that is localized in specific body cavities. The lung probably has been studied in greater detail than any other organ with respect to changes in pulmonary macrophage numbers and functions,[228] and although the number of pulmonary macrophages increases in pulmonary disorders, including cigarette smoking, such changes are less useful as diagnostic tools than the morphology and functions of macrophages recovered by lung lavage. For example, macrophages recovered by lavage in patients with pulmonary alveolar proteinosis are much larger than normal, and morphologic examination reveals that their cytoplasm is filled with lamellar bodies and structures with the appearance of tubular myelin as a result of the ingestion of lung surfactant.[229,230] Furthermore, such overburdened macrophages are unable to carry out phagocytosis in an efficient manner, which may impair lung defense mechanisms. In cigarette smokers, macrophages from the lung are larger than normal, contain more pigment in their cytoplasm, have fewer pseudopodia, and express more HLA-DR molecules (activation) than normal lung macrophages.[231–233] Thus, for most purposes, changes in macrophage numbers are not helpful in differential diagnosis, but their morphology and functions are useful in the evaluation of a few disorders. For example, macrophages from patients with cystic fibrosis have defective IgG opsonin and do not ingest *Pseudomonas* bacteria effectively.[234,235] In occupational lung disorders, one may identify particulate by ordinary or polarizing microscopy, and such analyses may permit the absolute identification of the cause for the pulmonary findings.[228] In sarcoidosis and idiopathic pulmonary fibrosis, alveolar macrophages are activated and secrete biologically active molecules such as growth factors for fibroblasts in idiopathic pulmonary fibrosis.[236–241] Hypersensitivity pneumonitis of certain types has been associated with foam cells,[242,243] and other lung diseases such as asthma and occupational exposures may show increased numbers of alveolar macrophages. Such increases, however, are nondiagnostic. The existing data related to changes in bronchoalveolar lavage specimens in human environmental and chemical exposures have recently been reviewed and can be consulted for further details.[244]

Several rare diseases are associated with monocyte abnormalities, and these include Chédiak-Higashi disease, chronic granulomatous disease, myeloperoxidase deficiency, osteopetrosis, and leukocyte adhesion deficiency.[51,245–248] Such disorders are characterized by either a defect in leukocyte motility or a disorder of phagocytic killing. Leukocyte adhesion deficiencies have been discussed previously and merit no additional treatment here, but Chédiak-Higashi disease is a rare autosomal recessive disorder characterized by abnormal leukocyte lysosomes. Morphologic abnormalities have been observed in neutrophils, monocytes, and lymphocytes from such patients, and in the monocyte, as in other leukocytes, there are giant cytoplasmic granules that may impede leukocyte chemotaxis.[249] No specific defect has been recognized to account for these lysosomal abnormalities, but there is speculation that it represents a generalized membrane defect. Similar disorders have been characterized in mink (Aleutian), cattle, and beige mice.

Osteopetrosis is an inherited disorder of bone in which the monocyte-derived osteoclasts are defective and bone resorption does not occur.[250,251] Unopposed bone accretion occurs in the absence of effective osteoclast activity.

Chronic granulomatous disease represents the expression of several different inherited disorders in which phagocytic cells can ingest particulate but are unable to initiate a respiratory burst.[252] This latter defect has been observed in neutrophils, monocytes, and eosinophils. The defective respiratory burst characteristic of the disorder leads to altered rates of bacterial and fungal killing, which makes such patients susceptible to recurrent infections with catalase-positive bacteria and fungi. Infections can occur in multiple organs, but the sites where mononuclear phagocytes reside (liver, spleen, lymph node, and lung) represent the tissues at highest risk for serious infection. Prolonged intracellular retention of microorganisms provides the stimuli for granuloma formation in the liver, lung, spleen, and lymph nodes. Because there is both an X-linked and autosomal recessive form of this disorder, more than one defect is responsible for the defective respiratory burst; hybrid

cells made from X-linked and autosomal recessive respiratory-burst-defective cells can generate a normal respiratory burst. Present data suggest that the X-linked defect resides in the gene or genes for the subunits of the cytochrome b component of NADPH oxidase, and the autosomal recessive form probably relates to the presence of a defective cytosolic factor essential for the triggering of NADPH oxidase activity. The complete story of the genetic deficiencies in this heterogenous disorder must await further biochemical studies of these defective cells.

Myeloperoxidase deficiency was thought to be an exceedingly rare disorder until automated cytochemistry was used to measure peroxidase activity in neutrophils.[253] In approximately 1 of 2000 healthy subjects, staining documented the absence of peroxidase activity in neutrophils and monocytes.[253] Most patients with deficient myeloperoxidase are healthy, but some individuals with complicating disorders (diabetes mellitus) have defective antifungal defenses and may have disseminated fungal infections with *Candida* and *Aspergillus fumigatus*.[160,254,255] In addition to the inherited forms of myeloperoxidase deficiency, acquired forms are observed in association with lead poisoning, pregnancy, Hodgkin disease, megaloblastic anemia, neuronal ceroid lipofuscinosis, and acute nonlymphocytic leukemia.[256–263] Myeloperoxidase deficiency is detected by examination of neutrophils and monocytes for peroxidase using either 3-amino-9-carbazole or 4-chloro-1-naphthol as substrates.[264,265] These histochemical stains permit a differentiation of eosinophil from neutrophil monocyte peroxidase, because an excess of eosinophils with their increased levels of peroxidase may disguise a neutrophil–monocyte peroxidase deficiency. Such myeloperoxidase-deficient cells also have an increased respiratory burst, with a resultant increase in the generation of increased superoxide radical and hydrogen peroxide.[266–269] Furthermore, such cells have an increased rate of oxygen consumption and hexose monophosphate shunt activity. These myeloperoxidase-deficient cells are unable to produce hypohalous acid and other halide-containing intermediates that have an effect on the cytotoxic reactions essential for microbicidal and fungicidal activities. The actual genetic lesion in the inherited form of myeloperoxidase deficiency has been characterized incompletely, and there may be heterogeneity within this inherited abnormality.

Phagocytic disorders have been reviewed in a comprehensive manner elsewhere. Those articles can be consulted for further details of these abnormalities.[252,270]

Both acquired and genetic disorders of lipid metabolism can give rise to foam cells that result from the ingestion of undigested lipids by monocytes or macrophages.[271] Storage lipids vary in their structure depending on the metabolic defect. The heritable lipid storage diseases include Gaucher, Nieman-Pick, Tay-Sachs, Sandhoff, Fabry, Wolman, Tangier, and Farber lipogranulomatosis.[272–276] The enzyme deficiency is different in each of these disorders, and foam cells are likely to be detected in bone marrow preparations or primary organs where lipid-laden macrophages or histiocytes are likely to be found, such as the spleen, liver, and lymph nodes. The diagnosis of these disorders depends on the clinical expression of the disease and laboratory confirmation of the enzymatic defect or stored lipid; details of such diagnostic studies can be found in standard texts dealing with inherited diseases.

A variety of disorders associated with increased levels of plasma cholesterol, triglyceride, and phospholipid concentrations also can be associated with foam cells. The hyperlipidemia associated with diabetes mellitus and glucose-6-phosphatase deficiency often contributes to the formation of foam cells, and patients with lipoprotein lipase deficiency and homozygous forms of familial hypercholesterolemia also may give rise to such foam cells. However, without special studies, these lipid-laden cells are indistinguishable from similar foam cells in glycolipid storage diseases.[271]

Inflammatory and malignant histiocytoses represent another expression of the multifaceted monocyte–macrophage series. Such disorders include the lipid storage diseases previously discussed, the inflammatory histiocytic disorders including Langerhans cell histiocytosis and its variants, familial and infectious hemophagocytic histiocytosis, sinus histiocytosis with massive lymphadenopathy, and malignant histiocytosis.[36,37,277–281].

As noted previously, Langerhans cells are present in lymph nodes, thymus, spleen, mucosa, and epidermis, where they represent a special type of macrophage with a typical "tennis racquet"–shaped inclusion, the Birbeck body. Specific markers for this cell type include the characteristic ultrastructural Birbeck body as well as adenosine triphosphatase, adenosine diphosphatase, and α-D-mannosidase activity; a protein marker, the β-chain of the neuroprotein S-100; and receptors for CD1 and peanut lectin. In Langerhans histiocytosis, cells with these characteristics are found in lesions of the skull, lung, skin, lymph nodes, spleen, and occasionally, the gastrointestinal tract and liver; such cells may eventually form granulomatous lesions that over time may become more xanthomatous and fibrotic. Limited lesions that are nonprogressive are common in male children, whereas chronic progressive disease has equal gender representation. Clinically, the disease may express itself as an expanding bone lesion with pain; an enlargement of the liver, lymph nodes, or spleen; or as

skin lesions. Biopsy of such lesions confirms the presence of pathologic Langerhans cells. Spontaneous improvement may occur without treatment, but glucocorticoids remain the primary treatment of the pulmonary manifestations. Chemotherapy is used for the generalized disease.

Familial hemophagocytic histiocytosis is a disorder of newborns who are frequently the products of consanguineous marriages. The disease is expressed most frequently as a hematologic disorder with pancytopenia and hepatosplenomegaly.[280] Marrow examination shows macrophages with ingested erythroid cells, and the cerebrospinal fluid often contains mononuclear cells, including macrophages. Despite the use of immunosuppressive agents, this disorder is fatal.

Hemophagocytic histiocytosis also may be associated with a variety of bacterial, viral, fungal, and protozoal infections in adults or children. Infections with Epstein-Barr virus, cytomegalovirus, herpes simplex, varicella zoster virus, adenovirus, mycobacteria, enteric bacteria, systemic babesiosis, and systemic leishmaniasis have all been implicated as vectors of this disorder.[278,279,281] In the adult, fever, malaise, and myalgia are associated with cytopenias of the erythroid series, platelets, and leukocytes, and children with this disorder often have hepatosplenomegaly and lymphadenopathy. Marrow macrophages usually are increased and often contain ingested erythroblasts, platelets, and rarely, neutrophils. Lymph node biopsies also demonstrate increased hemophagocytic histiocytes. It is important to document the antecedent viral infection by serum antibody titers to distinguish this disorder from a malignant histiocytosis. In the setting of immunosuppression, the disease may be fatal unless immunosuppressive drugs are stopped. Spontaneous recovery occurs in most cases.

Sinus histiocytosis with massive lymphadenopathy or the Rosai-Dorfman syndrome presents the frightening picture of discrete or adherent cervical lymphadenopathy that is painless and may be associated with a more generalized lymphadenopathy.[281,282] Such patients often have fever, elevated erythrocyte sedimentation rates, anemia, and polyclonal gammopathies (gamma type). Lymph nodes lesions also are present in a wide variety of systemic organs, and the most significant point in this disorder is that bone marrow evaluation is almost always unrewarding. However, lymph node pathology is diagnostic with its erythrophagocytosis, capsular fibrosis, and increase in phagocytic and paracortical veiled cells. Children with immunologic deficiencies are especially prone to develop this disorder, and the prognosis varies from spontaneous resolution to fatality. Treatment has little effect on the prognosis.

Malignant histiocytosis is a rare disorder that is sometimes difficult to distinguish from lymphoma, Hodgkin disease, and hemophagocytic histiocytic syndromes, because the pathologic expressions are similar.[283,284] Signs of a systemic disorder such as fever, weakness, and weight loss are almost always present, often associated with hepatosplenomegaly and lymphadenopathy. Anemia, leukopenia, and thrombocytopenia frequently are present, and bone marrow aspirates are only diagnostic in 50% of cases. Lymph node biopsy or pathologic examination of the spleen frequently are diagnostic, but an absolute diagnosis may not be made until postmortem examination. Both malignant- and benign-appearing histiocytes often are present in pathologic specimens. The atypia of histiocytes expressed as their pleomorphic appearance with nucleoli and the presence of mitotic figures must be sought carefully. Malignant histiocytes stain cytochemically for acid phosphatase and nonspecific esterase, but repeated tissue biopsies may be necessary for diagnosis. Multidrug regimens have resulted in a high frequency of complete remissions of this disease.

In summary, the monocyte–macrophage series of cells may provide useful clues to a variety of underlying diseases as a result of changes in the number of cells in the peripheral blood or body cavities. However, of greater significance as a diagnostic tool is the change in morphologic features or functions of the cells in this series; these changes may lead more directly to a specific diagnosis and permit more definitive approaches to characterize the prognosis and to undertake specific therapy.

REFERENCES

1. Stossel TP. Phagocytosis. N Engl J Med 1974;290:717–23, 774–80,833–9.
2. Root RK, Cohen MS. The microbicidal mechanisms of human neutrophils and eosinophils. Rev Infect Dis 1981;3:565–98.
3. Sharma SD, Remington JS. Macrophage activation and resistance to intracellular infection. Lymphokines 1981;3:181–212.
4. Unanue ER, Allen PM. The basis for the immunoregulatory role of macrophages and other accessory cells. Science 1987;236:551–7.
5. Van Furth R. Mononuclear phagocytes in inflammation. In: Vane JR, Ferreira SH, eds. Inflammation. Berlin: Springer-Verlag, 1978:68–108.
6. Van Furth R. Phagocytic cells: development and distribution of mononuclear phagocytes in normal steady state and inflammation. In: Gallin JI, Goldstein IM, Snyderman R, eds. Inflammation: Basic Principles and Clinical Correlates. New York: Raven Press, 1988:281–95.
7. Nichols BA, Bainton DF. Differentiation of human monocytes in bone marrow and blood: sequential formation of two granule populations. Lab Invest 1973;29:27–40.
8. Fedarko M, Hirsch JG. Structure of monocytes and macrophages. Semin Hematol 1970;7:109–24.
9. Cohn ZA, Benson B. The differentiation of mononuclear phagocytes: morphology, cytochemistry, and biochemistry. J Exp Med 1965;121:153–70.
10. Nathan CF, Murray HW, Cohn ZA. The macrophage as an effector cell. N Engl J Med 1980;303:622–6.
11. Golde DW. Disorders of mononuclear phagocyte proliferation, maturation and function. Clin Haematol 1975;4:705–21.
12. Nathan CF. Mechanisms of macrophage antimicrobial activity. Trans R Soc Trop Med Hyg 1986;77:620–30.
13. Edelson PJ. Intracellular parasites and phagocytic cells. Cell Biol Pathophysiol Rev Infect Dis 1982;4:124–35.
14. Metcalf D. The molecular biology and functions of the granulocyte-macrophage colony-stimulating factors. Blood 1986;67:257–67.
15. Zuckerman KS. Human erythroid burst-forming units: growth in vitro is dependent on monocytes, but not T lymphocytes. J Clin Invest 1981;67:702–9.
16. Hershko C. Storage iron regulation. In: Brown EB, ed. Progress in Hematology. Volume X. New York: Grune and Stratton, 1977:107.
17. Gordon S, Crocker PR, Morris L, Lee ZH, Perry VH, Hume DH. Localization and function of tissue macrophages. In: Biochemistry of Macrophages. Ciba Foundation Symposium 118. New York: John Wiley & Sons, 1986:54–67.
18. Gordon S, Keshaw S, Chung L-P. Mononuclear phagocytes: tissue distribution and functional heterogeneity. Curr Opin Immunol 1988;1:26–35.
19. Papadimitriou JM, Ashman RB. Macrophages: current views on their differentiation, structure, and function. Ultrastruct Pathol 1989;13:343–72.
20. Van Furth R. Origin and turnover of monocytes and macrophages. Curr Top Pathol 1989;79:125–50.
21. Jones EA, Summerfield JA. Functional aspects of hepatic sinusoidal cells. Semin Liver Dis 1985;5:157–74.
22. Van Furth R. Cellular biology of pulmonary macrophages. Int Arch Allergy Appl Immunol 1985;76(suppl 1):21–7.
23. Thorbecke GJ, Belsito DV, Bienenstock AN, Possick LE, Baer RL. The Langerhans cell, as a representative of the accessory cell system, in health and disease. Immunobiology 1984;168:313–24.
24. Springer TA, Unkeless JC. Analysis of macrophage differentiation and function with monoclonal antibodies. Contemp Top Immunobiol 1984;13:1–31.
25. Hopper KE, Wood PR, Nelson DR. Macrophage heterogeneity. Vox Sang 1979;36:257–74.
26. Raff HV, Picker LJ, Stobo JD. Macrophage heterogeneity in man: a subpopulation of HLA-DR-bearing macrophages required for antigen-induced T cell activation also contains stimulators for autologous-reactive T cells. J Exp Med 1980;152:581–93.
27. Shen HH, Talle MA, Goldstein G, Chess L. Functional subsets of human monocytes defined by monoclonal antibodies: a distinct subset of monocytes contains the cells capable of inducing the autologous mixed lymphocyte culture. J Immunol 1983;130:698–705.
28. Marder P, Hinson A, Russo C, Ferrone S, Ades E. Heterogeneity of human peripheral blood mononuclear cells detected by monoclonal antibodies to monomorphic determinants of human Ia antigens. Immunobiology 1984;167:483–94.
29. Dougherty GJ, McBride WH. Macrophage heterogeneity. J Clin Lab Immunol 1984;14:1–11.
30. Shellito J, Kaltreider HB. Heterogeneity of immunologic function among subfractions of normal rat alveolar macrophages. Am Rev Resp Dis 1984;129:747–53.
31. Hance AJ, Douches S, Winchester RJ, Ferrans VJ, Crystal RG. Characterization of mononuclear phagocyte subpopulations in

the human lung by using monoclonal antibodies: changes in alveolar macrophage phenotype associated with pulmonary sarcoidosis. J Immunol 1985;134:284–92.

32. Moreno J, Lipsky PE. Functional heterogeneity of human antigen-presenting cells: presentation of soluble antigens, but not self-Ia by monocytes. J Clin Immunol 1986;6:9–20.

33. Esa AH, Noga SJ, Donnenberg AD, Hess AD. Immunological heterogeneity of human monocyte subsets prepared by counter-flow centrifugation elutriation. Immunology 1986;59:95–9.

34. Pearson HA, Diamond LK. Chronic monocytic leukemia in childhood. J Pediatr 1958;53:259–70.

35. Bearman RM, Kjeldsberg CR, Pangalis GA, Rappaport H. Chronic monocytic leukemia in adults. Cancer 1981;48:2239–55.

36. Huhn D, Meister P. Malignant histiocytosis: morphologic and cytochemical findings. Cancer 1978;42:1341–9.

37. Carbone A, Micheau C, Cuilland JM, Carlu C. A cytochemical and immunohistochemical approach to malignant histiocytosis. Cancer 1981;47:2862–71.

38. Chan WC, Zaatari G. Lymph node interdigitating reticulum cell sarcoma. Am J Clin Pathol 1986;85:739–44.

39. Scriver CR, Beaudet AL, Sly WS, Valle D. The Metabolic Basis of Inherited Disease. Sixth Edition. New York: McGraw-Hill, 1989:1129–302,1623–839.

40. Winkelstein JA, Colten HR. Genetically determined disorders of the complement system. In: Scriver CR, Beaudet AL, Sly WS, Valle D, eds. The Metabolic Basis of Inherited Diseases. New York: McGraw-Hill, 1989:2711–37.

41. Rother K, Rother V. Hereditary and acquired complement deficiencies in animals and man. Prog Allergy 1986;39:1–397.

42. Mills EL. Mononuclear phagocytes in the newborn: their relation to the state of relative immunodeficiency. Am J Pediatr 1983;5:189–98.

43. Dale DC, Fauci AS, Wolff SM. Alternate-day prednisone: leukocyte kinetics and susceptibility to infections. N Engl J Med 1974;291:1154–8.

44. Cianciolo G, Hunter J, Silva J, Haskill JS, Synderman R. Inhibitors of monocyte responses to chemotaxins are present in human cancerous effusions and react with monoclonal antibodies to the P15(E) structural protein of retroviruses. J Clin Invest 1981;68:831–44.

45. Hill HR, Augustine NH, Rallison ML, Santos JI. Defective monocyte chemotatic responses in diabetes mellitus. J Clin Immunol 1983;3:70–7.

46. Smith PD, Okura K, Masur H, Lane HC, Fauci AS, Wahl SW. Monocyte function in the acquired immune deficiency syndrome: defective chemotaxis. J Clin Invest 1984;74:2121–8.

47. Altman LC, Furukowa CT, Klebanoff SJ. Depressed mononuclear leukocyte chemotaxis in thermally injured patients. J Immunol 1977;119:199–205.

48. Gordon DS, Hubbard M. Surface membrane characteristics and cytochemistry of the abnormal cells in adult acute leukemia. Blood 1978;51:681–92.

49. Salmon JE, Kimberly RP, Gibofsky A, Fotino M. Defective mononuclear phagocyte function in systemic lupus erythematosus: dissociation of Fc receptor-ligand binding and internalization. J Immunol 1984;133:2525–31.

50. Dana N, Todd RF III, Pitt J, Springer TA, Arnaout MA. Deficiency of a surface membrane glycoprotein (Mol) in man. J Clin Invest 1984;75:153–9.

51. Gallin JI. Phagocytic cells: disorders of function. In: Gallin JI, Goldstein IM, Snyderman R, eds. Inflammation: Basic Principles and Clinical Correlates. New York: Raven Press, 1988:493–511.

52. Fauci AS, Haynes BF, Katz P. Wegener's granulomatosis: prospective clinical and therapeutic experience with 85 patients for 21 years. Ann Intern Med 1983;98:76–85.

53. Bloom W, Bartelmez GW. Hematopoiesis in young human embryos. Am J Anat 1940;67:21–53.

54. Gilmour JR. Normal hemopoiesis in intrauterine and neonatal life. J Pathol 1942;52:25–55.

55. Keleman E, Calvo W, Fliedner TM. Atlas of Human Hemopoietic Development. Berlin: Springer-Verlag, 1979.

56. Quesenberry PJ. Hemopoietic stem cells, progenitor cells, and growth factors. In: Williams WJ, Beutler E, Erslev AJ, Lichtman MA, eds. Hematology. New York: McGraw-Hill, 1990:129–47.

57. Nicola NA. Hemopoietic cell growth factors and their receptors. Annu Rev Biochem 1989;58:45–77.

58. Pettenati MJ, LeBean LL, Lemons RS, et al. Assignment of CSF-1 to 5q 33.1: evidence for clustering of genes regulating hematopoiesis and for their involvement in the deletion of the long arm of chromosome 5 in myeloid disorders. Proc Natl Acad Sci U S A 1987;84:2970–4.

59. Crapper RM, Vairo G, Hamilton J, Clark-Lewis I, Shrader JW. Stimulation of bone marrow-derived and peritoneal macrophages by a T-lymphocyte-derived hemopoietic growth factor, persisting cell-stimulating factor. Blood 1985;66:859–65.

60. Fleischmann J, Golde DW, Weisbart RH, Glasson JC. Granulocyte-macrophage colony stimulating factor enhances phagocytosis of bacteria by human neutrophils. Blood 1986;68:708–11.

61. Villalta F, Kierszenbaum F. Effects of human colony-stimulating factor on the uptake and destruction of a pathogenic parasite *(Trypanosoma cruzi)* by human neutrophils. J Immunol 1986;137:1703–7.

62. Griffin JD. Clinical applications of colony-stimulating factors. Oncology 1988;2:15–21.

63. Finch CA. Erythropoiesis, erythropoietin, and iron. Blood 1982;60:1241–6.

64. Ogawa M, Porter PN, Nakahata T. Renewal and commitment to differentiation of hemopoietic stem cells (an interpretive review). Blood 1983;61:823–9.

65. Groopman JE, Molina J-M, Scadden DT. Hematopoietic growth factors: biology and clinical applications. N Engl J Med 1989;321:1449–59.

66. Evans SW, Rennick D, Farrar WL. Multi-lineage hematopoietic growth factor interleukin 3 and direct activators of protein kinase C stimulate phosphorylation of common substrates. Blood 1986;68:906–13.

67. Farrar W, Thomas TP, Anderson WB. Altered cytosol/membrane enzyme redistribution on Il-3 activation of protein kinase C. Nature 1985;315:235–7.

68. Sherr CF, Rettenmier CW, Sacca R, Roussel MF, Look AT, Stanley ER. The c-*fms* proto-oncogene product is related to the receptor for the mononuclear phagocyte growth factor, CSF-1. Cell 1985;41:665–76.

69. Sacca R, Stanley ER, Sherr CJ, Rettenmier CW. Specific binding of the mononuclear phagocyte colony stimulating factor CSF-1 to the product of the v-*fms* oncogene. Proc Natl Acad Sci U S A 1986;83:3331–5.

70. Rettenmeir CW, Sacca R, Furman WL, et al. Expression of the human c-*fms* proto-oncogene product (colony stimulating factor-1) receptor on the peripheral blood mononuclear cells and choriocarcinoma cell lines. J Clin Invest 1986;77:1740–6.

71. Bartocci A, Mastrogiannis DS, Migliorati G, Stockert RJ, Wolkoff AW. Macrophages specifically regulate the concentration of their own growth factor in the circulation. Proc Natl Acad Sci U S A 1987;84:6179–83.

72. Groopman JE, Golde DW. The histiocytic disorders: a pathophysiologic analysis. Ann Intern Med 1981;94:95–107.

73. Nichols BA, Bainton DF. Ultrastructure and cytochemistry of mononuclear phagocytes. In: van Furth R, ed. Mononuclear Phagocytes in Immunity, Infection, and Pathology. Oxford: Blackwell, 1975:17–55.

74. Bozdech MJ, Bainton DF. Identification of alpha napthyl butyrate esterase as a plasma membrane ectoenzyme of monocytes and as a discrete intracellular membrane bounded organelle in lymphocytes. J Exp Med 1981;153:182–95.

75. Saboori AM, Newcombe DS. Human monocyte carboxylesterase: purification and kinetics. J Biol Chem 1990;265:19792–9.

76. Suga M, Dannenberg AM Jr, Higuchi S. Macrophage functional heterogeneity in vivo: macrolocal and microlocal macrophage activation identified by double-staining tissue sections of BGG granulomas for pairs of enzymes. Am J Pathol 1980;99:305–24.

77. Van Furth R, Hirsch JG, Fedorko ME. Morphology and peroxidase cytochemistry of mouse promonocytes, monocytes and macrophages. J Exp Med 1970;132:794–812.

78. Werb Z. Phagocytic cells: chemotaxis and effector functions of macrophages and granulocytes. In: Sites DP, Stobo JD, Walls VJ, eds. Basic and Clinical Immunology. Sixth edition. Norwalk: Appleton and Lange, 1987:96–113.

79. Wright SD, Detmers PA. Adhesion-promoting receptors on phagocytes. J Cell Sci 1988;9(suppl):99–120.

80. Meuret G, Hoffmann G. Monocyte kinetic studies in normal and disease states. Br J Haematol 1973;24:275–85.

81. Baehner RB. Personal communication, 1990.

82. Hocking WG, Golde DW. The pulmonary-alveolar macrophage. N Engl J Med 1979;301:580–7.

83. Gale RP, Sparkes RS, Golde DW. Bone marrow origin of hepatic macrophages (Kupffer cells) in humans. Science 1978;201:937–8.

84. Van Waarde D, Hulsing-Hesselink E, van Furth R. Properties of a factor increasing monocytopoiesis (FIM) occurring in serum during the early phase of an inflammatory reaction. Blood 1977;50:727–41.

85. Sluiter W, Hulsing-Hesselink E, Elzenga-Classen I, et al. Macrophages as origin of the release of factor increasing monocytopoiesis. J Exp Med 1987;166:909–22.

86. Van Waarde D, Hulsing-Hesselink E, van Furth R. Humoral control of monocytopoiesis by an activator and an inhibitor. Agents Action 1978;8:423–37.

87. Boros DV. Granulomatous Inflammations. Prog Allergy 1978;24:183–267.

88. Adams DO. The granulomatous inflammatory response: a review. Am J Pathol 1976;84:164–91.

89. Epstein WL. Metal-induced granulomatous hypersensitivity in man. Adv Biol Skin 1969;11:313–35.

90. Epstein WL. Granulomatous hypersensitivity. Prog Allergy 1967;11:36–88.

91. Newcombe DS. The immunopathogenesis of pulmonary responses to environmental and chemical pollutants. In: Newcombe DS, Rose NR, Bloom JC, ed. Clinical Immunotoxicology. New York: Raven Press, 1982:203–75.

92. Parrillo JE, Fauci AS. Mechanisms of glucocorticoid action on immune processes. Annu Rev Pharmacol 1979;19:179–201.

93. Fauci AS, Dale DC. The effect of in vivo hydrocortisone on subpopulations of human lymphocytes. J Clin Invest 1974;53:240–6.

94. Fauci AS, Dale DC. Alternate day prednisone therapy and human lymphocyte subpopulations. J Clin Invest 1975;55:25–32.

95. Parrillo JE, Fauci AS. Mechanisms of corticosteroid action of lymphocyte subpopulations: III. Differential effects of dexamethasone administration on subpopulations of effector cells

96. Phillips SM, Zweiman B. Mechanisms in the suppression of delayed hypersensitivity in the guinea pig by 6-mercaptopurine. J Exp Med 1973;137:1494–510.

97. Gassmann AE, van Furth R. The effect of azathioprine (Imuran) on the kinetics of monocytes and macrophages during the normal steady state and an acute inflammatory reaction. Blood 1975;46:51–64.

98. Johnston CA, Russell AS, Kovithavongs T, Dasgupta M. Measures of immunologic and inflammatory responses in vitro in rheumatoid patients treated with methotrexate. J Rheumatol 1986;13:294–6.

99. Hu S-K, Mitcho YL, Oronsky AL, Kerwar SS. Studies on the effect of methotrexate on macrophage function. J Rheumatol 1988;15:206–9.

100. Snyderman R, Pike MC. Transductional mechanisms of chemoattractant receptors on leukocytes. In: Snyderman R, ed. Contemporary Topics in Immunobiology. New York: Plenum Press, 1984:1–28.

101. Kishimoto TK, Larson RS, Corbi AL, Dustin ML, Staunton DE, Springer TA. The leukocyte integrins. Adv Immunol 1989;46:149–82.

102. Snyderman R, Pike MC. Regulation of leukocyte function. Annu Rev Immunol 1984;2:257–81.

103. Snyderman R, Uhing RJ. Phagocytic cells: stimulus-response coupling mechanisms. In: Gallin JI, Goldstein IM, Snyderman R, eds. Inflammation: Basic Principles and Clinical Correlates. New York: Raven Press, 1988:309–23.

104. Wahl SM, Hunt DA, Wakefield LM, et al. Transforming growth factor type B induces monocyte chemotaxis and growth factor production. Proc Natl Acad Sci U S A 1987;84:5788–92.

105. Wiseman DM, Polverini PJ, Kang DW, Leibovich SJ. Transforming growth factor-beta (TGFB) is chemotactic for human monocytes and induces their expression of angiogenic activity. Biochem Biophys Res Commun 1988;157:793–800.

106. Snyderman R, Mergenhagen SE. Chemotaxis of macrophages. In: Nelson DS, ed. Immunobiology of the Macrophage. New York: Academic Press, 1976:323–46.

107. Postlethwaite AE, Arnold E, Snyderman R. Characterization of chemotactic activity produced in vivo by a cell-mediated immune reaction in guinea pig. J Immunol 1975;114:274–8.

108. Postlethwaite AE, Kang AH. Collagen- and collagen peptide-induced chemotaxis of human blood monocytes. J Exp Med 1976;143:1299–307.

109. Schiffman E, Corcoran BA, Wahl SM. N-formylmethionyl peptides as chemoattractants for leukocytes. Proc Natl Acad Sci U S A 1975;72:1059–62.

110. Meltzer MS, Stevenson MM, Leonard EJ. Characterization of macrophage chemotaxins in tumor cell cultures and comparison with lymphocyte-derived chemotactic factors. Cancer Res 1977;37:721–5.

111. Deuel TF, Senior RM, Huang JS, Griffin GL. Chemotaxis of monocytes and neutrophils to platelet-derived growth factor. J Clin Invest 1982;69:1046–9.

112. Senior RM, Griffin GL, Mecham RF. Chemotactic activity of elastin-derived peptides. J Clin Invest 1980;66:859–62.

113. Snyderman R, Smith CD, Verghese MW. Model for leukocyte regulation by chemoattractant receptors: roles of a guanine nucleotide regulatory protein and polyphosphoinositide metabolism. J Leuk Biol 1986;40:785–800.

114. Duncan R, Pratten MK. Pinocytosis: mechanism and regulation. In: Dean RT, Jessup W, eds. Mononuclear Phagocytes: Physiology and Pathology. Volume 11. Amsterdam: Elsevier, 1985:27–52.

mediating cellular cytotoxicity in man. Clin Exp Immunol 1978;31:116–25.

115. Bodmer JL. Membrane receptors for particles and opsonins. In: Dean RT, Jessup W, eds. Mononuclear Phagocytes: Physiology and Pathology. Amsterdam: Elsevier, 1985:55–78.

116. Mellman I, Koch T, Healey G, et al. Structure and function of Fc receptors on macrophages and lymphocytes. J Cell Sci 1988; 9(suppl):45–65.

117. Law SKA. C3 receptors on macrophages. J Cell Sci 1988; 9(suppl):67–97.

118. Ezekowitz RAB, Stahl PD. The structure and function of vertebrate mannose lectin-like proteins. J Cell Sci 1988; 9(suppl):121–33.

119. Goldstein JL, Brown MS, Anderson RGW, Russell DW, Schneider WJ. Receptor-mediated endocytosis: concepts emerging from the LDL receptor system. Annu Rev Cell Biol 1985;1:1–39.

120. Kaplan J, Buys SS. Macrophage surface receptors for soluble macromolecules. In: Dean RT, Jessup W, eds. Mononuclear Phagocytes: Physiology and Pathology. Amsterdam: Elsevier, 1985:79–90.

121. Unkless JC, Wright SD. Phagocytic cells: Fc and complement receptors. In: Gallin JI, Goldstein IM, Snyderman R, eds. Inflammation: Basic Principles and Clinical Correlates. New York: Raven Press, 1988:343–62.

122. Guyre PM, Morganelli PM, Muller R. Recombinant immune interferon increases immunoglobulin G Fc receptors on cultured human mononuclear phagocytes. J Clin Invest 1983;72:393–7.

123. Anderson JL, Guyre PM, Whitin JC, Ryan DH, Looney RJ, Fanger MW. Monoclonal antibodies to Fc receptors for IgG on human mononuclear phagocytes: antibody characterization and induction of superoxide production in a monocyte cell line. J Biol Chem 1986;261:12856–64.

124. Shen L, Guyre PM, Anderson CL, Fanger MW. Heteroantibody-mediated cytotoxicity: antibody to the high affinity Fc receptor for IgG mediates cytotoxicity by human monocytes that is enhanced by interferon-γ and is not blocked by human IgG. J Immunol 1986;137:3378–82.

125. Ceuppens JL, Baroja ML, Van Vaeck F, Anderson CL. Defect in the membrane expression of high affinity 72-kD Fc receptors on phagocytic cells in four healthy subjects. J Clin Invest 1988;82:571–8.

126. Wright SD, Silverstein SC. Tumor-promoting phorbol esters stimulate C3b and C3bi receptor-mediated phagocytosis in cultured human monocytes. J Exp Med 1982;156:1149–64.

127. Rosen H, Law SKA. The leukocyte cell surface receptor(s) for the iC3b product of complement. Curr Top Microbiol Immunol 1989;153:99–122.

128. Wright SD, Levin SM, Jong JTC, Chad Z, Kabbash LG. CR3 (CD11b/CD18) expresses one binding site for Arg-Gly-Asp-containing peptides and a second site for bacterial lipopolysaccharide. J Exp Med 1989;169:175–83.

129. Newman SL, Bucher C, Rhodes J, Bullock WE. Phagocytosis of Histoplasma capsulatum yeasts and microconida by human cultured macrophages and alveolar macrophages: cellular cytoskeleton requirements for attachment and ingestion. J Clin Invest 1990;85:223–30.

130. Mosser DM, Edelson PJ. The mouse macrophage receptor for C3bi (CR3) is a major mechanism in the phagocytosis of Leishmania promastigotes. J Immunol 1985;135:2785–9.

131. Payne NR, Bellinger-Kawahara CG, Horowitz MA. Phagocytosis of Mycobacterium tuberculosis by human monocytes is mediated by receptors for the third component of complement. Clin Res 1987;35:617A.

132. Schlesinger L, Horowitz MA. Phagocytosis of leprosy bacilli by human monocytes is mediated by complement receptors CR1 and CR3. Clin Res 1988;36:582A.

133. Payne NR, Horowitz MA. Phagocytosis of Legionella pneumophilia is mediated by human complement receptors. J Exp Med 1987;166:1377–89.

134. Wright SD, Jong MTC. Adhesion-promoting receptors on human macrophages recognize E. coli by binding to lipopolysaccharide. J Exp Med 1986;164:1876–88.

135. Wright SD, Detmers PA, Jong MTC, Meyer BC. Interferon-gamma depresses binding of ligand by C3b and C3bi receptors on cultured human monocytes, an effect reversed by fibronectin. J Exp Med 1986;163:1245–59.

136. Bohnsack JF, Kleinman HK, Takahashi T, O'Shea JJ, Brown EJ. Connective tissue proteins and phagocytic cell function: laminin enhances complement and Fc-mediated phagocytosis by cultured human phagocytes. J Exp Med 1985;161:912–23.

137. Pommier CG, Inada S, Fries LF, Takahashi T, Frank MM, Brown EJ. Plasma fibronectin enhances phagocytosis of opsonized particles by human peripheral blood monocytes. J Exp Med 1983;157:1844–54.

138. Wright SD, Craigmyle LS, Silverstein SC. Fibronectin and serum amyloid P component stimulate C3b- and C3bi-mediated phagocytosis in cultured human monocytes. J Exp Med 1983;158:1338–43.

139. Shaw DR, Griffin FM Jr. Phagocytosis requires repeated triggering of macrophage phagocytic receptors during particle ingestion. Nature 1981;289:409–11.

140. Karnovsky ML, Lazdims J, Simmons SR. Metabolism of activated macrophages at rest and during phagocytosis. In: van Furth R, ed. Mononuclear Phagocytes in Immunity, Infection, and Pathology. Oxford: Blackwell Scientific, 1975:423.

141. Loike JD, Kozler VF, Silverstein SC. Increased ATP and creatine phosphate turnover in phagocytosing mouse peritoneal macrophages. J Biol Chem 1979;254:9558–64.

142. Wright SD, Silverstein SC. Receptors for C3b and C3bi promote phagocytosis, but not the release of toxic oxygen from human phagocytes. J Exp Med 1983;158:2016–23.

143. Dean RT, Jessup W. The Zipper Model of Phagocytosis. In: Dean RT, Jessup W, eds. Mononuclear Phagocytes: Physiology and Pathology. Amsterdam: Elsevier, 1985:3–5.

144. Silverstein SC, Greenberg S, DiVirgilio F, Steinberg TH. Phagocytosis. In: Paul WE, ed. Fundamental Immunology. New York: Raven Press, 1989:710–20.

145. Fearon DT, Ahearn JM. Complement receptor type I (C3b/C4b receptor; CD35) and complement receptor type 2 (C3d/Epstein-Barr virus receptor; CD21). Curr Top Microbiol Immunol 1989;153:83–98.

146. Steinman RM, Cohn ZA. The metabolism and physiology of the mononuclear phagocyte. In: Zweifach BW, Grant L, McCluskey RT, eds. The Inflammatory Process. New York: Academic Press, 1974:449–510.

147. Cohn ZA. The activation of mononuclear phagocytes: fact, fancy and future. J Immunol 1978;121:813–6.

148. Karnovsky ML, Lazdims JK. Biochemical criteria for activated macrophages. J Immunol 1978;121:809–13.

149. North RJ. The concept of the activated macrophage. J Immunol 1978;121:806–9.

150. Adams DO, Hamilton TA. The cell biology of macrophage activation. Annu Rev immunol 1984;2:283–318.

151. Adams DO, Marino P. Activation of mononuclear phagocytes for destruction of tumor cells as a model for study of macrophage development. In: Gordon AS, Silber R, LoBue J, eds. Contemporary Topics in Hematology-Oncology. New York: Plenum Press, 1984:69–136.

152. Nathan CF, Prendergast TJ, Wiebe ME. Activation of human macrophages: comparison of other cytokines with interferon-gamma. J Exp Med 1984;160:600–5.

153. Weiser WY, Van Niel A, Clark SC, David JR, Remold HG. Recombinant human granulocyte/macrophage colony-stimulating factor activates intracellular killing of *Leishmania donovani* by human monocyte-derived macrophages. J Exp Med 1987;166:1436–46.

154. Reed SG, Nathan CF, Pihl DL, et al. Recombinant granulocyte/macrophage colony-stimulating factor activates macrophages to inhibit *Trypanosoma cruzi* and release hydrogen peroxide: comparison with interferon-gamma. J Exp Med 1987;166:1734–46.

155. Drysdale BE, Agarwal S, Shin HS. Macrophage-mediated tumoricidal activity: mechanisms of activation and cytotoxicity. Prog Allergy 1988;40:111–61.

156. Crawford RM, Finbloom DS, Ohara J, Paul WE, Meltzer MS. B-cell stimulatory factor-1 (interleukin-4) activates macrophages for increased tumoricidal activity and expression of Ia antigens. J Immunol 1987;139:135–41.

157. Nathan C, Yoshida R. Cytokines: interferon-γ. In: Gallin JI, Goldstein IM, Snyderman R, eds. Inflammation: Basic Principles and Clinical Correlates. New York: Raven Press, 1988:229–51.

158. Klebanoff SJ. Phagocytic cells: products of oxygen metabolism. In: Gallin JI, Goldstein IM, Snyderman R, eds. Inflammation: Basic Principles and Clinical Correlates. New York: Raven Press, 1988:391–444.

159. Meltzer MS, Nacy CA. Delayed-type hypersensitivity and the induction of activated, cytotoxic macrophages. In: Paul WE, ed. Fundamental Immunology. New York: Raven Press, 1989:765–77.

160. Diamond RD, Huber E, Haudenschild CC. Mechanism of destruction of *Aspergillus fumigatus hypae* mediated by human monocytes. J Infect Dis 1983;147:474–83.

161. Lehrer RI. The fungicidal mechanisms of human monocyte: I. Evidence for myeloperoxidase-linked and myeloperoxidase-independent candidacidal mechanisms. J Clin Invest 1975;55:338–46.

162. Locksley RM, Wilson CB, Klebanoff SJ. Role for endogenous and acquired peroxidase in the toxoplasmacidal activity of murine and human mononuclear phagocytes. J Clin Invest 1982;69:1099–11.

163. Tsunawaki S, Nathan CF. Enzymatic basis of macrophage activation. J Biol Chem 1984;259:4305–12.

164. Sasada M, Pabst MJ, Johnston RB Jr. Activation of mouse peritoneal macrophages alters the kinetic parameters of the superoxide-producing NADPH oxidase. J Biol Chem 1983;258:9631–5.

165. Dinarello CA. Cytokines: interleukin-1 and tumor necrosis factor (cachectin). In: Gallin JI, Goldstein IM, Snyderman R, eds. Inflammation: Basic Principles and Clinical Correlates. New York: Raven Press, 1988:195–208.

166. Durum SK, Oppenheim JJ. Macrophage-derived mediators: interleukin-1, tumor necrosis factor, interleukin-6, interferon, and related cytokines. In: Paul WE, ed. Fundamental Immunology. New York: Raven Press, 1989:639–61.

167. Pober JS, Gimbrone MA Jr, Lapierre LA, et al. Overlapping patterns of activation of human endothelial cells by interleukin-1, tumor necrosis factor and immune interferon. J Immunol 1986;137:1893–6.

168. Adams DO, Hamilton TA. The activated macrophage and granulomatous inflammation. Curr Top Pathol 1989;79:151–67.

169. Adams DO. Molecular interactions in macrophage activation. Immunol Today 1989;10:33–5.

170. Adams DO, Johnson WJ, Marino PA. Mechanisms of target recognition and destruction in macrophage mediated tumor cytotoxicity. Fed Proc 1982;41:2212–21.

171. Somers SD, Johnson WJ, Adams DO. Destruction of tumor cells by macrophages: mechanisms of recognition and lysis and their regulation. In: Herberman R, ed. Basic and Clinical Tumor Immunology. Netherlands, Martinus Nijhoff: 1986:69.

172. Adams DO, Cohen MS, Koren HS. Activation of mononuclear phagocytes for cytolysis: parallels and contrasts between activation for tumor cytotoxicity and for ADCC. In: Koren HS, ed. Macrophage Mediated Antibody-Dependent Cellular Cytotoxicity. New York: Marcel Dekker, 1983:43–52.

173. Murray HW. Cell-mediated immune response in experimental visceral leishmaniasis: II. Oxygen-dependent killing of intracellular *Leishmania donovani* amastigotes. J Immunol 1982;129:351–7.

174. Shurin SB, Stossel TP. Complement (C3)-activated phagocytosis by lung macrophages. J Immunol 1978;120:1305–12.

175. Chang YT, Neikirk RK. *Mycobacterium lepraemurium* and *Mycobacterium leprae* in cultures of mouse peritoneal macrophages. Int J Lepr 1965;33:586–603.

176. Kunkel SL, Chensue SW, Strieter RM, Lynch JP, Remick DG. Cellular and molecular aspects of granulomatous inflammation. Am J Resp Cell Mol Biol 1989;1:439–47.

177. Scales WE, Chensue SW, Otterness I, Kunkel SL. Regulation of monokine gene expression: prostaglandin E2 suppresses tumor necrosis factor but not interleukin-1 alpha or beta mRNA and cell-associated bioactivity. J Leuk Biol 1989;45:416–21.

178. Poulter LW, Seymour GJ, Duke O, Janossy G, Panayi G. Immunohistological analysis of delayed-type hypersensitivity in man. Cell Immunol 1982;74:358–69.

179. Platt JL, Grant BW, Eddy AA, Michael AF. Immune cell populations in cutaneous delayed hypersensitivity. J Exp Med 1983;158:1227–42.

180. Unanue ER. Macrophages, antigen-presenting cells, and the phenomenon of antigen handling and presentation. In: Paul WE, ed. Fundamental Immunology. New York: Raven Press, 1989:95–115.

181. Unanue ER, Cerottini J-C. Antigen presentation. FASEB J 1989;3:2496–502.

182. Chain BM, Kaye PM, Shaw M-A. The biochemistry and cell biology of antigen processing. Immunol Rev 1988;106:33–58.

183. Hackett CJ. Cell-mediated processing and presentation of T cell antigenic determinants. Curr Opin Immunol 1990;2:117–22.

184. Otten G. Antigen processing and presentation. Curr Opin Immunol 1990;2:204–9.

185. Swain SL. T cell subsets and the recognition of MHC class. Immunol Rev 1983;74:129–42.

186. Allen PM, Unanue ER. Differential requirement for antigen processing by macrophages for lysozyme-specific T cell hybridoma. J Immunol 1984;132:1077–99.

187. Ziegler HK, Unanue ER. Decrease in macrophage antigen catabolism by ammonia and chloroquine is associated with inhibition of antigen presentation to T cells. Proc Natl Acad Sci U S A 1982;78:175–8.

188. Springer TA, Dustin ML, Kishimoto TK, Marlin SD. The lymphocyte function-associated LFA-1, CD2, and LFA-3 molecules: cell adhesion receptors of the immune system. Annu Rev Immunol 1987;5:223–52.

189. Pernis B, Silverstein SC, Vogel HJ. Processing and presentation of antigens. New York: Academic Press, 1988:1–315.

190. Seshadri RS, Brown EJ, Zipursky A. Leukemic reticuloendotheliosis: a failure of monocyte production. N Engl J Med 1976;295:181–4.

191. Twomey JJ, Douglass CC, Sharkey O Jr. The monocytopenia of aplastic anemia. Blood 1973;41:187–95.

192. Treacy M, Lai L, Costello C, Clark A. Peripheral blood and bone marrow abnormalities in patients with HIV related disease. Br J Haematol 1987;65:289–94.

193. Peterson V, Hansbrough J, Buerk C, et al. Regulation of granulopoiesis following severe thermal injury. J Trauma 1983;23:19–24.

194. Den Ottolander GJ, van der Burgh FJ, Lopes Cardozo P. The Hemalog D automated counter in the diagnosis of hairy cell leukemia. Leuk Res 1983;7:309–20.

195. Tsokos GC. Immunomodulatory treatment in patients with rheumatic diseases: mechanisms of action. Semin Arthritis Rheum 1987;17:24–38.

196. Fahey JV, Guyre PM, Munck A. Mechanisms of antiinflammatory actions of glucocorticoids. Adv Inflammation Res 1981;2:21–51.

197. Rinehart JJ, Balcerzak SP, Sagone AL, LoBuglio AF. Effects of corticosteroids on human monocyte function. J Clin Invest 1974;54:1337–43.

198. Rinehart JJ, Sagone AL, Balcerzak SP, Ackerman GA, LoBuglio AF. Effects of corticosteroid therapy on human monocyte function. N Engl J Med 1975;292:236–41.

199. Rosenthal N, Abel HA. The significance of the monocytes in agranulocytosis (leukopenic infectious agranulocytosis). Am J Clin Pathol 1936;6:205–30.

200. Myhre EB, Braconier JH, Sjogren U. Automated cytochemical differential leukocyte count in patients hospitalized with acute bacterial infections. Scand J Infect Dis 1985;17:201–8.

201. Klemola E. Cytomegalovirus infection in previously healthy adults. Ann Intern Med 1973;79:267–8.

202. Gibson A. Monocytic leukemoid reaction associated with tuberculosis and a mediastinal teratoma. J Pathol Bacteriol 1946;58:469–75.

203. Flinn JW. A study of the differential blood count in 1000 cases of active pulmonary tuberculosis. Ann Intern Med 1929;2:622–36.

204. Daland GA, Gottlieb L, Wallerstein RO, Castle WB. Hematologic observations in bacterial endocarditis. J Lab Clin Med 1956;48:827–45.

205. Hill RW, Bayrd ED. Phagocytic reticuloendothelial cells in subacute bacterial endocarditis with negative cultures. Ann Intern Med 1960;52:310–9.

206. Rosahn PD, Pearce L. The blood cytology in untreated and treated syphilis. Am J Med Sci 1934;187:88–100.

207. Karayalcin G, Khanijou A, Kim KY, Aballi AJ, Lanzkowsky P. Monocytosis in congenital syphilis. Am J Dis Child 1977;131:782–3.

208. Brodsky I, Reiman HA, Dennis LH. Treatment of cyclic neutropenia in childhood. Am J Med 1965;38:802–6.

209. Zuelzer WW, Bajoghli M. Chronic granulocytopenia in childhood. Blood 1964;23:359–74.

210. Lang JE, Cutting HO. Infantile genetic agranulocytosis. Pediatrics 1965;35:596–600.

211. Spaet TH, Dameshek W. Chronic hypoplastic neutropenia. Am J Med 1952;13:35–45.

212. Cutting HO, Lang JE. Familial benign chronic neutropenia. Ann Intern Med 1964;61:876–87.

213. Sewell RL. Lymphocyte abnormalities in myeloma. Br J Haematol 1977;36:545–51.

214. Blom J, Nielsen H, Larsen SO, Mansa B. A study of certain functional parameters of monocytes from patients with multiple myeloma: comparison with monocytes from healthy individuals. Scand J Haematol 1984;33:425–31.

215. Ultmann JE. Clinical features and diagnosis of Hodgkin's disease. Cancer 1966;19:297–307.

216. Hurst DW, Meyer OO. Giant follicular lymphoblastoma. Cancer 1961;14:753–78.

217. Wiseman BK. The blood pictures in the primary diseases of the lymphatic system: their character and significance. JAMA 1936;107:2016–22.

218. Sexauer J, Kass L, Schnitzer B. Subacute myelomonocytic leukemia. Am J Med 1974;57:853–61.

219. Geary CG, Catovsky D, Wiltshaw E, et al. Chronic myelomonocytic leukemia. Br J Haematol 1975;30:289–302.

220. Kantarjian HM, Keating MJ, Walters RS, et al. Clinical and prognostic features of Philadelphia chromosome-negative chronic myelogenous leukemia. Cancer 1986;58:2023–30.

221. Castro-Malaspina H, Schaison G, et al. Subacute and chronic myelomonocytic leukemia in children (Juvenile CML). Cancer 1984;54:675–86.

222. Shaw MT. The distinctive features of acute monocytic leukemia. Am J Haematol 1978;4:97–103.

223. Linman JW, Bagby GC Jr. The preleukemic syndrome: clinical and laboratory features, natural course and management. Blood Cells 1976;2:11–31.

224. Jaworkowsky LI, Solovey DY, Rhausova LY, Udris OY. Monocytosis as a sign of subsequent leukemia in patients with cytopenias (preleukemia). Folia Hematol 1983;110:395–401.

225. Maldonado JE, Hanlon DG. Monocytosis: a current appraisal. Mayo Clinic Proc 1965;40:248–59.

226. Buchan GS, Palmer DG, Gibbins BL. The response of human peripheral blood mononuclear phagocytes to rheumatoid arthritis. J Leukocyte Biol 1985;37:221–30.

227. Budman DR, Steinberg AD. Hematologic aspects of systemic lupus erythematosus. Ann Intern Med 1977;86:220–9.

228. Newcombe DS, Terry PB. The immunopathogenesis of environmental and chemical exposures: the use of bronchoalveolar lavage for their detection. In: Newcombe DS, Rose NR, Bloom JC, eds. Human Immunotoxicity: Mechanisms and Controversies. New York: Raven Press, 1991.

229. Harris JO. Pulmonary alveolar proteinosis: abnormal in vitro function of alveolar macrophages. Chest 1979;6:156–9.

230. Singh G, Katyal SL, Bedrossian WM, Rogers RM. Pulmonary alveolar proteinosis: staining for surfactant apoprotein in alveolar proteinosis and in conditions simulating it. Chest 1983;83:82–6.

231. Barbers RG, Gong H, Tashkin DP, Oishi J, Wallace JM. Differential examination of bronchoalveolar lavage cells in tobacco cigarette and marijuana smokers. Am Rev Resp Dis 1987;135:1271–5.

232. Reynolds HY, Chretien J. Respiratory tract fluids: analysis of content and contemporary use in understanding lung disease. Dis Mon 1984;30:1–103.

233. Hunninghake GW, Gadek JE, Kawanami O, Ferrans VJ, Crystal RG. Inflammatory and immune processes in the human lung in health and disease: evaluation by bronchoalveolar lavage. Am J Pathol 1978;97:149–206.

234. Thomassen MJ, Boxerbaum B, Demko CA, Kuchenbrod PJ, Dearborn DG, Wood RE. Inhibitory effect of cystic fibrosis serum on pseudomonas phagocytosis by rabbit and human alveolar macrophages. Pediatr Res 1979;13:1085–8.

235. Fick RB, Naegel GF, Squier SU, Wood RE, Gee BL, Reynolds HY. Proteins of the cystic fibrosis respiratory tract: fragmented immunoglobulin G opsonic antibody causing defective opsonophagocytosis. J Clin Invest 1984;74:236–48.

236. Hunninghake GW. Release of interleukin-1 by alveolar macrophages of patients with active pulmonary sarcoidosis. Am Rev Resp Dis 1984;129:569–72.

237. Daniele RP, Danber JH, Rossman MD. Immunologic abnormalities in sarcoidosis. Ann Intern Med 1980;92:406–16.

238. Razma AG, Lynch JP III, Wilson BS, Ward PA, Kunkel SL. Expression of Ia-like (DR) antigen on human alveolar macrophages isolated by bronchoalveolar lavage. Am Rev Resp Dis 1984;129:419–24.

239. Hunninghake GW, Kawanami O, Ferrans VJ, Young RC Jr,

Roberts WC, Crystal RG. Characterization of the inflammatory and immune effector cells in the lung parenchyma of patients with interstitial lung disease. Am Rev Resp Dis 1981;123:407–12.

240. DuBois RM, Townsend PJ, Cole PJ, Haslam PL, Turner-Warwick M. Bronchoalveolar macrophages in sarcoidosis and cryptogenic fibrosing alveolitis. Clin Allergy 1981;11:409–19.

241. Robinson B, Gadek J, Fells G, Crystal RG. Increased plasminogen activator release by pulmonary alveolar macrophages in patients with chronic interstitial lung disease. Am Rev Resp Dis 1983;127(suppl):281.

242. Brun J, Dastugue B, Motta C, Jehan A, Molina C. Lipid analysis of bronchoalveolar lavage fluid from patients with sarcoidosis and hypersensitivity pneumonitis. In: Chretien J, Marsac J, Saltiel JC, eds. Sarcoidosis and Other Granulomatous Disorders. New York: Pergamon Press, 1983:659.

243. Reynolds HY. Bronchoalveolar lavage. In: Murray JF, Nadel JA, eds. Textbook of Respiratory Medicine. Philadelphia: W.B. Saunders, 1988:597–610.

244. Newcombe DS, Terry PB. Bronchoalveolar lavage and bronchial reactivity in humans associated with environmental and chemical exposures. In: Newcombe DS, Rose NR, Bloom JC, ed. Clinical Immunotoxicology. New York: Raven Press, 1992:277–337.

245. Blume RS, Wolfe SM. The Chediak-Hiyashi syndrome: studies in four patients and a review of the literature. Medicine 1972;51:247–80.

246. Baehner RL, Boxer LA. Morphological and biochemical alterations of polymorphonuclear neutrophil (PMN) leukocytes from patients with inborn errors of phagocytic function: a comprehensive review. In: Guttler F, Seakins JWT, Harkness RA, eds. Inborn Errors of Immunity and Phagocytosis. Baltimore: University Park Press, 1979:201–18.

247. Parry MF, Root RK, Metcalf JA, Delaney KK, Kaplow LS, Richar WJ. Myeloperoxidase deficiency: prevalence and clinical significance. Ann Intern Med 1981;95:293–301.

248. Nauseef WM, Root RK, Malech HL. Biochemical and immunologic analysis of hereditary myeloperoxidase deficiency. J Clin Invest 1983;71:1297–307.

249. Bainton DF. Phagocytic cells: developmental biology of neutrophils and eosinophils. In: Gallin JI, Goldstein IM, Snyderman R, eds. Inflammation: Basic Principles and Clinical Correlates. New York: Raven Press, 1988:265–80.

250. Ash P, Loutit JF, Townsend KMS. Osteoclasts derived from haematopoietic stem cells. Nature 1980;283:669–70.

251. Coccia PF, Krivit W, Cervemka J, et al. Successful bone marrow transplantation of infantile malignant osteopetrosis. N Engl J Med 1980;302:701–8.

252. Curnutte JT. Phagocytic defects. II: Abnormalities of the respiratory burst. Hematol Oncol Clin North Am 1988;2:189–334.

253. Forehand JR, Nauseef WM, Johnston RB Jr. Inherited disorders of phagocyte killing. In: Scriver CR, Beaudet AL, Sly WS, Valle D, eds. The Metabolic Basis of Inherited Disease. New York: McGraw-Hill, 1989:2779–801.

254. Lehrer RI, Cline MJ. Leukocyte myeloperoxidase deficiency and disseminated candidiasis. J Clin Invest 1969;48:1478–88.

255. Cech P, Stalder H, Widmann N, Rohner A, Miescher P. Leukocyte myeloperoxidase deficiency and diabetes mellitus associated with *Candida albicans* liver abscess. Am J Med 1979;66:149–53.

256. Caldwell KC, Taddeini L, Woodburn RL, Anderson GL, Lobell M. Induction of myeloperoxidase deficiency in granulocytes in lead-intoxicated dogs. Blood 1979;53:588–93.

257. El Maalem H, Fletcher J. Impaired neutrophil function and myeloperoxidase deficiency in pregnancy. Br J Haematol 1980;44:375–81.

258. Lehrer RI, Cline MJ. Leukocyte candidacidal activity and resistance to systemic candidiasis in patients with cancer. Cancer 1971;27:1211–71.

259. Lehrer RI, Goldberg LS, Apple MA, Rosenthal NP. Refractory megaloblastic anemia with myeloperoxidase-deficient neutrophils. Ann Intern Med 1972;76:447–53.

260. Bozdech MJ, Bainton DF, Mustacchi P. Partial peroxidase deficiency in neutrophils and eosinophils associated with neurological disease. Am J Clin Pathol 1980;73:409–16.

261. Bendix-Hansen K. Myeloperoxidase-deficient polymorphonuclear leukocytes: longitudinal study during preremission and remission phase in acute myeloid leukemia. Blut 1986;52:237–42.

262. Bendix-Hansen K, Kerndrup Q, Pedersen B. Myeloperoxidase-deficient polymorphonuclear leukocytes. VI: Relation to cytogenic abnormalities in primary myelodysplastic syndromes. Scand J Haematol 1986;36:3–10.

263. Bendix-Hansen K, Nielson HK. Myeloperoxidase-deficient polymorphonuclear leukocyte. II: Incidence in untreated myeloid leukemia, lymphoid leukemia, and normal humans. Scand J Haematol 1983;30:415–19.

264. Kaplow LS. Substitute for benzidine in myeloperoxidase staining. Am J Clin Pathol 1975;63:451.

265. Elias JM. A rapid sensitive myeloperoxidase stain using 4-chloro-1-naphthol. Am J Clin Pathol 1980;73:409–16.

266. Robertson CF, Thong YH, Hodge GL, Chency K. Primary myeloperoxidase deficiency associated with impaired neutrophil margination and chemotaxis. Acta Paediatr Scand 1979;68:915–9.

267. Cech P, Papathanassion A, Boreaux G, Roth P, Miescher PA. Hereditary myeloperoxidase deficiency. Blood 1979;53:403–11.

268. Klebanoff SJ, Hamon SB. Role of myeloperoxidase-mediated antimicrobial systems in intact leukocytes. J Reticuloendothel Soc 1972;12:170–96.

269. Stendahl O, Coble BI, Dahlgren C, Hed J, Molin L. Myeloperoxidase modulates the phagocytic activity of polymorphonuclear neutrophil leukocytes: studies with cells from a myeloperoxidase-deficient patient. J Clin Invest 1984;73:366–73.

270. Curnutte JT. Phagocytic defects. I: Abnormalities outside of the respiratory burst. Hematol Oncol Clin North Am 1988;2:1–179.

271. Beutler E. Lipid storage diseases. In: Williams WJ, Beutler E, Erslev AJ, Lichtman MA, eds. Hematology. New York: McGraw-Hill, 1990:886–94.

272. Barranger JA, Ginns EI. Glucosylceramide lipidoses: Gaucher disease. In: Scriver CR, Beaudet AL, Sly WS, Valle D, eds. The Metabolic Basis of Inherited Disease. New York: McGraw-Hill, 1989:1677–98.

273. Spence MW, Callahan JW. Sphingomyelin-cholesterol lipidoses: the Nieman-Pick group of diseases. In: Scriver CR, Beaudet AL, Sly WS, Valle D, eds. The Metabolic Basis of Inherited Disease. New York: McGraw-Hill, 1989:1655–76.

274. Sandhoff K, Conzelmann E, Neufield EF, Kabach MM, Suzuki K. The G_{mz} gangliosidoses. In: Scriver CR, Beaudet AL, Sly WS, Valle D, eds. The Metabolic Basis of Inherited Disease. New York: McGraw-Hill, 1989:1807–42.

275. Desnick RJ, Bishop DF. Fabry disease: α-galactosidase deficiency; Schindler disease: α-N-acetylgalactosaminidase deficiency. In: Scriver CR, Beaudet AL, Sly WS, Valle D, eds. The Metabolic Basis of Inherited Disease. New York: McGraw-Hill, 1989:1751–96.

276. Moser HW, Moser AB, Chen WW, Schram AW. Ceramidase deficiency: Farber lipogranulomatosis. In: Scriver CR, Beaudet AL, Sly WS, Valle D, eds. The Metabolic Basis of Inherited Disease. New York: McGraw-Hill, 1989:1645–54.

277. Komp DM. Langerhans cell histiocytosis. N Engl J Med 1987;316:747–8.

278. Reiner AP, Spivak JL. Hematophagic histiocytosis: a report of 23 new patients and a review of the literature. Medicine 1988;67:369–88.

279. Close P, Friedman D, Uri A. Viral-associated hemophagocytic syndrome. Med Pediatr Oncol 1990;18:119–22.

280. Ladish S, Poplack DG, Holiman B, Blaese RM. Immunodeficiency in familial erythrophagocytic lymphohistiocytosis. Lancet 1978;i:581–3.

281. Komp DM, Lichtman MA. Inflammatory and malignant histiocytosis. In: Williams WJ, Beautler E, Erslev AJ, Lichtman MA, eds. Hematology. New York: McGraw-Hill, 1990:895–902.

282. Rosai J, Dorfman RF. Sinus histiocytosis with massive lymphadenopathy: a newly recognized benign clinicopathologic entity. Arch Pathol 1969;87:63–70.

283. Rappoport H. Tumors of the hemopoietic system. Atlas of Tumor Pathology. Washington, D.C.: Armed Forces Institute of Pathology, 1966:49–63.

284. Kawahara E, Nakanishi I, Kurda Y, Morishita T. Fine needle aspiration biopsy of primary malignant fibrous histiocytoma of the lung. Acta Cytol 1988;32:226–30.

285. Gonwa TA, Picker LJ, Raff HV, Goyert SM, Silver J, Stobo JD. Antigen presenting capabilities of human monocytes correlates with their expression of HLA-DS, Ia determinant distinct from HLA-DR. J Immunol 1983;130:706.

286. Yasaka T, Mantich NM, Boxer LA, Baechner RL. Functions of human monocyte and lymphocyte subsets obtained by counter-current centrifugal elutriation: differing functional capacities of human monocyte subsets. J Immunol 1981;127:1515.

287. Norris DA, Morris RM, Sanderson RJ, Kohler PF. Isolation of functional subsets of human peripheral blood monocytes. J Immunol 1979;123:166.

11

Lymphocytes

Richard D. Leavitt, M.D.

THE IMMUNE SYSTEM

The immune system is a host-defense mechanism that provides for the specific recognition and elimination from the body of foreign proteins, pathogens, and altered host cells (discrimination of self and nonself) as well as enhancing resistance to subsequent challenges by the same offending agent (memory). Lymphocytes are the key component in this system, because they provide both specificity and memory. They also express gene products that permit the host to recognize an estimated 10^5 to 10^8 different antigenic determinants, control the cellular interactions required for the successful initiation and mediation of immunity, and provide for the passage of specific-antigen reactivity from one generation of cells to the next. In addition, lymphocytes control the intensity of immune responses as well as their specificity. Through cell–cell interactions and the secretion of soluble regulatory substances (i.e., the lymphokines), control is exerted directly over other effector and antibody-secreting lymphocytes; the activity of other accessory cells of immunity (i.e., the macrophages and neutrophilic leukocytes) is controlled indirectly either by the effects of secreted antibodies and lymphokines or the activation of the complement system or other mediators of inflammation. In turn, these accessory cells play a key role in the initiation and augmentation of the immune response by lymphocytes.

The Organization of the Immune System

Lymphocytes are dispersed throughout the body, circulating in the blood and lymph or migrating through the tissues, and they occur as resident populations in the organized tissues in lymph nodes and spleen as well as in association with gut, urogenital, and bronchial mucosa. Dispersed in the tissues, lymphocytes are better able to initiate and effect an immune response at the invasion site of a foreign antigen, and in organized lymphoid tissue, interaction between lymphocytes, accessory cells, and antigens facilitates the amplification of the immune response by the recruitment and proliferation of other effector cells. Two central lymphoid organs in humans, the thymus and the bone marrow, also play unique roles in differentiation, controlling the development of specialized lymphocyte subpopulations that have specific immune functions.

The lymphocytes that provide for the selective defense of the host belong to two distinct but morphologically indistinguishable functional classes: T and B lymphocytes. T lymphocytes mature in the thymus and then disseminate into peripheral tissues; there, they can react directly with antigens to generate specific effector cells essential for delayed-type hypersensitivity reaction, graft rejection, tumor suppression, and resistance to some intracellular organisms (cellular immunity). B lymphocytes originate in the bone marrow and then emigrate into peripheral lymphatic tissues, where they can interact with antigens and differentiate into plasma cells that secrete the specific immunoglobulins important in the defense against bacterial infections (humoral immunity). However, this division of labor between T

Part of this chapter appeared previously in Leavitt RD. Biological markers of differentiation in the diagnosis of leukemia and lymphoma. In: Mossa AR, Robson M, Schimpff SC, eds. Comprehensive Textbook of Oncology. Baltimore: Williams & Wilkins, 1985.

and B cells is not complete. Subpopulations of thymus-derived lymphocytes play important roles in regulating humoral and cellular immune responses (i.e., helper and suppressor T cells).

Usually, the initial exposure to a new antigen leaves behind an expanded number of resting, antigen-specific cells that can respond to the next exposure to that same antigen with greater proliferation, increased numbers of effector and regulatory cells, increased amounts of antibody, and increased secretion of a variety of lymphokines. The balance between augmentation and suppression of the immune response is determined by the nature of the exposure to the antigen and by the state of the host; through these regulatory mechanisms, lymphocytes control both the specificity and intensity of the host immune response.

With the recent expansion of knowledge about the components and function of the normal immune system,

a bewildering array of both clinical and laboratory manifestations of immune reactions has been described in human disease. Many can be attributed to physiologic changes produced by a normal immune system; others are a consequence of disordered immunity resulting in the breakdown of host defenses against environmental pathogens (immunodeficiency) (Table 11.1) or an immunologic assault on self-antigens (autoimmunity). Abnormal lymphocyte proliferation also may lead to an increase in the total lymphoid cell mass, enlargement of lymphoid organs, and infiltration of other organ systems (lymphoproliferative diseases). Illness results when cellular proliferation interferes with the function of infiltrated organs or causes secondary immunodeficiency or autoimmunity. Proliferating cells may be either malignant (leukemia or lymphoma) or benign (e.g., infectious mononucleosis), and in some cases, distinguishing between benign, premalignant, and malignant lymphopro-

TABLE 11.1. The Classification of Primary Immunodeficiency Diseases

Predominant Antibody Defects
    X-linked agammaglobulinemia
    X-linked hypogammaglobulinemia with growth hormone deficiency
    Autosomal recessive agammaglobulinemia
    Immunoglobulin deficiency with increased IgM (and IgG)
    IgA deficiency
    Selective deficiency of other immunoglobulin isotypes
    κ-Chain deficiency
    Antibody deficiency with normal γ-globulin levels or hypergammaglobulinemia
    Immunodeficiency with thymoma
    Transient hypogammaglobulinemia of infancy
    Common variable immunodeficiency with predominant B-cell defect
        Nearly normal B-cell number with $\mu^+ \delta^+$, without $\mu^+ \delta^+$, $\mu^+ \gamma^+$, γ^+, or α^+ cells
        Very low B-cell number
        $\mu^+ \gamma^+$ or γ^+ "Nonsecretory" B cells with plasma cells
        Normal or increased B-cell number with $\mu^+ \delta^+ \gamma^+$, $\mu^+ \delta^+ \alpha^+$, γ^+, and α^+ B cells
    Common variable immunodeficiency with predominant immunoregulatory T-cell disorder
        Deficiency of helper T cells
        Presence of activated suppressor T cells
    Common variable immunodeficiency with autoantibodies to B or T cells
Predominant Defects of Cell-Mediated Immunity
    Combined immunodeficiency with predominant T-cell defect
    Purine-nucleoside phosphorylase deficiency
    Severe combined immunodeficiency with adenosine deaminase deficiency
    Severe combined immunodeficiency
        Reticular dysgenesis
        Low T- and B-cell numbers
        Low T-cell and normal B-cell numbers (Swiss)
        "Bare lymphocyte syndrome"
    Immunodeficiency with unusual response to Epstein-Barr virus
Immunodeficiency Associated with Other Defects
    Transcobalamin 2 deficiency
    Wiskott-Aldrich syndrome
    Ataxia telangiectasia
    Third- and fourth-pouch/arch (DiGeorge) syndrome

Source: Rosen et al. 1984[1] Reprinted by permission of the New England Journal of Medicine.

liferation may be difficult or even impossible with present knowledge. However, despite the many unanswered questions, current knowledge of the astonishingly complex immune system does provide an essential framework for understanding and managing human disease.

Diversity in the Body's Lymphocyte Stores

Lymphocytes are the primary cells involved in immune responses. In normal animals, these cells are dispersed throughout the body in blood, lymph, lymph nodes, bone marrow, spleen, intestine, liver, lung, and skin. Their total mass has been estimated at 1% to 2% of body weight in most mammals (10^{12} cells, or 1 kg in humans).

Despite a rather uniform and nondescript appearance, this population displays a remarkable functional heterogeneity unseen in any other cell type. Although some 10^5 to 10^8 genes may code for antigenic recognition, evidence indicates that each lymphocyte expresses only one type of surface receptor and that this receptor can interact only with antigenic determinants exhibiting a closely related molecular structure. After engaging the specific antigen, the lymphocyte undergoes blast cell transformation and proliferates, forming a clone bearing the same surface receptor, and the clone can then differentiate into effector, regulatory, and memory cells specific for that antigen. Individual clones may vary in size from 1 to 10^6 cells, but the remarkable diversity provided by the entire lymphocyte population permits immune responses to a wide variety of foreign proteins and pathogens. These agents typically also possess multiple determinants of differing molecular structure.

This chapter approaches the complexity of the immune response in the following manner. First, the origin and development of the diverse types of lymphocytes and their functions will be considered. Next, the pattern of organization for efficient immune function of these cells in lymphoid tissues is described. Finally, both normal and abnormal lymphocytes as well as immune mechanisms are discussed.

THE DEVELOPMENT AND DIFFERENTIATION OF LYMPHOCYTES

Studies concerning the ontogeny of the immune system, whether in mice, chickens, or humans, have found a common pattern of development for the vertebrate immune system. Diversity in lymphocytes results from the proliferation and differentiation of precursor cells, independent of exposure to antigen, that successively become committed to different lines of differentiation. In humans, T-cell precursors differentiate within the thymus and B-cell precursors within the bone marrow, and when the immunocompetent and regulator cells appear, they already are committed to a particular antigenic specificity as well as a cell lineage and effector function that can be detected by the phenotypic markers expressed on their surface membranes.

The Differentiation of T cells during Embryonic Development

In human embryos, hematopoietic stem cells are present in the yolk sac after 2 weeks of gestation. Although most cells at this site are erythroid precursors, the stem cells probably are represented by large blast cells that lack immunocompetence and lymphocyte surface markers. The stem cells migrate to the hepatic sinusoids at 6 weeks of gestation, and this site gradually then becomes the major site of fetal hematopoiesis. By 8 weeks of gestation, cells from the fetal liver show proliferative responses when stimulated by allogeneic lymphocytes in mixed leukocyte cultures; however, they are not activated by phytohemagglutinin. Because this activation can be accompanied by the expression of T-cell surface markers, the precursor cells present at this early stage of development appear to be programmed to display some T-cell characteristics before thymic development begins. Shortly thereafter, the thymus develops from endoderm derived from the third branchial pouch, and its epithelial cells differentiate under the inductive stimuli provided by mesenchymal components. Soon after its appearance, the thymus is composed of multiple layers of epithelial cells linked by desmosomes; then, primitive lymphocytes infiltrate the gland by wedging themselves between adjacent epithelial cells and begin to proliferate, thus densely populating the cortex. At 12 weeks of gestation, the thymocytes express T-cell surface markers and can be activated in culture by mitogens. After this point, the lymph nodes, spleen, and bone marrow become populated by increasing numbers of morphologically identifiable lymphocytes having surface markers and mitogenic responses similar to those seen in mature cells.

The Thymus in T-cell Differentiation

At birth, the thymus is a pink, lobulated gland weighing from 10 to 15 g that lies in the anterior mediastinum; at this point, it lacks the afferent lymphatic vessels seen in peripheral lymph nodes. The thymus gradually increases in size to a maximum weight of 40 g in early childhood, then involutes after adolescence to form an ill-defined, lobulated structure that weighs 10 to 15 g that is infiltrated with fat in adult life.

The thymus exhibits the characteristic histology of an epithelial reticulum (Fig. 11.1). The dense population of proliferating lymphoid cells that is wedged between adjacent epithelial cells produces a honeycombing effect in the cortex, because the epithelial cells are distorted into irregular shapes. The medulla contains only a few lymphocytes, so the parenchymal cells in this zone display a more typical epithelial appearance. Hassall corpuscles, formed by concentric whorls of filamentous epithelial cells about a central cystic cavity, commonly are seen in humans, and thymic involution is characterized by a marked decrease in the number of infiltrating lymphocytes within the cortex even though the epithelium remains.

Studies of cellular traffic within the thymus of laboratory animals indicate that stem cells originating in the bone marrow move through the bloodstream and pass through the walls of blood vessels in the outer cortex to infiltrate the epithelial reticulum.[4] Within the gland, these cells proliferate rapidly, exhibiting mitotic indexes 10 times those seen in lymph nodes and a population-turnover time of from 24 to 36 hours; many of these cells

appear to die in situ during a process resembling the ineffective erythropoiesis seen in the bone marrow. During this intense period of proliferation that precedes any exposure to antigen, T cells are generated that are able to recognize the various antigenic determinants they later will encounter, and the surviving cells then assume a mature lymphocyte morphology and exit from the gland near the corticomedullary junction by moving back into postcapillary venules and efferent lymphatics. These emigrant cells pass through the blood and seed peripheral tissues where they carry out the various T-cell functions in immune responses. Although this antigen-independent proliferation and differentiation of lymphocytes within the thymus is greatest in young animals, there is evidence that these events continue, but at reduced rates, in the involuted thymus of adults.

Studies of cell surface markers have provided convincing evidence of T-lymphocyte differentiation within the human thymus as well.[5] A gradient in the degree of maturation exists from cortex to medulla. The earliest precursor forms, 0.5% to 5% of thymocytes, are found in the cortex, and these express the enzyme terminal deoxynucleotidyl transferase (TdT) but not the human "common thymocyte antigen" T-6 (cluster designation

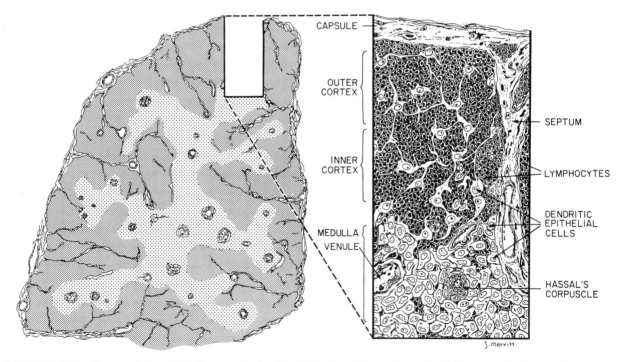

FIGURE 11.1.   The morphology of the thymus, showing the distribution of the cortex and medulla as seen in tissue sections at low magnification (*left*) and the appearance at higher magnification when the cortex is heavily infiltrated with differentiating and proliferating lymphocytes while the medulla is composed predominantly of epithelial cells with few infiltrating lymphocytes (*right*). *Source:* Weiss 1972[3]

CD1a). Also, some have acquired pan-T-cell antigens T-1 (CD5) and T-11 (CD2). Seventy-five percent of thymocytes are of the common cortical type (the next stage of differentiation), and all express the antigen T-6 (CD1a). The 10% to 15% of thymocytes in the medulla, which are the immediate precursors of peripheral T lymphocytes, have lost the enzyme TdT and the antigen T-6 (CD1a). The antigens that will mark distinct functional subpopulations in mature T cells (i.e., T-4 [CD4] for helper-inducer cells and T-5 and T-8 [CD8] for suppressor-cytotoxic cells) first appear together on the same cells in the thymic cortex, and subsequently, either antigen alone is expressed on the medullary thymocytes and mature peripheral T cells.

Several mechanisms have been proposed to explain T-cell differentiation within the thymus. The "finishing school" hypothesis suggests that the thymus provides a unique microenvironment where local inductive stimuli promote the proliferation and differentiation of T lymphocytes; the barrier about the blood vessels as well as the absence of afferent lymphatics in the thymus protect the immature cells from becoming tolerant to foreign antigens (but not self-antigens). Although this hypothesis is supported in part by repeated demonstrations that thymic grafts are more effective than thymic extracts in restoring full immunologic competence to thymectomized animals, the contribution of the thymic microenvironment to T-cell differentiation remains undecided.[6]

Several lines of evidence indicate that the thymus elaborates hormonal factors that determine T-cell differentiation and the functions of the various T-lymphocyte sublines in immune responses. Experiments during the 1960s demonstrated that both thymic grafts enclosed within cell-impermeable diffusion chambers as well as normal pregnancy could correct the immunologic deficits caused by thymectomy in animals.[7] Subsequently, crude extracts and partially purified polypeptides from thymic tissue were shown to induce the expression of specific T-cell differentiation markers in cultures of both marrow and spleen cells from thymectomized mice;[8] following such treatment, these cells were able to mediate graft-versus-host reactions, proliferate in response to allogeneic lymphocytes as well as nonspecific mitogens, and provide helper cells and probably T-cell–mediated cytotoxicity. A physiologic role for these agents is supported by observations that their injection into thymectomized animals can restore humoral and cellular immune responses and promote the proliferation of lymphocytes in peripheral lymphoid organs.

Several thymic hormones have been identified in humans. The biologically active peptides thymosin, thymopoietin, and thymic facteur serique (and possibly interleukin-7) can affect the growth and maturation of T cells. Their use as markers of disease and in treatment is under active investigation.[9,10]

Despite the evidence for a thymic hormone, there are still several puzzling aspects if the thymus is examined as a typical endocrine organ; for example, typical feedback controls of thymic function have not been identified. Also, lymphocyte mass, immunoglobulin levels, and both humoral and cellular immune responses are unaltered by engrafting from 1 to 30 additional syngeneic thymus glands into normal mice. Each of these grafts appears to function in complete autonomy, undergoing a typical cycle of growth and involution in correlation with the age of the donor. In addition, the cyclic pattern does not appear to be influenced either by the age of the recipient or the greatly augmented thymic mass provided by the adjacent grafts.[6]

The thymus cannot be considered completely autonomous, however. The initial phases of lymphocyte proliferation within those of neonatal animals require physiologic levels of somatotropic hormone; in the absence of such, both the thymus and peripheral lymphoid organs remain hypocellular. Pituitary changes and delayed sexual maturity are known to occur in thymectomized animals, but their genesis is obscure. In addition, absence of a functional thymus in mice reportedly is associated with decreased numbers of hematopoietic stem cells and the impaired ability of these cells to shift from G_0 phase to DNA synthesis. Because this defect can be corrected by injections of thymic extract, it has been suggested this approach might be useful for correcting pancytopenia in humans (particularly when associated with thymomas); however, this postulate has not yet been tested.

The Differentiation and Maturation of B Cells

Although B lymphocytes have only one biologic function (i.e., the synthesis and secretion of immunoglobulins), they comprise a heterogeneous cellular population. B lymphocytes produce antibody classes with very different functional properties and react specifically with literally thousands of different antigens. According to the currently favored germ line theory, all primordial B cells carry the full complement of genes required to make every possible antibody; however, owing to genetic rearrangement of the various separate genes coding for the variable (V), joining (J), and diversity (D) regions of the immunoglobulin molecule as well as random selection processes during early maturation, each cell expresses only the very limited portion of this information that is required to react with a single antigenic determinant.

In birds, the early differentiation and antigen-independent phases of cellular proliferation occur in a specialized lymphoepithelial organ termed *the bursa of Fabricius*. In humans, this structure does not exist, and B-cell differentiation is dispersed among hematopoietic tissue within the fetal liver, bone marrow, and spleen; peptide regulatory factors released by both T lymphocytes (lymphokines) and macrophages, thymic epithelium, and mast cells (cytokines) influence the maturation of human B cells at these sites (Table 11.2). The marrow is a site of rapid lymphocyte production, with estimated turnover times of 3 days, but this proliferation does not appear to be altered by depletion of the peripheral lymphocyte stores or depression of serum immunoglobulin levels.

B cells first appear in the marrow and hepatic sinusoids of human embryos at 7 weeks of gestation (Fig. 11.2). These lymphocytes contain cytoplasmic immunoglobulin, but for unknown reasons, they do not express this protein on their surfaces. At 9 weeks of gestation, lymphocytes with detectable surface IgM are present, and other cells then appear, bearing either IgD or both IgD and IgM on their membranes. The significance of IgD is unknown, but it may represent a fetal form of immunoglobulin. Thereafter, B cells bearing IgG and then IgA can be detected, and all of these cells proliferate and populate the various lymphoid tissues without maturing into plasma cells. The maturation sequence of IgM to IgG to IgA during embryonic development is governed by successive rearrangements

of the variable, joining, and diversity regions of the genes that code for immunoglobulin. The switch from IgM receptors to the other surface immunoglobulin classes during differentiation is independent of both antigen and T–helper cell activities.

The biologic significance of the prolonged delay between the initial synthesis of cytoplasmic IgM by early B cells and the subsequent emergence of reactive B lymphocytes that bear surface immunoglobulin receptors of the various classes is unclear. However, studies in fetal mice have shown that embryonic B cells expressing surface immunoglobulin bind the same diverse array of antigens, with avidities comparable to those found in B lymphocytes of mature animals.[12] A variety of experiments also have shown that organs excised during embryonic development are rejected when they are regrafted into the same recipients after maturation,[13] and from such evidence, it generally is believed that all mammals possess the genetic information required to produce lymphocytes reactive to self-antigens. These self-reactive cells probably arise constantly only to become either inactivated or tolerant.

The B-cell system appears highly susceptible to the induction of tolerance in the early phases of differentiation. The injection of heteroantibodies directed against isotypic, allotypic, or idiotypic determinants of immunoglobulin can lead to long-lasting inactivation of the B cells bearing these proteins on their membranes. In

TABLE 11.2.   Peptide Factors in the Regulation of Lymphocytes

Target Cell	Peptide Regulatory Factor	Source
Accessory cells (e.g., macrophages, dendritic cells)	Interferon-γ	T-cell
	Interleukin-1	Macrophage
	Tumor necrosis factor	T-cell
	Granulocyte-macrophage colony-stimulating factor	T-cell, mast cells
	Interleukin-4	T-cell, mast cells
T-lymphocytic activation and expansion	Interleukin-1	Macrophage
	Interleukin-2	T-cell
	Interleukin-4	T-cell, mast cells
	Interferon-γ	T-cell
	Interleukin-6	T-cell
	Interleukin-7 (possible)	T-cell
B-lymphocytic activation and expansion	Interleukin-1	Macrophage
	Interleukin-2	T-cell
	Interleukin-4	T-cell, mast cells
	Interleukin-5	T-cell, mast cells
	Interleukin-6	T-cell
	Interleukin-7	Thymic epithelium
	Interferon-γ	T-cell
Hematopoietic precursor cells	Granulocyte-macrophage colony-stimulating factor	T-cell, mast cells
	Interleukin-3	T-cell, mast cells
	Interleukin-4	T-cell, mast cells
	Interleukin-5	T-cell, mast cells

Source: Schrader 1991[11]

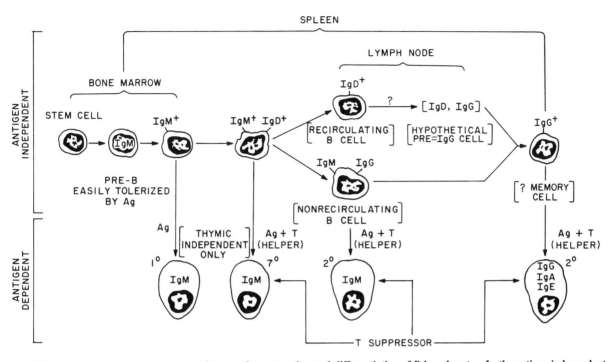

FIGURE 11.2.   A summary of current views on the maturation and differentiation of B lymphocytes. In the antigen-independent phase, B cells arising in the marrow initially express cytoplasmic IgM; the next stages in differentiation are represented by the appearance of B cells expressing surface IgM and then IgD. As maturation proceeds, the surface IgD may be lost as B cells switch from the expression of surface IgM to other immunoglobulin classes through unknown mechanisms. When stimulated by antigen (*Ag*) and appropriate helper cell interactions, the progeny of these cells bear surface immunoglobulin of the final clone selected for expression and mature into antibody-secreting plasma cells. *Source:* Anderson and Anderson 1984[2]

laboratory models, this tolerance is produced readily when the maturing B cells express only IgM, but it is more difficult to achieve after the IgD marker is expressed.[14] The reasons for this difference are not clear. Furthermore, while suppressor T cells with specificity directed against the challenging immunoglobulin can be formed in laboratory animals, it is unknown how anti-immunoglobulin injections could induce the formation of this suppressor population; this phenomenon has been cited widely as a mechanism for B-cell tolerance of self-antigens, which may be relevant to human disease.

THE STRUCTURE AND FUNCTIONS OF ORGANIZED PERIPHERAL LYMPHATIC TISSUES

Contact with both specific antigen and accessory cells is required for the further development of B cells into antibody-secreting plasma cells and of postthymic T cells into effector and regulatory T cells. Although it is possible that lymphocytes may engage antigens, un-

dergo cellular collaboration, and initiate immune responses virtually anywhere in the body, compelling arguments exist that the complex reticular meshwork, antigen-trapping capabilities, and the lymphatic and vascular connections of organized lymphatic tissue provide an efficient locus for immune reactions.

The lymphatic tissues in humans can be grouped into two major types: central and peripheral. The central lymphoid organs consist of the bone marrow and thymus, where stem cells give rise to proliferating and differentiating T and B lymphocytes through processes that are completely independent of antigenic stimulation. The peripheral lymphatic tissues include the lymph nodes, spleen, and lymphoid nodules dispersed beneath the mucous membranes of the respiratory, intestinal, and urogenital systems; lymphocytes preferentially accumulate within these tissues, where they undergo antigen-driven proliferation and maturation to produce the cells and secretory products for immune reactions. Variations in both the structure and location of these organized lymphoid tissues appear to represent specific adaptations that facilitate the host's mobilization of immune responses to pathogens invading distant tissue sites, the bloodstream, and mucous membranes.

The Recirculation of Lymphocytes

Although genetic diversity in both the T- and B-cell populations permits humans to respond to many different antigens, the development of a specific immune response requires the reacting lymphocytes to engage and bind the appropriate antigen with their surface receptors, and studies of nonimmune animals have shown that only a tiny minority of lymphocytes within a single lymph node are capable of reacting with a given antigenic determinant.[13] If these cells were static or their movements random throughout the body, then the likelihood of chance interactions between the reactive lymphocytes and the appropriate antigen would be very remote; however, this clearly is not the case in humans, where immunocompetent T and B cells continually recirculate between the blood and lymphatic tissues (Fig. 11.3). Long-lived lymphocytes that move through the blood show a unique "homing instinct" for lymph nodes and selectively attach to the luminal surfaces of high endothelial venules in the outer cortex.[15] These cells then emigrate across the venular wall by moving between the adjacent endothelial cells and enter the reticular meshwork; after variable periods of residence within the cortex, these lymphocytes then move back into the sinuses and exit by way of efferent lymphatics, passing through the thoracic duct and returning to the bloodstream. Then, they recirculate through other nodes in an identical fashion. Because the immunocompetent lymphocytes continually move through the antigen-binding meshworks of the lymph nodes, they provide a constant form of surveillance, and this probably enables a small depot of antigen to select a large number of antigen-sensitive cells from the body lymphocyte pool.

If an individual lymphocyte encounters an appropriate antigenic stimulus within the node, it can bind the antigen, interact with the other cell types, and give rise to a clonal burst of proliferating and mature lymphocytes that mediate immune responses. Many of these immature cells leave the stimulated node and disseminate to distant nodes, the spleen, and other tissues, where they can mature into specific effector and memory cells, thus providing systemic immunity to the inciting agent. A few of the B cells activated in this response also move into the medullary cords, where they mature into antibody-secreting plasma cells.

Both T and B lymphocytes emigrate from the same segments of high endothelial venules, but they are sorted by unknown mechanisms within the nodal parenchyma. The T lymphocytes establish residence in the deep cortex for relatively short intervals before moving out into the efferent sinuses. B cells emigrate to the superficial cortex and probably remain there for longer periods before exiting by way of the sinusoidal pathways. This migration pattern appears to permit both the T and B cells to interact with antigen-binding macrophages and to engage in cellular collaboration before segregating into their respective zones within the nodal cortex.

Other factors also influence the traffic patterns of lymphocytes in the body. The ability of T-cell subpopulations to recirculate appears to depend on their state of maturation (e.g., at least some effector T cells leave the circulation at random to enter sites of inflammation), and B lymphocytes display similar variations in their patterns of migration. The immature B cells appearing

---

FIGURE 11.3. Lymphocyte migration pathways in the body. Stem cells within the marrow differentiate into precursors of the T- and B-lymphocyte lines. This is followed by antigen-independent proliferation and differentiation within the marrow, generating mature B cells that emigrate from the narrow sinuses. Other stem cells form T-cell precursors that populate the thymus and differentiate into functional T cells. Mature lymphocytes of both classes are released continually into the bloodstream and circulate throughout the body, but they show little capacity to reaccumulate within the marrow and thymus. Small numbers of these cells emigrate from the blood into peripheral tissues, then pass into regional lymph nodes by way of afferent lymphatics. The majority of the long-lived T and B lymphocytes continually recirculate between blood and lymph by preferentially entering organized lymphatic tissue; some lymphocytes leave the blood and enter lymph nodes by selectively emigrating across the walls of specialized high endothelial venules. If these cells do not encounter an appropriate antigenic stimulus, they exit by way of efferent lymphatics and return by way of the thoracic duct to the blood where they continually repeat this mode of transit through other lymph nodes. Other recirculating lymphocytes are delivered directly into splenic sinusoids by arterial blood flow, and these cells move across the macrophage-rich marginal zone to enter the splenic white pulp, where they reside for varying periods before either re-entering the blood by moving back into the red pulp through "bridging zones" or exiting by way of splenic lymphatics. Many of the B and T lymphocytes produced during antigen-induced proliferation exhibit similar patterns of hematogenous dissemination into distant lymphoid organs, while other effector cells preferentially accumulate in sites of tissue inflammation. *Source:* Anderson and Anderson 1984[2]

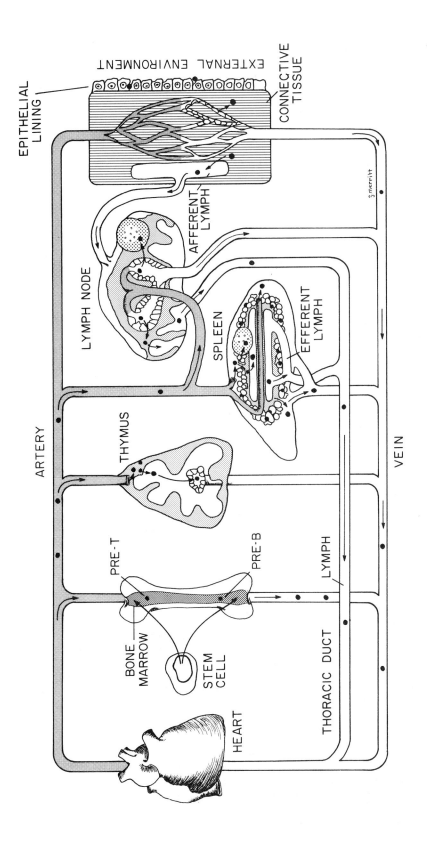

EPITHELIAL LINING

EXTERNAL ENVIRONMENT

CONNECTIVE TISSUE

AFFERENT LYMPH

LYMPH NODE

EFFERENT LYMPH

SPLEEN

THYMUS

ARTERY

PRE-T

PRE-B

VEIN

BONE MARROW

STEM CELL

LYMPH

THORACIC DUCT

HEART

j merritt

shortly after antigenic challenge may leave the node, but they frequently tend to lodge in the spleen and do not recirculate through the thoracic duct. Memory B cells that arise at the late stages after stimulation, however, do recirculate in the typical manner between the blood and lymph. Also, the B-cell precursors of IgA secretion possess distinct and quite different migration pathways in the mucosal immune system.

In nonstimulated animals, lymphocyte recirculation is characterized by a balanced flux of cellular traffic across the afferent and efferent terminals of lymphatic tissues, but this kinetic equilibrium is distorted rapidly in the regional nodes, which are draining sites of inflammation, infection, or antigenic challenge. The regional nodes show acute inflammatory changes, mast cell degranulation, edema, and increased blood flow within hours after such stimuli. There is also a rapid increase in lymphocyte accumulation unassociated with cellular replication within the node. Such nodal enlargement probably reflects the combined result of both increased lymphocyte traffic into the node and decreased cellular egress; these early changes are believed to be produced in part by secretory factors and lysosomal enzymes (released by macrophage activation) that alter lymphocyte surface adhesiveness and transit times within the node.[16] As this early sequestration of recirculating lymphocytes within the stimulated node clears, blast cell transformation and mitotic activity appear in the T- and B-cell zones of the cortex, reflecting the antigen-dependent clonal bursts of cellular proliferation. Because of such events, simple antigenic challenge can enlarge the regional node by four to six times its resting size, and a stimulated gland may require more than a month to return to its normal size.

The General Characteristics of Lymphocytes

When examined by standard microscopic techniques, the various subpopulations of T and B lymphocytes that occupy the peripheral lymphoid tissue and circulate in the blood and lymph possess remarkably similar size and morphologic characteristics.[3] The population of small lymphocytes that predominate in both peripheral blood smears and thoracic duct lymph obtained from normal individuals includes immunocompetent cells of both classes in interphase (G_0 or resting stage in the cell cycle). Their small size and lack of specialized cytoplasmic organelles may facilitate the recirculation of these cells between the bloodstream and lymphatic system; however, convincing evidence exists that other small lymphocytes represent differentiated T cells with both effector and regulatory functions. Similarly, most of the

large lymphocytes (those with more abundant cytoplasm and vesicular nuclei) that are found within the blood and lymph are the progeny of antigen-stimulated lymphoblasts of T- and B-cell lineage. They are intermediate stages of differentiation, but there also is evidence that some cells displaying this morphology are effector T cells that preferentially "home in" on sites of inflammation.

Small Lymphocytes

When examined by light microscopy, lymphocytes are oval cells, ranging from 5 to 12 μm in diameter, that exhibit an indented nucleus with dense chromatin and a scant rim of cytoplasm that stains pale blue with the Romanovsky stain. Their cytoplasm contains a few azurophilic granules and occasional vacuoles, and with histochemical staining, this cytoplasm also displays ribonucleoproteins, mitochondrial enzymatic activities, and some lysosomal hydrolase activity that, however, is less intense than that found in other leukocytes.

When scanning electron microscopy in used, circulating lymphocytes usually display numerous microvillus projections (mean length, 500 μm) but can exhibit a relatively smooth surface with a few ridge-like membrane ruffles (Fig. 11.4). These surface differences appear to reflect variations in the functional states of individual cells as well as changes introduced during processing or exposure to drugs such as vincristine and colchicine. Cell-to-cell contact, such as that employed in the formation of rosettes, can induce a lengthening and redistribution of the microvilli; therefore, the presence or absence of surface microvilli cannot be used to discriminate between T and B cells.

When studied by transmission electron microscopy, small lymphocytes typically display a dense, heterochromatic nucleus that contains some euchromatin. The nucleus is surrounded by a membrane possessing several nuclear pores, and the cytoplasm contains both free and clustered ribosomes and scant endoplasmic reticulum. A few lysosomes and vesicles are present and are usually most numerous in the Golgi complex. In addition, from two to six typical mitochondria may be seen in each thin section.

The organization of the lymphocyte cytoskeleton is still uncertain, but microtubules frequently are seen radiating from the centriolar region into the peripheral cytoplasm, where they follow a course parallel or tangential to the membrane. Direct linkage between the microtubules and the 5-μm thin filaments that form a continuous mat beneath the plasmalemma has not been

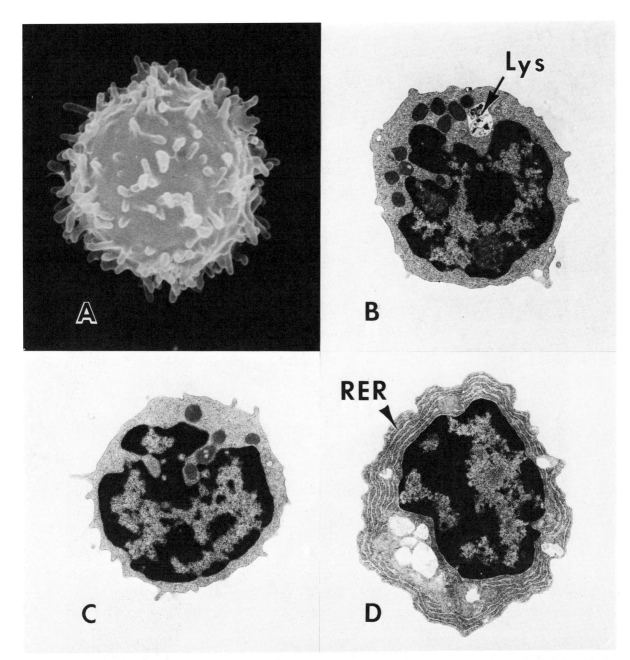

FIGURE 11.4. Thoracic duct lymphocytes. Scanning electron microscopy of both T and B lymphocytes may reveal microvilli (*A*) if the cells are collected from thoracic duct lymph and fixed at physiologic temperatures. T lymphocytes (*B*) and B lymphocytes (*C*) are virtually identical morphologically; however, when lymphocytes are separated by physical methods based on the affinity of specialized surface receptors on T or B cells, subtle differences in ultrastructure may be seen. Small T cells (*B*) have slightly more ribosomes in their cytoplasm than B cells, and T cells frequently contain two to three phagolysosomes at the centriolar end of the cells. Plasmacytoid lymphocytes (*D*) are found in small numbers in efferent lymph from normal animals. Following immunologic stimulation, the frequency of these preplasma cells may increase dramatically (× **10,000**). *Note:* Lys = lysosome; RER = rough endoplasmic reticulum. *Source:* Anderson and Anderson 1984[2]

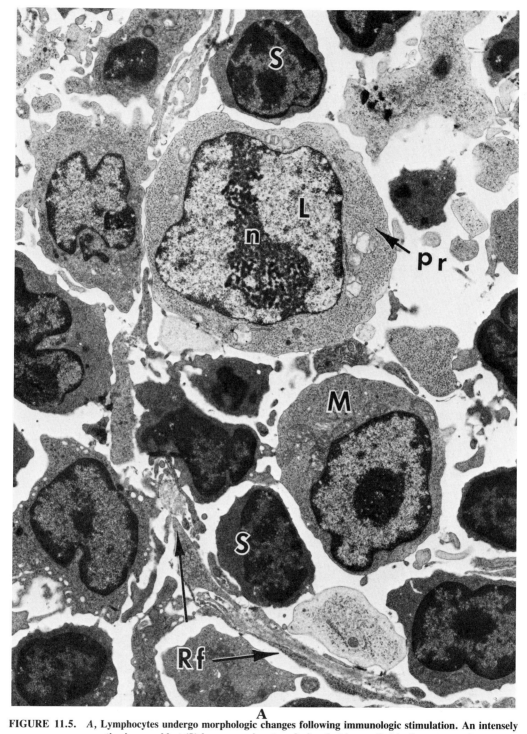

FIGURE 11.5. *A*, Lymphocytes undergo morphologic changes following immunologic stimulation. An intensely reactive immunoblast (*L*) has a prominent nucleolus that is uncoiled in the pattern of a nucleonema (*n*) in this electron micrograph. These cells are known to secrete lymphokines and other factors into the microenvironment, represented ultrastructurally by the presence of large numbers of polyribosomes (*Pr*) in the cytoplasm. An intermediate lymphocyte (*M*) has a

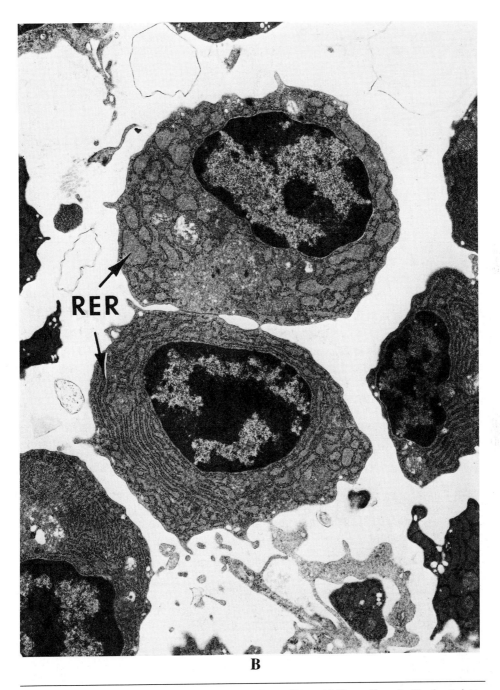

RER

B

prominent nucleolus and many free ribosomes, and these cells are highly motile and will migrate into other lymphatic tissues and sites of inflammation before continuing proliferation with differentiation into specific effector cells. A small lymphocyte (*S*) is the steady-state form of the cell, which is the precursor to *L* or may be the product of *M* when *M* is a T lymphocyte. *Note:* Rf = reticular fiber, which forms the microenvironment in which these lymphocytes were found. *B*, Intermediate lymphocytes derived from B-cell precursors divide and differentiate into plasma cells identified readily by their rough endoplasmic reticulum (*RER*) containing antibody for secretion. *Source:* Anderson and Anderson 1984[2] demonstrated. These filaments protrude into microvilli, and they form a central core of longitudinally oriented fibers.

Lymphoblasts

When stimulated by appropriate antigens or mitogens, small lymphocytes undergo a series of metabolic changes that are preparatory for division. They form large blast cells that rarely appear in normal blood and lymph, and ranging in diameter from 10 to 30 μm, these cells contain a large, vesicular nucleus and abundant basophilic cytoplasm that are recognized easily by light microscopy. With histochemistry, this cytoplasm shows heavy staining for ribonucleoprotein and increased acid hydrolase activities. Lymphoblasts also possess surface insulin receptors, protease and glycosyl transferase activities, and the capability of secreting plasminogen-activating factors as well as peptide regulatory factors (lymphokines) (Table 11.2), which are not seen in resting small lymphocytes.

When studied by transmission electron microscopy (Fig. 11.5A), lymphoblasts may exhibit the same microvillus projections seen in small lymphocytes, but the microvilli of lymphoblasts tend to decrease with time after stimulation. Other ultrastructural characteristics of the blast cell include a prominent nucleolus and loose euchromatin within the nucleus as well as an increase in cytoplasmic mass and organelles with numerous polyribosomes and a well-developed Golgi complex.

Transitional Atypical Lymphocytes

A small number of cells with size and morphologic characteristics between those of small lymphocytes and lymphoblasts are present in the blood and thoracic duct lymph of normal individuals, and because antigenic challenge and some infections can increase greatly their number, these cells are thought to be the progeny of proliferating blast cells, which are in varying stages of maturation as they pass through the blood. All of these cells display a prominent cytoplasm with variable amounts of polyribosomes, endoplasmic reticulum, vesicles, and Golgi development; however, only those with a well-developed endoplasmic reticulum have been shown to possess surface immunoglobulin markers and to exhibit antibody synthesis consistent with their ultimate maturation into plasma cells. This heterogeneous cellular population commonly is classified as atypical lymphocytes in clinical laboratories.

Large Granular Lymphocytes

Large granular lymphocytes containing large azurophilic granules represent a functionally distinct subset of lymphocytes with cytotoxic effector function that is independent of prior sensitization to antigen. Within the large granular lymphocyte population in normal human peripheral blood are cells that can mediate antibody-dependent cellular cytotoxicity through binding antibodies that are specific for either target antigens on malignant cells or cells infected with intracellular pathogens to their cell surface. Natural killer cells also can recognize and lyse target malignant or infected cells through a mechanism that requires neither an antigen-specific receptor nor the presence of a compatible major histocompatibility antigen. The number and activity of cells capable of this nonspecific cytotoxicity can be boosted by exposure to lymphokines (e.g., interleukin [IL]-2) and are termed *lymphokine-activated killer cells*.

Plasma Cells

Plasma cells represent the end stage of B-cell differentiation. These cells rarely are found in samples of blood and lymph, but they are one of the dominant lymphocyte populations in the spleen and lymph nodes. When studied by light microscopy, these oval cells range between 8 and 20 μm in diameter and exhibit an eccentric nucleus with condensed chromatin. They possess an abundant basophilic cytoplasm, and eosinophilic inclusions, a few vacuoles, and a perinuclear clear zone may be seen. When studied by electron microscopy, these cells can be distinguished readily by an extensive development and dilation of the rough endoplasmic reticulum (Fig. 11.5B). Although mature plasma cells are important in the synthesis and secretion of antibodies, they lack the surface immunoglobulin markers, prominent microvilli, and motility characteristics seen in other B cells.

The Separation of Lymphocytes by Physical Properties

Small lymphocytes have a density, negative net surface charge, surface adherence properties, and size that all differ from those of erythrocytes, granulocytes, monocytes, and macrophages; these properties can be exploited in the isolation of lymphocytes from the other cell types in mixed populations.[17] Lymphocytes usually can be separated from other blood cells by density, either using gradients of Ficol-Hypaque or other density gradient mixtures. Usually, lymphocytes isolated from normal blood in this way also contain from 5% to 20% monocytes; these can be removed partially by allowing the monocytes to adhere to glass or plastic and then gently rinsing free the nonadherent lymphocytes. Separation of lymphocytes from monocytes also can be done, but with more difficulty, on the basis of size, by differential sedimentation or centrifugal elutriation. Many T lymphocytes also are larger, denser, and more negatively charged than comparable B lymphocytes, but the considerable overlap in these properties limits their usefulness in separating B and T lymphocytes. Some T lymphocytes also are less adherent to glass bead and nylon wool columns than B lymphocytes, and cell separation by this technique can yield significantly enriched populations of T cells. However, the precise mechanism responsible for these differences is not well defined, and there is selective retention of an adherent T-lymphocyte subpopulation ("sticky T cells") by column fractionation procedures. Separation of T from B lymphocytes generally is done best by methods that are based on the presence of specific membrane receptors.

The Metabolism of Lymphocytes

Lymphocytes exhibit the same pathways for carbohydrate, fatty acid, protein, and lipid metabolism that are found in other somatic cells; however, there are some special features of nucleic acid metabolism in lymphocytes. As noted previously, thymocytes have high levels of TdT, which is a unique DNA polymerase that catalyzes the addition of deoxynucleoside monophosphates to preformed, single-stranded DNA without the direction of a nucleic acid template.[18] It is both an intracellular protein and a very specific marker for immature lymphoid cells. Its function is unknown, but high levels of TdT in thymocytes suggests that it may play a role in the generation of cells with diverse antigenic specificities by somatic mutation. TdT also is present, but at very low levels, in normal bone marrow.

Adenosine deaminase and purine nucleoside phosphorylase differ from TdT in that they are enzymes normally present in all mammalian cells. Congenital deficiency of either enzyme, however, leads to severe combined (both cellular and humoral) immunodeficiency;[1] other organ systems are unaffected by these deficiencies. In adenosine deaminase deficiency, toxic levels of deoxyadenosine that accumulate may be particularly toxic to lymphoblasts. In purine nucleoside phosphorylase deficiency, deoxyguanosine appears to be the toxic metabolite that accumulates. Attempts to correct these disorders by enzyme replacement have not been as successful as replacement of the abnormal stem cells through bone marrow transplantation.

The Responses of Lymphocytes to Ionizing Radiation and Chemotherapeutic Agents

Radiation, drugs, and biologic agents are used commonly to alter lymphocyte subpopulations to control a variety of human diseases. In general, humoral immune responses are more susceptible to radiation than are cellular immune responses; this has been attributed to a greater radiosensitivity in the B-cell precursors of antibody formation. However, such populations become less radiosensitive after antigen or mitogen stimulation, so this approach is of little benefit in the suppression of disease manifestations that are mediated by established humoral immunity.

Corticosteroid therapy causes a marked decrease in the absolute number of circulating lymphocytes (both T and B cells) in humans, and the remaining peripheral blood lymphocytes show reduced responses to mitogenic stimulation in tissue culture assays. These changes appear to result from altered migratory properties of the recirculating lymphocytes, which causes them to be redistributed in body tissues and depleted from the blood and lymphoid organs.[19] Although corticosteroids can produce direct lympholytic effects in some laboratory animals, mature human lymphocytes probably are not lysed by the usual therapeutic dosages (5 to 60 mg prednisone or its equivalent) employed in the clinical setting. The massive corticosteroid therapy that is used in managing such conditions as acute renal allograft rejection may produce cytolytic effects, but this has not been proven definitely.

Plasma cells appear to be equally resistant, and corticosteroid therapy has little effect on the synthesis of immunoglobulin. High dosages of corticosteroids administered over several days can produce a 20% lowering in serum IgG, which probably results from an increased catabolism of these proteins. The manifestations of both cellular immunity and delayed hypersensitivity reactions are susceptible to modification by corticosteroid therapy, and this is largely due to the capacity of corticosteroids to suppress capillary permeability, monocyte chemotaxis, and macrophage functions.

A variety of other drugs with general antimetabolite and cytotoxic activities, such as chlorambucil, methotrexate, and the nitrogen mustards, induce lymphopenia and are quite useful in the treatment of lymphoid neoplasms. Surprisingly, some agents also appear to have preferential effects on different lymphocyte populations. For example, cyclophosphamide produces a striking cellular depletion in the B-cell areas of the spleen and lymph nodes, and azathioprine inhibits rosette-forming T cells.

THE PROLIFERATION, MATURATION, AND COOPERATION OF LYMPHOCYTES IN IMMUNE RESPONSES

At birth, humans are well supplied with diverse populations of lymphocytes that have arisen by antigen-independent cellular proliferation and differentiation during fetal development. The number of these cells slowly increases during early growth, then levels off at relatively constant levels that are maintained throughout adult life. The lifespan of individual lymphocytes ranges from 4 days for some effector cells to more than 10 years for long-lived memory cells, and throughout life, the peripheral lymphoid organs are seeded with recently formed cells from the marrow and thymus to replenish T and B lymphocytes lost by senescence and end-stage differentiation. In addition, there is a dramatic shift in lymphopoiesis from these sites to the peripheral lymphatic tissues, where T and B cells continually undergo clonal bursts of proliferation and maturation in response to environmental antigens, and these antigen-driven responses are regulated by the remarkable series of genetic, cellular, biochemical, and humoral mechanisms that determine the type, intensity, and duration of each immune reaction.

The Response of Lymphocytes to Nonspecific Mitogens

Long-lived small lymphocytes as well as the cells of chronic lymphatic leukemia typically display low rates of respiration, absence of DNA synthesis, and minimal turnover of proteins, RNA, and lipids. Because these cells rarely divide under standard tissue culture conditions, they once were considered end-stage cells, but studies have demonstrated that they undergo blast cell transformation and mitosis when exposed to phytohemagglutinin.[20] Because of this characteristic response, small lymphocytes are now categorized as resting cells in the G_0 or early G_1 stage of the cell cycle.

Because antigens can induce identical cellular changes in small lymphocytes, it generally is assumed that both specific and nonspecific stimuli use common mechanisms to initiate the transformation of blast cells. The nonspecific mitogens have been particularly useful in defining metabolic changes associated with transformation; they induce larger numbers of altered cells than do conventional antigens that stimulate limited clonal proliferation in lymphocyte cultures.

Most antigens and nonspecific mitogens are believed to initiate the transformation of lymphocytes by acting as ligands that cross-link surface receptors, causing an influx of calcium into the cell within 45 seconds after binding has occurred.[21] The calcium ions appear to act in association with the cyclic nucleotides, triggering a series of metabolic changes, such as increased synthesis of RNA, protein, and DNA; increased utilization of glucose with augmented pyruvate, lactate, and glycogen production; and the appearance of several lysosomal

enzymatic activities. Synthesis of DNA is maximal at 3 days in mitogen-stimulated cultures, and this usually is followed by mitosis. Therefore, the activation of lymphocytes can be quantitated by using morphologic criteria, mitotic indexes, or a measurement of the cellular incorporation of radiolabelled DNA precursors. Also, many of the malignant cells in the acute lymphatic leukemias display the same morphologic, histochemical, and metabolic features as normal, activated lymphocytes.

Normal lymphocytes possess membrane receptors for a variety of polypeptide hormones and neurotransmitters, and their cytoplasm contains cyclic nucleotide cyclases and phosphodiesterases. This suggests that the function of lymphocytes is subject to neuroendocrine regulation similar to that demonstrated in other somatic cells. Evidence exists that cyclic adenosine monophosphate serves as an inductive signal in the differentiation of T- and B-cell precursors into mature cells,[22] and it has been postulated that the cyclic nucleotides regulate the subsequent functions of the mature cells. This is because cyclic adenosine monophosphate has a negative influence on the transformation of blast cells, direct cell lysis mediated by cytotoxic T cells, antibody release by plasma cells, and lymphocyte locomotion, while cyclic guanosine monophosphate promotes each of these events.

Antigen-Driven Proliferation and Maturation of T Cells

T cells with effector functions, and some of those with regulatory functions, have their functions directed by specific membrane receptors for antigen. When T lymphocytes encounter an antigen that binds specifically to their surface receptors, they undergo blast transformation that yields a progeny of helper, suppressor, or effector cells. Most of the mature lymphocytes are short lived and die through senescence in a few days. They mediate their specific functional roles by direct cellular contacts or the shedding of membrane-antigen complexes as well as secretion of low-molecular-weight proteins, and in addition, each clonal burst of proliferation also generates a few long-lived memory cells of each functional class that continually recirculate through peripheral lymphatic tissues. These cells provide heightened responses of the appropriate type on rechallenge with the appropriate antigen.

The nature of the T-cell receptor for antigen recently has been elucidated. It is a complex of molecules that is distinct from immunoglobulin. The T-cell antigen receptor is a heterodimer of either α-β or γ-δ chains that are closely associated with a signal transduction complex (CD3) on the cell surface.[23] The cluster designation

(CD) antigen CD3 is a common T-cell antigen consisting of five peptide subunits, and cross-linking of the CD3 complex by anti-CD3 antibody is capable itself of triggering T-cell proliferation. A similar polyclonal activation of T cells also can be triggered by nonspecific mitogens such as phytohemagglutinin and concanavalin A that bind to cell-membrane glycoproteins.

In the cases of antigen and polyclonal mitogens, T-cell proliferation is not simply the result of a triggering by the cross-linking of membrane receptors; the cooperation of a macrophage and an activated T cell also is required for the production of a macrophage product (IL-1 or leukocyte-activating factor). This in turn stimulates production by some activated T cells of a lymphokine (IL-2 or T-cell growth factor).[24] All activated T cells express a receptor for IL-2 and respond to its presence by undergoing both proliferation and maturation into fully functional effector and regulatory cells. The proliferation of these cells usually is limited by the cessation of IL-2 production, and this leads to the halting of proliferation as well as the disappearance of IL-2 receptors from the cell surface. It the production of IL-2 persists, however, or if exogenous IL-2 is added in tissue culture, then the receptor remains expressed and additional cycles of proliferation continue. Additional bioregulatory controls influence T-cell immune responses as well, and these probably involve networks of T-helper and T-suppressor cells similar to those operative for B cells.[25]

Drugs that Bind to Immunophilins

The transduction through the cytoplasm of the signal triggered by antigen binding to the T-cell receptor is not well understood, but it results in the activation of specific nuclear transcription factors. Two potent immunosuppressant drugs, cyclosporine and FK 506, are able to inhibit the transcription of early T-cell activation genes,[26] and both drugs block IL-2 secretion and expression of the IL-2 receptor on T cells, which inhibits the generation of cytotoxic T lymphocytes and thus blocks graft rejection.[27–29] Both drugs also bind with high affinity to separate cytoplasmic receptors (immunophilins) with enzymatic activity as prolyl peptidyl isomerases, and the relation of immunosuppressant action to the ability of these drugs to block the protein-folding activity of the enzyme is under active investigation.

Antigen-Driven Proliferation and Maturation of B Cells

Humoral immune responses begin when individual B lymphocytes encounter an antigen that binds to their specific immunoglobulin surface receptors. After receiving an appropriate "second signal," provided by the interaction with helper cells, these antigen-binding cells then undergo blast cell transformation and proliferation to generate a clonal progeny of mature plasma cells, which secrete specific antibody, and a few long-lived "memory cells" that possess the same capacity for antigenic recognition and cellular proliferation as the original parent cell. During this primary response, the immunoglobulin isotype synthesized by these self-replicating cells switches from IgM to either IgG, IgE, or IgA through mechanisms that are heavily dependent on interactions with T lymphocytes and macrophages. The generation of memory cells that bear the new surface immunoglobulin isotype generally is believed to account for the rapid and heightened production of non-IgM antibodies when the same antigen rechallenges the host (secondary or anamnestic immune response).

All levels of the humoral immune response, extending from antigen recognition, antigen processing, cellular cooperation, and cellular maturation to both antibody synthesis and secretion, are subject to precise genetic controls, and convincing evidence exists that the surface receptor for antigen on B lymphocytes is membrane-bound immunoglobulin possessing the same variable region combining sites as the antibodies secreted by this cell and its progeny. In the absence of structural genes coding for specific amino acid sequences in this variable region, B cells are unable to bind or synthesize antibodies against foreign determinants.

The mechanism by which antigen binding to these specific surface immunoglobulins initiates humoral immune responses is uncertain; however, polymeric antigens consisting of identical repeating units (e.g., bacterial lipopolysaccharide, dextran, pneumococcal polysaccharide) are known to bind to most B-cell surfaces and also evoke polyclonal DNA synthesis and immunoglobulin secretion without helper effects provided by other cells. Many of these thymus-independent antigens appear to function as nonspecific mitogens, but some may act as polyvalent determinants that aggregate specific immunoglobulin surface receptors and directly trigger IgM antibody responses. Indeed, direct antigenic stimulation of B cells has been offered as an explanation for the persistence of at least some IgM-antibody production by both athymic mice and humans.[17]

With most antigens, simple binding of the foreign determinant to the surface immunoglobulin receptor fails to result in B-cell stimulation unless T cells and macrophages provide helper effects. A variety of mechanisms have been proposed to explain the complex cellular interactions that trigger proliferation of antigen-binding B cells into a clone of mature plasma cells secreting antibodies of a different immunoglobulin class. Of particular interest are studies concerning both inbred animals and humans that indicate the ability of any given individual to mount effective immune responses against low dosages of some naturally occurring antigens is determined by genes encoded within the immune response region of the major histocompatibility locus.[30]

These gene products are expressed as nonimmunoglobulin macromolecules on the surfaces of T cells, B cells, and macrophages. These macromolecules regulate the cooperative interactions required to induce specific antibody formation, and according to current concepts, antigen-induced proliferation of T lymphocytes expressing the Lyl$^+$ phenotype (CD4 or T4$^+$ in humans), which mature into specific helper cells promote cellular collaboration. Such T cells are believed to bind antigen to their surfaces through specific receptors that are situated near the membrane components encoded for by the major histocompatibility complex; when the helper T cells interact with the surfaces of the appropriate B cells, it is postulated that the complex formed by the antigen-receptor immune response gene product must form an aggregate or focus to trigger clonal proliferation. These complexes also may be shed by the helper cells into the surrounding microenvironment, where they can either stimulate B cells directly or absorb onto macrophage surfaces to promote helper effects when these cells interact with B lymphocytes.

In addition, a number of nonspecific factors isolated from supernatants of mixed lymphocyte and mitogen-stimulated lymphocyte cultures have been reported to stimulate both polyclonal DNA synthesis and immunoglobulin secretion by B cells.[31] Such factors have been reported to act on T cells, B cells, and macrophages in different assay procedures (Table 11.2), and the biologic significance and clinical usefulness of such agents are under continued investigation.

Bioregulatory Control

The clonal burst of cellular proliferation and maturation that is produced by activated B cells is subject to a variety of bioregulatory control mechanisms. Although not supported by convincing proof, it has been suggested that genetic factors predetermine the total number of cellular divisions that any B cell can undergo, and end-stage maturation of B cells into plasma cells that are both heavily committed to immunoglobulin synthesis and incapable of any further division certainly plays a major role in limiting burst size as well. Nonspecific degradation and immune elimination of the stimulating antigen also may contribute to limiting immune responses, and because nascent antibodies possess a unique molecular structure in their variable region, it has been suggested that these may be recognized as foreign proteins and the immune response terminated by production of anti-antibodies.[32–34]

More recent studies indicate that both T lymphocytes and macrophages produce suppressor effects that are important in regulating the immune responses.[33] Specific suppression results from the antigen-driven proliferation and maturation of T lymphocytes exhibiting the Ly2$^+$3$^+$ phenotype (CD8 or T8$^+$ in humans), and these cells can inhibit humoral antibody responses to thymus-dependent antigens in a variety of in vitro and animal assay systems.[35] These T cells also release soluble substances that inhibit antibody formation, and such specific suppressor T cells have been shown to play an important role in blocking immune responses to single or multiple large doses of antigen (high-zone tolerance) and to interfere with the immunization produced by two closely related antigens (antigenic competition).[35] Several reports have shown that lymphocytes from both animals and patients with tumors can inhibit the generation of specifically cytotoxic lymphocytes directed against the tumor;[36] because this can lead to progressive tumor growth in immunized animals, it is widely held that specific T-cell suppressor effects may be an important contributor to the escape of human malignancies from immunologic control.[37] However, despite the obvious implications for therapy, this concept has not been firmly established as applicable in humans.

A wide variety of nonspecific immunosuppressors have been observed in other settings as well, and the best known clinical example of immunosuppression is the destruction of lymphoid cells by antimetabolites and alkylating agents. However, observations that both T-cells stimulated by concanavalin A and allogeneic histocompatibility antigens generate suppressor cells that interfere with the proliferation and differentiation of T and B effector cells are of greater biologic interest.[38] These suppressors appear to work by interacting with nonspecific helper factors, and this competitive inhibition can be overcome by adding more helper cells to the test system. Supernatants from mitogen-stimulated cultures also may contain a soluble factor (soluble immune response inhibitor) that absorbs onto macrophages and causes these cells to release a secondary product that inhibits B-cell responses. The biologic relevance of this factor as well as a variety of suppressor-macrophage effects that are produced by immunization with agents such as complete Freund adjuvant, bacille Calmette-Guérin organisms, *Corynebacterium parvum,* and pyran copolymers is still unknown; however, it is interesting that many of the agents now being used in clinical trials to augment human resistance to tumors are known to generate macrophage-suppressor activity in animal systems.

TABLE 11.3. Human Diseases Associated with Documented Increased Suppressor Cell Effects

Disease	Type of Suppressor	Manifestation
Malignancy		
Benign thymoma	T cell	Hypogammaglobulinemia
Multiple myeloma	Monocyte	Suppressed polyclonal immunoglobulin syntheses
Hodgkin disease	Monocyte with increased prostaglandin E_2 synthesis	Decreased T-cell responses
Solid tumors	? T cell	Suppressed antitumor immunity
	? Macrophage	Suppression of all T-cell responses
Congenital Disease		
X-linked agammaglobulinemia	T cell	Suppression of all B-cell responses
Selective IgA deficiency	T cell	Suppression of all IgA responses
Chronic mucocutaneous candidiasis	T cell	Suppression of T-cell response to *Candida* antigens and suppression of all T-cell responses
Acquired Defects		
Common variable agammaglobulinemia	T cell	Suppression of all B-cell responses
	? Humoral factor	
Disseminated fungal infections	T cell	Skin anergy and suppression of all T-cell responses
Disseminated tuberculosis	T cell and monocyte	Suppression of T- and B-cell responses
Disseminated coccidiodomycosis	T cell and monocyte	Suppression of T- and B-cell responses
Leprosy	T cell and monocyte	Suppression of T- and B-cell responses
Graft-versus-host disease	T cell	Suppression of T-cell responses

Source: Anderson and Anderson 1984[2]

One should use caution when interpreting the plethora of clinical reports that claim to show increased suppressor cell activity in numerous human diseases (Table 11.3). Many of these reports are based solely on demonstrations with in vitro cultures stimulated by mitogens or on the mixed leukocyte reaction, that cells or sera from patients can inhibit the activation of normal human lymphocytes. A variety of nonspecific factors (e.g., drugs) can produce identical effects, and these factors must be excluded by careful controls and the use of assay systems that measure both maturation and effector cell functions. In addition, some cells simply may die or else increase intracellular thymidine pools during culture, thus producing an artifactual inhibition of DNA synthesis from added precursors. Similarly, the monocytes and macrophages within such cultures can release enzymes, such as arginase, that both deplete essential growth factors and inhibit mitogenesis.

Studies of common variable hypogammaglobulinemia provide the best current evidence supporting a role for suppressor cells in the pathogenesis of human disease. Waldman et al.[39] demonstrated that some of these patients have a normal complement of B lymphocytes, but their cells failed to differentiate into plasma cells secreting antibody. Because peripheral blood lymphocytes from such patients suppressed the immunoglobulin production of normal lymphocytes that were stimulated with pokeweed mitogen, Waldman et al. concluded that this immunodeficiency resulted from enhanced, nonantigen-specific T-suppressor–cell ef-

fects. Similarly, the peripheral blood of patients with Hodgkin disease contains glass-adherent cells that inhibit the mitogenic responses of normal lymphocytes to phytohemagglutinin,[40] and this suppression appears to correlate with the increased prostaglandin E_2 secretion by suppressor cells and can be reversed by the addition of indomethacin, which inhibits prostaglandin synthetase.[40]

THE IDENTIFICATION OF SUBPOPULATIONS OF HUMAN LYMPHOCYTES

Functional Tests for Identifying Subpopulations

A number of antigens and nonspecific mitogens are useful in assessing the functions of lymphocyte subpopulations in vitro. Several plant lectins are known to react with specific oligosaccharide groupings and bind to cells that display the appropriate sugars on their surfaces, and in some instances (but certainly not all), these surface interactions initiate cellular transformation that leads to mitosis. Studies of murine lymphocytes have shown that both T and B cells express the same number of concanavalin A binding sites on their surfaces, but only T cells undergo mitogenic responses after reacting with this lectin. Similar observations of human lymphocytes indicate that lectins such as concanavalin A and phytohemagglutinin preferentially stimulate T cells while pokeweed mitogen primarily is a B-cell mitogen.

Protein A isolated from *Staphylococcus aureus* cell walls has been reported to function as a selective mitogen for B cells, but more recent studies have questioned this.[41] Also, although bacterial lipopolysaccharide is a very effective B-cell mitogen in mice, it is considerably less effective in eliciting transformation in human B lymphocytes.

Soluble antigens also can be used to stimulate lymphocyte transformation in tissue culture using blood from sensitized individuals. Most of the cells responding are of T-cell origin, and because only small numbers of specifically reactive lymphocytes are contained in such samples, the culture interval usually must be extended from 5 to 7 days to measure these responses adequately.

Mixed lymphocyte cultures are widely used for assessing lymphocyte responses to foreign histocompatibility antigens in vitro. In standard one-way reactions, normal lymphocytes are transformed by exposure to allogeneic lymphocytes (either heavily irradiated or pretreated with mitomycin to prevent their division during culture), and most of the cells responding in this assay are T cells, which can differentiate into populations showing regulator and cytolytic functions under appropriate conditions. A small number of macrophages must be present to obtain optimal lymphocytic proliferation with this assay. Also, B cells appear to be the most potent stimulators of these reactions, because they express higher densities of antigenic determinants from the HLA-D locus.

Each of these in vitro assays is believed to measure the functional ability of lymphocytes to proliferate following antigenic challenge, but lymphocytes can be suppressed by a wide variety of nonspecific factors in human serum (e.g., serum proteins, hormones, drugs, and antibodies). When care is taken to exclude such nonspecific effects, the assessment of both T- and B-cell activation can be a reliable diagnostic test, and if combined with surface marker techniques as well as tests that measure effector mechanisms such as lymphokine and antibody production, then the physiology of normal and disordered immune response in humans can be defined.

Antigens, Receptors, and Enzymes as Markers of Differentiation

Each cell at a different stage of differentiation or in a different lineage has its own unique repertoire of functions, tissue localization, migration patterns, cellular interactions, and regulatory factors that modulate its behavior. Ultimately, these properties are determined by which parts of the genome are active and which are unavailable for transcription. This unique functional state often can be recognized by morphologic features that are visible in polychrome stains by light microscopy; however, cells that are both functionally and developmentally distinct may be morphologically indistinguishable. The detection of a unique ensemble of biologic markers on the cell membrane may be the only practical means to identify these cells.

In the peripheral blood, resting T and B lymphocytes are morphologically identical even under the electron microscope. They can be distinguished easily, however, by detection of the unique antigens and receptors on their surface membranes;[17,42,43] for example, the peripheral blood B lymphocyte both synthesizes and displays immunoglobulin molecules on its surface that function as its antigen receptor. Morphologic features also may be an imprecise guide to a cell's state of differentiation. An antigen-triggered lymphocyte in the peripheral blood may share many "immature" morphologic features (large size, basophilic cytoplasm, open chromatin) with a lymphoblast in the marrow that is at a much earlier stage in normal lymphocyte differentiation. However, despite morphologic similarities, a peripheral blood B lymphocyte is distinct from its precursor in the marrow, because the peripheral blood B lymphocyte has immunoglobulin localized at the surface membrane. The B lymphoblast also may have immunoglobulin present, but it is localized to the cytoplasm and may be only an IgM heavy chain without a kappa (κ) or lambda (λ) light chain being present.

Thus, a cell is identified not only by the presence of a single marker but also by that marker's density, subcellular localization, and simultaneous expression with other markers. It is the combination of these features that describes the complete "immunologic phenotype" of a given cell type, and it is remarkable how many features of the normal phenotype also may be shared by both a malignant cell and the normal precursor from which it apparently arose. This forms the basis for the use of markers in diagnosing benign and malignant lymphoproliferative disorders.[42]

Many of the useful biologic markers of differentiation are antigens and receptors that can be detected at the cell surface.[17,43] This is partly due to technical factors that make it easier to detect cell surface macromolecules in intact cells; however, it also seems that some of the biologic functions that are specific to each stage of differentiation require that a cell express specific structures at the cell surface to perform those functions. It then is reasonable to expect that a cell surface adaptation is required to provide a specific receptor for binding to a soluble regulatory substance in the milieu or to recognize a cellular microenvironment to "home in" on or target antigen to attack. Certainly, the acquisition of new functions also requires the expression of new intracellular molecules and structures. However, an

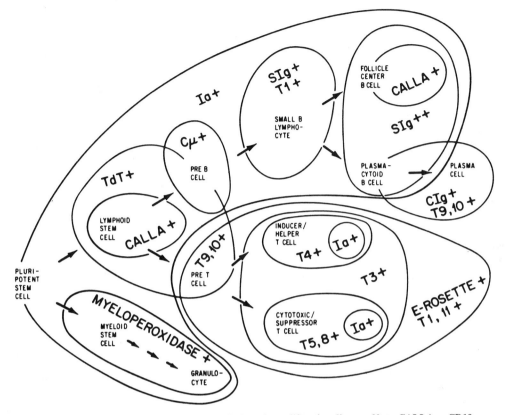

FIGURE 11.6. Lymphocyte surface markers in lymphoproliferative disease. *Note:* CALLA = CD10,
common acute lymphoblastic leukemia antigen; CIg = cytoplasmic immunoglobulin;
Cμ = cytoplasmic IgM heavy chain; SIg = surface immunoglobulin; TdT = terminal
deoxynucleotidyl transferase; Tn = monoclonal antiserum (T1 = CD5, T4 = CD8,
T8 = CD8, T9 = transferrin receptor CD71, T10 = CD38, T11 = CD2). *Source:*
Aisenberg 1983[42]

intracellular molecule, such as an enzyme, may be more
difficult technically to detect; moreover, intracellular
changes often are quantitative and not the new expression of a unique structure. Nevertheless, markers such
as cytoplasmic immunoglobulin and TdT can be extremely valuable in the study of acute lymphoblastic
leukemia. The most valuable biologic markers in the
study of normal human lymphocytes, leukemias, and
lymphomas have been cell surface or cytoplasmic immunoglobulin, cell surface receptors for macromolecules, and cellular antigens detected by monoclonal
antibodies.

Surface and Cytoplasmic Immunoglobulin

In many ways, the detection of the cellular expression
of immunoglobulin is a prototype for a biological
marker of differentiation (Fig. 11.6),[43,44] and with the
possible exception of hemoglobin, immunoglobulin is

the human protein having the best-understood structure,
function, cell biology, and genetics. The ability to
produce immunoglobulin, or antibody, is limited to one
cell lineage, the B lymphocyte. From the earliest commitment to B-cell differentiation, changes occur in the
genome that involve the synthesis of immunoglobulin.
The genes for human immunoglobulin heavy chain are
coded on chromosome 14, but the segments coding for
the constant and variable portions of the molecule are
physically separated on that chromosome. Before tran-
scribing the messenger RNA that will code for the mu
(μ) heavy chain of the IgM immunoglobulin molecule, a
pre-B cell first rearranges these sequences in the genome, thus bringing them into proximity (VJD rearrangement). Molecular probes of complementary DNA
can detect this rearrangement and, in effect, are the
earliest marker of B-cell differentiation. The application
of these techniques currently is restricted to the research
laboratory and will not be discussed further; in practice,

the earliest detectable evidence of B-cell differentiation occurs when these gene rearrangements lead to the synthesis of μ heavy chains of IgM in the cytoplasm (Fig. 11.6).[45]

Immunoglobulin molecules consist of subunits consisting of light and heavy polypeptide chain. The structure of the heavy chain identifies the immunoglobulin class as IgM, IgD, IgG, IgA, or IgE. There are only two classes of light chains, κ or λ; hybrid molecules with both light-chain types do not occur in nature.

Individual immunoglobulin molecules differ from one another in the amino acid sequence, especially over limited sequences (the "variable" and "hypervariable" regions of the light and heavy chain). This sequence variability gives unique binding characteristics to the antigen-binding segment (Fab fragment) of each antibody, and the antigen-combining site includes areas on both the light and heavy chain. The nonantigen-binding Fc fragment is common to other members of an immunoglobulin class, and cell receptors that bind immunoglobulin (Fc receptors) recognize this portion of the immunoglobulin molecule without respect to its antigen-binding specificity. This also is the region of the immunoglobulin molecule that activates and fixes serum complement components.

Unique immunoglobulin molecules are made by different clones of B lymphocytes, and the diversity of different antibodies that each individual makes is due to the generation of different cell clones during the early fetal development of the immune system. Each cell generated as well as all of its progeny are capable of producing antibodies with only one specificity (one cell, one antibody). Individual cells or clones of cells may change the class of heavy chain they produce, but they will maintain the same variable-region structure and antigen-binding specificity.

Individual clones of cells also continue to make only one light-chain type. During the process of generating antibody diversity, individual cells inactivate either the gene coding for κ light chain on chromosome 2 or the λ-coding gene on chromosome 22. The molecular mechanisms and adaptive advantage of this complex regulation are not known; nonetheless, this light chain inactivation remains stable in each B lymphocyte and its progeny. In virtually all reported cases of B-lymphocyte malignancies, only a single light-chain type is expressed, and in practice, the demonstration of only a single light-chain type in a lymphocyte population is presumptive evidence of a monoclonal proliferation of B lymphocytes. This is of great diagnostic value in cases of possible lymphoma or chronic lymphocytic leukemia, because it is possible to demonstrate such monotypic light-chain expression in most B-cell lymphomas and chronic leukemias. This is powerful evidence for the clonal origin of these malignancies, and it supports the more limited evidence available from both cytogenetic and glucose-6-phosphate dehydrogenase isoenzyme studies.

Because of the presence of surface immunoglobulin, B-cell leukemias and lymphomas also can be considered to be special cases in human malignancies in which a true "tumor-specific antigen" occurs. Of course, other normal B cells have surface immunoglobulins, but each B-cell clone makes only its own immunoglobulin with unique variable-region sequences. Because each B-cell leukemia or lymphoma is derived clonally from a single, normal B-cell progenitor, its surface immunoglobulin is unexpressed on other normal cells, and in a few cases, other antibodies have been produced that can distinguish these individual immunoglobulin molecule differences or "idiotypes." The use of "anti-idiotype" antibodies as tumor-specific immune therapy currently is under study, but striking improvement in at least one patient so treated has been reported.[46]

The Cellular Localization of Immunoglobulin

During B-lymphocyte development, immunoglobulin produced by the cell is present at different subcellular locations that are characteristic of each stage in maturation. As mentioned previously, the pre-B cell has immunoglobulin localized to the cytoplasm and may have only free-IgM heavy chain present; immunoglobulin is concentrated along smooth endoplasmic reticulum. Maturing B cells by definition are cells that begin to display immunoglobulin light and heavy chains on their surface. At the earliest stages, the heavy chain is μ of IgM, and the amount of cytoplasmic IgM either has begun to decrease or is undetectable. The immunoglobulin present is synthesized by the cell, contains either κ or λ light chain (but not both), is an integral part of the lymphocyte membrane, and is not merely absorbed passively on the surface. As differentiation proceeds, the concentration of surface immunoglobulin increases, and the heavy chain predominantly present changes usually from IgM (often with IgD) to IgA or IgG (Fig. 11.6). Only a few cells in the blood express IgE, and after antigen stimulation, B cells begin the transition to immunoglobulin-secreting plasma cells by decreasing their surface concentration of immunoglobulin and increasing its concentration in cytoplasm, especially along the rough endoplasmic reticulum where it is synthesized. This shift in immunoglobulin localization is synchronous with a morphologic change to a plasmacytoid lymphocyte with more abundant and basophilic cytoplasm. In the mature plasma cell, surface immunoglobulin is virtually absent, and there is a high concentration of cytoplasmic immunoglobulin destined for secretion.

Detecting Surface and Cytoplasmic Immunoglobulin and Other Antigens

The cellular expression of an antigen usually is detected using specific antibody and immunofluorescence techniques. Immunoglobulin molecules themselves can be recognized as antigens by other antibodies, so anti-immunoglobulin antibodies can be produced easily in other species. Such antibodies may be specific for all immunoglobulin molecules of one species or only a given light- or heavy-chain class, and these anti-immunoglobulin antibodies can be labelled and used as probes to detect antibody expressed on human cells (Fig. 11.7). Most conveniently, the antibody is labelled fluorescently with either fluorescein, phycoerythrin, or rhodamine dye; this "direct labelling procedure" usually provides a sufficiently bright "signal" that is seen easily under the fluorescence microscope or by the automated fluorescence-activated flow cytometer. Other labels, such as radioactive molecules, enzymes, or large particles that are visible under the light microscope, are used in special circumstances but are not as convenient for routine studies.

Cellular immunoglobulins also can be detected by an "indirect" technique. First, cells are treated with anti-immunoglobulin antibody that is unlabelled, and a second-step reagent is then used to detect the binding of the first antibody. This second-step reagent usually is a labelled anti-immunoglobulin antibody specific for the species of the first antibody but unreactive with human immunoglobulin. For example, one useful combination of reagents for detecting surface IgM might include goat-anti-human IgM (first antibody) and fluorescein-conjugated, rabbit-anti-goat immunoglobulin (second antibody).

The direct labelling procedure has the advantages of simplicity and uniformity of performance. There is less chance for nonspecific labelling than with the indirect technique, and high-quality, well-characterized reagents are available from a number of commercial sources. The sensitivity is sufficient to easily detect surface immunoglobulin in most cases. Thus, the direct method is the preferred technique for the detection of this antigen, and it also can be adopted conveniently for the detection of a number of other cellular antigens.

The indirect technique has several advantages that make it the preferred method in some cases, especially for the detection of some antigens other than surface immunoglobulin. Because several molecules of second

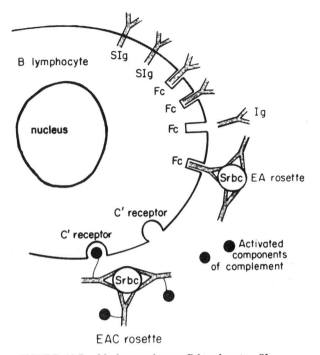

FIGURE 11.7. **Markers on human B lymphocytes.** *SIg* represents specific immunoglobulin molecules synthesized by a B cell, and Fc receptors bind the C-terminal portion of immunoglobulin molecules. This process can be visualized by tagging the Ig of the appropriate class (IgG) or subclass (IgG$_1$, IgG$_3$) with fluorescein. Alternatively, the Fc receptor may be identified by sensitizing the indicator cell (e.g., sheep red blood cells [*Srbc*] with antibodies of the appropriate subclass. Sensitized Srbc adherent to lymphocytes (or macrophages) are designated *EA rosettes*. C′ receptors are identified with antibody-sensitized Srbc incubated with complement (human or mouse), and the adherence of lymphocytes and macrophages to the indicator system are designated *EAC rosettes*. *Source:* **Rowlands and Danielle 1975**[43] **Reprinted by permission of the New England Journal of Medicine.**

antibody can bind to one molecule of first antibody bound to cell surface antigen, the opportunity exists to amplify the intensity of fluorescence, thus making it easier to detect antigens that are present in smaller numbers. Moreover, a single second antibody (e.g., a fluorescein-conjugated, goat-anti-mouse antibody) can be used with a variety of first antibodies from the same species, obviating fluorescein conjugation to each of the first antibodies. This is one reason why the indirect technique commonly is used when testing with a panel of mouse monoclonal antibodies.

Immunofluorescence Analysis and the Fluorescence-Activated Flow Cytometer

Immunofluorescence is the method most generally used for detecting antigens that are useful cell markers. Other labels, such as radioactivity, enzymes, or large particles, also can be useful in detecting certain cell markers, especially when cell surface receptors rather than antibody-defined antigens are sought, but immunofluorescence remains the most generally applicable method. Under the fluorescence microscope, fluorescein-labelled antibody bound to the cell surface is seen as a bright "apple-green" ring around the cell; phycoerythrin- or rhodamine-labelled cells are red. By placing a drop of cell suspension between the slide and coverslip, the percentage of cells staining with a fluorescent antibody can be counted conveniently. The fluorescence of many surface antigens is relatively faint, making it routinely necessary to reduce the background fluorescence by providing exciting illumination from above with an epifluorescence condenser; sensitivity is increased further by using high-quality optics, objectives, and filters. The operator switches between fluorescence and phase-contrast optics, recording the number of cells in each field that show detectable fluorescence, and the experienced technician also can discern a limited number of morphologic features under phase contrast, making it possible, for example, to count only the malignant cells in a complex cell mixture.

The fluorescence microscope has the advantages of convenience and relative economy; however, the number of cells or samples that can be counted is limited. Typically, 200 cells per sample are examined and can be scored only as negative or positive or, at most, brightly, moderately, or dimly positive. Both operator time and fatigue place a limit on the number of cells and samples that can be examined, and potentially valuable information concerning the density of antigens at the cell surface as well as smaller differences in the numbers of positive cells is lost.

The fluorescence-activated flow cytometer largely solves these problems.[47,48] It automatically counts large numbers of cells, sampling these statistically, and accurately measuring the distribution of both fluorescence intensity and antigen density on populations of cells. To a limited extent, it can make separate fluorescence measurements on different subpopulations of cells in complex mixtures by using light scatter to discern certain differences in cell morphology, and with the availability of new fluorescence dyes, it now is possible to make routine measurements of two different antigens

simultaneously without two separate light sources or complicated optical systems.

The heart of the flow cytometer is its optical system (Fig. 11.8). First, the optical system excites fluorescence of antibody-labelled cells by focusing a beam of monochromatic light, either from a laser or mercury arc-lamp source, on a passing stream of cells. Second, the fluorescence signal from a labelled antibody is detected by a photomultiplier ("fluorescence detector") tube that is placed at right angles to both the exciting beam and the stream of cells. Third, other light detectors simultaneously measure the passage of a cell within the beam by measuring the scatter of nonfluorescent light at narrow angles (0° to 10° "forward scatter") or a wide angle (90°). Narrow-angle scatter provides a measure of size, and wide-angle scatter measures granularity as well as other complex morphologic features.

The hydraulic system of the flow cytometer provides a steady stream of single cells that pass precisely between the beam of exciting light and the fluorescence and scatter detectors, and the analytic computer system records separately the measured values for each cell. Typically, each cell can have values recorded for the intensity of narrow-angle scatter, wide-angle scatter, and one or two colors of fluorescence. Flow cytometers often are referred to as "cell sorters" when they also are fitted with modules that allow individual cells to be physically separated (or sorted) on the basis of these physical properties.

Flow cytometry results usually are presented as frequency histograms; for example, the light scatter from cells isolated from normal peripheral blood by Ficoll-Hypaque can be shown as the number of cells with increasing values of narrow-angle light scatter (Fig. 11.9A). Because small or nonviable cells give a smaller light scatter, the peak at the far left of the histogram identifies platelets and dead cells. The largest cells in the preparation shown in Figure 11.9, monocytes, are in the peak at the far right. Narrow-angle scatter alone efficiently identifies the remaining cells in the center peak as lymphocytes, and even in more complex cell mixtures (such as whole blood in which red cells have been lysed), the combination of both narrow- and wide-angle light scatter displayed in a two-parameter histogram can be used to identify which cells are lymphocytes. The flow cytometer can be set to identify lymphocytes electronically and to measure only the fluorescence values from these cells (Fig. 11.9B); the percentage of fluorescence-positive cells in the "scatter-defined" lymphocytes is then calculated.

Clonal Excess

The potential analytic power of flow cytometry is demonstrated by using measurements of the surface

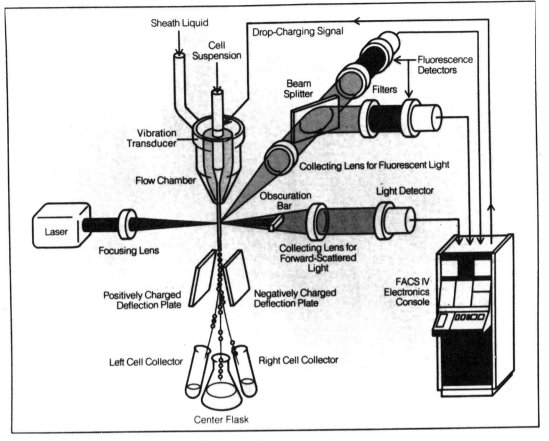

FIGURE 11.8. A fluorescence-activated flow cytometer.

immunoglobulin density to detect a "clonal excess" of malignant B lymphocytes in a mixture that may contain over 90% normal B lymphocytes.[49] An abnormal distribution of surface immunoglobulin densities is the key finding; if the malignant population has κ light chain in its surface immunoglobulin, then the normal shape of the surface immunoglobulin distribution curve still can be found in the λ light chain–bearing cells. However, these represent only the normal B-lymphocyte population, and in a normal population of B lymphocytes, the shapes of the frequency histograms for both κ and λ light-chain surface immunoglobulin distribution are congruent even though twice as many cells bearing κ as those bearing λ light chains are normally present. When malignant B lymphocytes bear an abnormally narrow distribution of κ-surface immunoglobulin, they distort the expected pattern of normal κ-positive cells, thus giving a skewed distribution as compared to the λ-positive cells.

The measurement of clonal excess has been demonstrated to have some clinical utility as well. Clonal excess has been shown to be present in the blood at the diagnosis of lymphoma, to disappear with treatment, and to reappear even before clinical relapse is evident; in some cases, clonal excess is detected even when lymphoma cells are not noted in the peripheral blood on conventionally stained smears. The general clinical utility of this test has not yet been confirmed by large, clinical trials, but such trials must be done before this procedure can be considered helpful in the diagnosis and follow-up examination of all patients with B-cell lymphoma.

Cell Surface Receptors for Macromolecules

Antibodies recognize a number of structures that are present on the cell surface, and some of these antigens have recognized functions. For example, cell surface immunoglobulin serves as the antigen receptor for B lymphocytes. Some structures, even though also detectable as antigens, were detected first by their ability to act as receptors and to bind other molecules in the environment. The nature of some of the ligands is known, as is

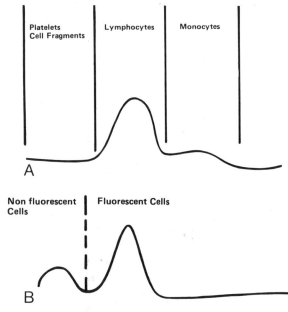

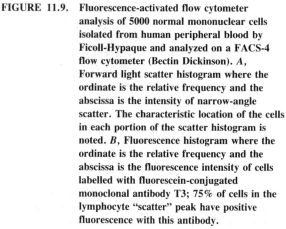

FIGURE 11.9.   Fluorescence-activated flow cytometer analysis of 5000 normal mononuclear cells isolated from human peripheral blood by Ficoll-Hypaque and analyzed on a FACS-4 flow cytometer (Bectin Dickinson). *A*, Forward light scatter histogram where the ordinate is the relative frequency and the abscissa is the intensity of narrow-angle scatter. The characteristic location of the cells in each portion of the scatter histogram is noted. *B*, Fluorescence histogram where the ordinate is the relative frequency and the abscissa is the fluorescence intensity of cells labelled with fluorescein-conjugated monoclonal antibody T3; 75% of cells in the lymphocyte "scatter" peak have positive fluorescence with this antibody.

the case with the receptors for the Fc fragment of immunoglobulin or the complement components, and some receptors are identified closely with certain lymphocyte functions and subpopulations but recognize structures whose function is not yet completely known.[17]

Sheep E-Rosette Receptors

Normal, mature human T lymphocytes have a receptor that binds normal sheep erythrocytes; however, the nature of the ligand, function of the receptor, and why it is specific for T lymphocytes still remain in question. (This receptor now is recognized with monoclonal antibodies as well.) At one time, it was clear to cellular

immunologists that most human peripheral blood lymphocytes without surface immunoglobulin (non-B cells) probably were functioning in a manner similar to the T lymphocytes found in mice; however, there were heterologous antisera in mice that recognized a common T-cell antigen, θ (now termed *Thy-1* and also present in mouse brain). No such antigen could be found in humans, and attempts to raise anti-T-cell sera were variously successful but usually were of low titer, had various cross-reactivities, or were not reproducible either within or between laboratories. Such reagents were unsuitable for the routine identification of T cells either in normal or abnormal samples.

A useful marker for human T cells became available once several laboratories observed that most non-B lymphocytes in normal blood bound red blood cells from sheep. Because cells with the receptor would bind added sheep red cells ("erythrocytes") in a ring about the cell, forming a "rosette," this is known as the *E-rosette assay*. Under carefully controlled conditions and using carefully standardized reagents, the E-rosette assay provides both a convenient and practical measure of T-lymphocyte numbers that can be done in any laboratory. Even malignant T lymphocytes such as those found in T-cell acute lymphoblastic leukemia can be recognized, but in many cases, the binding is less avid and fewer sheep red cells are bound. Attempts to increase the binding affinity by changing the assay conditions tend to decrease the specificity of the reaction; thus, as valuable as this assay has been for identifying T lymphocytes, the availability of specific T-cell antibodies may largely replace the E-rosette assay as a useful clinical test. Currently, the test still is valuable in identifying T cells when avid Fc receptor binding raises the possibility that an apparent antibody reaction may represent only nonspecific binding; the E-rosette assay is uninfluenced by the presence of Fc receptors.

Other Erythrocyte Receptors

Other species of erythrocytes also adhere to some subpopulations of human lymphocytes, and some lymphocytes will form E-rosettes with mouse, monkey, canine, and even autologous human red cells. The most useful of these has been the mouse E-rosettes. These are present on a small population of normal B lymphocytes, and they also are typically found on a high proportion of the B lymphocytes that occur in common B-cell chronic lymphocytic leukemia (CLL). As with sheep E-rosette receptors and T cells, the molecular basis of the binding and function of the receptor is unknown. Other markers also are available that are characteristic of common CLL and distinguish variant types of CLL, but it is not clear that demonstrating the presence of mouse E-rosettes provides any additional diagnostic or prognostic information.

Receptors for the Fc portion of the immunoglobulin molecule have been mentioned previously as a possible source of "nonspecific" binding of labelled antibodies (Fig. 11.7). Fc receptors are not lineage specific, and they occur on lymphocytes (both T and B cells), monocytes, and granulocytes. They are conveniently demonstrated using rosetting techniques, and sheep red cells (E) can be coated with anti-sheep red cell antibody (A). Cells with Fc receptors will form EA-rosettes with these antibody-coated cells under conditions where the uncoated erythrocytes will not. Usually, the binding is strong and the formation of EA-rosettes easily demonstrated after short incubation periods at room temperature. Simultaneous controls are performed with erythrocytes not coated with antibody to demonstrate that E-rosettes do not form under these conditions.

The demonstration of Fc receptors has not been of great use in the classification of leukemias and lymphomas, but there is one possible exception. Under the proper conditions, T cells can be shown to have rather low-affinity receptors for the Fc portion of either IgG or IgM, and functional studies of normal T cells have shown that cells with receptors for IgM (Fcμ) function as helper T cells during immunoglobulin synthesis by B cells. T cells with Fc receptors for IgG (Fcγ) function as suppressor cells. The assay is somewhat laborious, first requiring the isolation of E-rosetting T cells and then the demonstration of Fc receptors with either IgM- or IgG-coated red cells, but Fcγ receptors have been found on both normal natural killer cells (CD16) and the cells in some patients with T-cell variant of CLL, especially those variants characterized by neutropenia and recurrent infection. Cells from Sézary syndrome as well as the cutaneous T-cell lymphomas sometimes have Fcμ receptors, and these results agree with the independent determination of $T_{suppressor}$ and T_{helper} phenotype in these entities using monoclonal antibodies, which provide a more convenient and reliable method for this determination.

Cell surface receptors exist that can recognize the components of complement and their fragments when they are fixed to cells, tissues, or other surfaces, and at least three classes of complement receptors (CR1, CR2, and CR3) are recognized on the basis of their binding specificity for certain complement fragments (Table 11.4). CR1 receptors recognize C3b, C4b, and C5b fragments. They are found on B lymphocytes, monocytes, macrophages, and neutrophils; on normal erythrocytes, receptors with the same specificity are known as "immune adherence" receptors. CR2 receptors recognize C3d (and also the C3d portion in its immediate

precursor molecule, C3bi), and CR2 receptors are present on normal B lymphocytes. CR3 receptors recognize the C3bi molecule but not its C3d-containing portion and are present on neutrophils, monocytes, and macrophages.

Previously, these receptors were best detected by rosetting techniques. Sheep erythrocyte (E) and antibody (A) complexes are allowed to fix complement (C) under conditions where the lytic phase of the complement reaction is inactive. Cells with complement receptors will form "EAC-rosettes" with these antibody- and complement-coated erythrocytes under conditions where EA- or E-rosettes do not form. The different classes of complement receptors can be distinguished further by preparing stable cellular intermediates of the reactants in the complement system, but again, the procedures are laborious, require meticulous controls, and are ill-fitted to the routine study of clinical material.

Using rosetting techniques, measuring complement receptors has limited use; however, the study of complement receptors may become significantly easier if recently developed antibodies to complement receptors become generally available. A mouse monoclonal antibody to human CR1 has been reported, as well as heterologous antiserum to CR2. It is likely that three monoclonal antibodies to cluster determinant CD11b, (OKM-1, Mac-1, and Leu-15 widely used because of their reactivity with myeloid cells, monocytes, and macrophages) are specific for an antigen on CR3 (C3bi), and this provides a good example of the development of a monoclonal antibody on the basis of its specificity for a cell population with later discovery of the functional significance of the antigenic structure.

There are a host of other receptors for defined macromolecular structures on the surface of hematopoietic and lymphoid cells as well. Chemotactic cells (monocytes and granulocytes) bear receptors for chemotactic factors such as the formylated oligopeptides (e.g., F-*met-leu-phe*) that are common components on bacterial cell membranes.[50] Cell adhesion receptors that mediate cell homing to tissues may be recognized by monoclonal antibodies (e.g., CD57), and activated T cells express a

TABLE 11.4. **Complement Receptors**

Receptor Type	Components Bound	Cell Type
CR1	C3b	B lymphocyte
	C4b	Macrophage
	C5b	Neutrophil, human erythrocyte
CR2	C3d	B lymphocyte (CD21)
	C3bi (C3d part)	
CR3	C3bi (not C3d)	Macrophage (CD11b), neutrophil

receptor for the lymphokine IL-2 (also known as *T-cell growth factor*) which in turn is necessary for sustaining the proliferation of T cells.[24] This IL-2 receptor also is expressed on some T-cell leukemia–lymphomas that are highly associated with a human T-cell leukemia virus (HTLV-1); the receptor reportedly is recognized by a monoclonal antibody called *Tac* as well.[51] Epstein-Barr virus, the cause of common infectious mononucleosis, binds specifically to receptors on B cells, presumably explaining the specificity of this viral infection for these cells.[52] (In typical infectious mononucleosis, the B cells are virus infected, but the atypical lymphocytes in the peripheral blood that are characteristic of this disorder actually are the reactive, but not the virus-infected, T cells.)

Monoclonal Antibodies That Detect Cellular Antigens

Monoclonal antibodies are the first products of modern genetic engineering to find wide clinical applicability. They have made possible the routine use of cell surface markers as a diagnostic test,[53] and useful markers have been developed for acute leukemia. The recognition of not only T cells themselves but also functional subsets of T cells is now possible using a wide variety of commercially available antibodies. Because of the clinical applicability of these products, commercial interest has been keen, and industry now supplies a steady flow of new and potentially valuable monoclonal antibodies to the marketplace.

A monoclonal antibody consists of identical immunoglobulin protein molecules that are all produced by a single clone of cells. As mentioned in the discussion of normal differentiation, each B cell and its progeny are committed to producing one unique immunoglobulin molecule; the genetic material coding for this molecule is rearranged so that only an immunoglobulin molecule of a single specificity can be produced. Monoclonal antibodies are produced in quantity using the techniques of molecular biology to selectively expand the numbers and antibody production of only this clone of cells, and many antibodies are now routinely produced in this way and have specificities, high affinities, and consistency that before was impossible.

Cells that make monoclonal antibodies are derived from mixed populations of B cells that are producing polyclonal antibody in response to in vivo immunization. Spleen cells, which contain a high proportion of antibody-producing cells, typically are isolated from a mouse that has been immunized to an antigen; the antigen may have been highly purified or just one of a number the mouse was exposed to by the injection of whole cells. The production of a useful monoclonal antibody then requires a series of steps as illustrated in Figure 11.10. First, some of the antibody-producing cells are given the capacity for prolonged growth in tissue culture by transferring to them genetic material from a mouse myeloma cell line that no longer produces its own immunoglobulin; this is done by inducing fusion of cell membrane through a variety of chemical or physical treatments. Generally, only a small fraction of the cells (less than 1 in 10,000) are successfully fused and yield viable hybrid progeny; however, successful fusions result in cells with some of the genetic material from both the immunized B lymphocyte and the myeloma cell. The subsequent steps in the production of a monoclonal antibody are designed to isolate and identify hybrid cells derived from the successful fusion of an immune B cell and myeloma cell ("hybridomas") that continue to proliferate and produce a useful antibody.

In tissue culture, hybridoma cells increase in numbers, but the unsuccessfully fused cells do not. This is because of the properties of the parent fusion partners. The parent myeloma cell line is chosen for its capacity for sustained growth in tissue culture and, usually, also as an ascites tumor in mouse peritoneal cavity. Successfully fused spleen cells acquire this capacity with the genetic material from the myeloma cells, and those spleen cells that do not acquire the material survive for only a short period in tissue culture. The hybridoma also is given a genetically determined proliferative advantage over the parent-myeloma-cell fusion partner; the myeloma cells chosen for fusion are deficient in the enzyme hypoxanthine phosphoribosyl transferase and are selectively killed when myeloma cells and hybridomas are grown in a medium containing hypoxanthine, aminopterin, and thymidine. Subsequently, individual clones of cells are grown from surviving hybridoma cells and the clones tested to determine which have maintained their ability to synthesize and secrete antibody. The most difficult and laborious part of the procedure is determining which clones actually are producing the specific antibody of interest. Each new antibody requires a new strategy for large-scale screening of possible clones of interest, followed by specific and rigorous testing to determine the properties of both the antibody and its antigen. Success is often unpredictable, and a number of fusions and screenings, requiring months, may be necessary.

Monoclonal antibodies that reliably identify subpopulations of normal T lymphocytes now are generally available (Table 11.5). Some antibodies available from different commercial sources are products of different fusion and screening strategies, but they still identify the same cell surface antigen if not the identical epitope (i.e., the local area of the antigen to which the antibody specifically binds). Also, different antibodies may be

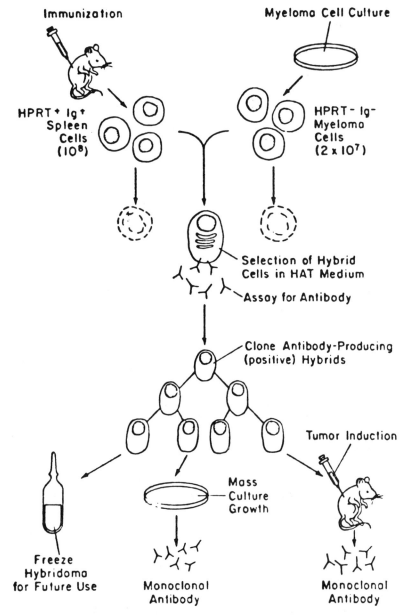

FIGURE 11.10. Mouse myeloma cells that no longer produce their own immunoglobulin (*Ig*) and lack hypoxanthine phosphoribosyl transferase (*HPRT*) activity are fused to spleen cells from an immunized mouse. The hybrid cells are selected in a medium containing hypoxanthine, aminopterin, and thymidine (*HAT*). The unfused myeloma cells are killed by the HAT medium, whereas the unfused spleen cells do not grow in tissue culture. Source: Diamond 1981[53] Reprinted by permission of the New England Journal of Medicine.

TABLE 11.5. Monoclonal Antibodies to Human Lymphocyte Antigens

	Cluster of Differentiation	Commercial Source	Description	Normal Blood Lymphocytes, %
Group I	CD5			
OKT1		Ortho	Pan-T cell	65 to 80
Leu-1		Bectin-Dickinson	Common B-cell CLL	
T101		Boehringer		
Lyt-2		New England Nuclear		
Group II	CD2			
OKTII		Ortho	Pan-T cell	75 to 85
T11		Coulter	E-rosette receptor	
Leu-5		Bectin-Dickinson		
Lyt-3		New England Nuclear		
Group III	CD3			
OKT3		Ortho	Pan-T cell	65 to 80
T3		Coulter	Mitogenic	
Leu-4		Bectin-Dickinson	Antigen receptor	
Group IV	CD4			
OKT4		Ortho	T-helper-inducer	35 to 55
T4		Coulter		
Leu-3		Bectin-Dickinson		
Group V	CD8			
OKT8		Ortho	T cytotoxic-suppressor	20 to 40
T8		Coulter	Natural killer cells	
Leu-2		Bectin-Dickinson		
OKT5		Ortho		
Group VI	CD1a			
OKT6		Ortho	Thymocytes	0
Leu-6		Bectin-Dickinson		
Group VII				
BA-1		Boehringer	Pre-B cells, B cells	—
BA-2		Boehringer	Pre-B cells (variable)	
B-1	CD20	Coulter	Pre-B cells (variable), B cells	5 to 15
Leu-12	CD19	Bectin-Dickinson	B cells	5 to 15
Leu-16	CD2b	Bectin-Dickinson	B cells	5 to 15
Leu-14	CD22	Bectin-Dickinson	B cells	5 to 15
Leu-20	CD23	Bectin-Dickinson	B cells	< 10
Group VIII				
Leu-11	CD16	Bectin-Dickinson	Natural killer cells, IgG Fe receptor	8 to 22
Leu-7	CD57	Bectin-Dickinson	T-cell subset	13 to 27
Leu-19	CD56	Bectin-Dickinson	Natural killer cells, cytotoxic T-cell subset	9 to 21

useful in identifying the same subpopulations of cells but may detect entirely different antigens; thus, the antibodies Leu-1, T101, OKT1, and Lyt-2 all react with a common 65,000 MW antigen present on all peripheral blood T cells. Other antibodies also detect additional independent "pan-T cell" antigens present on the same cells; thus, Leu-5, OKT11, T11, and Lyt-3 identify a structure that is identical with the receptor for sheep E-rosettes. OKT3, T3, and Leu-4 identify a common antigen that may be part of the T-cell receptor for antigen and also stimulate resting T cells to proliferate. While there may be some difference in the affinity of these various monoclonal antibodies, the use of any one can all but replace the E-rosette test for T lymphocytes.

Monoclonal antibodies reliably identify functional subsets and differentiation stages of T cells as well. There is a different cell surface antigen phenotype defined by monoclonal antibodies for the successive stages of maturation from medullary to cortical thymocyte and to mature peripheral blood T cell; even more important has been the demonstration that cell surface antigens identify lymphocyte subpopulations that normally are responsible for certain T-cell functions. The monoclonal antibody OKT4 (as well as Leu-3 and others) identify $T_{helper-inducer}$ cells that normally cooperate with B cells in the induction of antibody synthesis and also augment ("help") the antibody synthesis stimulated by polyclonal B-cell activators (e.g., pokeweed mitogen). The antibody OKT8 (as well as T8, Leu-2, and others) identify T$_{suppressor-cytotoxic}$ cells that inhibit antibody synthesis by B cells or have cytotoxic effector function. Further subsets of these subpopulations, with different functions, may be identified by the simultaneous expression of other antigens such as TQ1, which is equivalent to Leu-8.

The orderliness of identifying functional subsets by surface membrane phenotype can be beguiling, but it is potentially misleading. The function of a cell cannot be assumed automatically from its cell surface antigen phenotype; the correspondence between surface membrane phenotype and function usually has only been established for the predominant cell having this function in normal peripheral blood. Other minor subpopulations with different markers also may have a similar function, and their function can become important under certain circumstances and in response to certain stimuli. For example, the suppressor cell that results from stimulation of normal lymphocytes by concanavalin A, paradoxically, has a T4$^+$ phenotype. Moreover, the surface phenotype of a malignant lymphocyte does not necessarily predict that it has the same functional capacity as its normal counterpart. Only some cases of Sézary syndrome have shown T$_{helper}$ activity, but most share the T$_{helper}$ phenotype of T4$^+$.[54] As a rule, surface membrane phenotype is more likely than normal function to be conserved in malignant transformation.

The major stages of B-cell differentiation are marked by shifts in both the expression and the cellular location of immunoglobulin. Monoclonal antibodies reactive with other B-cell surface antigens also recognize different stages in normal B-cell differentiation. Small numbers of pre-B cells with cytoplasmic immunoglobulin are present in normal bone marrow (1% to 2% of nucleated cells),[45] but they are more frequent in fetal marrow (10.3% of nucleated cells), liver (4.5%), spleen (0.9%), lymph node (2.9%), and blood (0.2%), in which they largely do not appear after birth. Typically, pre-B cells are BA-1$^+$ (> 75%) and variably BA-1$^-$ or B1$^+$. They also lack both complement receptors and Fc receptors. Most are Ia$^+$, but fewer than 5% express chronic acute lymphoblastic leukemia antigen (CALLA) or TdT. The surface immunoglobulin-bearing B cells also have the antigens BA-1 and B1 as well as Ia, but they lack BA-2, CALLA, and TdT. The pan-T-cell antigens largely are not expressed on B cells, but with one important exception. The pan-T-cell antigen of 65,000 MW, which is recognized by the family of antibodies OKT1, Leu-1, and T101, is present on a very small population of B cells in fetal bone marrow and in normal adult tonsil and lymph node. These cells are important because they are the likely parent cells of common B-cell chronic lymphocytic leukemia as well as

some B-cell lymphomas that "anomalously" express this ordinarily T-cell antigen.[55,56]

Major Histocompatibility Complex Antigens

The major histocompatibility antigens have been studied extensively because of their role as targets for transplant rejection, but a larger role for these antigenic structures exists with their participation in a number of immune reactions. A number of immune functions are now known to be "major histocompatibility complex–restricted," that is, occurring only between immune and accessory or target cells that share a common major histocompatibility complex antigen. The type 1 major histocompatibility complex antigens mediate strong rejection of tissue grafts, are present on a broad range of human tissues, and are coded by the region of chromosome 6, HLA-A, -B, and -C. There is a great deal of polymorphism in these structural genes that is responsible for the individuality of the HLA antigens, but there also is strong structural homology. Monoclonal antibodies to the shared "backbone" of the molecules have been developed, and these are broadly reactive to the HLA-A, -B, or -C antigens of all individuals. The HLA-D or -DR (for D-related) antigens are the human class II antigens; they probably are the human equivalent of the mouse Ia antigen and mediate, for example, cooperation between the monocyte and lymphocyte. Monoclonal antibodies that are broadly reactive with all HLA-DR antigens but not with HLA-A, -B, or -C antigens also are widely available; they detect HLA-DR antigen on the precursors of all hematopoietic cells as well as on most B cells (except plasma cells), thymocytes, some activated T-cells, and most granulocytes. Unlike mice, virtually all human monocytes and macrophages have Ia antigen. Also, interferon-γ and -β, which in mice seem to augment the induction of an immune response by increasing the percentage of monocytes that are Ia$^+$, may act in humans by increasing the amount of Ia antigen expressed.

THE MECHANISMS OF LYMPHOCYTOSIS AND LYMPHOPENIA

No adequate techniques are available to assess accurately the total lymphocyte stores or the relative size and cellular turnover of the various T- and B-cell subpopulations in humans. The size of the lymph nodes can be estimated by palpation as well as radiologic and lymphangiographic techniques, but in each instance, the finding of enlarged lymph nodes must be interpreted with clinical knowledge to determine whether the changes in size result from inflammation, infection, tumor metastases, granulomatous disease, or a lymphoproliferative disorder. Frequently, such questions can be resolved only by lymph node biopsy and culture.

In most patients, the presence of a disorder of the proliferation, function, or number of lymphocytes is first considered only if there is an infection where peripheral blood smears reveal alterations in both lymphocyte morphology and number. Significant deviation from the usual lymphocyte counts of 2000 to 4000 cells/mm^3, with 70% T cells and 20% B cells as observed by rosetting or immunofluorescence techniques, merits further study with several considerations kept in mind. Approximately 80% of the lymphocytes normally present in the peripheral blood are long-lived, recirculating T and B cells. Although significant numbers of effector cells and immature lymphocytes are being mobilized continuously from stimulated nodes throughout the body, these cells rapidly sequester in peripheral tissue, and because of this short transit time, these cells usually account for only a small percentage of the total blood lymphocyte population even in situations where foreign proteins stimulate multiple lymph nodes. Transient elevation or depression of the blood lymphocyte counts may result from altered lymphocyte migration patterns rather than altered rates of lymphopoiesis.

Lymphopenia Caused by Altered Cellular Traffic

Abnormalities in the traffic patterns of recirculating lymphocytes may cause lymphopenia (Table 11.6), and increased blood cortisol levels due to stress or corticosteroid therapy frequently cause transient lymphopenia. Following a single, large dose of hydrocortisone, the levels of T and B lymphocytes in the blood fall to less than 500 cells/mm^3 within 4 hours, then slowly return to normal values between 12 and 24 hours. This effect is due to a fully reversible alteration in the traffic pattern of recirculating lymphocytes that causes them to sequester in the bone marrow and other tissues; however, the precise biochemic basis for this change in cellular traffic is unknown.

Some viral diseases are associated with a similar type of transient lymphopenia, and long-lived T lymphocytes exhibit specific surface receptors for influenza, myxoviruses, and paramyxoviruses. During systemic infection, these viruses attach to sialic acid residues on the lymphocyte glycocalyx; when they elute, the viruses destroy the receptor site, releasing sialic acid. Because of the loss of this surface carbohydrate, the recirculating T cells preferentially sequester in the hepatic sinuses until their membranes are repaired by resynthesis and then resume their normal patterns of migration through the blood.[57] The persistence and extent of this lymphopenia vary with the viremic phase of the particular infection, but animal studies have established that enzymatic stripping of the sialic acid from lymphocyte surfaces by brief exposure to neuraminidase can block cellular recirculation for 18 to 24 hours.[58]

Disseminated granulomatous diseases such as miliary tuberculosis, coccidioidomycosis, leprosy, and some types of Hodgkin disease occasionally are accompanied by the loss of long-lived T and B lymphocytes from the peripheral blood. Several reports have suggested that lymphopenia results from the sequestration of recirculating lymphocytes within the lymph nodes and spleen due to a mechanical obliteration by granulomas of the normal traffic pathways. Lymphopenia also may be caused by the release of secretory products from activated macrophages, thus altering lymphocyte motility and adhesiveness as well as causing a nonspecific lymphocyte "trapping" similar to that described in antigen-stimulated lymph nodes.[59] Disseminated lymphomas and leukemias may produce similar disruption of lymphocyte traffic when the lymph nodes and spleen are massively infiltrated with neoplastic cells.

The lymphocyte loss syndromes are frequent causes of profound lymphopenia (Table 11.7), and these syndromes result from congenital defects, mechanical blockade, or increased pressure and fluid flow within the intestinal lymphatics that results in the continual loss of both lymph and recirculating lymphocytes into the intestinal lumen. Because the long-lived T and B cells

TABLE 11.6. **Lymphopenia Caused by Abnormalities in the Traffic of Recirculating Lymphocytes**

Cause	Site of Redistribution
Corticosteroids	Sequester in marrow
Myxoviruses and paramyxoviruses	Sequester in liver
Disseminated granulomas	Sequester in spleen and nodes
Protein-losing enteropathies	External loss

Source: Anderson and Anderson 1984[2]

TABLE 11.7. **Diseases Associated with the Lymphocyte Loss Syndrome**

Protein-Losing Enteropathies
  Constrictive pericarditis
  Tricuspid regurgitation
  Mediastinal fibrosis
  Whipple disease
  Regional enteritis
  Intestinal lymphangiectasia
Thoracic Duct Lesions
  External thoracic duct fistulas
Thoracic Duct Rupture with Chylous Ascites

Source: Anderson and Anderson 1984[2]

are replenished at slow but relatively constant rates that are not accelerated in response to depletion, the end result is a profound lymphopenia with impairment of both cellular and humoral immunity. However, these defects can be repaired if the loss of lymphocytes can be terminated.

There have been several attempts at using thoracic duct drainage to deplete mechanically the recirculating lymphocyte pool as well as alter immune responses in humans. Although patients with severe rheumatoid disease have been reported to show significant clinical improvement during lymph drainage, they relapsed shortly after the fistulas were closed. Short-term thoracic duct fistulas both initiated before and maintained for brief intervals after transplantation also have been reported to enhance renal allograft survival in animals and humans;[60] however, this cumbersome procedure entails considerable morbidity and has not gained widespread acceptance in human organ transplantation programs. A less traumatic method for depleting lymphocytes is chronic leukapheresis using continuous-flow centrifugation, but the populations of lymphocytes removed from the blood in this procedure are not identical to those in thoracic duct lymph.

Lymphopenia Caused by Altered Cellular Turnover

Although rarely seen in the United States, the most common cause of lymphopenia worldwide is malnutrition (Table 11.8). Severe starvation of both children and

adults has been shown to cause thymic involution, depletion of thymus-dependent zones in lymphatic tissues, reduction of recirculating T cells in the peripheral blood, skin anergy, and defective responses of cultured blood lymphocytes to T-cell mitogens. The mechanisms responsible for these changes are uncertain, but all of the defects can be corrected by refeeding. The variable lymphopenic states seen in occasional patients with chronic diarrhea or with the severe cachexia of end-stage malignancy may be of similar etiology as well.

Congenital defects in the maturation of stem cells into B and T cells as well as the absence of thymic hormones are rare causes of lymphopenia, and they usually are recognized in early childhood. These defects include congenital thymic aplasia, Swiss-type agammaglobulinemia, Nezelof syndrome, Wiskott-Aldrich syndrome, and primary lymphopenic aggamaglobulinemia (Table 11.1).[1] Because of the long lifespan of recirculating T and B cells, patients with aplastic anemia due to acquired stem cell or microenvironmental defects may display relatively normal or slightly reduced blood lymphocyte levels throughout the course of their illness.

Some severe viral infections are associated with a modest lymphopenia manifested by a reduction in identifiable B lymphocytes and, occasionally, by an increase in null cells (unclassifiable by surface marker techniques). These changes appear to result from the ability of measles, varicella, polio, and lactic dehydrogenase viruses to both infect and destroy B cells carrying surface receptors for these viral agents. The lympholytic

TABLE 11.8. Abnormalities in Lymphocyte Turnover

Cause	Mechanism
Starvation	Uncertain
Congenital	Defect in stem cell maturation into T and B cells
Congenital thymic aplasia	
Swiss-type agammaglobulinemia	
Nezelof syndrome	
Wiskott-Aldrich syndrome	
Primary lymphopenic agammaglobulinemia	
Virus infections	Lysis of infected lymphocytes
Acquired immunodeficiency syndrome	
Measles	
Varicella	
Polio	
Lactic dehydrogenase virus	
Autoimmune	Destruction of antibody-coated lymphocytes in spleen
Systemic lupus erythematosus	
Felty syndrome	
Therapeutic agents	
Alkylating agents (cyclophosphamide)	Cross-linking DNA
Antilymphocyte serum	Complement-mediated lysis

Source: Anderson and Anderson 1984[2]

events are more pronounced within organized lymphatic tissues, and it may take weeks for the B-cell population to return to normal levels as the restoration rate by marrow precursors is so slow. Because B cells normally account for only a small percentage of the blood lymphocytes, the magnitude of the lymphocyte lysis may not be apparent from simple examination of blood smears and rosetting cells.

The acquired immune deficiency syndrome (AIDS) also causes lymphopenia, especially of T_{helper} cells, that is unique in its severity, progression, and irreversibility. The immune defect results in the occurrence of opportunistic infections, most often *Pneumocystis carinii* pneumonia, as well as cancers such as Kaposi sarcoma and Burkitt lymphoma.[61,62] Human immunodeficiency virus (HIV-1), a retrovirus related to the human T-cell leukemia virus is the etiologic agent of AIDS,[63–65] and HIV-1 is transmissible by sexual contact or parenterally. There are a variety of immune abnormalities in AIDS involving both T and B cells, and the most consistent and predictably progressive abnormality in the blood is the marked lowering of T_{helper}-cell numbers (< 600 cells/mm^3) and of the ratio of $T_{helper}:T_{suppressor}$ cells (usually < 1.0). Abnormal T-cell subpopulation numbers help to support the diagnosis of AIDS, but this is not a specific finding. Other viral infections, such as Epstein-Barr virus and cytomegalovirus, also may cause transient, similar abnormalities. Moreover, abnormal T-cell subpopulations may occur in otherwise healthy male homosexuals or in the presence of lymphadenopathy and other unexplained illness in members of groups that are at risk for AIDS. The diagnosis of infection with HIV-1 rests on viral studies, including serology and viral culture, but studies of lymphocyte populations, especially CD4 cell numbers also may be of importance prognostically.

A variable degree of lymphopenia has been observed in association with splenomegaly, and in conditions such as systemic lupus erythematosus and Felty syndrome, lymphopenia probably results from the splenic destruction of lymphocytes bearing isoantibodies on their surfaces. The lymphopenia appearing in some patients with portal hypertension has never been explained adequately, but this simply may reflect increased lymphocyte sequestration within the interstices of the enlarged spleen.

A variety of drugs and biologic agents also can produce lymphopenia.[66] Alkylating agents such as cyclophosphamide that cross-link DNA produce cell death in both interphase and mitosis, and this lowers both the T- and B-cell mass in the body. However, the slower regeneration of the B-cell series appears to explain the preferential effects of cyclophosphamide on humoral immunity. Azathioprine and methotrexate therapy usually have little effect on the total blood lymphocyte count, but they may decrease the number of both medium and large lymphocytes that move through the circulation. Heterologous antiserum, raised by immunizing horses or rabbits with human thymocytes, possesses antibodies specific for T-cell determinants after other cross-reacting antibodies are removed by the appropriate absorption techniques; administered to achieve immunosuppression in humans, this antithymocyte serum causes a profound T-cell lymphopenia due to the cytolytic effects mediated by complement. In addition, such an antiserum may alter the lymphocyte traffic patterns through mechanisms that are poorly understood (i.e., blindfolding of the lymphocyte surface receptors).

Lymphocytosis Caused by Altered Recirculation Patterns

In normal individuals, the rate of lymphocyte entry into and exit from the blood is relatively constant; however, this equilibrium can be disrupted by mecha-

TABLE 11.9. The Causes of Lymphocytosis

Condition	Cause	Mechanism
Abnormalities in the traffic of lymphocytes	*Bordetella pertussis*	Block attachment to high endothelial venules
	Adenoviruses	Block attachment to high endothelial venules
	Heparin	Block attachment to high endothelial venules
	Dextran	Block attachment to high endothelial venules
Abnormalities in lymphocyte turnover	Immunoproliferative disorders	Proliferation of neoplastic cells that do not "home in" to lymph nodes
	Systemic infection	Antigen-driven proliferation and mobilization of lymphocytes
	Diffuse inflammation	Antigen-driven proliferation and mobilization of lymphocytes
	Virus infections	Replication of virus-infected cells followed by immune response to virus expressed on infected cell surface
	Autoimmune disease	Lack of suppressor cell control over antigen-driven lymphopoiesis

Source: Anderson and Anderson 1984[2]

TABLE 11.10. Human Diseases Associated with Documented Decreased Suppressor Cell Effects

Disease	Type of Suppression	Manifestation
Hashimoto thyroiditis	Decreased T suppressor	Autoantibodies
Rheumatoid arthritis	Decreased T suppressor	Increased antibody response
Systemic lupus erythematosus	Decreased T suppressor	Increased antibody response

Source: Anderson and Anderson 1984[2]

nisms that prevent the recirculating lymphocytes in the blood from both recognizing and attaching to the high endothelial venules in lymph nodes (Table 11.9). Such a blockade can rapidly elevate the blood level of both small T and B lymphocytes to from 20,000 to 30,000 cells/mm³, thus producing a simultaneous reduction in cellularity within the peripheral lymph nodes. This mechanism clearly accounts for the striking elevation in the number of blood lymphocytes that display a completely normal morphology during either spontaneous infections or immunization with killed vaccines of *Bordetella pertussis*. In addition, an identical blood picture can be seen in both children and young adults with an acute febrile illness thought to be caused by adenoviruses, and in these cases of acute infectious lymphocytosis, the striking elevation in the blood lymphocyte count may persist for 2 to 3 weeks and then resolve in a phase that is accompanied by a transient peripheral blood eosinophilia. Although the mechanisms are not entirely clear, animal studies suggest that *B. pertussis* secretes a product that alters the lymphocyte membrane, thus preventing their attachment to lymph node venules.[67] These surface changes are insufficient to cause lymphocyte sequestration in other vascular beds; however, recovery of normal recirculation patterns is presumed to require shedding of the altered surface components and resynthesis of membrane receptors.

Although less convincing, evidence exists that high-dose heparin and dextran therapy in animals produces a similar lymphocytosis that results from a blockade of lymphocyte entry into the lymph nodes as well as the simultaneous mobilization of cells from the peripheral lymphatic tissues.[68] The evidence that these changes in traffic result from coating anions is still indirect. There have been no reports of a similar lymphocytosis in humans, but it is quite possible that these transient blood changes simply have been overlooked in the clinical setting.

Lymphocytosis Caused by Altered Turnover of Lymphocytes

In addition to the lymphoproliferative disorders discussed in other chapters, several situations exist where a transient lymphocytosis results from the increased production and/or release of cells from the peripheral lymphatic tissues (Table 11.8). In both animals and humans, systemic infections and immunizations can augment the antigen-driven proliferation and mobilization of lymphocytes in both the nodes and the spleen; if these stimuli are widespread and sustained, increased lymphocyte traffic through the circulation can be detected by routine laboratory techniques. However, when smears containing increased numbers of atypical lymphocytes are evaluated, it should be remembered that both blast and plasma cells rarely are present in peripheral blood when the stimulus is inflammation or antigens.

A modest lymphocytosis has been observed to persist for years in some patients with systemic lupus erythematosus and other putative autoimmune disorders (Table 11.10); such patients appear to be at higher risk for the subsequent development of lymphomas and lymphatic leukemias. Because similar findings have been observed in New Zealand black mice, it has been suggested that such individuals have a deficiency in T-cell suppressor activity that permits unbridled and prolonged stimulation of the B-cell system, thus facilitating the emergence of a malignant clone by spontaneous mutation.[69] This thesis has not been proven, however, and the entire sequence could be explained equally well by processes such as oncogenic virus infections.

Infectious Mononucleosis*

The most common cause of an absolute lymphocytosis with an increased number of atypical lymphocytes in the circulation is infectious mononucleosis, a disorder caused by Epstein-Barr virus (EBV). EBV is a lymphotropic, double-stranded DNA virus of the herpes family that shares the characteristics of latency and endogenous reactivation in common with other herpesviruses.[70] Only those B lymphocytes that have surface immunoglobulin, are capable of secreting immunoglobulin, and contain surface receptors for the third component of

---

*This section was written by Jerry L. Spivak, M.D.

complement (C3) are susceptible to invasion by this virus.[71] The EBV receptor on the B lymphocyte appears to be associated closely with the C3 receptor (CR2), but these receptors may not be identical.

Serologic studies indicate that EBV is disseminated widely in humans; where living conditions are primitive and at the lower socioeconomic strata of industrialized nations, infection with EBV occurs at an early age, most often in a mild or asymptomatic form.[72] The peak age for infection in individuals of higher socioeconomic status is 14 to 24 years,[73] and while the classic clinical syndrome of infectious mononucleosis is seen most often in this age group, it must be emphasized that infections with EBV in this age group can be subclinical. Also, in contrast to EBV, infection with another virus of the herpes group, cytomegalovirus, is more common in patients over 24 years of age.[73] By the age of 40 years, most individuals have been exposed to EBV; clinical infectious mononucleosis is rare in these patients, but occasional cases (often with atypical manifestations) are observed.[74] With the widespread use of immunosuppressive agents, reactivation of EBV is being recognized now with increasing frequency, and it may be responsible for clinical problems encountered in patients receiving immunosuppressive therapy, such as renal transplant recipients,[75] or those in patients with AIDS.[76]

The incubation period for EBV ranges from 4 to 7 weeks depending on whether the virus is transmitted parenterally or by oral contact. EBV is present in the oropharyngeal secretions of from 10% to 20% of asymptomatic, seropositive individuals, thus providing a source for dissemination of the virus in the general population.[77] Among patients with immunosuppression, the incidence of oropharyngeal excretion of EBV is approximately 50%.[77]

The major clinical features of infectious mononucleosis are fever, pharyngitis, lymphadenopathy, splenomegaly, palatal exanthem, periorbital edema, and hepatocellular dysfunction.[78] In patients older than 40 years, the incidence of adenopathy is reduced, hepatic dysfunction is more severe, and the febrile period is prolonged.[74] Tonsillectomy may minimize the degree of pharyngeal involvement.

The hallmark of infectious mononucleosis is an absolute lymphocytosis with more than 15% atypical lymphocytes (Fig. 11.11). The lymphocytosis begins during the first week of the illness, reaches a peak during the second or third week, and declines thereafter, returning to normal after 2 to 8 weeks.[79] Studies of peripheral blood lymphocytes indicate that, early in the course of the illness, an increase in B lymphocytes is followed by an increase in T lymphocytes and, in particular, by the T-cell suppressor/cytotoxic subpopulation.[79-81] The

atypical lymphocytes may be either B or T cells, but they most often are T cells.

Infection with EBV is associated with a polyclonal increase in immunoglobulin production. IgM viral capsid antigen (VCA) antibodies are the first virus-specific antibodies to appear, reaching a peak during the first 2 weeks and declining rapidly thereafter.[82] These are followed by the development of IgG VCA antibodies and, subsequently, antibodies to early antigen. IgG antibodies against EBV nuclear antigen arise several months after the onset of clinical illness, and unlike the IgM antibodies, these IgG antibodies persist in the circulation for life.[82]

The characteristic sheep red cell agglutinating heterophil antibody associated with infectious mononucleosis is an IgM that develops during the first 2 weeks of the illness. It appears slightly after the IgM VCA antibody,[82] and it can be detected for 1 to 2 months. The nature of the antigen that stimulates heterophil antibody production during EBV infection is unknown; however, the distinctive cross-reactivity of these heterophil antibodies with beef red blood cells but not with antigen derived from guinea-pig kidney provides the diagnostic test for distinguishing the heterophil antibodies of infectious mononucleosis from those of other acute infectious or inflammatory disorders. In general, an unabsorbed heterophil sheep erythrocyte agglutination titer of 1:224 or more suggests the presence of infectious mononucleosis, as does a titer of antibody against beef red cells of 1:40 or more. On occasion, false-positive responses may occur in patients with other illnesses, but these individuals generally lack the other characteristic features or hematologic abnormalities that are associated with an acute EBV infection. A false-negative heterophil antibody test also can occur in children with EBV infections.[83]

In addition to specific antibodies against EBV and heterophil antibodies, the production of other antibodies has been identified in patients with infectious mononucleosis. Some of these other antibodies may be responsible for complications occurring during the course of the illness, and they include anti-i antibodies, lymphocytotoxins, and smooth muscle antibodies.[84]

Infectious mononucleosis usually is an acute, self-limited illness, with resolution over a 3- to 4-week period. Other than fever and malaise, pharyngitis generally is the most distressing problem to the patient, and it may produce substantial pain and dysphagia. In some instances, airway obstruction develops, but this responds rapidly to a short course of prednisone at a dose of 40 mg/day. Streptococcal infection also may complicate the pharyngitis.

Infectious mononucleosis is due to an infection of B lymphocytes by EBV, but the marked suppressor/

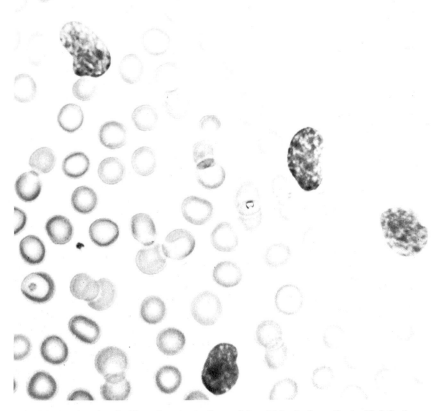

FIGURE 11.11.   Atypical lymphocytes in the peripheral blood of a patient with infectious mononucleosis. *Source:* **Anderson and Anderson 1984[2]**

cytotoxic T-lymphocyte response to this infection can result in the impairment of cellular function in organs other than the lymphatic system. Impairment of hepatic function sufficient to cause jaundice occurs in approximately 15% of patients,[85] and hematologic abnormalities include hemolytic anemia, agranulocytosis, thrombocytopenia, and on rare occasions, aplastic anemia. Hyperuricemia is not uncommon, particularly in males,[86] and Guillain-Barré syndrome, transverse myelitis, and meningoencephalitis are seen occasionally, as are myocarditis and pneumonitis. Immunologic abnormalities in addition to increased antibody production include impaired cell-mediated immunity with cutaneous anergy, ampicillin-induced skin reactions, and agammaglobulinemia. Fetal complications are rare, but these have occurred as a consequence of airway obstruction, unrecognized splenic rupture, and fulminant hepatitis. In patients with an impaired immune response, fatal EBV infections also have been documented. This may take the form of an overwhelming infection or the development of a lymphoma; the latter appears to be a

feature of the peculiar, X-linked recessive lymphoproliferative syndrome of males.[87,88]

When the appropriate clinical hematologic and serologic abnormalities are present, the establishment of the diagnosis of infectious mononucleosis usually is no problem. When the typical clinical picture is associated with a negative heterophil agglutinin test, other infectious agents that should be considered include HIV, cytomegalovirus, rubella virus, adenovirus, and *Toxoplasma* species.[89,90]

Substantial evidence has accumulated that suggests EBV may be oncogenic in humans. The virus is oncogenic in New World primates, causing malignant lymphoma in cotton-top marmosets,[91] and the EBV genome is found in nasopharyngeal carcinoma tumor cells as well as the tumor cells of African Burkitt lymphoma.[92] The presence of high VCA-antibody levels in patients with Burkitt lymphoma long before development of the tumor itself is strong evidence supporting the possibility that the virus is involved with pathogenesis of this lymphoma.[92] Reports concerning the development of lymphoma in patients with immune deficiencies who have been infected with EBV also support the contention that this virus can be oncogenic in humans.[61,87,92,93]

MARKERS IN THE STUDY OF LYMPHOID MALIGNANCIES

Both acute and chronic leukemias and lymphomas are malignancies that arise from normal hematopoietic cells at different stages of differentiation.[42] In principle, any normal hematopoietic precursor cell is a potential target for neoplastic transformation if it has the proliferative to self-renew and give rise to more differentiated progeny, and the resulting malignant cells may retain a number of the parent cell's properties, including morphology, proliferative potential, and tissue localization, while acquiring the capacity for sustained, uncontrolled proliferation. One approach to the leukemias and lymphomas is to classify them according to their presumed cell of origin; this has utility because cells of apparently similar origin often have similar clinical features, response to therapy, and prognosis. A system based on the malignant cells' biologic properties gives the clinician a unified, rational, and useful classification for an otherwise bewildering variety of leukemias and lymphomas.

Leukemia-Associated Antigens

Common acute lymphoblastic leukemia antigen (CD10) was first detected by conventional heteroantisera, but its routine clinical use awaited the availability of monoclonal antibodies to CD10 (J-5, BA-3, and anti-CALLA).[42,94–97] The antigen detected is a cell surface glycoprotein with a molecular weight of 100,000, and it is present in 80% of the patients with non-T-cell acute lymphoblastic leukemia (ALL). It is not a tumor-specific antigen and is expressed on some normal pre-B cells as well as increased numbers of cells in regenerating bone marrow. It is not specific for ALL, because it also is present in 30% to 50% of patients with chronic myelogenous leukemia in blast crisis and in some cases of acute "biphenotypic" leukemias that also have myeloid differentiation markers. It also is not specific for leukemia or even undifferentiated lymphomas. Burkitt lymphoma, lymphoblastic lymphoma, and other B-cell non-Hodgkin lymphomas may be CALLA[+] (Fig. 11.6).

The enzyme found in lymphoid precursors both in normal marrow and normal thymocytes, TdT, is an important marker of ALL.[18,98] Clinical experience with TdT was developed largely with an assay for its enzymatic activity. A newer immunofluorescence technique

has advantages over that radioassay, because the new technique requires small numbers of cells (as few as 100 to 1000), is quick, and is very sensitive to even small numbers of positive cells. It is especially valuable in determining if TdT is limited to a subpopulation of cells. On the other hand, the radioassay is a true measure of enzymatic activity and generates a wider range of values that may be of some diagnostic value; however, large numbers of cells are required (at least 20 million) as well as more expensive radiolabelled reagents and the oligonucleotide initiator substrate. Radioactivity detection techniques also are more expensive and slower. The entire radioassay requires approximately 8 hours, instead of only 2 hours for the immunoassay, and in one study that directly compared the two techniques, the immunoassay was preferred for these reasons as long as both the preparation and the storage of cells was meticulous before the assay. Also, some false positives (7.8%) and false negatives (9%) occurred. Radioenzymatic assay is recommended when the clinical features or therapeutic response vary from immunoassay results; this might occur if the cytochemical features (myeloperoxidase or Sudan Black positivity)[99] or a lack of cytolytic response to vincristine and prednisone therapy suggest the presence of acute nonlymphocytic leukemia.

As with CALLA, TdT is not absolutely specific for leukemia and can occur in a small number of cells within normal and regenerating marrow;[100] however, it is a highly sensitive test. In one series of 100 patients with ALL, 96 patients were TdT[+].[98] ALL is TdT[+] in adults or children whether null, pre-B, pre-T, or T cell in type; a case of TdT[+] B-cell ALL has also been reported as well. TdT also has provided evidence for the involvement of two cell lineages in more cases of acute leukemia than any other marker. Approximately 30% of patients with chronic myelogenous leukemia blast crisis (but never during chronic phase) have TdT[+] cells, and approximately 5% of acute nonlymphocytic leukemic cells are TdT[+]. TdT[+] cells also have been found in acute leukemia following myeloproliferative disorders such as myeloid metaplasia with myelofibrosis and polycythemia vera; conventional wisdom would have expected an acute leukemia to involve a myeloid stem cell. Such biphenotypic leukemias may indicate that two stem cells from different lineages have undergone leukemic transformation.

Acute Lymphoblastic Leukemia and Lymphoblastic Lymphoma

The marker phenotypes of ALL follow closely, if not absolutely faithfully, the phenotypes of the corresponding cells of early, normal lymphocyte differentiation.[42,96,97] With successive stages of differentiation, there is an orderly appearance and disappearance of markers; common or "null cell" ALL (actually early pre-B-cell ALL, as shown by gene probes) is the earliest stage, with TdT$^+$, CALLA$^+$, Ia$^+$, and no T- or B-cell markers (55% of patients with ALL). Pre-B-cell ALL (20% of cases) has cytoplasmic IgM and usually is BA-1$^+$ and TdT$^+$ as well as sometimes B1$^+$ or CAL-LA$^+$.[45] B-cell ALL is surface IgM$^+$, BA-1$^+$, B1$^+$, usually cytoplasmic immunoglobulin$^+$, but CALLA$^-$ and TdT$^-$. The cells typically are vacuolated, with the French-American-British classification L-3 (Burkitt-type ALL [5% of cases]).

T-cell ALL is defined by the presence of a T-cell marker, usually of the OKT1/T101 group (20% of cases),[97,101,102] but only about 50% of patients have the E-rosette receptor. T-cell ALL can be divided into pre-T-cell (only T10$^+$), common thymocyte (T10$^+$ and T6$^+$), and mature thymocyte type (T10$^+$ and T3$^+$). T-cell ALL has typical clinical features and a poorer prognosis, which also distinguish it from common ALL. The presence of T-cell markers in ALL is more common among adolescent boys, and they predict a high probability of mediastinal involvement, lower response to conventional treatment, and earlier relapse in the marrow, testicle, or central nervous system. The number of long-term disease-free survivors is low; thus, the choice of more intensive treatment for ALL with T-cell markers is justified and may alter the usually poor outcome of this disease.

It is unclear that the subtypes of T-cell ALL differ in clinical behavior. In fact, the closely related lymphoblastic lymphoma may have markers that are indistinguishable from those of T-cell ALL, and the recognition of this lymphoma has been aided greatly by the demonstration of TdT, which is present in almost every case (a TdT$^-$ case has been reported, however). The clinical course is typical, but after an initial period of predominantly nodal and thymic involvement, this lymphoma may evolve into a clinical entity that is indistinguishable from T-cell ALL having dominant involvement of the bone marrow and early invasion of the central nervous system with meningeal involvement.

Proliferative Disorders of Peripheral T Cells

The T-cell lymphomas (those other than lymphoblastic lymphoma) as well as the chronic T-cell leukemias are derived from normal precursors that represent lineages of postthymic development. They are less common than the B-cell lymphomas and chronic leukemias, and several of these T-cell disorders have both clinical presentations and histologic pictures that are associated with a consistent marker phenotype.[42,54,103] Sézary syndrome and the cutaneous T-cell lymphomas are all of T$_{helper/inducer}$-cell origin; some also have demonstrable helper cell activity. No difference in phenotype has been reported between the Sézary syndrome, in which there are large numbers of circulating malignant T-cells, and the more predominantly cutaneous and infiltrative disease of mycosis fungoides. Most are of the phenotype pan-T$^+$ (including the OKT1, OKT3, and OKT11 groups) and are T$_{helper/inducer}$-cell$^+$ (e.g., OKT4 or Leu-3), thymocyte$^-$ (OKT6$^-$), TdT$^-$; all are B-cell$^-$.

Adult T-cell leukemia-lymphoma is an important and newly recognized syndrome. It is unusual because of a high tendency for geographic clustering, and although rare in the United States, it is common in the West Indies and endemic in areas of Japan. The reason for the geographic clustering almost certainly is the high association of this entity with a transmissible agent, HTLV-1. This is a type-C human retrovirus similar to tumor viruses studied in animals. This virus often can be recovered from the cells, and viral antigens are displayed on the cell surface. High levels of antibody also are found in close contacts. There is a typical clinical picture, but the clinical scope of HTLV-associated T-cell lymphomas now is recognized as perhaps much broader. There usually is a moderately aggressive clinical course with visceral involvement and frequent skin lesions and hypercalcemia. The malignant cells have lobulated or deeply indented nuclei, and markers consistently show a phenotype of pan-T-cell$^+$ (e.g., T1$^+$, T3$^+$, T11$^+$) and T4$^+$ (or Leu-3$^+$). The T-cell growth factor receptor, Tac, is present and appears to be induced by the virus. Common thymocyte antigen T6 is absent, but cortical thymocyte antigen T10, also found on other proliferating cells, is present.

T$_{suppressor/cytotoxic}$ surface markers (e.g., T8 or Leu-2) are always absent, but a number of cases "paradoxically" have cells with suppressor activity for antibody synthesis. Despite the presence of the T$_{helper/inducer}$ phenotype, helper activity is absent, which suggests that the normal cell of origin for this malignancy may be related to the concanavalin A–induced suppressor cell that is T4$^+$.

Several lymphoproliferative disorders of small lymphocytes are of T-cell origin, but they are very uncommon. T-cell chronic lymphocytic leukemia makes up at most 1% to 3% of all CLL cases. Few of these disorders have had extensive marker and functional studies performed, but the T8$^+$ variant with neutropenia and high incidence of infection has been reported. Some authors decline to call this a "leukemia," however, and designate it only as a T$_{suppressor}$ lymphocytosis. Hairy-cell leukemia most often is a B-cell disorder, but an unusual

T-cell variant as well as an apparent mononuclear phagocyte (true histiocyte) origin have been reported. Some cases of diffuse small cell, T-zone, and Lennert lymphomas (all not always well classified in conventional schemas) are of T-cell origin.

The "histiocytic" lymphomas of the older Rappaport classification now are recognized as being of lymphoid origin. The Lukes and Collins classification recognizes them as large cell lymphomas with morphologic features that are highly predictive of either B-cell origin (more common) or T-cell origin (more rare).[103,104] The large cell lymphomas of intermediate grade (by the new International Working Formulation) and the high-grade immunoblastic sarcoma also are both lymphomas that are more commonly B cell than T cell in origin.

The vast majority of non-Hodgkin lymphomas and chronic lymphoid leukemias are of B-cell origin,[42] and they typically display immunoglobulin on their surface and have a monotypic light chain of either κ or λ as discussed earlier. The B cell of the lymph node follicle center is thought to be the origin of all nodular lymphomas (small, mixed, or large cell), most large cell lymphomas, and many poorly differentiated and diffuse small cell lymphomas (Fig. 11.6).

Burkitt lymphoma also is of B-cell origin, and surface or cytoplasmic immunoglobulin is demonstrated readily. Moreover, a typical translocation in Burkitt lymphoma involves loci on chromosomes and genes coding for either immunoglobulin light chains (chromosome 2 or 22) or heavy chains (chromosome 14). There is a high association of this tumor with EBV as well, especially in the endemic African cases, which corresponds well to the known B-cell specificity of that virus.

The immunoglobulin-secreting lymphomas clearly are of B-cell origin as well. Histologically, Waldenström macroglobulinemia is a well-differentiated lymphoma of small plasmacytoid lymphocytes with both surface and cytoplasmic immunoglobulin. Multiple myeloma is a malignancy of plasma cells with cytoplasmic and secretory immunoglobulin, and it illustrates that a malignancy which in fact arises from cells near the end of a differentiation pathway still can be morphologically immature and at times even appear "undifferentiated."

Is there any clinical importance to the presence of lymphocyte markers? When histologic appearance is sufficient for classification, does the knowledge of lymphoid markers add to the prognostic information? To date, only a few studies have attempted to address this question. Bloomfield et al.[103] confirmed the observations of others that patients with B-cell lymphomas generally had longer survival than those with T-cell lymphomas, and they additionally observed that patients with "null" cell lymphomas, without demonstrable surface immunoglobulin or E-rosette formation, had the

worst survival of all. Also, in a careful study limited to patients with large cell lymphomas, Warnke et al.[104] found a contradictory result. Those having lymphomas with surface immunoglobulin had the shortest survival, and those with lymphomas without surface immunoglobulin but believed to be of B-cell origin by morphologic criteria not only had better survival but a high rate of long-term, disease-free survival (90%) following chemotherapy as well. These earlier studies need to be repeated on different patient populations and should include testing with the newer monoclonal antibody techniques for the detection of T- and B-cell antigens.

Chronic B-Cell Leukemias

The marker studies of common B-cell chronic lymphocytic leukemia (at least 90% of all CLL cases) are so characteristic as to be diagnostic of CLL or its lymphomatous counterpart, diffuse well-differentiated lymphocytic lymphoma.[42,55,56] Monotypic light-chain surface immunoglobulin is present, usually in low concentration, and the heavy chain generally is IgM, often with IgD. The surface immunoglobulin is situated abnormally in the membrane and does not "cap" or migrate to one or two poles of the surface membrane as it does in normal cells that are treated with anti-immunoglobulin molecules. (This difference from the normal cells will not be noted if reactions are always carried out with the metabolic inhibitor sodium azide present, which is common practice to facilitate the reading of surface immunoglobulin patterns and prevent loss of the label from the cell surface.) In addition, the cells paradoxically also show the presence of the ordinarily pan-T-cell antigen that is detected by the family of antibodies OKT1, Leu-1, and T101; the presence of both this antigen and monotypic surface immunoglobulin, without the presence of other pan-T-cell markers (e.g., E-rosette or OKT3) is virtually diagnostic of these disorders as well as some lymphoma cases of intermediate differentiation. No benign proliferation of lymphocytes will display uniformly this ensemble of markers, although a few normal cells, especially in the lymph nodes, can be found with this phenotype. Other markers of B-cell differentiation (e.g., complement receptors, Ia antigen) are present as well.

Other surface antigen phenotypes of CLL are associated with different clinical features. Bright rather than faint surface immunoglobulin often is associated with a serum paraprotein or urinary Bence Jones protein (a clinical course that perhaps is more like Waldenström macroglobulinemia) and with the appearance of more plasmacytoid lymphocytes. The lack of the paradoxic T-cell antigen on morphologically diagnostic CLL cells often is associated with nephrotic syndrome and albuminuria but not Bence Jones proteinuria, and the clinical course in these individuals may not be as indolent as that in common CLL.

Hairy-cell leukemia usually is a B-cell disorder, and as in other B-cell malignancies, this is demonstrated convincingly by the presence of surface immunoglobulin with monotypic light chain. An occasional case also has been associated with a serum immunoglobulin paraprotein of the same light-chain type. Hairy-cell leukemia can be distinguished from common CLL and other B-cell lymphomas, which also may have a leukemic phase, by several features. Hairy-cell leukemia has both a characteristic cellular morphology and histologic appearance in the bone marrow and spleen. Histochemical stains are helpful as well, because hairy-cell leukemia has acid phosphatase present whose activity persists after treatment with tartrate (tartrate-resistant acid phosphatase, isoenzyme 5). B-cell CLL probably arises from a normal cell that is at a differentiation stage just after the antigen-responsive B cell yet earlier than the follicular center B cell of lymph nodes; the origin of the B-cells of hairy-cell leukemia is less certain. Interestingly, several investigators have found a "paradoxic" T-cell antigen on true B-cell hairy-cell leukemia—the T-cell growth factor receptor, Tac; however, it is not known if T-cell growth factor supports the growth of these cells.

MEDIATORS OF IMMUNE RESPONSE

The prime function of normal antigen-driven lymphopoiesis is to generate cells that provide the mechanisms for both recognizing and eliminating foreign substances from the body. These effector responses generally are divided into two types: humoral immunity that is provided by specific immunoglobulins, and cellular immunity that is mediated by specifically sensitized T lymphocytes interacting directly with the antigen. Although this is still a useful classification, the traditional boundaries between cellular and humoral immunity have blurred after demonstrations of the interactions between T and B lymphocytes and their specific mediators in most immune responses. Furthermore, subpopulations of mononuclear cells that cannot be classified readily as either lymphocytes or monocytes are known now to play important roles in host defense through cell-mediated mechanisms that are independent of immunity (natural killer cells).

Specific antibody and the heterogeneous populations of effector lymphocytes can both engage and selectively eliminate foreign substances in their own right, but these effector systems include mechanisms for amplifying these reactions by activating phagocytic cells as well as the kinin, complement, and clotting systems. Without the participation of such nonspecific inflammatory mechanisms, the effectiveness of antibody and immune lymphocytes in host defense would be compromised severely.

The Complement System

The complement system (Fig. 11.12) is the primary mediator of the cell lysis and inflammation produced by humoral immunity. This system consists of 14 different proteins that are present as inactive precursors in normal plasma. When activated by an appropriate stimulus, these components interact with one another in a carefully regulated sequence of protein–protein and enzyme–substrate interactions that generate biologically active products. Five of these proteins (C1q, C1r, C1s, C4, and C2) belong to the classic complement pathway, which is activated by antigen–antibody complexes. Three proteins (B, D, and properdin) provide for the nonspecific activation of the complement cascade by the alternate pathway. The remaining six (C3 and C5 through C9) serve as the final common pathway for activation initiated by both immune complexes and nonspecific mechanisms, and these latter proteins mediate cytolytic functions by damaging the membranes of bacteria, fungi, viruses, and altered host cells. In addition, the enzymatic cleavage of both C3 and C5 generates active fragments that promote opsonization, leukocyte chemotaxis, histamine release from mast cells, and the activation of B lymphocytes and macrophages.

In normal individuals, C1 circulates as a large macromolecule formed by three discrete proteins (C1q, C1r, C1s) bound by Ca^{2+} ions. The C1q molecule is similar chemically to collagen, and it consists of six bundles of three polypeptide chains each that are arranged in a triple helix. Peripheral globular subunits in these chains form binding sites that interact with the Fc regions of immunoglobulin, and because C1q is activated only when it binds with two adjacent IgG molecules (or with one molecule of polymeric IgM), this protein appears to be designed specifically to focus the complement effect on cell surfaces and to maximize interactions between the evanescent, short-lived split products.

Following attachment of the C1 macromolecule to immunoglobulins, the C1r component activates C1s into proteolytic activity so that a bimolecular complex which binds to biologic membranes is formed from the C2 and C4 globulins. The formation of the C42 complex is not efficient, and many molecules lose their labile binding sites and diffuse away from the site as inactive products. However, some C42 attaches to the membranes, thus forming a proteolytic enzyme that can attack the next

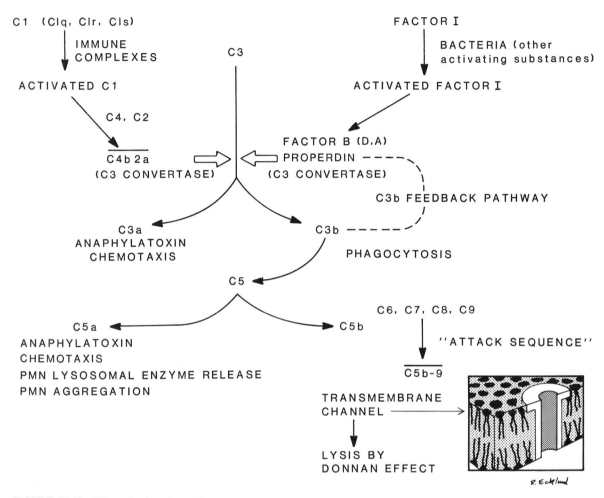

FIGURE 11.12. The activation of complement cascade by both classic and alternate pathways. *Note:* **PMN = neutrophil.**
Source: **Anderson and Anderson 1984[2]**

component, C3, and generate both inflammatory mediators and membrane attack mechanisms.

The alternate pathway of complement activation includes a group of proteins that were classified originally within the properdin system that become activated by nonimmunologic interactions with endotoxin, yeast, lipopolysaccharides, and enzymes. These agents interact with factor B and factor D (an enzyme normally present in blood) to generate B_b, which attacks C3 to activate the final common pathway; this alternate sequence of activation probably runs continuously at low levels in normal individuals but is controlled by an inhibitor unless the activated C3b component is bound to cell surfaces. In some patients, an autoantibody that is directed against new determinants on this B_bC3b complex acts to stabilize the enzyme, thus blocking feedback controls and allowing C3 cleavage to continue until exhaustion (nephritogenic factor seen in patients with hypocomplementemic mesangiocapillary nephritis).

The enzymes activated by both the classic and the alternate pathways cleave the globulin protein C3 into two fragments. The smaller split product (called C3a) is released into the microenvironment where it causes histamine release from mast cells and serves as a chemoattractant for phagocytic leukocytes; loss of this peptide exposes new sites on the larger remaining fragment (C3b), which permits the fragment to bind to the membrane adjacent to the original immunoglobulin-C42 site. This generates a C423 complex that cleaves C5 into two fragments, and again, the smaller peptide C5a diffuses away and serves as both a chemoattractant for leukocytes and an activator of macrophages and B lymphocytes. The large C5b fragment combines reversibly with C6, forming an activating enzyme that reacts with C7 to yield a trimolecular complex which can attach to bacterial, mammalian cell, and liposomal membranes. This results in the additional assembly of the complement components C8 and C9 within the membrane, where they form transmembrane channels that resemble flanged pipes of 10-μm diameter when viewed by electron microscopy. These channels are large enough to permit the passage of small molecules, fluids, and ions between the cell and its external environment, but they are too small to allow the exchange of macromolecules. Also, because of the Donnan effect, water enters through these channels and causes the cell to swell and burst.

Both complement pathways have been shown to lyse bacteria, viruses, fungi, protozoa, erythrocytes, and a variety of mammalian cells by the same membrane attack mechanism; however, the susceptibility of these targets to lysis varies from the vulnerability of erythrocytes that can be destroyed by a "single hit" to the complete resistance of other cells despite the activation of multiple complement sites on their surfaces. This difference may reflect cellular repair mechanisms or the lack of binding sites for late components in the cascade. Also, membrane modulation, wherein antibody alters the distribution of surface antigens into arrangements that prevent complement attachment or cause their shedding before complement activation occurs, has been proposed as one means by which tumor cells escape destruction by specific antibodies.[105]

Due to its unique properties, the complement cascade provides a highly integrated system that capitalizes on the immune recognition provided by antibody to mediate cell lysis. This system also provides for the activation of nonspecific inflammatory mechanisms through reactions that are regulated by feedback controls; thus, both the localization and the extent of inflammation are appropriate for the insult evoked by the foreign pathogen.

Complement deficiency rarely is seen in humans. Only 140 cases of hereditary complement deficiency diseases have been reported in the literature, and none involved the alternate pathway (Table 11.11). The heritable disorders of the C1q, C1r, C1s, C4, and C2 components usually are not manifested by increased

susceptibility to bacterial infections, because the alternate pathway remains functional. However, all of these patients have displayed systemic lupus erythematosus or similar syndromes, and it has been suggested that this could reflect an underlying chronic viral infection. Three cases of C3 deficiency have been described in humans, and each was complicated by severe and recurrent bacterial infections as would be expected from disruption of the final common pathway of complement activation.[105] Some 24 cases of variable deficiencies in the C5 through C9 components have been studied, but only a few exhibited clinical manifestations that are associated with autoimmune diseases. Patients lacking C6 through C8 are of particular interest, because at least half suffered from repeated *Neisseria* infections that caused gonorrhea and meningitis.[106] Such findings suggest that the lytic activity of complement may be particularly important in the defense of human hosts against these bacterial strains.

In normal individuals, the control mechanisms provided by serum inhibitors, rapid decay, and limited diffusion of the activated complement components are quite effective. Because of this, the regulatory system carries out its normal functions of amplifying inflammation induced by immune complexes or activators of the alternate pathway in virtually all clinical settings where complement has been implicated in disease pathogenesis.

The diseases of the immune complex produce a variety of clinical manifestations depending on the particular clearance system affected when the complement system is activated. In most instances, antigen–antibody complexes are removed rapidly by phagocytic macrophages in the liver, lung, and spleen; however,

TABLE 11.11.   Inherited Disorders of the Complement System

Deficiency	Clinical Manifestation
C1q	Immunodeficiency and hypogammaglobulinemia
C1r	Systemic lupus erythematosus and glomerulonephritis
C4	Systemic lupus erythematosus
C2	Systemic lupus erythematosus, glomerulonephritis, and Henoch-Schönlein purpura
C3	Repeated infections with pyogenic bacteria
C5	Systemic lupus erythematosus and pyogenic infections
C6	Repeated infections with *Neisseria* species
C7	Raynaud phenomenon and infections with *Neisseria* species
C8	Systemic lupus erythematosus and repeated infections with *Neisseria* species
C1 inactivator	Hereditary angioneurotic edema

Source: Anderson and Anderson 1984[2]

chronic infections or repeated exposures to some antigens can result in the deposition of circulating complexes within renal glomeruli. It still is uncertain whether this localization results from the binding of complexes to the C3 receptors that are known to be present at this site or from simple mechanical sieving effects that cause the complexes to lodge in the basement membrane. In other situations, complexes of IgA and complement are deposited in the glomerular mesangium, but the antigens and mechanisms responsible for this localization pattern are unknown. It is possible to demonstrate circulating immune complexes in the blood of these patients by means of binding assays with radiolabelled C1q, but their serum complement levels may be normal, low, or even elevated as the synthesis of complement proteins is increased markedly by inflammation.

The hemolytic anemia induced by IgM antibodies (cold agglutinins) provides another prototype for involvement of the classic complement pathway in human disease. In such anemias, the IgM antibodies and complement combine with the C3b receptors on erythrocytes, causing the red cells to adhere to Kupffer cells within hepatic sinusoids. However, in contrast to IgG antibodies, this IgM binding does not provide an effective stimulus for phagocytosis, and it permits C3b inactivation by serum enzymes to release erythrocytes coated with C3d (Coombs-positive cells) back into the circulation. These cells are less likely to be damaged and gradually become protected from immune destruction as the cycle is repeated and more surface sites become saturated with C3d.

Hereditary angioneurotic edema is the best-known example of an inherited disorder that involves complement activation by the classic pathway. In this autosomal recessive disease, patients experience recurrent episodes of erythema marginatum rheumaticum, edema, and abdominal pain with clinical signs suggestive of peritonitis, and radiologic examination of the upper gastrointestinal tract may reveal edematous folds in the intestines. These folds appear to produce pain by stretching visceral surfaces, but there rarely is progression to frank necrosis. Such patients have low serum levels of the C1 inhibitor that normally participates in regulating the activation of the complement, kinin, and clotting systems; because this is a recessive trait, it generally is believed these low levels of C1 inhibitor result from the inheritance of one gene coding for a normal product and another coding for a nonfunctional protein. The resulting low levels of inhibitor permit uncontrolled consumption of the first complement components (yielding low C4 and C2 levels), but other regulators rapidly inactivate the final pathway so that patients maintain normal levels of C3 during severe attacks. These episodic bouts of pain and swelling do not respond to epinephrine therapy, but the entire symptom complex can be controlled by treatment with androgens, which appear to augment synthesis of the functional inhibitor coded for by the single normal gene.

The alternate complement pathway may be activated and contribute to human diseases by several different mechanisms. Paroxysmal nocturnal hemoglobinuria appears to result from the development of an abnormal clone of erythroid precursors in the bone marrow, which express membrane abnormalities capable of inducing cell lysis by activating the alternate pathway; because this membrane defect arises in the pluripotent stem cell, the clonal progeny of platelets and leukocytes are sensitive to damage by complement as well. The biochemical defect appears to be an abnormality that involves the glycosyl-phosphatidylinositol-membrane anchoring of the proteins responsible for modulating the effects of complement,[107] and it should be emphasized that these patients do not exhibit detectable changes in the circulating levels of C3. Overwhelming bacterial septicemia and the extracorporeal circulation of blood through the membrane oxygenators used in bypass surgery also can activate the alternate complement pathway, and for reasons that are not understood, the C5a generated by these reactions causes both bacteria and leukocytes to sequester within the pulmonary vasculature. Infections with some streptococcal strains result in the formation of autoantibodies directed against determinants on the B_bC3b complex, which causes uncontrolled activation of the alternate pathway (nephritogenic factor) and results in the depletion of serum C3 levels and the lodging of activated complement components in the kidney where they produce glomerulonephritis. Because C4 levels are normal in such patients, laboratory findings can be useful in differentiating this disease from the nephritis produced by circulating immune complexes where both C3 and C4 levels are depressed.

Mediators of Cellular Immunity

Generally, it is agreed that cell-mediated immunity plays important roles in the host defense against mycobacterial and fungal infections, chemically modified somatic cells, viral-infected cells, allografts, and malignant cells expressing tumor antigens. This system provides for both specific recognition of the foreign agent by immune T lymphocytes as well as the elaboration and activation of a variety of nonspecific factors that collaborate in destroying the inciting pathogen. Because of the close similarities and functional overlap between the mediators of cellular and humoral immunity, some effector responses are carried out by macrophages and B lymphocytes.

Antigen-driven proliferation of T lymphocytes generates two different populations of effector cells; in addition to providing helper effects during evolving immune responses, T cells expressing the Ly1$^+$ phenotype (T4$^+$ in humans) mature into effector lymphocytes capable of secreting soluble factors (lymphokines) that help mediate cellular immunity. The T-lymphocyte subpopulations that bear CD8 surface markers (T8$^+$ in humans) cause direct target cell lysis. These effector cells are mobilized from lymphatic tissues but do not recirculate; instead, they appear to leave the circulation at random to enter peripheral tissues and sites of inflammation. If they encounter the appropriate antigen during this random migration, the T cells cooperate to produce lysis of the offending agent, and this response is amplified when the CD4$^+$ lymphocytes secrete lymphokines that cause circulating leukocytes to marginate along the surfaces of adjacent blood vessels and establish chemotactic gradients that direct the migration of leukocytes into the inflammatory site. Other lymphokines appear to arrest the migration of macrophages at this site and enhance their phagocytic, bactericidal, and killer properties. This can be combined with a similar activation of B lymphocytes in the area, thus yielding a typical delayed-type hypersensitivity response where the vast majority of the infiltrating cells lack immunologic specificity.

From in vitro models of this reaction, it now is generally agreed that when CD4$^+$ lymphocytes engage specific antigens or immune response gene determinants on a target cell surface, these lymphocytes are triggered to secrete several discrete polypeptides that produce the inflammatory effects described.[108] These mediators are characterized best by means of descriptive terms related to their various biologic activities. It still is uncertain how many distinct mediators are involved in these cellular immune reactions; however, lymphokine production is not restricted to T lymphocytes expressing the CD4$^+$ marker. Convincing evidence exists that B cells elaborate identical factors when they are activated by antigen–antibody complexes,[109] and in some settings, B lymphocytes may be the prime mediators of cellular immune responses.

The properties of some of the better characterized lymphokines can be summarized briefly.[110] For instance, macrophage chemotactic factor (12,500 MW) is a heat-stable polypeptide elaborated by immune lymphocytes that is selectively chemotactic for both monocytes and macrophages. This agent produces chemotactic effects by combining with macrophage surface receptors that are different from those binding other chemoattractants such as C5a and the formyltripeptides. Sensitized lymphocytes reacting with antigen also secrete slightly different proteins (25,000 to 50,000 MW), which are selectively chemotactic for eosinophils and

basophils, and these chemoattractants are thought to contribute to the inflammatory response in cutaneous basophilic hypersensitivity reactions.

Migration inhibition factor, a protein of 65,000 MW, alters macrophage surfaces, thus causing increased intercellular surface adhesion. Although this process impedes cellular locomotion for several hours, it is fully reversible; after 24 hours, the cells may resume normal or increased rates of motility.

Macrophage activation factors (Table 11.2) are a poorly defined mixture of substances, including monocyte-macrophage colony-stimulating factor, migration inhibition factor and interferon-γ, that appear to convert normal macrophages into killer cells with enhanced bactericidal and tumoricidal activities. The precise mechanisms responsible for these changes (which may take several days to appear) still are unknown, but the activated macrophages show increased metabolic activities, rapid spontaneous motility, as well as increased adherence and spreading on glasses surfaces. These factors are believed to play an important role in augmenting nonspecific host resistance to tumors, and they may be similar to the osteoclast-activating factor secreted by lymphocytes that increases both the number and activity of the specialized macrophage population (osteoclasts) that is engaged in bone resorption. Some of these actions are also mediated by interferon-α, -β, and -γ.

After challenge with antigen, sensitized lymphocytes also have been found to release mitogenic factor (20,000 MW), which induces nonsensitized lymphocytes to divide and elaborate lymphokines. This nonspecific recruitment appears analogous to that produced by the plant lectins, and it probably plays an important role in the amplification of all delayed-type hypersensitivity reactions where dividing cells are found within the local lesions. Stimulated lymphocytes also produce interferon-γ that may contribute to host defense against the spread of viral infections.

Immune T lymphocytes lyse target cells by two distinct mechanisms that are independent of the complement system (Fig. 11.13).[111] When CD4$^+$ effector cells engage specific antigens, they secrete a protein (45,000 MW) that causes slow and nonspecific lysis of nonlymphoid cells in the immediate microenvironment. Although lymphotoxin appears to be a relatively weak cytotoxic agent in its own right, this factor greatly enhances and accelerates the direct target cell lysis mediated by CD8$^+$ cytotoxic T-lymphocytes, and because rapid diffusion or inactivation limits the cytotoxic effects of lymphotoxin to relatively short ranges, it has been suggested that interactions between immune response gene products may concentrate helper T-lymphocytes either on or near the target cell surface. Such cell surface interactions probably resemble those in-

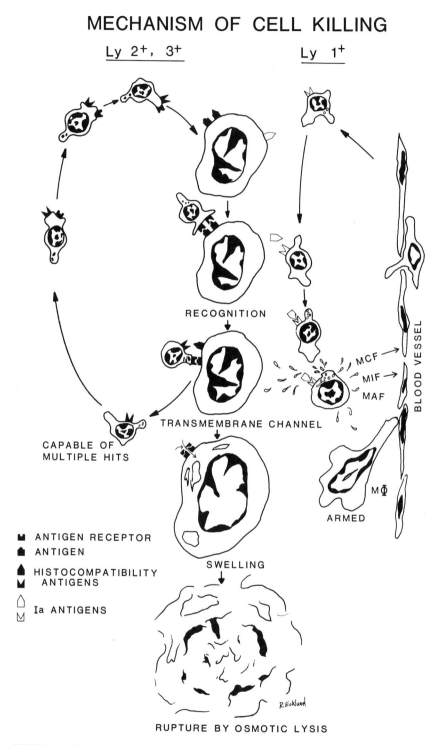

MECHANISM OF CELL KILLING

Ly 2$^+$, 3$^+$ Ly 1$^+$

RECOGNITION

TRANSMEMBRANE CHANNEL

CAPABLE OF
MULTIPLE HITS

MCF
MIF
MAF

BLOOD VESSEL

MΦ

ARMED

■ ANTIGEN RECEPTOR
◆ ANTIGEN
◆ HISTOCOMPATIBILITY
◹ ANTIGENS
◻ Ia ANTIGENS

SWELLING

R. Ecklund

RUPTURE BY OSMOTIC LYSIS

**FIGURE 11.13.   Postulated mechanisms by which T lymphocytes mediate target cell
lysis.** *Note:* **MAF = macrophage-activating factor; MCF = macrophage
chemotactic factor; MIF = macrophage-inhibiting factor.** *Source:*
Anderson and Anderson 1984[2]

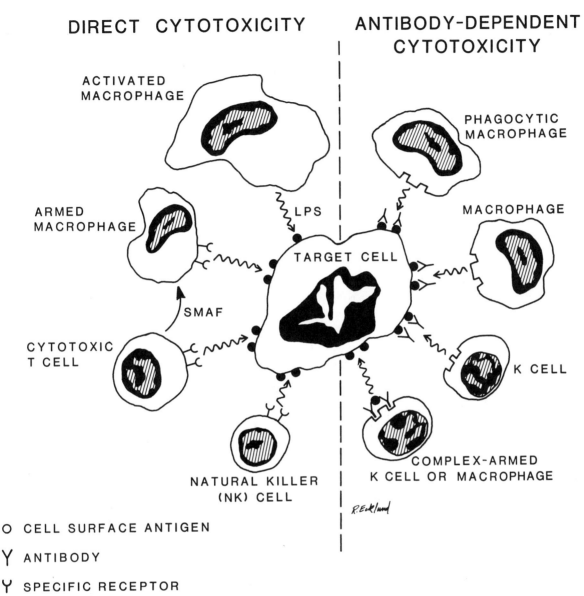

DIRECT CYTOTOXICITY

ANTIBODY-DEPENDENT CYTOTOXICITY

ACTIVATED MACROPHAGE

PHAGOCYTIC MACROPHAGE

ARMED MACROPHAGE

LPS

TARGET CELL

MACROPHAGE

SMAF

CYTOTOXIC T CELL

K CELL

NATURAL KILLER (NK) CELL

COMPLEX-ARMED K CELL OR MACROPHAGE

R. Ecklund

O CELL SURFACE ANTIGEN

Y ANTIBODY

Y SPECIFIC RECEPTOR

⊔ Fc RECEPTOR

FIGURE 11.14. **Proposed mechanisms for the induction of cell-mediated cytotoxicity.** *Note:* **LPS = bacterial lipopolysaccharide (endotoxin); SMAF = specific macrophage arming factor.** *Source:* **Anderson and Anderson 1984[2]**

volved in the helper-cell effects, and they do not require identity between other membrane determinants encoded within the major histocompatibility locus.

The direct target cell lysis mediated by CD8[+] immune lymphocytes requires intimate contact between the membranes of both cell types. Because convincing evidence exists that these membrane interactions require

both cells to express the same surface antigens coded by the major histocompatibility locus,[112] lymphocytolysis appears to have evolved as a defense mechanism designed specifically to eradicate virally infected, chemically modified, or malignant cells that arise within the host. Current concepts hold that T-cell killing requires "dual recognition" in which the CD8[+] lymphocytes must bind to two distinct determinants expressed on the target cell membrane (i.e., histocompatibility and viral antigens); in this system, sharing of the immune response region gene products that are necessary for other cellular interactions is insufficient to promote target cell lysis.[29]

The exact mechanisms by which cytotoxic lymphocytes mediate target cell lysis still are controversial; this killing mechanism cannot be attributed to antibody, complement, or lymphotoxin bound to the lymphocyte surface. Evidence indicates that membrane recognition results in the exposure of special hydrophobic peptides on the killer cell surface,[113] and during intercellular contact, these are believed to be inserted into adjacent segments of the target cell membrane, where they form ion channels and cause cell swelling and rupture analogous to that produced by complement. Continued intercellular contact is not required after the membrane channels are formed, so the cytotoxic lymphocytes can move away and engage other target cells in repetitive cycles of recognition, attachment, and lysis.

Other Forms of Cell-Mediated Cytotoxicity

Other cell types use a variety of mechanisms to induce target cell lysis. Macrophages, B lymphocytes, and small mononuclear cells that cannot be classified readily as either lymphocytes or monocytes (natural killer and killer cells) possess surface receptors for immunoglobulin,[114] and when specific antibody binds to these receptors, the cells become "armed" with a specific immunologic recognition mechanism that permits them to interact with target cells bearing the appropriate antigenic determinants. Conversely, antibodies may bind directly with antigens on the target cell membrane, exposing Fc portions of the immunoglobulin molecules at these sites; this exposure permits all three cell types to interact with the antibody-coated target cells. Both events can culminate in target cell destruction without assistance from the complement system (Fig. 11.14).[115] Macrophages destroy the targets through the combined effects of phagocytosis and lysosomal enzyme secretion, and B lymphocytes and killer cells probably cause cell lysis by creating transmembrane channels. Together, these forms of target cell destruction have been classified as antibody-dependent, cell-mediated cytotoxicity (ADCC).

A few nonlymphoid cells are capable of causing direct cytotoxicity in the absence of antibody; the best known examples are the macrophages that become activated by exposure to lymphokines, endotoxin, and adjuvants. In addition to their increased metabolism and motility, these cells show enhanced bactericidal activities as well

as a unique ability to destroy tumor cells yet spare normal somatic cells. The mechanisms responsible for this selective recognition and tumor killing are unknown despite numerous attempts to use this phenomenon in the adjuvant therapy of human malignancies. In other settings, cytotoxic T lymphocytes may shed their surface receptors for antigen, and these can be absorbed onto the macrophage surfaces to provide such cells with a specific recognition mechanism that allows them to engage and destroy target cells.

Another small, mononuclear cell of unknown lineage that bears Fc surface receptors may be an exceedingly important defense mechanism against malignant disease.[116] When isolated from normal animals and humans, these cells have been shown to lyse virtually all tumor lines and viral-infected cells in tissue culture without producing any detectable alterations in the normal cells. The mechanisms by which these "natural killer cells" both recognize and destroy the various target cell populations are still unknown. The natural killer cells are distributed in the blood, spleen, and lymph nodes, but they rarely are found in the bone marrow and thymus.[117] They have been ascribed various functions in immunosurveillance against tumor cells, protection against viral infections, regulation of hematopoiesis, and mediation in the rejection of bone marrow allografts. Of particular interest are reports that the activity of these cells is greatly increased by viral infections, immunization with bacille Calmette-Guérin and *Corynebacterium parvum* organisms, and interferon therapy,[118] and because interferon has been reported to be useful in eradicating solid tumors in animals, there are strong suspicions this antitumor effect may be mediated by natural killer cells. If this proves correct, then future immunotherapy for tumors may allow the manipulation of this cell population.

REFERENCES

1. Rosen FS, Cooper MD, Wedgwood RJP. Primary immunodeficiencies, I and II. N Engl J Med 1984;311:235–42,300–10.
2. Anderson ND, Anderson AO. Lymphocytes. In: Spivak JL, ed. Fundamentals of Clinical Hematology, 2nd Ed. Philadelphia: Harper & Row, 1984:175–220.
3. Weiss L. The Cells and Tissues of the Immune System: Structure, Functions, Interactions. Englewood Cliffs, NJ: Prentice-Hall, 1972.
4. Mosier DE, Cohen PL. Ontogeny of mouse T-lymphocyte functions. Fed Proc 1975;34:137.
5. Rheinherz EL, Kung PC, Goldstein G, et al. Discrete stages of human intrathymic differentiation: analysis of normal thymocytes and leukemic lymphoblasts of T-cell lineage. Proc Natl Acad Sci U S A 1980;77:1588–92.
6. Metcalf D. The nature and regulation of lymphopoiesis in the normal and neoplastic thymus. In: Wolstenholme GEW, Porter

R, eds. Ciba Foundation Symposium on the Thymus: Experimental and Clinical Studies. Boston: Little, Brown and Co., 1966:242.

7. Osoba D, Miller JFAP. The lymphoid tissues and immune response of neonatally thymectomized mice bearing thymic tissues in Millipore diffusion chambers. J Exp Med 1964;119:117.

8. Weissman IL. Differentiation of thymus cells. Fed Proc 1975;34:141.

9. Trainin N. Thymic hormones and the immune response. Physiol Rev 1974;54:272.

10. Trainin N, Pecht M, Handzel ZT. Thymic hormones: inducers and regulators of the T-cell system. Immunol Today 1983;4:16–21.

11. Schrader JW. Peptide regulatory factors and optimization of vaccines. Mol Immunol 1991;28:295–9.

12. Miller RG, Phillips RA. Development of B-lymphocytes. Fed Proc 1975;34:145.

13. Triplett EL. On the mechanism of immunologic self-recognition. J Immunol 1962;89:505.

14. Watson JD. The origins of lymphocyte diversity. Cold Spring Harbor Symp Quant Biol 1977:41.

15. Gowans JL, Knight EJ. The route of a re-circulation of lymphocytes in the rat. Proc R Soc Biol 1964;159:257.

16. Frost P, Lance EM. The cellular origin of the lymphocyte trap. Immunology 1974;26:175.

17. Marchalonis JJ. The Lymphocyte: Structure and Function. New York: Marcel Dekker, 1977.

18. McCaffrey R, Lilquist A, Sallan S, et al. Clinical utility of leukemia cell terminal transferase measurements. Cancer Res 1981;41:4814–20.

19. Spry CJF. Inhibition of lymphocyte recirculation by stress and corticotropin. Cell Immunol 1972;4:86.

20. Stobo JD. Phytohemagglutinin and concanavalin A: probes for murine "T" cell activation and differentiation. Transplant Rev 1972;11:60.

21. Loor F. Structure and dynamics of the lymphocyte surface in relation to differentiation, recognition and activation. Prog Allergy 1977;23:1.

22. Katz DH, ed. Lymphocyte Differentiation, Recognition and Regulation. New York: Academic Press, 1977.

23. Reinherz EL, Meur SC, Schlossman SF. The delineation of antigen receptors on human T-lymphocytes. Immunol Today 1983;4:5–8.

24. Ruscetti FW, Gallo RC. Human T-cell growth factor: regulation of growth and function of T-lymphocytes. Blood 1981;57:379–94.

25. Ward PA, Offen CD, Montgomery JR. Chemoattractants for leukocytes, with special reference to lymphocytes. Fed Proc 1971;30:1721.

26. Schreiber SL. Chemistry and biology of the immunophilins and their immunosuppressive ligands. Science 1991;251:283.

27. Tutschka PJ, Benchorner WE, Allison AE, et al. Use of cyclosporin A in allogeneic bone marrow transplants in the rat. Nature 1979;280:148.

28. Nonspecific immunosuppression-immunosuppressive drugs: cyclosporin A. Transplant Proc 1983;15:433–556.

29. The Canadian Multicenter Transplant Study Group. A randomized clinical trial of cyclosporine in cadaveric renal transplantation. N Engl J Med 1983;309:809–15.

30. Levitt HO, ed. Ir Genes and Ia Antigens. New York: Academic Press, 1978.

31. Feldman M. Current concepts of the antibody response: heterogeneity of lymphoid cells, interactions and factors. Cold Spring Harbor Symp Quant Biol 1976;41:113.

32. Jerne NK. The Immune System: A Web of V-Domains. Harvey Lectures, Series 70. New York: Academic Press, 1976.

33. Richter PH. A network theory of the immune system. Eur J Immunol 1975;5:350.

34. Bona CA, Pernia B. Idiotypic networks. In: Paul WE, ed. Fundamental Immunology. New York: Raven Press, 1984:577–92.

35. Diener ED, Feldman M. Relationship between antigen and antibody-induced suppression of immunity. Transplant Rev 1972;8:76.

36. Hellstrom KE, Hellstrom I. Lymphocyte-mediated cytotoxicity and blocking serum activity to tumor antigens. Adv Immunol 1974;18:209.

37. Baldwin RW, Price MR. Tumor antigens and tumor-host relationships. Annu Rev Med 1976;27:151.

38. Tadkuma T, Pierce CW. Mode of action of a soluble immune response suppressor (SIRS) produced by concanavalin A activated spleen cells. J Immunol 1978;120:481.

39. Waldman TA, Broder S, Blaese RM, et al. Role of suppressor T-cells in pathogenesis of common variable hypogammaglobulinemia. Lancet 1974;ii:609.

40. Goodwin JS, Messner RP, Bankhurst AD, et al. Prostaglandin-producing suppressor cells in Hodgkin's disease. N Engl J Med 1977;297:963.

41. Vyas GN, Stiles DP, Brecher G, eds. Laboratory Diagnosis of Immunologic Disorders. New York: Grune & Stratton, 1975.

42. Aisenberg AC. Cell lineage in lymphoproliferative disease. Am J Med 1983;74:680.

43. Rowlands DT, Danielle RP. Surface receptors in the immune response. N Engl J Med 1975;293:26–32.

44. Marchalonis JJ. Lymphocyte surface immunoglobulins. Science 1975;190:20.

45. Cooper MD. Pre-B cells: normal and abnormal development. J Clin Immunol 1981;1:81–9.

46. Miller RA, Maloney DG, Warnke R, et al. Treatment of B-cell lymphoma with monoclonal anti-idiotype antibody. N Engl J Med 1982;306:517–22.

47. Melamed MR, Mullaney PF, Mendelsohn, ML, eds. Flow Cytometry and Sorting. New York: John Wiley & Sons, 1979.

48. Leavitt RD. Biological Markers of Differentiation in the Diagnosis of Leukemia and Lymphoma. In: Comprehensive Textbook of Oncology. Baltimore: Williams and Wilkins, 1986.

49. Ligler FS, Smith RB, Kettman JR, et al. Detection of tumor cells in the peripheral blood of nonleukemic patients with B-cell lymphoma: analysis of "clonal excess." Blood 1980;55:792–801.

50. Schiffman E, Corcoran BA, Wahl SM. N-Formylmethionyl peptides as chemoattractants for leucocytes. Proc Natl Acad Sci U S A 1975;72:1059.

51. Leonard WJ, Depper JM, Uchiyama T, et al. A monoclonal antibody that appears to recognize the receptor for human T-cell growth factor: partial characterization of the receptor. Nature 1982;300:267–9.

52. Jondal M, Klein G. Surface markers on human B and T lymphocytes: II. Presence of Epstein-Barr virus receptors on B lymphocytes. J Exp Med 1973;138:1365.

53. Diamond BA. Monoclonal antibodies. N Engl J Med 1981;304:1345.

54. Haynes BF, Metzgar RS, Minna JD, et al. Phenotypic characterization of cutaneous T-cell lymphoma. N Engl J Med 1981;304:1319–23.

55. Koziner B, Gebhard D, Denny T, et al. Characterization of B-cell type chronic lymphocytic leukemia cells by surface markers and a monoclonal antibody. Am J Med 1982;73:802–7.

56. Dillman RO, Beauregard JC, Lea JW, et al. Chronic lymphocytic leukemia and other chronic lymphoid proliferations: surface marker phenotypes and clinical correlations. J Clin Oncol 1983;1:190–7.

57. Woodruff JJ, Woodruff JF. Virus-induced alterations of lym-

phoid tissues: IV. The effect of Newcastle disease virus on the fate of radiolabeled thoracic-duct lymphocytes. Cell Immunol 1974;10:78.

58. Woodruff JJ, Gesner BM. The effect of neuraminidase on the fate of transfused lymphocytes. J Exp Med 1969;129:551.

59. Hoeprich PF, ed. Infectious Diseases: A Modern Treatise of Infectious Processes, 2nd Ed. New York: Harper & Row, 1977.

60. Fish J. Supplemental report on the thoracic-duct drainage for immunosuppression. Transplant Proc 1972;4:467.

61. Gottlieb MS, Groppman JE, Weinstein WM, et al. The acquired immunodeficiency syndrome. Ann Intern Med 1983;99:208–20.

62. Ziegler JL, Beckstead JA, Volberding PA, et al. Non-Hodgkin's lymphoma in 90 homosexual men: relation to generalized lymphadenopathy and the acquired immunodeficiency syndrome. N Engl J Med 1984;311:565–70.

63. Leavitt RD. Searching for the cause of acquired immune deficiency syndrome. Eur J Clin Microbiol 1984;3:79–84.

64. Popavic M, Sarngadharan MG, Read E, et al. Detection, isolation, and continuous production of cytopathic retroviruses (HTLV-III) from patients with AIDS and pre-AIDS. Science 1984;224:497–500.

65. Klatzmann D, Barre-Sinoussi F, Nugeyre MT, et al. Selective tropism of lymphadenopathy-associated virus (LAV) for helper-induced T lymphocytes. Science 1984;225:59–63.

66. Bach JF. The Mode of Action of Immunosuppressive Agents. New York: North Holland, 1975.

67. Morse SI, Morse JH. Isolation and properties of the leukocytosis- and lymphocytosis-promoting factor of *Bordetella pertussis*. J Exp Med 1976;143:1483.

68. Bradfield JWB, Born GVR. Inhibition of lymphocyte recirculation by heparin. Nature 1969;222:1183.

69. Barthold DR, Kysela S, Steinberg AD. Decline in suppressor T-cell function with age in female NZB mice. J Immunol 1974;112:9.

70. Henle W, Henle G, Lennette ET. The Epstein-Barr virus. Sci Am 1979;241:48.

71. Jondal M, Klein G, Oldstone MBA, et al. Surface markers on human B and T lymphocytes: VII. Association between complement and Epstein-Barr virus receptors on human lymphoid cells. Scand J Immunol 1976;5:401.

72. Henle G, Henle W, Clifford P, et al. Antibodies to Epstein-Barr virus in Burkitt's lymphoma and control groups. J Natl Cancer Inst 1969;43:1147.

73. Evans AS. Infectious mononucleosis and related syndromes. Am J Med Sci 1978;276:325.

74. Horwitz CA, Henle W, Henle G, et al. Clinical and laboratory evaluation of elderly patients with heterophil antibody positive infectious mononucleosis. Am J Med 1976;61:333.

75. Cheeseman SH, Henle W, Rubin RH, et al. Epstein-Barr virus infection in renal transplant recipients. Ann Intern Med 1980;93:39.

76. Brix DL, Redfield RR, Tosato G. Defective regulation of Epstein-Barr virus infection in patients with acquired immunodeficiency syndrome (AIDS) or AIDS-related disorders. N Engl J Med 1986;314:874–9.

77. Miller G. Epstein-Barr herpesvirus and infectious mononucleosis. Prog Med Virol 1975;20:84–112.

78. Hoagland RJ. The clinical manifestations of infectious mononucleosis: a report of two hundred cases. Am J Med Sci 1960;240:20.

79. Mangi RJ, Niederman JC, Kellehei JE, et al. Depression of cell-mediated immunity during acute infectious mononucleosis. N Engl J Med 1974;291:1149.

80. DeWaele M, Thielemans C, Van Camp BKG. Characterization

of immunoregulatory T cells in EBV-induced infectious mononucleosis of monoclonal antibodies. N Engl J Med 1981;304:460.

81. Rickinson AB, Crawford D, Epstein MA. Inhibition of the *in vitro* outgrowth of Epstein-Barr virus transformed lymphocytes by thymus-dependent lymphocytes from infectious mononucleosis patients. Clin Exp Immunol 1977;28:72.

82. Henle W, Henle GE, Horwitz CA. Epstein-Barr virus specific diagnostic tests in infectious mononucleosis. Hum Pathol 1974;5:551.

83. Ginsburg CM, Henle W, Henle G, et al. Infectious mononucleosis in children. JAMA 1977;237:781.

84. Anonymous. Immunopathology of infectious mononucleosis. Lancet 1973;ii:712.

85. Horwitz CA, Burke MD, Grimes P, et al. Hepatic function in mononucleosis induced by Epstein-Barr virus and cytomegalovirus. Clin Chem 1980;26:243.

86. Cowdry SC. Hyperuricemia in infectious mononucleosis. JAMA 1966;196:319.

87. Purtilo DT, Szymanski I, Bhawan J, et al. Epstein-Barr virus infections in the X-linked recessive lymphoproliferative syndrome. Lancet 1978;i:798.

88. Sullivan JL, Byron KS, Brewster FE, et al. X-linked lymphoproliferative syndrome: natural history of the immunodeficiency. J Clin Invest 1983;71:1765–78.

89. Horwitz CA, Henle W, Henle G, et al. Heterophil-negative infectious mononucleosis and mononucleosis-like illnesses. Am J Med 1977;63:947.

90. Cooper DA, Maclean P, Finlayson R, et al. Acute AIDS retrovirus infection. Lancet 1985;i:537–40.

91. Miller G. Biology of Epstein-Barr virus. In: Klein G, ed. Viral Oncology. New York: Raven Press, 1980:713.

92. de-The G. Role of Epstein-Barr virus in human diseases: infectious mononucleosis, Burkitt's lymphoma, and nasopharyngeal carcinoma. In: Klein G, ed. Viral Oncology. New York: Raven Press, 1980:769.

93. Robinson JE, Brown N, Andman W, et al. Diffuse polyclonal B cell lymphoma during primary infection with Epstein-Barr virus. N Engl J Med 1982;302:1293.

94. Ritz J, Nadler LM, Bhan AK, et al. Expression of common acute lymphoblastic leukemia antigen (CALLA) by lymphomas of B-cell and T-cell lineage. Blood 1981;58:648–52.

95. Ritz J, Pesando JM, Notis-McConarty J, et al. Use of monoclonal antibodies as diagnostic and therapeutic reagents in acute lymphoblastic leukemia. Cancer Res 1981;41:4771–5.

96. Kersey JH. Lymphoid progenitor cells and acute lymphoblastic leukemia: studies with monoclonal antibodies. J Clin Immunol 1981;1:201–7.

97. Schroff RW, Foon KA, Billing RJ, et al. Immunologic classification of lymphocytic leukemias based on monoclonal antibody-defined cell surface antigens. Blood 1982;59:207–15.

98. Schumacher HR, Haider Y, Miller WM, et al. Terminal-deoxynucleotidyl transferase (TdT): serial observations on patients with leukemia. Am J Med Sci 1983;286:18–24.

99. Li C-Y. Immunocytochemical techniques for identifying leukemias. Mayo Clin Proc 1984;59:185–8.

100. Brusamolino E, Isernia P, Lazzarino M, et al. Clinical utility of terminal deoxynucleotidyl transferase and adenosine deaminase determinations in adult leukemia with a lymphoid phenotype. J Clin Oncol 1984;2:871–80.

101. Bernard A, Boumsell L, Reinherz EL, et al. Cell surface characterization of malignant T cell from lymphoblastic lymphoma using monoclonal antibodies: evidence for phenotypic differences between malignant T cells from patients with acute lymphoblastic leukemia and lymphoblastic lymphoma. Blood 1981;57:1105–10.

102. Koziner B, Gebhard D, Denny T, et al. Analysis of T-cell differentiation antigens in acute lymphatic leukemia using monoclonal antibodies. Blood 1982;60:752–7.

103. Bloomfield CD, Gajl-Peczalska KJ, Frizzera G, et al. Clinical utility of lymphocyte surface markers combined with the Lukes-Collins histologic classification in adult lymphoma. N Engl J Med 1979;301:512.

104. Warnke R, Miller R, Grogan T, et al. Immunologic phenotype in 30 patients with diffuse large-cell lymphoma. N Engl J Med 1980;303:293–300.

105. Nicolson GL. Transmembrane control of the receptors in normal and tumor cells: II. Surface changes associated with transformation and malignancy. Biochem Biophys Acta 1976;458:1.

106. Alper CA, Block KJ, Rosen FS. Increased susceptibility to infection in a patient with type II essential hypercatabolism of C3. N Engl J Med 1973;288:143.

107. Davitz MA, Low MG, Nussenzweig V. Release of decay-accelerating factor (DAF) from the cell membrane by phosphatidylinositol-specific phospholipase C (PIPLC). J Exp Med 1986;163:1150–61.

108. David JR. Lymphocyte mediators and delayed-type hypersensitivity. N Engl J Med 1973;288:143.

109. Vyas GN, Stites DP, Brecher G, eds. Laboratory Diagnosis of Immunologic Disorders. New York: Grune & Stratton, 1975.

110. David JR, David RR. Cellular hypersensitivity and immunity: inhibition of macrophage migration and the lymphocyte mediators. Prog Allergy 1972;116:300.

111. Gately MK, Mayer MM, Henrey CS. Effect of antilymphotoxin in cell-mediated cytotoxicity: evidence of two pathways, one involving lymphotoxin and the other requiring intimate contact between the plasma membranes of killer and target cells. Cell Immunol 1976;27:82.

112. Doherty PC, Blanden RV, Zinkernagel RM. Specificity of virus-immune effector T-cells for H-2 K or H2D compatible interactions: implications for H-antigen diversity. Transplant Rev 1976;29:89.

113. Mayer MM. Mechanism of cytolysis by lymphocytes: a comparison with complement. J Immunol 1977;119:1195.

114. Perlman P. Cellular immunity: antibody-dependent cytotoxicity (K cell activity). Clin Immunobiol 1976;3:107.

115. Miller JL, Humphreys RE, Mann DL. Lack of association of human "B cell" antigens and FC receptor activity of antibody-dependent cytotoxic lymphocytes. J Immunol 1976;117:491.

116. Herberman RB, Holden HT. Natural cell-mediated immunity. Adv Cancer Res 1978;27:305.

117. Kiessling R, Wigzell H. An analysis of the murine NK cell as to structure, function, and biological relevance. Immunol Rev 1979;44:165.

118. Djeu JY, Heinbaugh JA, Holden HT, et al. Role of macrophages in the augmentation of mouse natural killer cell activity by poly I:C and interferon. J Immunol 1979;122:182.

12

The Spleen

Edward R. Eichner, M.D.

The spleen has long intrigued mankind. Hippocrates detailed its anatomy in 421 B.C., yet 600 years later and reflecting his times, Galen called it the organ of mystery. No longer the organ of mystery, the spleen is today the organ of paradox: it is expendable, yet its absence can predispose to fatal infection.

What, then, is the function of the spleen? Simply put, the spleen is the key filter of the blood and a "lymph gland" of the bloodstream. The unique circulation of the spleen makes it a sophisticated filter, and its meshwork of macrophages and lymphocytes enables it to initiate the immune response to blood-borne bacteria or other particulate antigens that it traps.

PHYSIOLOGY

Six vital functions of the spleen are:

1. clearance of microorganisms and particulate antigens;
2. synthesis of immunoglobulin, tuftsin, and properdin;
3. embryonic and extramedullary hematopoiesis;
4. providing a "training camp" for reticulocytes;
5. destruction of effete or abnormal red blood cells; and
6. removal of antigen–antibody complexes.

The unique circulation of the spleen makes it the main site for clearance of poorly opsonized microorganisms and the initial site for synthesis of specific IgM antibody. The liver clears the bulk of well-opsonized bacteria from the blood, but the spleen, a more elegant filter,

is more efficient in removing poorly opsonized bacteria (Fig. 12.1).[1]

An experiment in rabbits with plastic microspheres too large to pass through the pores in the venous sinuses proved the fundamental anatomic point that underlies the singular splenic microcirculation: only 10% of blood in the arterial capillaries empties directly into venous sinuses. Ninety percent of the blood entering the spleen is dumped into the "open circulation" of the red pulp and then forced into the sinuses. This means the blood cells and other particles contained in the blood are required to percolate along the fine meshwork of the splenic cords, until they can squeeze through tiny 0.5 to 2.5 μm pores between endothelial cells that line the walls of the venous sinuses, enter the venous circulation, and leave the spleen. This meandering microcirculation allows time for splenic phagocytes to remove even poorly opsonized bacteria.[2]

The microcirculation of the spleen also facilitates the immune response to intravenous particulate antigens. When blood enters the spleen, the soluble antigens are skimmed off, with much of the plasma, to enter the right-angled arterioles that supply the germinal centers of the white pulp, but the particulate antigens first lodge in the red pulp and are transported across the marginal zone into the germinal center where IgM antibody response begins. When the splenic microcirculation is impaired, as in sickle cell anemia, or when the spleen has been removed, the antibody response to intravenous antigen is blunted and serum IgM levels fall.[3]

Tuftsin and properdin, two plasma proteins that serve as opsonins and fall in concentration after splenectomy, are synthesized in the spleen. For example, children

221

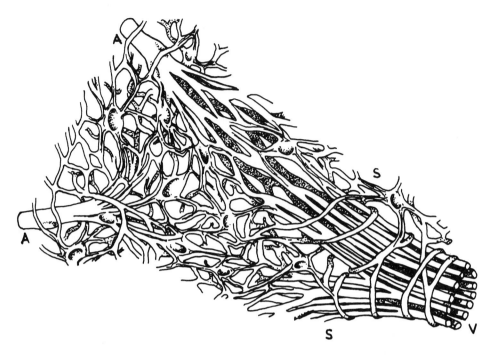

FIGURE 12.1.   A diagrammatic representation of the structure of the spleen. Blood enters the spleen by way of the arterioles or small arteries (*A*) and then flows into the sinuses (*S*), which form a mesh of vascular spaces. Blood cells pass slowly through the sinuses and enter the veins (*V*) through the slits between the endothelial (vascular lining) cells of the venous walls. The blood then drains from the spleen by way of the splenic veins (*V*). *Source:* Eichner 1989[39]

with sickle cell anemia have subnormal levels of properdin and abnormal alternate pathway activity, thus impairing their opsonization of pneumococci and placing them at risk for fatal pneumococcemia; however, normal children after splenectomy have normal pneumococcal serum opsonizing activity. While partial deficiencies of tuftsin and properdin may be minor risk factors after splenectomy or in functional asplenia, it seems likely that the integrity of the singular microcirculation of the spleen is crucial to the survival of the nonimmune patient with pneumococcemia.[4]

The spleen also carries out hematopoiesis in utero, and in a classic example of the dictum that ontogeny recapitulates phylogeny, the human fetus produces blood cells in numerous extramedullary sites that in lower vertebrates remain organs of hematopoiesis. At 5-months' gestation, however, the human switches to strictly medullary hematopoiesis and shuts down synthesis in extramedullary locations such as the spleen, presumably because the microenvironment ("soil") changes. These sites of embryonic hematopoiesis do become active again in agnogenic myeloid metaplasia, but the reasons for this are unclear at present.

The spleen is a major site for clearance of immune complexes, and impairment of splenic removal of heat-damaged or IgG-sensitized red cells labelled with chromium 51 has been shown in patients with active systemic lupus erythematosus, rheumatoid arthritis, Goodpasture syndrome, and other vasculitides. This defect in reticuloendothelial function is thought to be caused by the saturation of the splenic macrophage Fc receptors by immune complexes and can be reversed by plasma exchange, which removes enough immune complexes to "unblock" the reticuloendothelial blockade. A general defect in splenic function, however, is not a universal feature of active lupus. One group of investigators studying patients with lupus and without clinical nephritis found normal splenic function in most, despite high titers of circulating immune complexes. This area undoubtedly will receive more attention in the near future.[5,6]

The sophisticated splenic filter, which receives 5% of the blood volume per minute, makes the spleen a "training camp" for reticulocytes, which the spleen retains (Fig. 12.2). During their sojourn in the spleen, these cells are molded, pitted, and if abnormal, culled

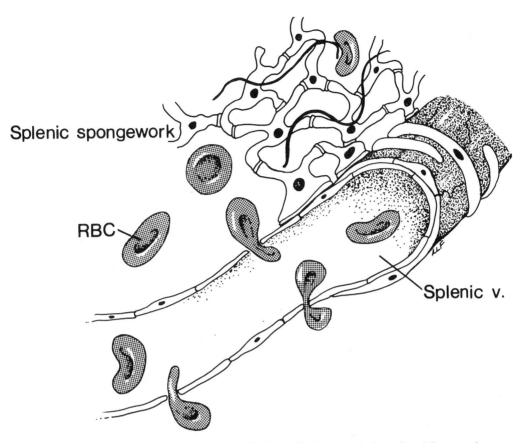

Splenic spongework

RBC

Splenic v.

FIGURE 12.2. **A schematic representation of red blood cells leaving the splenic meshwork by squeezing between endothelial cells of the splenic veins' walls.** *Source:* **Eichner 1989**[39]

out. The spleen also reduces the membrane surface area by one third, which converts red cells from targets into biconcave disks. It removes surface craters, pits from normal red cells, any Howell-Jolly bodies (nuclear remnants), Heinz bodies (denatured hemoglobin), or Pappenheimer bodies (iron granules), and culls out any acanthocytes (spur cells) that may be present. The new red cells, now free of debris, are then released from the spleen and possess the necessary deformability to circulate the microvasculature for 4 months.

These normal splenic functions enable the spleen to remove senescent or abnormal blood cells. Spherocytes, fixed sickled cells, and hemoglobin C cells are too rigid to pass through the splenic pores easily, and any blood cell coated with IgG antibody is attacked and often destroyed by splenic macrophages with Fc surface receptors. For this reason, the spleen is the predominant organ of cell destruction in autoimmune hemolytic anemia, autoimmune thrombocytopenic purpura, and probably Felty syndrome as well. The spleen also is able to remove parasites, such as the malarial organism, from red cells.

Is the spleen a reservoir? In many mammals, the answer is yes. When a horse races, for example, its spleen contracts to provide a timely autotransfusion; similarly, the Weddell seal can dive underwater for an hour because its spleen stores gallons of blood and ejects oxygen-rich red cells during the dive. In humans, however, the spleen is hardly a reservoir. The normal human spleen holds only about 50 ml of blood (20 ml of packed red cells), or only 1% of the total blood volume. Accordingly, although recent research showed that the human spleen does contract during all-out exercise and owing to a surge in adrenalin,[7] it ejects negligible numbers of red and white cells in the process. In contrast, the normal spleen holds 30% of the circulating mass of platelets at any given time, so splenic release of pooled platelets contributes to the thrombocytosis seen transiently after exercise.

SPLENOMEGALY

The size of the spleen is not always a reliable guide to splenic function. Likewise, palpable spleens are not

TABLE 12.1. The Mechanisms of Splenomegaly

Mechanism	Common Examples
Work hypertrophy	
Immune response	Subacute bacterial endocarditis, infectious mononucleosis, Felty syndrome
Red cell destruction	Spherocytosis, thalassemia major
Venous congestion	Cirrhosis, splenic vein thrombosis
Myeloproliferation	Chronic myelocytic leukemia, myeloid metaplasia
Infiltration	Sarcoidosis, amyloidosis, Gaucher disease
Neoplasia	Lymphoma, chronic lymphocytic leukemia, metastatic cancer
Miscellaneous causes	Cysts, hemangiomas, arteriovenous malformations

always abnormal, and abnormal spleens are not always palpable. Patients with low diaphragms have palpable but normal-sized spleens, as do 3% of healthy first-year college students and almost 5% of hospitalized patients.[8,9] In contrast, clinical splenomegaly is noted rarely in idiopathic (autoimmune) thrombocytopenic purpura despite the avid destruction of antibody-coated platelets by the spleen.

What is the best bedside maneuver to gauge the size of the spleen? Recently, the clinical assessment of splenomegaly was studied in 118 hospitalized patients who underwent ultrasound testing.[10] Forty-three had splenomegaly, and 75 did not. The optimal process seemed to be percussing Traube semilunar space for dullness and palpating for splenomegaly in the supine or right lateral decubitus position. (Traube space is defined here as the area delineated superiorly by the sixth rib, laterally by the midaxillary line, and inferiorly by the left costal margin.)

In that study, the percussion of Traube space for the "splenic dullness" that suggests splenomegaly was more accurate in lean than obese patients, and no one method of palpation was superior to another. Specifically, right lateral decubitus palpation, considered by many as the optimal maneuver to detect splenomegaly, added nothing when performed after supine palpation, and palpation was more accurate in lean than obese patients as well.

Table 12.1 presents the mechanisms of splenomegaly and common diseases in each category. The most common cause of splenomegaly is "work hypertrophy" from immune response and/or the destruction of red cells. Subacute bacterial or viral diseases also can cause splenomegaly by immune-response work hypertrophy, as can immunologic diseases such as systemic lupus erythematosus and Felty syndrome. Work hypertrophy from continued red cell destruction is the main cause of splenomegaly in patients with lifelong hemolytic anemias. Cirrhosis and splenic vein thrombosis produce splenomegaly by venous congestion, and splenomegaly

in the myeloproliferative diseases occurs both because of extramedullary hematopoiesis in agnogenic myeloid metaplasia and polycythemia vera and because of the splenic circulation of the massively expanded young-myeloid population in chronic myelocytic leukemia. Splenomegaly sometimes results when the spleen is infiltrated by granulomatous tissue or by amyloid, or when the reticuloendothelial cells are stuffed with an indigestible lipid (e.g., glucocerebroside in Gaucher disease).

Even severe, longstanding hypertriglyceridemia (as in patients with type IV hyperlipoproteinemia and diabetes) can cause splenomegaly, along with hepatomegaly that may create diagnostic confusion; correcting the hypertriglyceridemia shrinks the enlarged, fatty spleen.[11] There are neoplastic causes of splenomegaly as well, such as lymphoma, chronic lymphocytic leukemia, and rarely, metastatic cancer, and splenomegaly also may arise from cysts, hemangiomas, or other malformations.

In the United States, relatively few diseases now cause giant splenomegaly (10 times or more the usual upper-limit-of-normal of approximately 200 gm) as a presenting or early feature; the largest spleens (up to 5000 gm) are usually from the myeloproliferative disorders (agnogenic myeloid metaplasia and chronic myelocytic leukemia). Hairy-cell leukemia (leukemic reticuloendotheliosis) is a newly recognized cause of giant splenomegaly and striking hypersplenism. Isolated splenic lymphoma also causes giant splenomegaly, and earlier reports of this disorder probably include some patients with hairy-cell leukemia. Occasionally, hypersplenism is the presenting feature of Gaucher disease. In the tropics, giant splenomegaly (tropical splenomegaly) is seen from a unique hyperimmune response to malaria in which serum IgM levels are notably elevated. A counterpart, idiopathic nontropical splenomegaly, occurs in rare individuals with no obvious cause of splenomegaly at diagnosis, but one 10-year follow-up of 10 such patients showed that 4 developed typical splenic lymphoma. The far-advanced stages of chronic lymphocytic leukemia and polycythemia vera often cause considerable splenomegaly, as does long-standing thalassemia major, and rare causes of giant splenomegaly include sarcoidosis, in which hypersplenism may be a presenting or major feature and seems to correlate with disseminated disease,[12] as well as chronic congestive splenomegaly.

HYPERSPLENISM

When does splenomegaly become hypersplenism? Classically, hypersplenism means:

1. splenomegaly;

2. any combination of anemia, leukopenia, and/or thrombocytopenia;
3. compensatory bone marrow hyperplasia; and
4. improvement after splenectomy.

Even within this narrow framework, however, different diseases cause slightly different forms of hypersplenism. Furthermore, an enlarged spleen can cause problems for the patient without meeting the just-stated definition of hypersplenism. Thus, hypersplenism perhaps could be redefined to mean that the spleen in question is doing more harm than good; examples of diseases in which massive splenomegaly causes symptoms without fulfilling the strict definition of hypersplenism are chronic myelocytic leukemia and agnogenic myeloid metaplasia. Table 12.2 lists other "modern-day" prototype hypersplenism diseases in which it can be seen that diverse pathophysiologic mechanisms are involved. Hairy-cell leukemia may cause hypersplenism, because its unique lymphocyte, which probably arises in the bone marrow, is relatively rigid and unable to pass easily through the splenic pores. Splenic histology in this disease shows massive congestion of the red pulp, so the characteristic pancytopenia may occur because of a "traffic jam" in the red pulp.[13]

Cirrhosis and splenic vein thrombosis cause pancytopenia, because the normal splenic pool of blood cells is enlarged. Normally, the spleen pools approximately 30% of blood platelets (approximately 20 ml of red cells) and an unknown but probably marginal fraction of granulocytes. When the spleen is greatly enlarged, however, there is considerably more pooling of these blood cells (e.g., up to one third of the red cell mass), and pancytopenia may result. When the mechanism of the hypersplenism is simple pooling, as in congestive splenomegaly, the leukopenia often is characterized by a "balanced" diminution, so the ratio of polymorphonuclear leukocytes to lymphocytes and monocytes remains

normal. Also, the leukocytes may be available when needed in times of stress, so the risk of infection is not as great. These features contrast sharply with the severe relative granulocytopenia and frequent infections of the hypersplenism in Felty syndrome.

Gaucher disease causes pancytopenia by increased pooling, increased reticuloendothelial cell function with phagocytosis of platelets, and a dilutional anemia (seen also in certain other varieties of giant splenomegaly) in which a flow-induced portal hypertension expands the portal vascular space. This causes a decreased effective intravascular volume, stimulates the renin-angiotensin-aldosterone system, and leads to an accelerated rate of albumin synthesis and an expansion of the plasma volume.[14]

The newly described syndrome of hypersplenism in patients with renal hemodialysis apparently results from "combined" work hypertrophy. The reticuloendothelial system of the spleen is hypertrophied because of accelerated red cell destruction, perhaps attributable in part to the uremic defect in the red cell hexose monophosphate shunt. The immune system of the spleen is hypertrophied as well, apparently because of repeated viral infections including hepatitis and/or repeated antigenic challenge from blood transfusion or during dialysis.[15]

Felty syndrome, the triad of chronic deforming rheumatoid arthritis, splenomegaly, and granulocytopenia which occurs in up to 1% of patients with rheumatoid arthritis, may represent a unique variant of hypersplenism in which the spleen acts mainly as a giant lymph node. There are at least four current theories for the granulocytopenia of Felty syndrome:

1. decreased marrow granulopoiesis,
2. increased margination of granulocytes in the peripheral blood,
3. increased splenic sequestration of granulocytes, and
4. antigranulocyte antibodies.

There are neutrophil kinetic data supporting the concept of increased marginal pooling of granulocytes, and there also is a report of suppressor T cells that inhibit marrow granulopoiesis. One investigator showed that granulocytes in Felty syndrome are coated with immunoglobulin that may be either an antigranulocyte antibody or part of an immune complex adsorbed to granulocytes. The spleen seems to be a site of production for this immunoglobulin in that titers fall after splenectomy.[16]

SPLENIC RUPTURE

Pathologic or spontaneous rupture of the spleen is a well-known complication of acute infectious disease, notably malaria, typhoid, and infectious mononucleo-

TABLE 12.2. Hypersplenism in Various Diseases

Disease	Most Likely Mechanism
Hairy-cell leukemia	Retention of hairy cells in red pulp ("traffic jam")
Cirrhosis: splenic vein thrombosis	Increased pooling of blood cells
Felty syndrome	Immune system work hypertrophy
Thalassemia major	Reticuloendothelial system work hypertrophy
Renal dialysis splenomegaly	Immune and reticuloendothelial system work hypertrophy
Gaucher disease	Increased pooling and flow-induced dilutional anemia
Agnogenic myeloid metaplasia	Extramedullary hematopoiesis

sis.[17] In infectious mononucleosis, splenic rupture usually occurs in the second or third week of illness, when the spleen is enlarged, with weakness of the capsule, trabeculae, and vascular wall. Rupture can occur spontaneously or with minimal trauma, and the most common symptom is abdominal pain that usually begins in the upper left quadrant and radiates to the left shoulder. Symptoms, physical findings, and the results of routine radiography, spleen scan, and even peritoneal tap, however, vary depending on the amount and the site of bleeding, and normal diagnostic findings do not rule out the diagnosis. Probably the best diagnostic test is selective splenic angiogram although computed tomography can also be diagnostic. Delayed rupture can occur after trauma or cardiac massage, but scrutiny of such reports suggests that many instances really are delayed recognition of immediate rupture. Spontaneous rupture is less common in the acute and chronic leukemias and is especially uncommon in the lymphomas, although one article reviewed 10 such instances and included patients with histiocytic lymphoma and Hodgkin disease.[18] Spontaneous rupture is sometimes the presenting feature of a hematologic malignancy,[18] and spontaneous splenic rupture has also been reported in amyloidosis and in paroxysmal nocturnal hemoglobinuria.

SPLENIC ABSCESS

A large review of splenic abscess pointed out that most patients fall into one of four categories:

1. septicemic involvement, usually from subacute bacterial endocarditis;
2. seeding from peritonitis, perforation of the bowel, or abdominal surgery;
3. sickle cell hemoglobinopathies, in which case the abscess may instead represent a cavitary infarct; and
4. disease in contiguous organs (such as cancer of the stomach or colon or a gastric ulcer).

Most patients have sudden or gradual pain and tenderness of the upper left quadrant along with fever and leukocytosis after a latent period of days to weeks from the apparent resolution of antecedent infection or trauma. Sometimes, however, the abscess may be relatively covert. Diagnosis can be made by spleen scan and confirmed by a positive gallium scan, and the treatment is splenectomy and suitable antibiotic coverage.[19]

SPLENECTOMY

Splenectomy may be indicated to control or stage the basic disease in patients with hereditary spherocytosis,

autoimmune thrombocytopenia or hemolysis, or Hodgkin disease. Because the spleen is the main organ of red cell destruction in hereditary spherocytosis, splenectomy controls but does not cure this disease; the patient lives a normal life despite spherocytes in the blood. Similarly, the spleen also is the dominant organ of cell destruction and a source of antibody production in autoimmune thrombocytopenia and autoimmune warm hemolytic anemia. In these disorders, splenectomy offers good control of the disease in up to 70% of patients, although low-grade destruction of the blood cells continues in other reticuloendothelial organs such as the liver. In Hodgkin disease, the spleen is removed as part of the staging laparotomy, and this brings a risk of lethal septicemia, especially in children. One study showed that almost 10% of 200 children splenectomized for Hodgkin disease developed fulminant bacteremia. Partial splenectomy for staging, however, is fraught with false-negative results. Also, it has been learned that therapeutic irradiation of the spleen in patients with Hodgkin and non-Hodgkin lymphomas can produce splenic atrophy with lethal pneumococcal septicemia.[20]

Several diseases that commonly cause severe and chronic hypersplenic symptoms may require therapeutic splenectomy. A review of infections in hairy-cell leukemia concluded that at least 40% of patients develop serious infections; bacterial infections were linked with granulocytopenia and opportunistic fungal and tuberculous infections with corticosteroid therapy.[21] With chemotherapy improving, however, splenectomy has a shrinking role in hairy-cell leukemia. Splenectomy for Felty syndrome has long been a debatable subject; a clinicopathologic study of 27 patients showed optimistic long-term results from splenectomy, with only 12% of the patients having persistent or recurrent granulocytopenia and with recurrent infections a major problem in only 1%.[22] While it is not unanimous, and it is likely that granulocytes of patients with Felty syndrome also have functional defects that may not be influenced by splenectomy, the majority opinion holds that splenectomy is the treatment of choice for patients with Felty syndrome and a long history of leg ulcers or substantial and recurrent infections. Splenectomy at least remains the standard against which to test newer proposed therapies, such as the use of testosterone, lithium, or gold.

Splenectomy also has been performed at times for advanced agnogenic myeloid metaplasia because of repeated splenic infarcts and rapid red cell destruction, and therapeutic splenectomy often is required in long-standing thalassemia major. It seems likely, however, that high-transfusion regimens coupled with effective iron-depletion regimens such as continuous subcutaneous infusion of chelating agents will largely prevent severe hypersplenism and sharply reduce the need for therapeutic splenectomy in thalassemia major. Studies of splenectomy for the palliation of advanced chronic myelocytic and chronic lymphocytic leukemia have shown only marginal gains and with substantial postoperative complications; the role of splenectomy in these diseases remains controversial. As mentioned earlier, the data from several groups suggest that 5% to 10% of chronically hemodialyzed patients with uremia develop pancytopenia and marked increases in transfusion requirements because of a poorly understood hypersplenism. Therapeutic splenectomy increasingly is being performed in such patients. Finally, splenic vein thrombosis, usually caused by pancreatic disease, is a cause of hypersplenism and variceal bleeding that can be cured by splenectomy.

The clinician should ponder several practical questions before recommending therapeutic splenectomy. Is hypersplenism really the cause of the patient's anemia, leukopenia, and/or thrombocytopenia? How severe is the hypersplenism? Are any symptoms coming from the spleen per se? Is the anemia incapacitating? Is the neutropenia causing infections? Is thrombocytopenia causing important bleeding or only purpura? What are the alternatives to splenectomy, and what is the risk of waiting? These concerns are discussed further in a recent article on the clinical indications for splenectomy.[23]

HYPOSPLENISM

Severe hyposplenism is a potentially lethal condition. This was established by Dameshek when he reported a case of nontropical sprue and hyposplenism that was first suspected because of Howell-Jolly bodies and target cells in the peripheral blood smear; additional clues to hyposplenism in the peripheral smear are the presence of acanthocytes and siderocytes. After splenectomy, there are long-term changes in the complete blood cell count that also serve as hematologic clues to the asplenic state. Granulocytosis occurs immediately after splenectomy and is replaced in several weeks by long-lived lymphocytosis and monocytosis, which fits the observation that the normal spleen selectively removes lymphocytes and monocytes from the blood. Thrombocytosis occurs immediately after splenectomy, but within a few weeks, the platelet count usually returns to high-normal levels. However, if the patient has a continuing hemolytic or sideroblastic anemia with the concomitant active bone marrow, or if the patient has an underlying myeloproliferative disease, the postsplenectomy thrombocytosis may be severe and sustained, with platelet counts exceeding 1 million/mm^3.

These hematologic clues should lead the physician to suspect hyposplenism. Confirmatory tests include splenic scan, quantitation by interference phase microscopy of red cell surface pits and craters (which are increased postsplenectomy), and the determination of splenic uptake of heat-damaged radiolabelled red cells.

The prototype of hyposplenism is the child with sickle cell anemia who is vulnerable to overwhelming and often fatal pneumococcemia. Ironically, the child is at greatest risk when the spleen is enlarged, not later when it is atrophic from "autosplenectomy." Children with sickle cell anemia and enlarged spleens have functional asplenia, and transfusion temporarily can reverse this phenomenon, presumably by restoring splenic circulation and phagocytic activity to normal by reducing the load of fixed sickled cells.[24] As the child grows older, the spleen shrinks because of repeated infarcts, but the child gains immunity to the different serotypes of pneumococcus and can rely more on the liver for the clearance of blood-borne pneumococci. However, fatal pneumococcemia has occurred in teenagers with sickle cell anemia, and transient splenic hypofunction has been reported during a painful crisis in a 22-year-old patient with hemoglobin SC.

A wide variety of conditions and spleen sizes are associated with hyposplenism. Atrophic spleens may be noted in ulcerative colitis, celiac disease, dermatitis herpetiformis, thyrotoxicosis (Graves disease), hemorrhagic thrombocytopenia, as a result of therapeutic irradiation, and after radiocontrast studies with thorium dioxide (Thorotrast). The spleen may be of normal size or enlarged in sickle cell anemia, sarcoidosis, amyloidosis, and with the use of high-dose corticosteroids.

In the category of atrophic spleens, the classic association has been with celiac sprue or idiopathic steatorrhea, with more than 50 cases reported. Up to 40% of patients with either celiac sprue or dermatitis herpetiformis have evidence for hyposplenism on peripheral blood smear or by splenic uptake studies. Although the mechanism of hyposplenism in these disorders remains unknown, it has been linked with the generalized lymphoreticular atrophy noted in celiac sprue and with the autoimmune theory of the pathogenesis of celiac sprue. A review of hyposplenism with sprue suggests that the risk of pneumococcemia is not great; perhaps enough splenic activity remains to defend against bacteremia.

In one study, hospital patients were screened for Howell-Jolly bodies and target cells on peripheral blood smear. Six of the 12 patients had celiac sprue, 2 had discoid lupus, and 2 had Graves disease. There are now at least 5 reported cases of hyposplenism of mysterious mechanism in Graves disease, and clear-cut hyposplenism has been documented in 3 of 8 patients with hemorrhagic thrombocythemia, a relatively well-defined myeloproliferative disease in which the major abnormality is an excessive production of megakaryocytes and platelets. In this disease, splenic atrophy can occur because of repeated infarcts from large aggregates of platelets.

There also are several reports of splenic atrophy and one report of fatal pneumococcemia in patients who had received thorium dioxide as a radiocontrast agent. The α-irradiation from this long-lived isotope that remains in the reticuloendothelial cells causes fibrosis and atrophy of the spleen and also can cause liver cancer, and therapeutic irradiation (but not chemotherapy) in patients with Hodgkin disease has been shown to have a 30% to 40% risk of inducing splenic atrophy.

Although patients with ulcerative colitis do not have hyposplenism at diagnosis, about 40% develop it during the disease, and the hyposplenism waxes and wanes with the activity of the colitis. Hyposplenism becomes severe when pancolitis develops, and this probably helps to explain the link between notable thrombocytosis and active ulcerative colitis. When patients with pancolitis and hyposplenism require colectomy, there is a high risk of immediate postoperative septicemia that on occasion is pneumococcal and fatal. Hyposplenism rarely is seen in association with regional enteritis, and the mechanism of severe hyposplenism in aggressive ulcerative colitis remains a mystery.[25]

Hyposplenism also has been described in 5 of 70 patients with systemic lupus erythematosus. Two of these patients had definite splenic atrophy, and one died of overwhelming pneumococcemia.[26]

As noted previously in children with sickle cell anemia, hyposplenism (or functional splenia) occurs even with a normal-sized or large spleen. Fatal pneumococcemia has been documented in an apparently healthy woman who at autopsy had a 300-g spleen totally replaced by granulomatous tissue from sarcoidosis. Also, 2 of 35 patients with light-chain myeloma had evidence of hyposplenism from amyloidosis on peripheral smear and splenic scan, which may account in part for the risk of repeated pneumococcal infections and pneumococcemia in multiple myeloma.[27] Finally, the reported effect of high-dose corticosteroids in blocking splenic monocyte destruction of antibody-coated platelets and red cells in autoimmune thrombocytopenic and hemolytic states suggests that high-dose corticosteroid therapy in general may impair splenic phagocytic activity and increase the risk of overwhelming bacteremia.

Recent research has described a new syndrome, functional asplenia after bone marrow transplantation, as a late complication of extensive and chronic graft-versus-host disease. In one report, 6 of 15 bone marrow–graft recipients developed functional asplenia in the months after transplant; this late complication of allogeneic bone marrow transplantation is thought to increase the risk of bacterial infections.[28]

The Risk of Fulminant Bacteremia

The hyposplenic state is potentially lethal because of the risk of fulminant bacteremia.[29] This risk is greatest in young children who are splenectomized, especially during the first 2 years after surgery (80% of cases) and when the disorder that required splenectomy is a disease of the reticuloendothelial system such as thalassemia major, histiocytosis X, or the Wiskott-Aldrich syndrome (20% risk of septicemia). The high risk in children splenectomized during the staging laparotomy for Hodgkin disease has been mentioned, but there is a low yet significant risk even in normal subjects who have incidental splenectomy. Recently, more than 50 cases of serious and often fatal postsplenectomy septicemia have been reported in adults, many of whom had splenectomies for trauma, and although the actual risk of fulminant bacteremia in these normal subjects remains unknown, some have estimated it to be as high as 1% per year after splenectomy. The longest interval between incidental splenectomy and bacteremia has been 31 years. In the typical syndrome, a previously healthy, normal adult develops a high fever, usually after a brief and mild upper respiratory infection, and within hours develops shock and disseminated intravascular coagulation that often proves fatal. It is speculated that the nasopharynx is the site of infection and that perhaps a synergistic viral infection is needed to convert an asymptomatic carrier state of a pathogenic pneumococcus into a fulminant bacteremia. In the fulminant syndrome, blood levels of pneumococci (sometimes meningococcus or *Haemophilus influenzae*) reach extraordinary proportions, seen only in patients with hyposplenism, and their capsular polysaccharides trigger bacterial shock and disseminated intravascular coagulation. The peripheral blood smear reveals telltale signs of vacuolated polymorphonuclear leukocytes, thrombocytopenia, and even pneumococci that are both free and within polymorphonuclear leukocytes.[30]

Classic examples of this tragic syndrome are still reported, for example, a 25-year-old man whose spleen had been removed nine years earlier after a motorcycle accident. Entirely healthy, and despite splenosis, this man developed pneumococcemia from a cryptic focus and progressed from influenza-like symptoms to septic shock and death within 24 hours.[31]

The true risk of postsplenectomy sepsis in adults, however, remains unclear. One population study suggested that the risk is low. This study was of 193 adults in Rochester, Minnesota, who underwent splenectomy during a 25-year period ending in 1979; the incidence of any type of serious infection after splenectomy was only one infection for every 14 person-years of follow-up. Patients with the highest risk of infection were those who had splenectomy for cancer and those who had chemotherapy, irradiation, or immunosuppressive therapy. Patients who had splenectomy for trauma had the lowest risk of infection. Only two cases of fulminant sepsis (one fatal) occurred during 1090 person-years of follow-up.[32]

The threat of fatal pneumococcemia after splenectomy for trauma may be reduced because of the "born-again" spleen, or splenosis, which had been demonstrated in approximately half of the subjects (both children and adults) previously splenectomized for trauma and which can be detected as early as 1.5 years after surgery. Presumably, these "minispleens" function well enough to protect against fatal pneumococcemia. This has led to the suggestion that certain patients should receive splenic autotransplants at the time of splenectomy;[33] however, splenosis does not guarantee protection.[34]

Also, in this era of widespread use of computerized tomography, one should know that splenosis on this scan can be mistaken for metastatic tumor implants. This consequently can confuse the diagnostic evaluation.[35]

The Risk of Septicemia

Possible approaches to reducing the threat of lethal septicemia are:

1. performance of fewer splenectomies after splenic trauma,
2. immunization with bacterial vaccines,
3. treatment of high fever as a medical emergency,
4. prophylactic administration of penicillin for selected patients, and
5. performance of splenic autotransplants for selected patients.

Fewer splenectomies probably should be done after splenic trauma. In fact, the management of splenic trauma is moving toward nonsurgical means in some cases and toward surgical repair in others analogous to the surgical management of liver trauma.

Splenic autotransplantation also is being used, and about 100 cases had been reported as of 1987. One study assessed splenic reticuloendothelial function 2 to 5 years after splenectomy (with or without autotransplantation), splenic repair, or partial splenectomy. Reticuloendothelial function was best preserved by partial splenectomy or splenic repair; however, autotransplantation (25 to 30 g of splenic slices in an extraperitoneal pocket) preserved some splenic function when compared with splenectomy alone.[36]

Bacterial vaccines should be used in patients with hyposplenism. Significant protection from pneumococcemia in children with sickle cell anemia who were followed for 2 years after receiving an octavalent pneumococcal vaccine has been noted. Although there have been some failures of protection in children with sickle cell disease, the commercial pneumococcal vaccine (Pneumovax) should be given to these children, to those splenectomized for Hodgkin disease, to adults after incidental splenectomy (asplenic hosts respond normally to subcutaneous immunization), and probably to patients having diseases associated with hyposplenism. All of these patients also might be given the vaccines for types A and C meningococcus and, when they become available, vaccines for type B meningococcus and *H. influenzae*.

Because the pneumococcal vaccine has not yet been proved effective in children under 2 years of age, perhaps prophylactic penicillin should be given for those 2 years to infants born with sickle cell anemia. One also could recommend prophylactic penicillin for patients with ulcerative colitis and hyposplenism who are to undergo colectomy. Asplenic subjects or those with diseases linked with hyposplenism who develop fevers without obvious sites of infection should be treated as medical emergencies; they should immediately see a physician, who should obtain cultures and treat them expectantly for pneumococcemia with intravenous penicillin. Perhaps an aggressive approach to such patients will save lives by eliminating pneumococci from the bloodstream before the lethal chain of events begins.[37]

A recent comprehensive review of asplenia and infection noted the evolving attitudes toward splenectomy. The surgical approach to splenic trauma shifted from routine splenectomy toward maximal splenic preservation with the recognition of postsplenectomy sepsis, but it now is shifting back slightly with recognition of the risks of attempts at splenic repair accompanied by hemorrhage and transfusion. The review also noted that computed tomographic scanning and/or ultrasonography can be useful in the diagnosis and monitoring of splenic trauma or spontaneous rupture. Arguing that common sense and the available information suggest that splenectomy should not be done for trivial reasons, it called for a balanced approach to surgery for splenic injury, but neither should enthusiasm for splenic salvage make the salvage procedure itself life-threatening. The review also argued that splenic implants are reasonable, if they can be done safely, when the spleen cannot safely be preserved; however, patients with implants still may be at risk for fatal sepsis.[38]

Asplenic patients who received the original 14-valent pneumococcal vaccine now should get the current 23-valent vaccine, and perhaps should be revaccinated every few years. Although penicillin prophylaxis commonly is used for pediatric patients in the initial years after splenectomy, experts seem to agree that long-term penicillin prophylaxis for asplenic adults is not firmly supported at present; on the other hand, early antibiotic therapy for any febrile illness–perhaps even self-treatment beginning at home—is prudent.

One must remember that neither splenic transplant nor pneumococcal vaccination is fail safe. Fatal sepsis has been reported in each setting, and indeed, there is no substitute for the intact spleen. Also, no current test reliably tells us whether a given asplenic patient belongs to the small group who will develop overwhelming sepsis or to the much larger group who will never experience serious infectious morbidity.[38] With this in mind, it is important to educate both the patient and caregiver as to the warning signs of infection in the hope that early antibiotic therapy will save lives.

REFERENCES

1. Schulkind ML, Ellis EF, Smith RT. Effect of antibody upon clearance of I[125]-labelled pneumonococci by the spleen and liver. Pediatr Res 1967;1:178.
2. Chen L-T. Microcirculation of the spleen: an open or closed circulation? Science 1978;201:157.
3. Gavrilis P, Rothenberg SP, Guy R. Correlation of low serum IgM levels with absence of functional splenic tissue in sickle cell disease syndromes. Am J Med 1974;57:542.
4. Johnston RB Jr. Increased susceptibility to infection in sicle cell disease: review of its occurrence and possible causes. South Med J 1974;67:1342.
5. Lockwood CM, Worlledge S, Nicholas A, et al. Reversal of impaired splenic function in patients with nephritis or vasculitis (or both) by plasma exchange. N Engl J Med 1979;300:524.
6. Elkon KB, Sewell JR, Ryan PFJ, et al. Splenic function in non-renal systemic lupus erythematosus. Am J Med 1980;69:80.
7. Froelich JW, Strauss HW, Moore RH, McKusick KA. Redistribution of visceral blood volume in upright exercise in healthy volunteers. J Nucl Med 1988;29:1714–8.
8. McIntyre OR, Ebauch FG Jr. Palpable spleens in college freshmen. Ann Intern Med 1967;66:301.
9. Sullivan S, Williams R. Reliability of clinical techniques for detecting splenic enlargement. BMJ 1976;4:1043.
10. Barkun AN, Camus M, Green L, et al. The bedside assessment of splenic enlargement. Am J Med 1991;91:512–8.
11. Small JM, Moatamed F, Deiss A, Wilson DE. Diabetic lipemia with fatty splenomegaly culminating in unnecessary splenectomy. West J Med 1987;147:196–8.
12. Kataria YP, Whitcomb ME. Splenomegaly in sarcoidosis. Arch Intern Med 1980;140:35.
13. Eichner ER. Splenic function: normal, too much and too little. Am J Med 1979;66:311.
14. Hess CE, Ayers CR, Sandusky WR, et al. Mechanism of dilutional anemia in massive splenomegaly. Blood 1976;47:231.
15. Higgins MR, Grace M, Ulan RA, et al. Anemia in hemodialysis patients. Arch Intern Med 1977;137:172.
16. Spivak JL. Felty's syndrome: an analytical review. Johns Hopkins Med J 1977;141:156.
17. Aung MK, Goldberg M, Tobin MS. Splenic rupture due to infectious mononucleosis. JAMA 1978;240:1752.
18. Andrews DF, Hernandez R, Grafton W, et al. Pathologic rupture of the spleen in non-Hodgkin's lymphoma. Arch Intern Med 1980;140:119.
19. Chun CH, Raff MJ, Contreras L, et al. Splenic abscess. Medicine 1980;59:50.
20. Dailey MO, Coleman CN, Kaplan HS. Radiation-induced splenic atrophy in patients with Hogkin's disease and non-Hodgkin's lymphoma. N Engl J Med 1980;302:215.
21. Bouza E, Burgaleta C, Golde DW. Infections in hairy-cell leukemia. Blood 1978;51:851.
22. Laszlo J, Jones R, Silberman HR, et al. Splenectomy for Felty's syndrome. Arch Intern Med 1978;138:597.
23. Eichner ER. Indications for splenectomy. Surg Rounds 1989;12:52–63.
24. Pearson HA, Cornelius EA, Schwartz AD, et al. Transfusion-reversible functional asplenia in young children with sickle-cell anemia. N Engl J Med 1970;183:334.
25. Ryan FP, Smart RC, Holdsworth CD, et al. Hyposplenism in inflammatory bowel disease. Gut 1978;19:50.
26. Dillon AM, Stein HB, English RA. Splenic atrophy in systemic lupus erythematosus. Ann Intern Med 1982;96:40.
27. Stone MJ, Frenkel EP. The clinical spectrum of light chain myeloma. Am J Med 1975;58:601.
28. Kahls P, Panzer S, Kletter K, et al. Functional asplenia after bone marrow transplantation. Ann Intern Med 1988;109:461–4.
29. Pearson HA. Splenectomy: its risks and its roles. Hosp Pract 1980;15:85.
30. Kitchens CS. The syndrome of post splenectomy fulminant sepsis: case report and review of the literature. Am J Med Sci 1977;274:303.
31. Stryker RM, Orton DW. Overwhelming postsplenectomy infection. Ann Emerg Med 1988;17:161–4.
32. Schwartz PE, Sterioff S, Mucha P, et al. Postsplenectomy sepsis and mortality in adults. JAMA 1982;248:2279–83.
33. Pearson HA, Johnston D, Smith KA, et al. The born-again spleen: return of splenic function after splenectomy for trauma. N Engl J Med 1978;198:1389.
34. Rice HM, James PD. Ectopic splenic tissue failed to prevent fatal pneumococcal septicaemia after splenectomy for trauma. Lancet 1980;i:565.
35. White JD, West AN, Priebat DA. Splenosis mimicking an intra-abdominal malignancy. Am J Med 1989;87:687–90.
36. Traub A, Giebink GS, Smith C, et al. Splenic reticuloendothelial function after splenectomy, spleen repair, and spleen autotransplantation. N Engl J Med 1987;317:1559–64.
37. Dickerman JD. Splenic defenses against infection. Hosp Pract 1980;15:1.
38. Styrt B. Infection associated with asplenia: risks, mechanisms, and prevention. Am J Med 1990;88:33–42.
39. Eichner ER. Splenectomy: changing roles and challenging consequences. New Developments in Medicine 1989;4(2):65–71.

13

Leukemia

Janice P. Dutcher, M.D., and Peter H. Wiernik, M.D.

The diseases classified as *leukemias* are characterized by a neoplastic proliferation of one or more of the blood-forming cellular elements. If left untreated, all forms of leukemia ultimately are fatal, although the duration of life may vary from only a few days in some patients with acute leukemia to two or three decades in some with chronic lymphocytic leukemia. Infiltration of the bone marrow by leukemic cells eventually results in granulocytopenia, thrombocytopenia, or anemia; death usually results from complications of this myelophthisic process.

CLASSIFICATION

The different forms of leukemia usually are classified according to both morphologic and clinical criteria. The first classification is based on the cell line affected, that is, whether or not the neoplastic cells are lymphoid or myeloid in appearance. The second categorization is into *acute* or *chronic leukemia*, based on the patient's expected longevity with the disease as well as the maturity of the leukemic cells. With the therapy currently available, however, the expected longevity of some patients with acute leukemia approaches that of some who have chronic leukemia—in the range of several years—thus blurring this latter distinction. Nevertheless, distinguishing acute from chronic leukemia is still worthwhile because of other differences in the manifestations of these diseases and their management.

The acute leukemias are characterized by proliferation in the bone marrow of cells that are almost indistinguishable from normal, immature hematopoietic cells.

In the untreated state, these leukemic cells enter the bloodstream (Fig. 13.1) and usually become the predominant leukocyte, eventually also invading other organs. If the patient is not treated, death occurs on average approximately 3 months after diagnosis of the illness, but the course of the disease can vary considerably. Only rarely does a patient survive longer than 1 year without effective therapy.

The acute leukemias are commonly divided into *acute lymphocytic leukemia* (ALL) and *acute nonlymphocytic* or *acute "myelogenous" leukemia* (AML). Because of differences in the age groups commonly affected by these illnesses, and because the drugs used in treatment and the response to them differs significantly, this division is a useful one. Each major group is divided into morphologically defined subtypes; for example, AML subtypes include myelocytic, myelomonocytic, monoblastic or monocytic, and progranulocytic leukemias, erythroleukemia, and some rarer types. To systematize our thinking about the myeloid and lymphoid acute leukemias, a morphologic classification system has been developed, and this system, the French-American-British classification, provides both standard morphologic criteria for subtype diagnosis as well as a basis for international communication regarding acute leukemia.[1,2] The acute lymphocytic, acute myelocytic, and acute myelomonocytic leukemias are the most commonly occurring types.

The chronic leukemias are characterized by the abnormal proliferation of initially mature-looking leukocytes in the bone marrow and other organs, with life expectancy usually measured in years rather than months. Division of the chronic leukemias into *chronic lympho-*

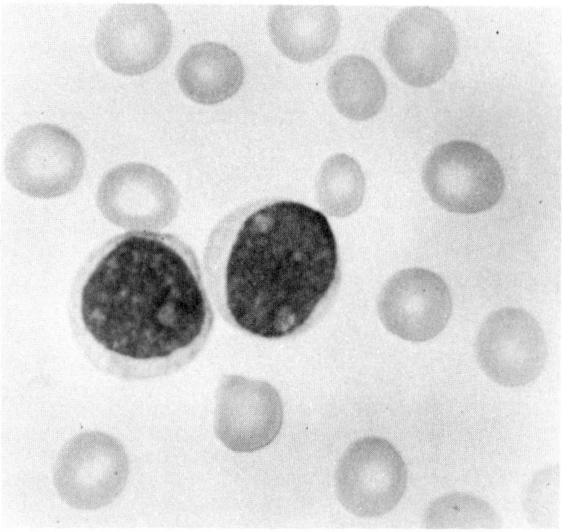

FIGURE 13.1. Circulating leukemic myeloblasts.

cytic leukemia (CLL) and *chronic myelocytic leukemia* (CML) is based on the predominant cell type usually seen in the peripheral blood. It should be noted that CML is characterized by increased numbers of neutrophils and band forms as well as of myelocytes, and CML also is one of the variant myeloproliferative syndromes, distinguished by its unique cytogenetic and certain clinical characteristics. Also, CLL has several subtypes that have been subdivided and classified.[3]

HISTORY

The symptoms and signs of leukemia—pallor, weakness, fever, hemorrhage, and lymphadenopathy—have been reported in the literature since the time of Hippocrates, but leukemia was not recognized as a disease until the period from 1839 to 1845. At this time, the first careful microscopic observations by Donne and postmortem and clinical examinations by Virchow were completed.[4,5] Virchow named the disease leukemia because he considered the blood of a patient with a high white blood cell count to be whitish in appearance; he subsequently was able to divide the leukemias into those with lymphadenopathy and those without. Ehrlich's cellular blood stains, first developed in 1877 when he was a medical student, allowed the recognition of a lymphocytic, myelocytic, and acute form, but only in 1900, when Naegeli first described the myeloblasts, were acute leukemias divided into myelocytic and lymphocytic forms. The monocytic (Schilling) variety of acute leukemia was initially described in 1913 by Reschad and Schilling-Torgau.

The evolution and use of radiotherapy in the 1920s provided the first effective means of palliation for patients who had chronic leukemias. The first effective therapy for the acute leukemias was discovered in the late 1940s, when glucocorticosterioids and antifolic acid preparations produced the first remissions in ALL. The subsequent development of multidrug chemotherapy for acute leukemia as well as the innovation of prophylactic meningeal leukemia treatment in childhood acute lymphoblastic leukemia now have improved the prognosis such that a substantial proportion of these patients have been disease-free for more than a decade, and are probably cured. Therapy of the other leukemias lags behind that of childhood ALL to various degrees, and it is hoped that the substantial strides in treating the childhood disease will result in progress treating the other leukemias.

EPIDEMIOLOGY

The incidence of all types of leukemia in the United States is approximately 68 per one-million people annually.[6,7] Leukemia occurs worldwide with an annual mortality rate of 30 to 70 deaths per one-million people, a lesser variation than is seen for many other cancers. Mortality from leukemia tends to be highest in Israel and the Scandinavian countries and lowest in Chile and Japan.[8] The lower mortality in Japan appears mainly to be the result of a markedly reduced incidence in chronic lymphatic leukemia in this population.[8] In the United States, overall leukemia mortality tends to be lower in nonwhites than in whites, and slightly more than one half of these deaths are caused by acute leukemias.[6,7,9]

It is difficult to develop an exact frequency distribution of the various types of leukemia, because statewide and national statistics on leukemia tend to be quite unreliable in distinguishing cell types. Also, large series of patients reported by various referral centers may not be representative of the true pattern overall. Therefore, the type of leukemia that occurs most commonly is uncertain.

All types of leukemia tend to be more common in males than in females, regardless of race and age. The male/female ratio is especially high for CLL (2:1),[8] and in very young children, the gender incidence is almost the same.

Age does have a marked influence on the type of leukemia seen.[8,10] Leukemia is the most commonly diagnosed malignancy in the pediatric population, accounting for 32% of all new cancer cases yearly in children. This is caused predominantly by the high incidence of ALL, which comprises 80% to 90% of cases in those under 15 years of age. This acute leukemia accounts for almost half the deaths as well, and it is the leading cause of death from malignancy in this population. Conversely, CLL accounts for most cases in the geriatric population. Ninety percent of CLL cases occur in patients over 50 years of age, and approximately two thirds of these patients are over the age of 60.[11]

ETIOLOGY

The etiology of most leukemias is still uncertain, although many factors have been implicated as predisposing to its development. These include radiation, chemicals, genetic factors, and viruses.

Radiation

The leukemogenic effect of ionizing radiation in laboratory animals has been well documented.[12] Similarly, ionizing radiation is the agent most clearly associated with an increased risk of all leukemias except CLL in humans. Most of these have been cases of the acute and chronic myelocytic types, and before the institution of protective measures, radiologists sustained as much as a tenfold increase in mortality caused by leukemia compared with other physicians and the general population.[13] Survivors of the atomic bombings of Hiroshima and Nagasaki were found to have a dose-related increase in the incidence of leukemia, with those less than 1500 meters from the epicenter of the explosion having the highest incidence and those beyond 2000 meters having no increase in incidence.[14–16] The first cases of leukemia in this population were noted 2 years after exposure. The peak incidence was between 5 and 7 years after exposure, but a persistent increase was noted as long as 20 years afterward.

A similarly increased incidence of leukemia also has been noted in patients treated with therapeutic partial-body irradiation for ankylosing spondylitis, patients with malignant lymphomas, children who have received radiation for lymphoid hyperplasia, and patients treated with radioactive iodine for thyroid cancer.[17–25] With the increased use of combined radiation and cytotoxic drug therapy (also possibly leukemogenic), particularly for the treatment of malignant lymphomas, subsequent cases of acute leukemia have been described.[20,22,26–28]

It still is uncertain whether a threshold dose of radiation exists below which there is no accompanying increased risk of developing leukemia. There seems to be no convincing evidence that current doses of radiation used in radiodiagnostic studies increase the risk of leukemia in adults, and studies on the effects of fetal exposure in utero to radiation from either diagnostic radiographic procedures or atomic-bomb explosions have conflicting results.[15,29–31] If a threshold dose exists, then ionizing radiation overall probably is only a minor factor in causing leukemia. If, however, any exposure increases the risk of leukemia even slightly, it may be a major causative agent, and recent reports associating low-dose electromagnetic radiation emanating from power lines and household appliances with acute leukemia are being investigated.[32]

Chemicals

Long-term exposure to numerous chemicals has been implicated in the development of some cases of myelogenous leukemia, both chronic and acute.[33] Long-term occupational exposure to benzene has long been associated with an increased incidence of leukemia,[34–36] and AML also has been reported after marrow aplasia following exposure to chloramphenicol and phenylbutazone. Some cytotoxic chemotherapeutic agents, including the alkylating agents, have been found to be carcinogenic both in animals and in humans,[37] and patients with myeloma, ovarian tumors, lymphomas, lung cancer, brain tumors, and even CLL treated for long periods of time (18 months to 4 years) with various alkylating agents have been reported subsequently to have developed AML.[20,22,37–42] The exact risk from long-term treatment with these drugs is still undetermined, however, because AML may represent a part of the natural history of these diseases, manifest only in those with long survival times.

Genetic Factors

Many cytogenetic abnormalities have been described in leukemia patients. In addition, a few families have been described with a higher incidence of CLL than can be ascribed to chance. Three families in particular have been studied in which two or more members with CLL also had an inherited abnormality of chromosome 21 (Christchurch chromosome).[43,44] Similarly, a 20-fold increase in the incidence of acute leukemia (lymphoid or myeloid) has been reported in children with Down syndrome (trisomy 21), and there is an increased risk of Down syndrome among siblings of children who have acute leukemia.[45–47] Thus, it may be that a significant part of the genetic information for leukocyte growth and differentiation is carried on this chromosome. Other heritable diseases such as Bloom syndrome, Fanconi constitutional aplastic anemia, and ataxia-telangiectasia also are associated with excessive chromosomal breakage (but with less specificity than the aberrations discussed earlier) as well as with an increased incidence of acute leukemia.[48–50]

The results from studies of leukemia in twins also suggest a genetic predisposition to the disease in some circumstances. If one member of a pair of monozygotic (identical) twins develops leukemia, the other has a strikingly high risk (one chance in five) of doing so as well.[51] In these instances, the disease usually appears within a few months. Results of another study showed that monozygotic twins have a 12-fold greater risk of concordant leukemia than do dizygotic (fraternal) twins.[52]

Also of interest are recent findings of cytogenetic abnormalities in almost all cases of acute leukemia.[53,54] These findings have been associated with specific subtypes of AML and ALL with prognostic implications, and this will be discussed specifically with each disease.

Viruses

It is well known that viruses can cause leukemia and related lymphoreticular neoplasms in vertebrates. These viruses may be directly leukemogenic when inoculated, or they may lie dormant and be passed on through the ova or through milk and other secretions to a future generation which then may manifest the disease.[55] Many environmental and genetic factors appear to help determine whether an infected animal will develop leukemia and, if so, what type; among these are the strain of the host, the quantity of inoculum, as well as the age, sex, hormonal and immunologic status of the animal, and the presence of environmental carcinogens or exposure to radiation.[56,57]

Conclusive evidence that viruses can cause common leukemia in humans is still lacking, despite good evidence for their leukemogenic activity in animals, including subhuman primates. The strongest evidence thus far is based on several molecular biologic observations, beginning with the discovery of an RNA-dependent DNA polymerase (reverse transcriptase) in avian sarcoma and murine leukemia viruses.[58,59] The presence of this enzyme in these type C viruses (a group of RNA viruses that can be leukemogenic in fowl and mammals, including subhuman primates) allows them to synthesize DNA that subsequently can be inserted into the infected cell's genome, then allowing viral genetic information to be passed on through normal cell replication.[55] Thus, this enzyme can provide the capability to produce more viruses and to maintain a neoplastic state under the proper conditions.

Reverse transcriptase that is biochemically and immunologically similar to that of mammalian type C viruses has been identified in some human leukemic cells and also in normal-appearing leukocytes from leukemic patients in complete remission.[60–64] This enzyme now has been shown to be absent in fresh leukocytes of normal subjects (including those with nonneo-

plastic leukocytosis) and in normal lymphocytes transformed to lymphoblasts by phytohemagglutinin.[60,65] Results of an investigation of two sets of identical twins, one having leukemia in each, showed that the patients' DNA contained leukemia-specific polynucleotide sequences; these sequences could not be found in the DNA of the healthy identical twins.[66] This suggests that the leukemia-related genetic information was an acquired characteristic not passed through the germ line. Electron microscope studies and classic virologic infectivity studies largely have failed to produce convincing evidence for the presence of complete type C viral particles in human leukemic cells and cell cultures, because lack of confirmation and failure to exclude possible contaminating infections confuse the picture.[67,68]

There is, therefore, evidence that the components related to type C RNA tumor virus, which are found in both leukemic and normal cells of those with leukemia, may be clues to a closely related but perhaps incompletely expressed human leukemia virus. However, at present, there is no demonstration of infectivity of these viral components and postinfection development of leukemia, and it is noteworthy that all of the possible etiologic factors discussed previously, including ionizing radiation and cytotoxic chemotherapy, are characterized by abnormalities of genetic information. It is quite possible this may be a final common pathway in the development of these diseases.

Recently, a new type of leukemia has been diagnosed that is associated strongly with the presence of retrovirus, human T-cell leukemia virus (HTLV-I).[69,70] This disease, termed *T-cell leukemia*, is an aggressive form of lymphoma/leukemia, and HTLV-I appears to be etiologic.[69,70] HTLV-I is a retrovirus that produces reverse transcriptase, infects T-cells at a consistent location on a given chromosome, and is able to transform T-cells in tissue culture.[71,72] This suggests an acquired process involved in the development of leukemia, and it appears to be the first human malignancy that is proven to be virally induced.

ACUTE LEUKEMIAS

Acute Lymphocytic Leukemia

Although ALL does occur in adults, it predominantly is a disease of children. Fortunately, in childhood, it is a disease that has been most responsive to various manipulations of specific treatment modalities (i.e., changes in the drugs available for use and their combination) and to combinations of treatment modalities (i.e., incorporation of craniospinal irradiation and intrathecal drug therapy into the total treatment design), so the possibility of cure now exists for a substantial number of these children.

CLINICAL MANIFESTATIONS. The onset of ALL usually is acute and without prodromal preleukemic symptoms. Only a few days to weeks pass from the time of initial symptoms in most patients to consultation with a physician. Fatigue, petechiae or other evidence of hemorrhage, fever, infection, as well as bone and joint pain are common initial complaints and, as with AML, are related to the replacement of normal hematopoietic elements in the bone marrow by the abnormal leukemic cells. Physical examination can be normal; however, moderate hepatosplenomegaly and infiltration of other organs, which produces lymphadenopathy (usually non-tender), are quite common and occur in at least 75% of patients.[73-75] Sternal tenderness occurs in over 60%, as do petechiae or ecchymoses, but severe gastrointestinal hemorrhage, epistaxis, and hematuria are much less common. Liver function generally is not affected by the leukemic infiltration.

LABORATORY FINDINGS. The total leukocyte count is elevated ($> 10,000$ cells/mm^3) in about 60% of patients.[73-75] Less than 15% of patients have extreme leukocytosis ($> 100,000$ cells/mm^3), and approximately 25% have leukopenia ($< 5,000$ cells/mm^3). Leukemic lymphoblasts usually predominate in the differential count at the expense of neutrophils and other normal leukocytes, except in some patients with leukopenia who may have few or no circulating lymphoblasts (aleukemic leukemia). Cerebral hemorrhage caused by extreme leukocytosis ($> 150,000$ blasts/mm^3) also is an occasional occurrence, although the smaller lymphoblasts seem less prone to leukostasis than myeloblasts. Despite the presence of thrombocytopenia, cerebral hemorrhage is much less common in ALL than AML.[73,74] Leukemic meningitis and cranial nerve palsies due to nerve infiltration by leukemic blasts are quite common in ALL, although usually late occurrences, and the frequency increases with duration of the disease. It is not unusual for patients in hematologic remission to develop these complications if no prophylactic therapy is given. Thrombocytopenia and anemia are almost always present at diagnosis; the latter is primarily a manifestation of the failure of red blood cell production and, to some extent, of blood loss if significant hemorrhage is present.

Hyperuricemia and the resulting urate nephropathy occasionally may be present before treatment, but these are much more likely to be precipitated by the initiation of chemotherapy, when massive lysis of leukemic cells occurs. This complication usually is prevented easily by adequate hydration and administration of the xanthine oxidase inhibitor allopurinol before chemotherapy begins.

Radiographic films of the chest occasionally show hilar or mediastinal adenopathy, and osteolytic lesions or periosteal infiltration usually is demonstrable in patients with bone pain. A radiolucent metaphyseal line (clinically asymptomatic) caused by altered growth associated with the onset of ALL commonly is demonstrable as well (Fig. 13.2). Bone infarcts, a less frequent cause of bone pain, usually are not visualized radiographically early in their evolution.[76-78]

The diagnosis of acute leukemia cannot be made on the basis of peripheral blood examination alone; suspicion of acute leukemia necessitates a bone marrow examination. Wright-stained smears of marrow from patients with ALL typically show diffuse infiltration by a predominance of lymphoblasts. Most previously untreated patients have over 50% lymphoblasts; a differential count of bone marrow cells showing less than 30% abnormal cells makes a diagnosis of acute leukemia less likely. Lymphoblasts characteristically have a high nuclear/cytoplasmic ratio. The nuclei are not indented or folded, and the number of nucleoli is low (i.e., one or two). Azurophilic granules rarely are seen, and Auer bodies are absent. The cells of the granulocyte series usually are reduced in numbers, although different stages of both lymphocytic and granulocytic maturation, including mature cells, can be seen. Patients with larger, more primitive lymphoblasts tend to respond less well than do those with more differentiated leukemic cells.[79,80] On occasion, leukemic blasts may be so primitive in appearance that they lack distinguishing lymphoid or myeloid characteristics; these patients are designated as having *acute undifferentiated* or *stem cell leukemia*. Their management is the same as that of patients with AML.

Special cytochemical staining with periodic acid-Schiff reagent usually results in a reddish-pink positive cytoplasmic reaction in at least 5% of the leukemic blasts in patients with ALL; only mature neutrophils are stained in patients who have other leukemias, including acute undifferentiated leukemia.[2,74,75] The staining of the blasts tends to be clumped in nature rather than diffuse, as is the case with mature cells. Sudan black and peroxidase stains give negative results.

Terminal deoxynucleotidyl transferase (TdT) is a useful enzyme marker found in the blast cells of most patients who have acute lymphoblastic leukemia. This enzyme can be detected by a simple immunofluorescent method.[81,82] TdT is not found in mature, well-differentiated lymphocytes or in the majority of myeloblasts. Therefore, it is a useful marker for lymphoblastic malignancy, and the finding of TdT-positive cells during

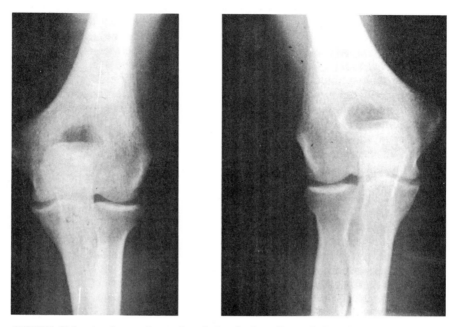

FIGURE 13.2. An abnormal metaphyseal plate in the radius and ulna of a child with acute lymphocytic leukemia.

presumed remission may signify the presence of residual leukemia cells.[83,84] In addition, however, a certain percentage of CML patients develop blast crisis consisting of TdT-positive blasts, and mixed-lineage AML may express TdT in addition to myeloid antigens.[85,86]

Newer diagnostic techniques using monoclonal antibodies and fluorescence-activated cell sorters allow a determination of the maturation stage of the leukemic blasts by identifying cell surface antigens expressed at different stages of maturation. Lymphoid blast cells are thus defined as being of B-cell or T-cell origin, and the exact stage of development can then be delineated by the pattern of immunologic markers (Fig. 13.3).[87,88] This information has prognostic significance in ALL and is now used to plan treatment approaches.

On occasion, the marrow cellularity is so great that marrow aspiration is unsuccessful. When such a "dry tap" occurs, it is imperative to perform a marrow biopsy with touch preparations of the biopsy specimen. The pathologist usually can recognize replacement of normal marrow by abnormal cells in the hematoxylin-eosin–stained sections; staining the touch preparations with Wright stain, however, is more useful in identifying the specific type of leukemia. Chromosomal analysis of the leukemic cells frequently shows an abnormal karyotype, and certain recurrent chromosomal abnormalities have been seen in ALL, including the Philadelphia chromo-

some and abnormalities of chromosome 14. This latter abnormality also has been seen in other B-cell malignancies.[89] Also of interest, many patients with ALL are hyperdiploid, which confers a better prognosis, whereas hypodiploid and diploid patients often have structural abnormalities detected by the newer banding techniques.[90]

DIFFERENTIAL DIAGNOSIS. The diagnosis of ALL usually is not difficult. Anemia, granulocytopenia, and thrombocytopenia usually are present at the time of initial presentation, and even if leukemic cells are not recognizable in the peripheral blood, bone marrow studies to investigate the cytopenias will reveal the true neoplastic nature of the disease. Peripheral lymphocytosis occurs in infectious mononucleosis, infectious lymphocytosis, pertussis, and to a lesser degree in other viral illnesses such as infectious hepatitis and varicella. The bone marrow, however, is less affected in these conditions and does not show infiltration with immature cells. Anemia and thrombocytopenia also should be less prominent than in ALL, although an autoimmune anemia, thrombocytopenia, or both can accompany infectious mononucleosis on occasion. Mononucleosis can be characterized by the presence of lymphoblast-like cells in the peripheral blood, and these cells tend to be less uniform than those of leukemia and are rarely seen

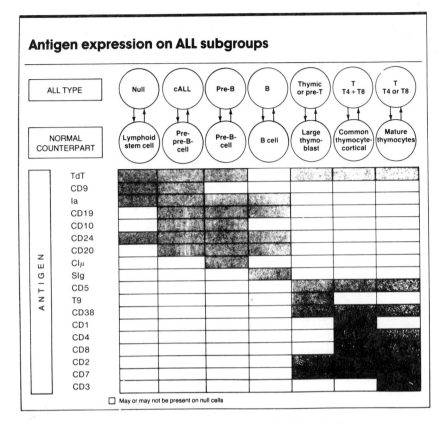

FIGURE 13.3. Antigen expression on acute lymphocytic leukemia subgroups.

in the marrow. A heterophile antibody test for mononucleosis also should be helpful in clarifying the situation.

In childhood ALL, poor prognostic features include elevated white blood cell count at diagnosis, lymphadenopathy, male gender, and impairment of normal hematologic parameters.[74,91,92] However, the mere development of ALL in an adult confers a poor prognosis; therefore, therapy of adult ALL continues to be more intensive than that used in all but poor-prognosis cases of childhood ALL. Identification of the lymphoblasts as being T-cell–derived confers a particularly poor prognosis and warrants intensive treatment.[91,92] T-cell ALL is seen most frequently in adolescent males and often is accompanied by a mediastinal mass.

A more difficult differential diagnosis, especially in an adult with suspected ALL, is *prolymphocytic leukemia.* Quite rare in children, this entity is characterized by the presence of poorly differentiated lymphocytes that may have prominent nucleoli. Although the clinical evolution of the disease tends to be more rapid than in CLL, it is rarely so abrupt as to suggest ALL. The typical lymphoblasts in ALL have less cytoplasm than

the cells of prolymphocytic leukemia and the nuclear chromatin is more delicate and the nucleoli less clearly discernible in lymphosarcoma cells.[74,75] Occasionally, patients with solid tumors such as Ewing sarcoma, embryonal rhabdomyosarcoma, or neuroblastoma may have bone marrow infiltration with tumor cells similar to those of ALL;[74] lack of other clinical features of ALL, particularly circulating lymphoblasts, as well as the presence of other features of the various solid tumors should suggest the correct diagnosis.

Acute Myeloid Leukemia

Acute myeloid leukemia characteristically affects people in middle age, although the disease can occur at any age. AML is subdivided on the basis of clinical and laboratory features into a number of variants: acute myelomonocytic, acute myelocytic, acute monocytic, and acute progranulocytic leukemia, as well as erythroleukemia (Di Guglielmo syndrome). The general management is the same for these subgroups, and there is some difficulty in distinguishing among them. Therefore, caution is necessary in assessing and accepting opposing opinions about their characteristic features and response to therapy. Myelocytic leukemia is distinguished from the myelomonocytic type by the absence of monoblasts in the former. On the other hand, some investigators have suggested there is no sharp demarcation between the very common myelomonocytic (Naegeli-type) leukemia with its abundance of both myeloblasts and monocytoid blasts and the rare pure monocytic (Schilling-type) leukemia; rather, these investigators suggest there is a continuum of morphologic variation from mostly granulocytic with a few monocytoid cells at one end to all monocytoid cells at the other. However, the greater degree of tissue infiltration (e.g., gingival hyperplasia, leukemia cutis) and more recent cytochemical specificities of the monocytoid blasts in the Schilling type of AML seem adequate to define the subgroup.[93] Acute progranulocytic leukemia is characterized by a marked predominance of progranulocytes rather than myeloblasts in the bone marrow and by a characteristic hemorrhagic tendency caused by disseminated intravascular coagulation in addition to thrombocytopenia. This disseminated intravascular coagulation syndrome is produced by release of the granules of the progranulocytes, which contain a tissue factor that triggers the coagulation process.[94,95] Erythroid abnormalities occur to some extent in all types of ANLL and the distinction between erythroleukemia and other acute leukemias rests chiefly on the marked megaloblastosis and predominance of erythroblasts in the marrow and blood of patients who have this rare variant.[96,97]

At present, the significance of identifying the subgroups is more to recognize the complications that tend to occur with some varieties and the differences required in immediate supportive management rather than in the ultimate responsiveness to chemotherapy. All of these variants respond fairly similarly to current chemotherapy. Nevertheless, research into the subtleties and pathogenesis of these differences is being pursued, because this ultimately may be of value in defining type-specific therapy.

CLINICAL MANIFESTATIONS. The basic clinical presenting manifestations of AML are similar to those of ALL, and again, they are related to the same replacement process of the normal marrow elements by leukemic blasts. The onset of AML can be as abrupt as that of ALL, with severe prostration from acute infection or hemorrhage (Fig. 13.4), or it may be somewhat more gradual, with low-grade fever or recurring episodes of infection or hemorrhage. In most instances, organ infiltration is less prominent than in ALL. Splenomegaly and lymphadenopathy are not uncommon but are generally

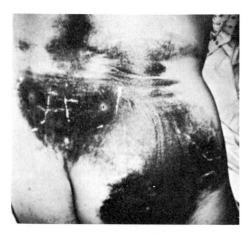

FIGURE 13.4. A severe hemorrhage into the flanks and buttocks of a patient with acute myelomonocytic leukemia and disseminated intravascular coagulation.

less remarkable than in ALL, and a normal physical examination is not unusual. Gingival hyperplasia caused by leukemic infiltration is limited almost exclusively to patients with acute monocytic and acute myelomonocytic leukemia,[98,99] and these hyperplastic gums often are inflamed, infected, or necrotic, and are very prone to bleeding (Fig. 13.5). Skin lesions also tend to be common in acute monocytic leukemia and somewhat less so in myelomonocytic leukemia;[98,99] typical lesions vary from macules or maculopapules to raised petechiae, exfoliative dermatitis, and even frank tumorous infiltrations (Fig. 13.6). Occasionally, localized tumor masses may arise in bones or soft tissues in patients with AML, and because of the presence of large quantities of the enzyme myeloperoxidase, these tumors often appear green on the cut surface, hence the term *chloromas*. More recently, the fact that many of these lesions are not colored has led to the application of the term *granulocytic sarcoma*. These tumors most commonly occur subperiosteally around the orbit, skull, sternum, rib, and proximal long bones; less frequently in the soft tissues of the breast, nodes, ovary, and dura; and rarely in other organs.[100,101] They also occasionally can precede other manifestations of the disease by months, thereby confusing the diagnosis greatly (Fig. 13.7).

LABORATORY FEATURES. The general hematologic manifestations of AML (i.e., anemia, thrombocytopenia, and leukocytosis) are similar in frequency and degree to those of ALL. When leukocytosis occurs (approximately one third of patients), it usually is characterized by an increased number of leukemic cells

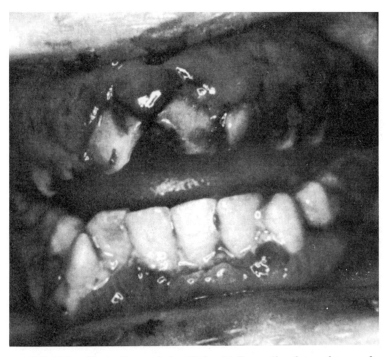

FIGURE 13.5. Gingival hyperplasia with local inflammation, hemorrhage, and necrosis in a patient with acute monoblastic leukemia.

and may become an emergency.[102] Circulating nucleated red blood cells are more common in AML than ALL; however, severe thrombocytopenia is less common in AML than ALL.[73,103]

Although the anemia usually seen in ALL is normochromic and normocytic in type, the marrow erythroblasts tend to be megaloblastoid in appearance. Administration of folate, vitamin B_{12}, or other nutritional factors fails to correct the anemia. Hemorrhage caused by thrombocytopenia usually is not severe unless the platelet count is less than 20,000 cells/mm^3. Patients who have AML, and especially those who have acute progranulocytic leukemia, may have a severe hemorrhagic diathesis known as *disseminated intravascular coagulation,* characterized not only by thrombocytopenia but also by hypofibrinogenemia, decreased concentrations of factor V, and elevated levels of fibrin split products.[104]

The serum and urinary muramidase (lysozyme) levels in most patients with acute monocytic and myelomono-

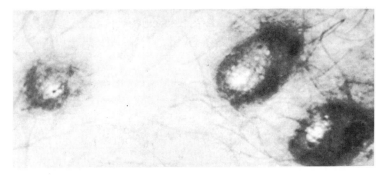

FIGURE 13.6. Tumorous leukemic skin infiltrates a patient with acute monoblastic leukemia.

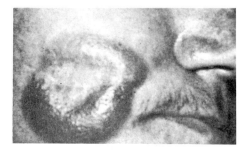

FIGURE 13.7. A granulocytic sarcoma on the cheek of a 35-year-old woman who did not manifest acute nonlymphocytic leukemia until 10 months after the appearance of this lesion.

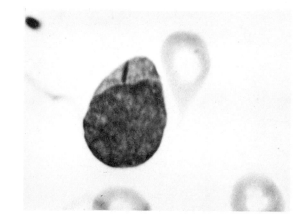

FIGURE 13.8. A myeloblast containing an Auer body.

cytic leukemia also tend to be high, whereas in other varieties of AML and ALL, they tend to be low or normal.[93] The highest serum and urinary muramidase levels tend to occur in those with monocytic leukemia. Patients with heavy muramidasuria also can develop a renal tubular defect that results in hypokalemia, hyperkaliuria, and azotemia.[105,106] Occasionally, patients who have acute monocytic or myelomonocytic leukemia also have other protein abnormalities such as increased polyclonal plasma immunoglobulin concentration.[107]

The diagnosis of AML, as with ALL, rests primarily on demonstrating increased numbers of blast cells in the blood and bone marrow. However, unlike ALL, in which lymphoblasts are almost always the predominant marrow cells seen at diagnosis, some AML patients can present with relatively few marrow blasts. If Auer bodies (rod- or needle-shaped azurophilic cytoplasmic structures) are present in any of the blasts (Fig. 13.8), the leukemia is almost certainly acute myelocytic or myelomonocytic;[1,93,98] thus, a thorough search should always be made for these. Typical myeloblasts are visible when stained with Wright stain, and these are fairly large and have abundant cytoplasm. The nuclear chromatin is finely disbursed, and multiple (three to five) nucleoli are visible. Progranulocytes are common in myelocytic leukemia, and the more mature granulocytes also may have abnormalities, such as the pseudo-Pelger-Huët anomaly. Hypogranular neutrophils and eosinophils may be noted.[1] The abnormal cells of monocytic leukemia resemble large histiocytes, with an abundance of light-blue cytoplasm and numerous azure granules, digestive vacuoles, and a large, indented, irregularly shaped, and often convoluted or folded nucleus. Myelomonocytic leukemia usually has mixed features from both the myelocytic and monocytic types, with two or more abnormal cell lines seen in the marrow, and when more than half of the leukemic cells are

progranulocytes, the diagnosis of acute progranulocytic leukemia is applied.[94,95,104]

Erythroleukemia typically presents with anemia, a few circulating and nucleated red blood cells, and bizarre megaloblastic erythroblasts predominating in the marrow.[1,96,97] In this rare disorder, changes in the red cell series overshadow the myeloblasts and, on occasion, may be seen before a demonstrable increase in myeloblasts is noted. Multinucleated bizarre erythroblasts and ringed sideroblasts are characteristic, as is their reaction to periodic acid-Schiff stain, that is, producing large clumps or blocks of cytoplasmic periodic acid-Schiff–positive material.[1] As the disease progresses, myeloblasts often become more prominent and lead to the development of more typical acute myelocytic or myelomonocytic leukemia.

To refine our diagnostic acumen, other tests have been developed to help differentiate ALL and the subgroups of AML; among these are the cytochemical stains, such as periodic acid-Schiff (gives a positive reaction in ALL and erythroleukemia), Sudan black, and peroxidase (usually positive in cases of acute myelocytic and myelomonocytic leukemia), as well as various esterase stains for myelomonocytic and monocytic leukemia.[1,93,98] In general, these seem to be most helpful in confirming a strongly suspected diagnosis.

Immunophenotyping using monoclonal antibodies against antigens present at varying stages of myeloid or monocytoid maturation usually confirms the morphologic impression.[108] A truly undifferentiated AML has neither morphologic nor immunophenotypic features to allow better characterization. Additionally, with the advent of monoclonal antibodies and fluorescence-activated cell sorters technology, the existence of biphenotypic and mixed-lineage leukemias has been identified and is not uncommon.[85,86]

TABLE 13.1. Specific Cytogenetic Abnormalities Associated with Specific Leukemias

Subtype of Myeloid Leukemia	Cytogenetic Abnormality	Prognosis
Acute myeloid leukemia with differentiation	t(8;21)	Good
Acute promyelocytic leukemia	t(15;17)	Good
Acute myelomonocytic leukemia with eosinophilia	inversion 16	Good
Acute myelomonocytic leukemia	t(4;11)	Poor
Secondary acute leukemia	−5, −7	Poor

Chromosomal abnormalities are seen frequently in AML, and these are enhanced by the use of newer banding and cell culture techniques.[53,54] These abnormalities may be present in the blasts of the majority of leukemic patients,[54] and a number of specific translocations have been associated with specific leukemia phenotypes (Table 13.1) and have prognostic importance.[109] In general, chromosomal translocations are associated with a better prognosis than are chromosomal deletions, and a normal karyotype carries a better prognosis than one with multiple abnormalities.[110] An interesting and very strong association (nearly 100%) has been found in acute progranulocytic leukemia with the characteristic translocation of t(15;17).[111] This association is even more interesting because this subtype of leukemia is unique in that it almost always can be made to differentiate into mature granulocytes when stimulated during in vitro cultures with compounds such as vitamin A derivatives (i.e. retinoic acid).[112,113] Subsequently, recent reports have shown clinical responses of a majority of patients with acute promyelocytic leukemia treated by oral *trans*-retinoic acid.[114–117] In addition, the gene for the retinoic acid receptor is located on chromosome 17.[118]

DIFFERENTIAL DIAGNOSIS. Leukemoid reactions, or nonneoplastic elevations of the leukocyte count, rarely are characterized by a large number of circulating blast cells. Appropriate microbiologic evaluation should help to eliminate such infections as tuberculosis or meningococcemia. The case reports of patients having tuberculosis and large numbers of marrow myeloblasts are subject to some question, because it is possible that these patients actually may have had coincident AML rather than a leukemoid reaction.[119,120]

Bone marrow metastasis from oat cell carcinoma of the lung may be difficult to differentiate morphologically from AML, but the clinical background should make the distinction fairly easy. Diffuse histiocytic lymphoma with marrow invasion may present more of a problem because of its monocytoid features and tendency to invade the skin and other organs. Gingival hyperplasia, however, is much more characteristic of monocytic leukemia; retroperitoneal adenopathy, characteristic of diffuse histiocytic lymphoma, is most unusual in monocytic leukemia. Malignant lymphoma with hepatosplenomegaly and marrow involvement but without lymphadenopathy, although rare, may be indistinguishable clinically from monocytic leukemia.

Regardless of the cause, aplastic anemia in a regenerative phase can be associated with a bone marrow picture very similar to that of AML, with a predominance of myeloblasts. An astute history of prior drug or toxin exposure, suspicion of the marrow's true status, and the "test of time" to demonstrate further regeneration help to distinguish the disorders. Occasionally, patients having aplastic anemia subsequently develop AML.

Erythroleukemia is particularly difficult to diagnose, and it may be confused with sideroblastic anemia, paroxysmal nocturnal hemoglobinuria, or primary refractory anemia, all of which themselves can terminate in AML. It has been suggested these actually all may be early forms of erythroleukemia.[121]

UNUSUAL FORMS OF AML

Myelodysplasia. This term is a descriptive one that encompasses a variety of marrow abnormalities, some of which evolve into acute leukemia. These include refractory anemia with excess blasts (RAEB) or RAEB in transformation. These sometimes are termed *smouldering leukemia*, and the pre-existing anemia often is termed *preleukemia*.

Myelodysplasia that evolves into leukemia is a clonal disorder, often with karyotypic abnormalities. Patients with RAEB present with anemia, thrombocytopenia, and obvious abnormalities of all cell lines, and although some maturation is present in the myeloid series beyond the promyelocyte stage, there are clear abnormalities compatible with leukemia in the marrow.

Not all myelodysplastic marrows progress to acute leukemia, but a very high incidence of RAEB and RAEB in transformation do.[122–124] Attempts to determine which patients will develop frank leukemia have included studies of their karyotypes and in vitro colony growth of their marrow cells.[125,126] Chromosomal analysis has been very helpful in this regard, identifying an abnormality called 5q-, a deletion of a long arm of chromosome 5.[127,128] During the stable phase, karyotypes show only 5q-, but with progression to leukemia, additional karyotypic abnormalities develop.[128] Response to treatment when these patients develop AML has been poor uniformly; they tend to die of infection whether or not the leukemia is treated. Recently, however, more aggressive treatment has been investigated that may prove helpful,[129] and biologic agents as well as hematopoietic growth factors also are being explored as therapy for this entity.

Eosinophilic Leukemia. Abnormal eosinophils often are present in small numbers in both AML and CML. There also is evidence to suggest that in some AML patients, cells appearing to be eosinophils are actually neoplastic neutrophils containing abnormal granules.[130]

Although called *eosinophilic leukemia*, the clinical presentation of extreme eosinophilia (possibly over 100,000 cells/mm^3) appears to be part of a spectrum of disorders termed *hypereosinophilic syndromes*.[131–133] The eosinophils in such patients usually are mature cells with segmented nuclei, and chromosomal analyses are normal. The clinical manifestations include peripheral and marrow eosinophilia, hepatosplenomegaly, and often cardiac infiltration that leads to arrhythmias, angina, or congestive heart failure;[134] there may be neurologic dysfunction as well. Review articles have described the spectrum of the disease,[131,132] and one study proposed a clinical and hematologic grading system to predict the clinical course and help determine the need for early therapy.[131,132] Treatment of the hypereosinophilic syndrome depends on the severity of the disease. Patients are observed with minimal organ involvement, but with progressive involvement, either steroids or the combination of steroids and cytotoxic therapy are necessary. This disorder rarely progresses to a disease similar to AML.

Mast Cell Leukemia. Urticaria pigmentosa is a disease of unknown etiology characterized by a maculopapular, predominately truncal rash that is represented histologically by infiltration of mast cells in large numbers into the affected skin.[135,136] Exaggerated wheal-and-flare reactions resulting in dermographia usually are demonstrable, and patients occasionally develop systemic mastocytosis, that is, infiltration of the liver, spleen, gastrointestinal tract, and other organs with mast cells. Hemorrhagic tendencies often develop in the terminal stages.

Plasma Cell, Basophilic, and Megakaryocytic Leukemia. These forms tend to occur as end stages in other diseases rather than de novo. Basophilic and megakaryocytic leukemia evolve as variants of CML or other myeloproliferative states.[137,138] Peripheral plasmacytosis rarely occurs as a terminal or presenting feature of myeloma; it usually is a grave prognostic event.[139,140]

Plasma cell leukemia can arise de novo and may precede or exist separately from myeloma. It is a distinct clinical entity, with severe anemia, hepatosplenomegaly, and leukocytosis. Bony lesions are less common than in myeloma, and the production of M components is related to the maturity of the plasma cells.[141,142] Transmission electron microscopy has proven helpful in making the correct diagnosis in patients presenting with leukemia,[142] but the response to treatment with glucocorticoids and an alkylating agent is poor.

Therapy and Management of the Acute Leukemias

The best time to achieve the longest remission and the possible cure of acute leukemia by maximal cell kill is when the disease is first diagnosed, because cells that survive the first attack of treatment generally are more resistant to subsequent therapy with drugs that were initially effective. Thus, the first remission achieved usually is the longest, with subsequent remissions becoming shorter and more difficult to maintain. The use of combinations of effective drugs rather than single drugs generally has improved the response rate in acute leukemia, but without a sensitive method to predict the combinations, sequencing, and order that will achieve maximal cell kill with minimal side effects, most regimens are empiric and tend to be rather complex. Meaningful comparisons between different series often are difficult because of differences in patient selection, age of patients, prior therapy, criteria for evaluability of patient material, and variability in measuring duration of remission and survival. Because none of these therapies has been uniformly successful as yet, no standard treatment regimens have been established, and investigators still are trying to improve on current results with comparative clinical trials. Whenever possible, it is advisable for patients to be treated by physicians well-versed in the complex management of these diseases and therapeutic regimens.

PRIMARY TREATMENT OF ACUTE LYMPHO-CYTIC LEUKEMIA. The most successful current induction regimens for ALL are based on the use of vincristine and prednisone. Remission rates of 80% to 90% for children and 50% to 60% for adults are reported using combinations of these drugs.[74,75] Remissions last only a few months if therapy is discontinued after induction, but subsequent use of drugs such as 6-mercaptopurine and methotrexate in a continuous-treatment regimen with periodic reinforcing doses of vincristine and prednisone every 4 to 12 weeks has lengthened remissions progressively.

In adults and children with poor prognostic features, the use of combination chemotherapy and the addition of an anthracycline drug for induction therapy has improved both the remission induction rate and duration.[75,143–149] The recent Berlin Childhood Acute Lymphoblastic Leukemia Therapy Study[150] used very intensive induction and maintenance treatment, and this produced a 5-year continuous remission in 60% of children treated. The treatment of adult ALL has not yet matched these results; however, newer and more intensive approaches appear to improve outcome.[143–149] Current therapy for ALL consists of several phases, including remission induction, cytoreduction, and maintenance.[146,150–153] Maintenance therapy has improved survival substantially; however, the optimal duration of maintenance therapy is not yet precisely known. Unfortunately, rare, late relapses still occur.

Without specific therapy for the central nervous system (CNS), approximately one half of all affected children develop leukemic meningitis (infiltration of the meninges and brain); often, this is the initial manifestation of relapse. Such patients manifest headaches, irritability, vomiting, changes in personality, meningism, papilledema, and cranial nerve palsies.[154] It is suspected that this failure results from a sequestration of leukemic cells in a pharmacologic sanctuary beyond the blood–brain barrier, and because of this high incidence of leukemic meningitis, regional therapy with craniospinal irradiation (to the entire brain, retinas, and upper cervical cord) has been combined with intrathecal methotrexate following attainment of remission.[154,155] It is unclear that such a combined approach is necessary, however, because use of intrathecal methotrexate alone or systemic high-dose methotrexate may be as effective.[151,156,157] Concern regarding long-term CNS dysfunction with a combined-modality approach has led to greater interest in using chemotherapy alone as CNS prophylaxis; CNS prophylaxis has contributed substantially to long-term disease-free remission and survival.

It has not yet been established at what point therapy should be discontinued. Because most relapses occur within 3 years, treatment has been shortened to 3 years without detriment in some studies.[150]

Also, because adults with ALL are considered poor-prognosis patients, often with fewer favorable clinical characteristics, intensification of therapy with bone marrow transplantation is a consideration. This is usu-

ally recommended for patients with very poor prognosis (i.e., Philadelphia chromosome and ALL) or for those in second remission. Current data do not show any advantage over chemotherapy in first remission.[158]

PRIMARY TREATMENT OF ACUTE MYELOGENOUS LEUKEMIA. The treatment of AML continues to improve. Numerous drugs are effective as single agents to induce remission. The first highly successful combination regimen that was developed used the two most active single agents, daunorubicin (an anthracycline) and cytosine arabinoside; a remission rate of 65% or better is achieved consistently with this combination.[159,160] The median duration of remission ranges from 10 to 25 months, with approximately 30% of complete remissions lasting 2 or more years, and some have added 6-thioguanine to this induction regimen with good, although not better, results.[161,162]

In the past 5 to 10 years, several new chemotherapeutic agents have added to the armamentarium against AML, and to some degree ALL. These include mitoxantrone, an anthraquinone that appears to be noncross-resistant,[163,164] and idarubicin, an anthracycline with an active metabolite that makes it a more effective induction agent.[165,166] Both are given with cytosine arabinoside. In addition, a regimen of high-dose cytosine arabinoside appears to be effective in inducing remission, particularly in patients developing resistance to anthracyclines.[167]

Once achieving remission, patients with AML will relapse readily if left untreated;[168] therefore, postremission therapy is considered essential in AML as well as ALL. However, the success of such an approach appears to be related to the intensity, ranging from ALL-type outpatient maintenance[168] to intensive prolonged maintenance[169–171] to intensive short-course consolidative therapy[172–174] to bone marrow transplantation.[175] The latter three approaches appear to be equally effective, with more than 50% of patients remaining in remission after 2 years.

Prophylactic CNS therapy does not appear to be necessary to prevent meningeal leukemia in the majority of patients with AML. The use of a continuous infusion of cytosine arabinoside during induction treatment and the use of subcutaneous cytosine arabinoside during maintenance therapy, both of which produce continuous therapeutic CNS drug levels, may be the reason the incidence of CNS leukemia in AML has not risen in long-term survivors.[176,177]

Because of the relatively poor overall prognosis in AML, bone marrow transplantation has been advocated as a potential cure. Recipients must be selected carefully by age and availability for an HLA-matched sibling, although unrelated transplants are being used more frequently. The major complications of transplantation are infection and graft-versus-host disease,[178] and both the remission duration and the survival of patients undergoing bone marrow transplantation in first remission are not significantly different at present from those of a similar group treated with intensive postremission chemotherapy alone.[103,170–175] The role of bone marrow transplantation in high-risk patients and second remission is now being defined.

SUPPORTIVE CARE. The supportive care of patients with acute leukemia is as important as specific systemic therapy for the disease itself. Certain emergencies may exist at the time of the diagnosis of acute leukemia that require treatment before intensive systemic antileukemia therapy is instituted. Other problems arise during treatment, but all require rigorous evaluation and intensive management.

Intracerebral Leukostasis. Occasionally patients with AML, and rarely those with ALL, who have greatly elevated leukocyte counts often die rather suddenly from intracerebral hemorrhage as opposed to the subarachnoid or subdural bleeding more characteristic of patients who have thrombocytopenia.[179] Pathologic examination of the brains of these patients has led to the conclusion that leukostasis from the high leukemic blast concentrations ruptured the cerebral microvasculature; this probably accounts in part for the poor prognosis in patients with AML who have high initial white blood cell counts ($> 150,000$ blasts/mm^3). Immediate administration of small doses of cranial radiation (300 to 600 rads) to resolve such leukostatic foci as well as therapy with hydroxyurea to lower quickly the white blood cell count in such patients have resulted in almost total elimination of this problem.[180]

Hemorrhage. Platelet transfusions employed prophylactically in patients with fewer than 20,000 platelets/mm^3, regardless of clinical bleeding, have improved significantly the poor prognosis associated with thrombocytopenia on presentation.[181] Bleeding may occur at higher platelet levels if the platelet count is falling rapidly, and this should be handled similarly. Pooled random-donor platelets usually are adequate initially for most patients; however, many patients will develop resistance to such platelets at some time in their usage. There does not, however, appear to be a dose-response relationship determining the rate of alloimmunization.[182,183] For this reason, the physician should observe and assess each individual patient for response to random-donor platelets;[184] if the patient becomes alloimmunized, transfusions of HLA-matched platelets often can be successful in either preventing or stopping thrombocytopenic hemorrhage.[185,186] It is also feasible to remove, freeze, and store platelets from some patients in remission for their own use during subsequent treatment cycles.[187,188]

Thrombocytopenic hemorrhage usually is capillary in nature, leading to the development of petechiae. At times, patients present with ecchymotic hemorrhage and bleeding from needle-puncture sites (Fig. 13.2), which are more suggestive of a dysfunction of coagulation factors and typical of disseminated intravascular coagulation. A coagulation profile, including measurements of prothrombin time, partial thromboplastin time, fibrinogen, and fibrin split products, should be performed for any patient with such disproportionate bleeding. If this is compatible with intravascular coagulation, even if no evidence of hemorrhage is present, low-dose heparin therapy should be started immediately at a loading dose of 50 U/kg, followed by 100 to 200 U/kg over each 24-hour period; the serum fibrinogen is a useful value to follow for response. This therapy usually results in definite improvement within 24 to 48 hours.[189,190] Also, as stated previously, DIC frequently is associated with acute promyelocytic leukemia.

Infection. The most frequent cause of death among adult patients with acute leukemia is infection, and some of these occur before there is an adequate chance to respond to chemotherapy. Any patient with febrile granulocytopenia must be considered to have a life-threatening infection until proven otherwise, and after appropriate cultures and physical examination, the physician should institute empiric broad-spectrum antibiotic therapy immediately. Appropriate changes can be made in antibiotics when baseline cultures identify a specific organism;[191–193] if no organism is cultured, the patient's clinical response to empiric antibiotic therapy should be used as the guide to changing or discontinuing antibiotics. It is of utmost importance to be aware that patients with granulocytopenia may not show localized signs or symptoms of inflammation and that fever can be the only evidence of a life-threatening infection. Frequent chest radiographs and daily physical examinations similarly are vital in the diagnosis of pneumonia, the most common serious infection in patients with acute leukemia.[193] The second most common infection, and probably the most common cause of gram-negative septicemia in these patients, is the perianal or perirectal lesion.[193] Also, with the increasing use of venous access catheters, gram-positive organisms from catheter-related infections have become much more common. These organisms have been identified in as many as 30% of documented bacteremias.[193]

Fungal infections are becoming more common as well, due in part to the greater effectiveness and suppressive effects of current broad-spectrum antibiotics and perhaps also because patients with granulocytopenia are being maintained for longer periods of time.[192] Candida and Aspergillus species remain the most common pathogens, and amphotericin B remains the major antifungal antibiotic.

Some patients, especially those with persistent granulocytopenia, develop progressive infections despite the early institution of appropriate antibiotic therapy. Granulocytes from normal ABO group–compatible donors have been collected by centrifugation and leukapheresis and then transfused into these patients to control their infections.[194] At least 10^{10} granulocytes should be transfused daily, beginning as early in the course of infection as feasible. The dose of granulocytes administered is vitally important in obtaining a good clinical response, and therapeutic granulocyte transfusions, when given appropriately and in adequate doses, are beneficial in at least one third of infected patients with granulocytopenia who have not responded to appropriate antibiotics. Granulocyte transfusions have been used less frequently in recent years because of more effective antibiotics and a general acceptance of the concept of empiric antibiotic therapy. The use of granulocyte colony-stimulating factors in this situation currently is being studied.

Unlike platelet transfusions, however, prophylactic granulocyte transfusions have not been shown to be universally helpful. Although they do seem to prevent infection, an increasing number of transfusion reactions and pulmonary infiltrates may result.[195,196]

In addition, various forms of reverse isolation in Life Islands or in Laminar Air Flow rooms both with or without oral nonabsorbable antibiotics have been used to try to prevent the acquisition of pathogens by patients with leukemia, thereby decreasing the incidence of infections.[197,198] Although infections have been reduced during induction therapy, investigations conflict as to whether this resulted in a higher remission rate. It is unclear which aspect of such infection prevention is most beneficial to patients with the cytotoxic chemotherapy currently used; it is clear, however, that all patient isolation techniques have resulted in fewer serious infections during treatment of granulocytopenic leukemia.

Tissue Infiltration. Leukemic infiltration of virtually every organ in the body has been described. Such infiltrates are most common in children with ALL and in adults with myelomonocytic leukemia but can occur with any acute leukemia, and symptoms of organ dysfunction attributable directly to leukemic cell infiltration are generally lacking, except in the case of leukemic meningitis. Low-dose radiation therapy usually will eradicate leukemic foci in most locations, such as the mediastinum in children with gross mediastinal adenopathy and respiratory distress from ALL; the retina when funduscopic examination shows leukemic retinal exudates or hemorrhages; or cranial nerves when cranial nerve palsies caused by leukemic infiltration of a nerve occur. Intrathecal chemotherapy with methotrexate should be employed if a lumbar puncture reveals meningeal leukemia, and maintenance treatment with periodic intrathecal methotrexate should be continued after the spinal fluid is cleared of leukemic cells.[199] Because of the superior response of systemic AML to cytosine arabinoside, the intrathecal use of this drug may be tried in patients with AML who develop leukemic meningitis or in patients with ALL and leukemic meningitis that is refractory to intrathecal methotrexate.[200,201]

Prognosis

The average survival of a patient with untreated ALL is only 3 months. With improved chemotherapy and control of meningeal leukemia, over 90% of children and 70% of adults with ALL now achieve remission, and there are several reports indicating that over 50% of children live beyond 5 years.[74,92,150] Because many of these children have been disease-free and off therapy for several years, it appears likely that some may be cured; however, a much longer follow-up period is necessary to see if their lifespan approaches normal. For adults with ALL, median survival is reported at over 16 months for those who respond to treatment and 13 months for all patients.[75,146–149,151,152]

The prognosis of patients with AML is becoming more optimistic, and current regimens are able to produce remission in over 60% of patients. The median duration of first remission is between 6 and 25 months, and the average survival is approaching 2.5 years compared with 3 months for nonresponding and untreated patients.[170,171,173–175] Nevertheless, a scant 30% of patients have achieved disease-free survival of 5 years or more. Obviously, continued research is necessary.

CHRONIC LEUKEMIAS

Chronic Myelocytic Leukemia

Chronic myelocytic leukemia primarily affects adults between the ages of 30 and 50 years, but in a series of 113 patients, one third were more than 60 years of age.[202] CML is characterized by an abnormal overproduction and accumulation of granulocytic precursors in the marrow, spleen, and blood. Cytogenetic and morphologic abnormalities are seen in both the red cell and platelet series as well as in the white cells, so the disease actually is a panmyelosis and can be grouped with the myeloproliferative diseases such as myeloid metaplasia with myelofibrosis and polycythemia vera.

The natural history of CML can be divided into two fairly distinct phases. In the chronic or early phase, the disorder is myeloproliferative with accumulation of neutrophils and granulocytic precursors. Clinical manifestations of the disease are readily controlled during this phase, which usually is of 2- to 3-years' duration. The terminal phase is characterized by increasing refractoriness to chemotherapy with either progressive myeloproliferation or myelofibrosis or, more commonly, a transition to a state called *blast crisis* that resembles AML both clinically and pathologically.[203–205]

CLINICAL MANIFESTATIONS. As many as 20% of patients with CML are diagnosed when asymptomatic; in these patients, an abnormal white blood cell count is found during examination for other reasons. More commonly, patients complain of fatigue that has progressed over several weeks to months and often of anorexia and weight loss. Fever is uncommon in this disease until the terminal phase. Symptoms relating to splenomegaly are common, and there may be a feeling of fullness or heaviness or of a dragging sensation in the upper left quadrant of the abdomen. The discovery of an abdominal mass may cause the patient to see a physician, and occasionally, a patient may complain of sternal tenderness. Less frequently, the physician may be consulted because of symptoms of anemia, pain caused by splenic infarction, hemorrhagic or thrombotic manifestations, or rarely, an attack of gout.

The most common physical findings at the time of diagnosis are pallor, sternal tenderness, and splenomegaly. Sternal tenderness can be elicited in most patients, and other bones may be tender as well. Because of extramedullary hematopoiesis, the spleen is palpable in nearly all patients, and the organ may be quite large or, not infrequently, even massive. Splenic infarction tends to be more common in CML than in other types of leukemia, and it usually is heralded by severe pain in the upper left quadrant, with splenic tenderness on palpation. A friction rub may be heard over the spleen.

LABORATORY FINDINGS. Invariably, the leukocyte count is elevated; it is usually over 50,000 cells/mm^3 and may be as high as 500,000 cells/mm^3. Symptomatic patients generally have white blood cell counts greater than 75,000 cells/mm^3. Differential white blood cell counts show a predominance of all degrees of immature and mature granulocytes (Fig. 13.9), but myeloblasts rarely exceed 5%. Eosinophils and basophils may be

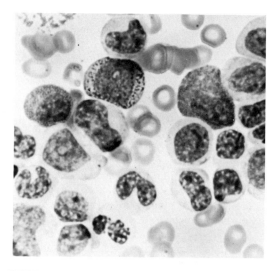

FIGURE 13.9.   A peripheral blood smear from a patient with chronic myelocytic leukemia.

increased, and bone marrow aspiration often is difficult because of marrow hypercellularity. Marrow fat usually is scant, because it has been replaced by cells, 80% to 90% of which are granulocytic precursors. These are found in approximately the same distribution as in the peripheral blood, with only a slight shift in distribution toward immature forms. Megakaryocytes usually are increased markedly, and in 25% of needle-biopsy specimens from patients with CML, some degree of fibrosis is initially demonstrable by reticulin stain.

Anemia of varying degrees may be present, and thrombocytosis is seen in approximately one half of patients at diagnosis, sometimes with associated thrombotic and hemorrhagic complications. Occasionally, patients present with thrombocytopenia; this finding becomes more frequent as the disease progresses.

Leukocyte alkaline phosphatase activity in the neutrophils usually is decreased or absent, but it can become normal or even elevated with intercurrent infection, inflammation, or the onset of blast crisis.[206,207] Uric acid levels characteristically are elevated, as are the levels of serum vitamin B$_{12}$, vitamin B$_{12}$-binding protein, transcobalamin I, and serum lactic dehydrogenase.

Approximately 90% of patients with the clinical and hematologic features of CML have a unique and characteristic chromosome (Philadelphia). This abnormality consists of a translocation of chromosomal material from the long arm of chromosome 22 to chromosome 9.[208] The Philadelphia chromosome is found in all marrow cell lines but not in skin, lymphocytes, or connective tissue, suggesting this abnormality is an acquired defect of a stem cell common to the red cells, platelets, and granulocytes. The Philadelphia chromosome persists throughout the course of the disease and rarely is affected by therapy.

Molecular biologic techniques have demonstrated that the 9;22 translocation involves movement of an oncogene, c-*abl*, in approximation with the *bcr* segment.[209] This complex codes for a new protein with tyrosine kinase activity that may be a factor in the proliferative nature of this disease.[210] Using molecular biologic techniques, patients with the clinical picture of CML can be demonstrated to have the translocation even if a Philadelphia chromosome is not apparent.

The 10% of patients with other characteristic features of CML but no Philadelphia chromosome usually follow an atypical course. They are less responsive to therapy, and they usually have a shorter survival then Philadelphia chromosome–positive patients.[211,212] They usually are older, and they may have lymphadenopathy and a peripheral moncytosis. One subgroup has neither a Philadelphia chromosome nor the *bcr/abl* translocation demonstrated.

DIAGNOSIS AND DIFFERENTIAL DIAGNOSIS. The diagnosis of CML can be made easily and accurately in most patients by examining a well-stained peripheral blood smear. The impressive leukocytosis with the characteristic shift to immature granulocytes and the abundant eosinophils and basophils suggest the diagnosis of CML. The presence of splenomegaly in most cases will help to distinguish CML from leukemoid reactions but not from other myeloproliferative syndromes. In leukemoid reactions caused by infections or neoplasms, a normal or elevated leukocyte alkaline phospatase level and absence of the Philadelphia chromosome also would be expected. Characteristically, the CML patient is relatively well at the time of diagnosis, whereas most patients with leukemoid reactions have underlying disease associated with various signs and symptoms.

Myeloid metaplasia with myelofibrosis, a morphologically similar myeloproliferative syndrome, is sometimes difficult to distinguish from CML. Splenomegaly, leukocytosis, and thrombocytosis are characteristic of both disorders. In myeloid metasplasia, however, the bone marrow biopsy should reveal marked fibrosis, the leukocyte alkaline phosphatase level is normal or high, and there is no Philadelphia chromosome.

Patients about whom the suspicion of CML is raised solely by an elevated leukocyte count initially may present a problem in diagnosis. Their white blood cell counts may only be mildly elevated, that is, in the range of 15,000 cells/mm^3 to 20,000 cells/mm^3, with perhaps a mild shift to immature forms. Although the leukocyte alkaline phosphatase level may not be reduced in these

patients, demonstration of a Philadelphia chromosome usually is possible and greatly facilitates diagnosis. Also, molecular biologic techniques can be used to demonstrate the *bcr/abl* translocation.

TREATMENT. Treatment of the chronic phase of CML essentially involves controlling both the level of the white blood cell count and the size of the spleen. This is done relatively easily by using oral agents such as busulfan or hydroxyurea. This approach does not alter the transformation of the disease. Of the two agents, hydroxyurea has gained popularity because it has less long-term toxicity.[213,214] If the patient is a potential candidate for bone marrow transplant, hydroxyurea is preferable to avoid possible pulmonary toxicity from busulfan.

Before therapy, all patients should be adequately hydrated and started on allopurinol. This is both because of the initial presence of hyperuricemia (presumably caused by the increased cell turnover in the granulocytic population) and the impending release of more purine metabolites during chemotherapy.

If hydroxyurea is used, the starting dose is 1000 to 1500 mg daily, which is continued until the white blood cell count falls below 15,000 cells/mm^3, and weekly monitoring of the blood count allows dose adjustments. Unlike busulfan, there is often rapid rebound of the white blood cell count once hydroxyurea administration is stopped.

Busulfan also can be used, at a starting oral dose of 4 mg/m^2 daily. There is a delayed onset of effect with this drug as well as a continued fall in white blood cell count for 1 to 2 weeks after therapy has been halted. Therefore, white blood cell counts are monitored weekly, and drug doses are reduced or stopped when the white blood count falls below 15,000 cells/mm^3. Busulfan then can be reinstituted at a lower dose to maintain a white blood cell count near 10,000 cells/mm^3 until the spleen is no longer palpable.

The diagnostic features of the disease, including splenomegaly, thrombocytosis, abnormal white cell differential count, and anemia, return to normal in over 60% of patients, and control of the leukocyte count is achieved in over 90% with therapy. The leukocyte alkaline phosphatase level also may rise to normal in some patients; however, the Philadelphia chromosome almost always persists. Most physicians discontinue therapy when maximal clinical benefit is attained, because continued small maintenance doses do not seem to prolong the controlled state but rather increase the risk of side effects. When clinical manifestations of the disease reappear, usually in several weeks to several months, therapy is restarted using the original regimen, but successive remissions characteristically are shorter and harder to achieve.

In the one fourth of patients with initial marrow fibrosis, this process is generally progressive, and eventually, may result in a picture indistinguishable from that of myeloid metaplasia with myelofibrosis. In these patients in whom the attendant hypocellularity of the bone marrow makes it difficult to continue administering effective doses of chemotherapeutic agent, the prognosis is poor.[215]

In another, smaller group of patients, the disease simply becomes refractory to continued oral chemotherapy. It becomes impossible to control the leukocyte count without unacceptable myelosuppression, especially thrombocytopenia in the case of busulfan. In the absence of frank transformation to blast crisis, hydroxyurea (0.5 to 2.0 g/day orally) may be able to control the proliferative aspects of the disease at this time;[214] hydroxyurea seems to have a "platelet-sparing" property.

Recently, interferon-α has been used to control the proliferative aspects of the chronic phase of CML. There also is evidence that the Philadelphia chromosome can be modified and, in some cases, eliminated by interferon therapy.[216] It is not yet clear whether these effects will reduce or delay the development of blastic crisis, but those patients with complete suppression of the Philadelphia chromosome have longer duration of the chronic phase.

The use of interferon-α in the treatment of chronic phase CML has provided new insights into the disease. In a recently published series involving 96 patients, 73% achieved a hematologic remission, and 19% had complete suppression of the Philadelphia chromosome.[217] Eleven patients had durable, complete cytogenetic responses for between 6 to more than 45 months.[217] The molecular analysis of this suppression has shown the complete disappearance of the bcr/abl translocation in many cases,[216] and this suggests a reversal of the cytogenetic abnormality that may accelerate or initiate the disease process.

In the majority of patients, CML eventually enters a blast crisis, typified by replacement of the mature granulocytic elements in both the peripheral blood and marrow by myeloblasts and progranulocytes, thus producing a picture indistinguishable from that of AML. Additional cytogenetic abnormalities, such as a double Philadelphia chromosome, as well as peripheral basophilia may accompany or precede this change.[208,218]

Because the natural history of CML culminates in a blastic phase that remains a major therapeutic dilemma, recent innovations in the treatment of CML have included attempts to prolong the chronic phase or to eliminate the Philadelphia chromosome–positive clone during that phase. These attempts include the use of intensive multiagent chemotherapy for induction and maintenance to produce a reduction in marrow Philadel-

phia chromosome–positive cells; however, the rate of blastic transformation in such studies is not lower than in groups treated less intensively.[219] Whether interferon therapy will alter this where true absence of the Philadelphia chromosome has been documented is as yet unknown.

Another innovative, and perhaps more promising, approach is the use of bone marrow transplantation following sublethal chemotherapy and total-body irradiation. At least in some patients transplanted during the chronic phase, it appears that the malignant clone is eradicated.[220] However, marrow transplantation has not been successful in the later stages of CML.

The blast crisis phase of CML generally is unresponsive to therapy. Vincristine and prednisone have been reported to produce clinical remission in 20% of patients with CML in blast crisis, particularly those whose karyotypes became hypodiploid during the transformation to blast crisis and who have a lymphoid morphology.[208]

The cellular marker TdT appears to identify cells of a lymphoid nature, and it may be used as an indicator of the potential benefit of treatment with vincristine and prednisone.[221,222] One caution is that in CML, not all TdT-positive blasts appear to be lymphoid, and those that do not are less likely to respond to this treatment.[223] Any benefit obtained from vincristine and prednisone is brief, however, and does not appear to influence overall survival.[223]

Intensive combination chemotherapy for blast crisis, similar to that used in AML, has been used with occasional success.[224–226] A few patients who present with blast crisis and no prior chronic phase seem to repond to this type of therapy and revert to a chronic phase; however, despite attempts at intensive treatment including preparation for bone marrow transplantation, the blastic phase remains an extremely resistant disease. On average, fatal complications occur only 2 months after blast crisis begins.

PROGNOSIS. Despite good symptomatic therapy for the chronic phase of CML, the median survival of patients with this disease continues to hover between 2.5 and 3.5 years, the same as that reported in the early 1920s. Most patients are comfortable and able to function well until the onset of blast crisis, but no means have yet been developed to prevent the appearance of this terminal transformation.

Chronic Lymphocytic Leukemia

Chronic lymphocytic leukemia is a disease primarily of the elderly and middle-aged. It is characterized by accumulation in the blood, lymphoid organs, and bone marrow of long-lived but functionally inactive, mature-appearing small lymphocytes. A mild to severe immunologic dysfunction also typifies this disease. There usually is hypogammaglobulinemia, but autoimmune hemolytic anemia and increased delayed hypersensitivity reactions, such as to insect bites, often are seen as well.

The exact relationship of CLL to the other lymphoproliferative diseases is somewhat uncertain at present because of the similarity of CLL to well-differentiated lymphocytic lymphoma. The recognition of cell surface markers for distinguishing T and B cells, however, has delineated both T-cell–derived and B-cell–derived CLL.

CLINICAL FEATURES. The onset of CLL is so insidious that at least 25% of patients are asymptomatic at diagnosis; the disease is suggested by abnormal findings on a blood cell count performed during a routine examination for evaluation of an unrelated illness. Patients in whom CLL is diagnosed when asymptomatic are on the average 4 years younger than patients who are symptomatic at diagnosis,[227] and this suggests there may be an average interval of at least 4 years between the onset of recognizable disease and the initial manifestation of symptoms.

The most common presenting symptom is malaise, possibly with fatigueability, and loss of appetite and weight as well as a low-grade fever with night sweats also are fairly common. Occasionally, patients will present with a complicating infection as the first indication of the underlying disorder. An appreciable number of patients may consult a physician because of lymphadenopathy or splenomegaly without other symptomatology.

In the absence of infection, the major initial physical findings are related to the infiltration of the liver, spleen, and lymph nodes by the leukemic cells, thus enlarging these organs. Cervical and supraclavicular adenopathy are seen most commonly, with axillary and inguinal node enlargement also being quite frequent. Palpable retroperitoneal enlargement is uncommon, but lymphangiograms demonstrate frequent involvement of the retroperitoneal nodes, particularly in patients with inguinal adenopathy.[227] Such enlargement can be associated with either gastrointestinal or genitourinary complaints. Enlarged hilar nodes may be seen on chest radiographs. The typical lymphadenopathy in CLL is firm, relatively fixed, and nontender. Moderate splenomegaly is present in 75% of patients, and 25% will have a moderately enlarged liver.[228]

Although generalized leukemia cutis is rare, skin manifestations are more common in CLL than in any

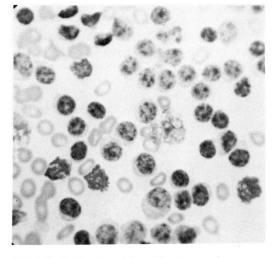

FIGURE 13.10. A peripheral blood smear from a patient with chronic lymphocytic leukemia.

other type of leukemia. They often consist of nonspecific leukemids, that is, various rashes in which a biopsy fails to show any leukemic infiltration. Scattered maculopapular or vesicular lesions, which can be intensely pruritic, also are common, and these latter lesions show lymphocytic infiltration of the basal epidermis and dermis. Herpes zoster also commonly occurs and may become generalized. Finally, it should also be noted that a small but significant proportion of patients will have a normal physical examination.

LABORATORY FINDINGS. The peripheral blood examination reveals a characteristic absolute lymphocytosis with primarily small, mature, and rather uniform lymphocytes (Fig. 13.10). Smudge cells are common, a large lymphoblast with nucleoli or an indented nucleus occasionally may be seen. The total white blood cell count generally is not as high as in CML, with about one third of patients having counts exceeding 100,000 cells/mm[3].[227,228] The granulocyte and platelet counts often are normal at diagnosis, but bone marrow examination shows spotty or diffuse infiltration by the same small lymphocytes seen in the peripheral blood. The pattern of marrow infiltration appears to have prognostic significance in that a nodular or interstitial as opposed to a diffuse pattern is associated with a more indolent clinical course;[229] however, the blood lymphocyte count correlates poorly with the degree of organ infiltration.[230]

Mild anemia initially may be present in about one half of patients with CLL.[227,228,230] This usually is normocytic and normochromic in type, with a normal or low reticulocyte count and a normal to slightly decreased red cell lifespan, suggesting that reduced red cell production is present. Hemolytic anemia can occur at any time in the course of the disease, and it may be associated either with a positive or negative Coombs test. About 20% of patients manifest this latter phenomenon at some time during the course of their disease.

Chronic lymphocytic leukemia appears to be a process of accumulation rather than overproduction of long-lived lymphocytes; the rate of cell production often is only slightly augmented, if at all.[231] These cells are predominantly of the B-cell type, and in most cases, they appear to be coated with a monoclonal immunoglobulin of the IgM or IgD type.[232,233]

B cells are necessary for immunoglobulin production. However, leukemic B cells appear to be unable to function normally because hypogammaglobulinemia usually is present initially and becomes progressively worse as the disease develops. Circulating antibody response to antigenic challenge with vaccines also has been shown to be depressed. Hypogammaglobulinemia has been observed to precede the onset of hematologic abnormalities in CLL,[227,228] and the reduction in circulating antibodies leads to an increased susceptibility to infection that is the major cause of morbidity and death in patients with CLL.

Although gross tests of cell-mediated immunity—for example, delayed cutaneous hypersensitivity to antigens such as tuberculin—are unimpaired, more sensitive tests show that both the absolute number of T cells and the percentage of T cells that react to antigen or phytohemagglutinin stimulation are reduced. These values may return to normal with successful treatment.

Most other laboratory tests are normal. There is no typical cytogenetic abnormality, and levels of both serum vitamin B_{12} and its binding proteins are in the normal range.

DIAGNOSIS AND DIFFERENTIAL DIAGNOSIS. The patient with CLL usually presents little diagnostic difficulty. Most have blood lymphocyte counts that persistently exceed the ranges expected in lymphocytosis from most other causes, and most have palpable enlargement of lymphoid tissue.

Persistent lymphocytosis with normal-appearing lymphocytes is rare in diseases other than CLL. Infectious lymphocytosis, a disease usually occurring in children and thought to be of viral etiology, occasionally affects adults, but unlike those in mononucleosis, lymphocytes in this disease appear normal, similar to those in CLL. The lymphocytosis is transient, and blood cell counts should return to normal after several weeks.

Chronic infections, particularly tuberculosis, may be associated with absolute lymphocytosis, particularly as the patient recovers from the illness. Absolute lymphocyte counts in these circumstances usually are less than 10,000 cells/mm³, while absolute lymphocyte counts in patients with CLL typically are higher. Patients with chronic infections usually have elevated immunoglobulin levels in contrast to patients who have CLL, and if lymphadenopathy is present, a lymph node biopsy should suffice to distinguish a leukemoid reaction from CLL.

Lymph node biopsy cannot distinguish between CLL and well-differentiated lymphocytic lymphoma. This malignant lymphoma occasionally occurs with organomegaly and lymphocytosis indistinguishable from that in CLL. It seems likely the two represent different parts of the spectrum in the same disease. In both cases, the normal nodal architecture is replaced by a diffuse infiltrate of small lymphocytes.

An attempt to clinically stage patients with CLL has been proposed, based on the concept that CLL is a disease of progressive lymphocyte accumulation, and it appears to be clinically useful in determining prognosis.[230,234] The stages include:

Stage 0—Bone marrow and blood lymphocytosis only,
Stage I—Lymphocytosis with enlarged nodes,
Stage II—Lymphocytosis with enlarged spleen or liver or both,
Stage III—Lymphocytosis with anemia, and
Stage IV—Lymphocytosis with thrombocytopenia.

In a study of 125 patients, the stage was found to be a reliable predictor of survival whether it was used at diagnosis or during the course of the disease. This staging system has been useful in sorting out different categories of patients, and may help to direct and evaluate therapy more effectively.[228,230,235]

TREATMENT. The course of CLL is quite variable, and although there are various therapeutic regimens that will improve most signs and symptoms of the disease, none is curative at present. In view of this as well as the finding that a sizeable proportion of patients are asymptomatic at diagnosis and continue that way for many years, it generally has been recommended that therapy be withheld until there is significant disease activity in the form of cytopenia, unexplained weight loss, unexplained fever (usually more than 2 weeks in duration), rapidly enlarging or painful lymph nodes or spleen, hemolytic anemia, skin involvement, or recurrent infections. Bothersome, isolated lymph node enlargement can be treated with local radiation therapy. Similarly, symptomatic splenomegaly can be treated effectively with splenic irradiation, which is often accompanied by general improvement in the disease manifestations.

Standard systemic therapeutic agents consist primarily of the alkylating agents such as chlorambucil, and corticosteroids. Chlorambucil is begun traditionally at a dose of 0.1 to 0.2 mg/kg/day orally, with the dose titrated according to the clinical response and the degree of suppression of normal myeloid elements. The major clinical benefit is usually discernible at the end of 12 weeks of therapy, by which time some improvement in all measurable disease parameters will have occurred in approximately two thirds of patients. In approximately 10% of patients, the physical examinations will be normal, with the disappearance of symptomatology, return of a normal blood count, and reduction in marrow lymphocytes sufficient to qualify as "complete remission."

Based on the observation that leukemic lymphocytes proliferate less rapidly than normal myeloid elements, it has been suggested that less myelosuppression may be obtained by giving chlorambucil orally in a dose of 0.4 to 0.8 mg/kg once every 2 weeks.[236] Results with this regimen suggest it is more effective than daily oral administration and causes less myelosuppression; mild nausea and vomiting occurred somewhat more frequently with this regimen but were easily controlled. In addition, a few patients resistant to continuous chlorambucil responded to the intermittent schedule.

Corticosteroids have a marked lymphocytolytic effect without myelosuppression, and they may be especially useful when given with chlorambucil to patients having advanced disease, extensive bone marrow involvement, and resultant anemia, granulocytopenia, or thrombocytopenia. A study of patients who had advanced disease (stages III and IV) compared different dose schedules of chlorambucil both with or without prednisone.[237] Improved benefit was seen using high-dose intermittent chlorambucil, and in patients with advanced disease, both combination regimens were more effective than prednisone alone.[237] In patients with less advanced but active disease, however, it was unclear whether the addition of prednisone to chlorambucil was superior to chlorambucil alone, and this has been the subject of active investigation.[238] Prednisone usually is given orally in a dose of 20 to 30 mg/day, or a dose of 60 to 80 mg/day is given orally for 5 days every 2 weeks.[238] This latter schedule may reduce the risk of infection and other side effects from steroid therapy. During the early weeks after steroid therapy is begun, it is not unusual to see further lymphocytosis even while adenopathy and splenomegaly are disappearing. Subsequently, the white blood cell count also will decline, usually by the end of the sixth week of treatment. Corticosteroid therapy is mandatory for autoimmune hemolytic anemia, and it may be life-saving in that instance.

Treatment is maintained at least until the maximal benefit has been achieved, usually a minimum of 12 weeks. Peripheral blood counts are monitored weekly until they are stable, then every 2 weeks during treatment. Discontinuation of therapy until symptoms reappear may be possible in a small percentage of patients whose disease is completely or almost completely controlled, but most will require constant treatment. In addition, studies using combination chemotherapy similar to that used with lymphoma patients having advanced disease have been completed, and although preliminary results are encouraging,[239,240] one study showed no added benefit of aggressive combination chemotherapy.[241]

Infections should be treated quickly, vigorously, and as specifically as possible. The clinical index of suspicion should be especially high in patients who are on steroid therapy or granulocytopenic, because their ability to signal infections will be vastly impaired. Prophylactic intravenous gamma globulin has been demonstrated to be useful in preventing bacterial, and not nonbacterial, infections in hypogammaglobulinemic patients with CLL.

The serum uric acid level generally is normal at diagnosis, however, allopurinol and adequate hydration when therapy is started will minimize any chance of urate nephropathy accompanying a massive lymphocytolysis.

In addition to chemotherapeutic agents, thymic irradiation, splenic irradiation, and total-body irradiation have been successful in achieving clinical remissions in patients with CLL.[242–245] These techniques are still being compared with standard treatment such as the administration of chlorambucil, and are not currently recommended for general use. Toxicity has been a limiting factor.[244]

Recently, several new findings have prompted consideration for earlier and more aggressive treatment of selected patients with CLL. First, although the median age has stayed essentially the same, younger patients with CLL (<50 years of age) are coming more frequently to medical attention; this has prompted an evaluation of more aggressive treatment options, such as may be used in non-Hodgkin lymphoma, including bone marrow transplantation. Second, the recent utilization of new chemotherapeutic agents with very different mechanisms of action, adenosine deaminase inhibitors such as pentostatin and 2-chlorodeoxyadenosine[246–248] as well as a new purine analogue, fludarabine,[249,250] has altered the therapeutic response, including increased numbers of durable complete remissions after relatively brief therapy. These agents, however, may increase the risk of infection. Thus, therapeutic goals may change in CLL as improved therapy develops.

PROGNOSIS. The median survival of patients with CLL varies from less than 4 to 6 years.[7,227] The prognosis of the disease appears to be related to the extent of organ infiltration at the time of diagnosis; the median survival thus varies from 2 years in patients with anemia and thrombocytopenia to 10 years in those with only lymphocytosis and adenopathy.[228] The principal cause of death in patients with CLL is infection.

Because these patients are in an older age group and thus are subject to numerous other illnesses, it perhaps is not surprising that 25% of patients with CLL die of unrelated diseases, and attempts to improve the immune status have not been particularly successful. Infusions of gamma globulin can reduce the incidence of bacterial infection,[251] and while expensive, these infusions may be useful in patients with recurring bacterial infections. On the other hand, 75% of these patients do eventually die of their leukemia, and some of the small percentage of complete remissions have included patients in whom depressed immunoglobulin levels returned to normal after various treatments. Current studies are aimed at the question of whether a more aggressive approach to this disease may be warranted.

REFERENCES

1. Bennett JM, Catovsky D, Daniel MT, et al. Proposals for the classification of the acute leukaemias. Br J Haematol 1976;33:451.
2. Bennett JM, Catovsky D, Daniel MT, et al. The morphologic classification of acute lymphoblastic leukaemia: concordance among observers and clinical correlations. Br J Haematol 1981;47:553.
3. Bennett JM, Catovsky D, Daniel MT, et al. The French-American-British (FAB) Cooperative Group proposals for the classification of chronic (mature) B and T lymphoid leukemia. J Clin Pathol 1989;42:567.
4. Dameshek W, Gunz FW. Leukemia. New York: Grune & Stratton, 1974.
5. Hayhoe FGJ, Cawley JC. Acute leukemia: cellular morphology, cytochemistry, and fine structure. Clin Haematol 1972;1:49.
6. National Cancer Institute. 1987 Annual Cancer Statistics Review. NIH Publications, 2788-2789. Washington, DC: U.S. Department of Health and Human Services, 1988.
7. Alderson M. The epidemiology of leukemia. Adv Cancer Res 1980;31:1.
8. Levin DL, Devesa SS, Godwin JD, Silverman DT. Cancer Rates and Risks. Washington, DC: U.S. Government Printing Office, 1974.
9. McPhedran P, Heath CW Jr, Garcia JS. Racial variations in leukemia incidence among the elderly. J Natl Cancer Institute 1970;45:25.
10. Brinker H. Population-based age and sex-specific incidence rates in the 4 main types of leukaemia. Scand J Haematol 1982;29:241.
11. Cutler SJ, Axtell L, Heise H. 10,000 cases of leukemia: 1940–1962. J Natl Cancer Inst 1967;39:993.
12. Kaplan HS. The role of irradiation in experimental leukemogenesis. Natl Cancer Inst Monogr 1964;14:207.
13. March HC. Leukemia in radiologists, ten years later: with review of pertinent evidence for radiation leukemia. Am J Med Sci 1961;242:137.
14. Bizzozero OJ, Johnson KG, Ciocco A. Leukemia in Hiroshima and Nagasaki. N Engl J Med 1966;274:1095.
15. Brill AB, Tomonaga M, Heyssell RM. Leukemia in man following exposure to ionizing radiation: summary of findings in Hiroshima and Nagasaki and comparison with other human experience. Ann Intern Med 1962;56:590.
16. Heyssell RM, Brill AB, Woodbury LA, et al. Leukemia in Hiroshima atomic bomb survivors. Blood 1960;15:313.
17. Court-Brown WM, Doll R. Mortality from cancer and other causes after radiotherapy for ankylosing spondylitis. BMJ 1965;2:1327.
18. Ezdinli EZ, Sokal JE, Aungst CW, Kim U, Sandberg AA. Myeloid leukemia in Hodgkin's disease: chromosomal abnormalities. Ann Intern Med 1969;71:1097.
19. Lowenbraun S. Transformation of reticulum cell sarcoma to acute leukemia. Cancer 1971;27:579.
20. Sahakian GJ, Alj-Mondihry H, Lacher MB, Connolly CE. Acute leukemia in Hodgkin's disease. Cancer 1974;33:1369.
21. Steinberg MH, Geary CG, Crosby WH. Acute granulocytic leukemia complicating Hodgkin's disease. Arch Intern Med 1970;125:496.
22. Weiss RB, Brunning RD, Kennedy BJ. Lymphosarcoma terminating in acute myelogenous leukemia. Cancer 1972;30:1275.
23. Donnell JF, Brereton HD, Greco FA, Gralnick HR, Johnson RE. Acute nonlymphocytic leukemia and acute myeloproliferative syndrome following radiation therapy for non-Hodgkin's lymphoma and chronic lymphocytic leukemia: clinical studies. Cancer 1979;44:1930.
24. Murray R, Heckel P, Henzelmann LH. Leukemia in children exposed to ionizing radiation. N Engl J Med 1959;261:585.
25. Lilienfeld AM. Epidemiological studies of the leukemogenic effects of radiation. Yale J Biol Med 1966;39:143.
26. Rosner F, Grunwalk H. Hodgkin's disease and acute leukemia. Report of eight cases and review of the literature. Am J Med 1975;58:339.
27. Cadman EC, Capizzi RL, Bertino JR. Acute nonlymphocytic leukemia: a delayed complication of Hodgkin's disease therapy. Analysis of 109 cases. Cancer 1977;40:1280.
28. Blayney DW, Longo DL, Young RC, et al. Decreasing risk of leukemia with prolonged follow-up after chemotherapy and radiotherapy for Hodgkin's disease. N Engl J Med 1987;316:710.
29. Graham S, Levin ML, Lilienfeld AM, et al. Preconception, intrauterine, and postnatal irradiation as related to leukemia. Natl Cancer Inst Monogr 1966;19:347.
30. Hoshino T, Kato H, Finch SC, Hrubec Z. Leukemia in offspring of atomic bomb survivors. Blood 1967;30:719.
31. MacMahon B. Prenatal x-ray exposure and childhood cancer. J Natl Cancer Inst 1962;28:1173.
32. Savitz DA, Wachtel H, Barnes FA, et al. Case-control study of childhood cancer and exposure to 60-H_z magnetic fields. Am J Epidemiol 1988;128:21.
33. Mitelman F, Brandt L, Nilsson PG. Relation among occupational exposure to potential mutagenic/carcinogenic agents, clinical findings, and bone marrow chromosomes in acute non-lymphocytic leukemia. Blood 1978;52:1229.
34. Rawson RZ, Parker F Jr, Jackson H Jr. Industrial solvents as possible etiologic agents in myeloid metaplasia. Science 1941;93:541.

35. Vigliani EC, Saito G. Benzene and leukemia. N Engl J Med 1964;27:872.
36. Aksoy M, Erdem S. Follow-up study on the mortality and development of leukemia in 44 pancytopenic patients with chronic exposure to benzene. Blood 1978;52:285.
37. Casciato DA, Scott JL. Acute leukemia following prolonged cytotoxic agent therapy. Medicine 1979;58:32.
38. Kyle RA, Pierre RV, Bayrd ED. Multiple myeloma and acute myelomonocytic leukemia. N Engl J Med 1970;283:1121.
39. Kaslow RA, Wisch N, Glass JL. Acute leukemia following cytotoxic chemotherapy. JAMA 1972;219:75.
40. Cohen RJ, Wiernik PH, Walker MD. Acute nonlymphocytic leukemia associated with nitrosourea chemotherapy: report of two cases. Cancer Treat Rep 1976;60:1257.
41. Zarrabi MH, Grunwald MW, Rosner F. Chronic lymphocytic leukemia terminating in acute leukemia. a review. Arch Intern Med 1977;137:1059.
42. Genuardi M, Zollino M, Serra A, et al. Long-term cytogenetic effects of antineoplastic treatment in relation to secondary leukemia. Cancer Genet Cytogenet 1988;33:201.
43. Gunz FW, Fitzgerald PH, Adams A. An abnormal chromosome in chronic lymphocytic leukemia. BMJ 1962;2:1097.
44. Gunz FW, Veale AMO. Leukemia in close relatives: accident or predisposition? J Natl Cancer Inst 1969;42:517.
45. Stewart A, Webb J, Hewitt D. A survey of childhood malignancies. BMJ 1985;1:1495.
46. Wald N, Borges WH, Li CC, Turner JH, Harnois MC. Leukemia associated with monogolism. Lancet 1961;i:228.
47. Miller RW. Down's syndrome (monogolism), other congenital malformations and cancers among sibs of leukemic children. N Engl J Med 1963;268:393.
48. Sawitsky A, Bloom D, German J. Chromosomal breakage and acute leukemia in congenital telangiectatic erythema and stunted growth. Ann Intern Med 1966;65:487.
49. Bloom GE, Warner S, Gerald PS, Diamond LK. Chromosomal abnormalities in constitutional aplastic anemia. N Engl J Med 1966;274:8.
50. Hecht R, Koler RD, Rigas DA, et al. Leukemia and lymphocytes in ataxia-telangiectasia. Lancet 1966;ii:1193.
51. MacMahon B, Levy MA. Prenatal origin of childhood leukemia: evidence from twins. N Engl J Med 1964;270:1082.
52. Zuegler WW, Cox DE. Genetic aspects of leukemia. Semin Hematol 1969;6:228.
53. Rowley JD, Golomb HM, Vardiman J. Nonrandom chromosomal abnormalities in acute nonlymphocytic leukemia in patients treated for Hodgkin disease and non-Hodgkin lymphomas. Blood 1977;50:759.
54. Yunis JJ, Bloomfield CD, Ensrud K. All patients with acute nonlymphocytic leukemia may have a chromosomal defect. N Engl J Med 1981;305:135.
55. Jarrett WFH. Annotation: viruses and leukaemia. Br J Haematol 1973;25:287.
56. Rowe WP, Hartley JW, Landes MR, Pugh WE, Teich N. Noninfectious AKR mouse embryo cell lines in which each cell has the capacity to produce infectious murine leukemia virus. Virology 1971;46:866.
57. Weiss RA, Fris RR, Katz E, Vogt PK. Induction of avian tumor viruses in normal cells by physical and chemical carcinogens. Virology 1971;46:920.
58. Baltimore D. Viral-dependent DNA polymerase in virions of RNA tumor viruses. Nature 1970;226:1209.
59. Temin H, Mutzutani S. RNA-dependent DNA polymerase in virions of Rous sarcoma virus. Nature 1970;226:1209.
60. Baxt W, Hehlmann R, Spiegelman S. Human leukemic cells contain reverse transcriptase associated with a high-molecular-weight virus-related RNA. Nature 1972;240:72.
61. Gallo RC, Miller N, Saxinger W, Gillespie D. Primate RNA tumor virus-like DNA synthesized endogenously by RNA-dependent DNA polymerase in virus-like-particles from fresh human acute leukemic blood cells. Proc Natl Acad Sci U S A 1973;70:3219.
62. Gallo RC, Yang SS, Ting RC. RNA-dependent DNA polymerase of human actue leukemia cells. Nature 1970;228:927.
63. Todaro GJ, Gallo RC. Immunological relationship of DNA polymerase from human acute leukemia cells and primate and mouse leukemia reverse transcriptase. Nature 1973;244:206.
64. Viola MV, Frazier M, Wiernik PH, McCredie KB, Spiegelman S. Reverse transcriptase in leukocytes of leukemic patients in remission. N Engl J Med 1976;294:75.
65. Bobrow SN, Smith RG, Reitz MS. Stimulated normal human lymphocytes contain ribonuclease-sensitive DNA polymerase distinct from viral RNA-dependent DNA polymerase. Proc Natl Acad Sci U S A 1972;69:3228.
66. Baxt W, Yates JW, Wallace JH Jr. Leukemia-specific DNA sequences in leukocytes of the leukemic members of identical twins. Proc Natl Acad Sci U S A 1973;70:2629.
67. Gallagher RE, Gallo RC. Type C RNA tumor virus isolated from cultured human acute myelogenous leukemia cells. Science 1975;187:350.
68. Gallagher RE, Salahuddin Z, Hall WI, McCredie KB, Gallo RC. Growth and differentiation in culture of leukemic leukocytes from a patient with acute myelogenous leukemia and re-identification of type C virus. Proc Natl Acad Sci U S A 1975;72:4137.
69. Catovsky D, Greaves MF, Rose M, et al. Adult T-cell lymphoma-leukemia in blacks from the West Indies. Lancet 1982;i:639.
70. Uchiyama T, Yodoi J, Sagawa K, et al. Adult T-cell leukemia: clinical and hematologic features in 16 cases. Blood 1977;50:481.
71. Poiesz BJ, Ruscetti FW, Gazdar AF, et al. Detection and isolation of type-C retrovirus particles from fresh and cultured lymphocytes of a patient with cutaneous T-cell lymphoma. Proc Natl Acad Sci U S A 1980;77:7415.
72. Yamamoto N, Okada M, Koyanagi Y, et al. Transformation of human leukocytes by co-cultivation with an adult T-cell leukemia virus producer line. Science 1982;217:737.
73. Boggs DR, Wintrobe MM, Cartwright GE. The acute leukemias: an analysis of 343 cases and review of the literature. Medicine 1962;41:163.
74. Mckenna SM, Baehner RL. Diagnosis and treatment of childhood acute lymphocytic leukemia. In: Wiernik PH, Canellos GP, Kyle RA, Schiffer CA, eds. Neoplastic Diseases of the Blood, Second Edition. New York: Churchill Livingstone, 1991:231–52.
75. Hoelzer DF. Diagnosis and treatment of adult acute lymphocytic leukemia. In: Wiernik PH, Canellos GP, Kyle RA, Schiffer CA, eds. Neoplastic Diseases of the Blood, Second Edition. New York: Churchill Livingstone, 1991:253–74.
76. Kundel DW, Brecker G, Bodey GP, Brittin GM. Reticulum fibrosis and bone infarction in acute leukemia: implications for prognosis. Blood 1964;22:526.
77. Nies BA, Kundel DW, Thomas LB, Freireich EJ. Leukopenia, bone pain and bone necrosis in patients with acute leukemia. Ann Intern Med 1965;62:698.
78. Thomas LB, Forkner CE Jr, Frei E III, Besse BE, Stabeneau JR. The skeletal lesions of acute leukemia. Cancer 1961;14:608.
79. Lee SL, Kopel S, Glidewell O. Cytomorphological determinations of prognosis in acute lymphoblastic leukemia of children. Semin Oncol 1976;3:209.
80. Miller DR, Krailo M, Bleyer WA, et al. Prognostic implications of blastic cell morphology in childhood acute lymphoblastic

leukemia: a report from the Children's Cancer Study Group. Cancer Treat Rep 1985;69:1211.

81. Sarin PS, Anderson PN, Gallo RC. Terminal deoxynucleotidyl transferase activities in human blood leukocytes and lymphoblast cell lines: high levels in lymphoblast cells lines and in blast cells of some patients with chronic myelogenous leukemia in acute phase. Blood 1976;47:11.

82. Pangalis GA, Beutler E. Terminal transferase in leukemia of adults. Acta Haematol 1979;62:199.

83. Coleman MS, Greenwood MF, Hutton JJ, Bollum FJ, Lampkin B, Holland P. Serial observations on terminal deoxynucleotidyl transferase and lymphoblast surface markers in acute lymphoblastic leukemia. Cancer Res 1976;36:120.

84. Bregni M, Siena S, Neri A, et al. Minimal residual disease in acute lymphoblastic leukemia detected by immune selection and gene rearrangement analysis. J Clin Oncol 1989;7:338–43.

85. Gucalp R, Paietta E, Weinberg V, Papenhausen P, Dutcher JP, Wiernik PH. Terminal transferase expression in acute myeloid leukaemia: biology and prognosis. Br J Haematol 1991;77:48.

86. Ball ED, Davis RB, Griffin JD, et al. Prognostic value of lymphocyte surface markers in acute myeloid leukemia. Blood 1991;77:2242–50.

87. Greaves MF. Analysis of the clinical and biologic significance of lymphoid phenotypes in acute leukemia. Cancer Res 1981;41:4752.

88. Paietta E, Wiernik PH. Acute versus chronic leukemia cells: is phenotyping a good prognostic indicator? Diagnostic Medicine Nov/Dec 1984, 1.

89. Rowley JD. Chromosome abnormalities in acute lymphoblastic leukemia. Cancer Genet Cytogenet 1979;1:263.

90. Pui CH, Carroll AJ, Raimondi SC, et al. Clinical presentation, karyotypic characterization and treatment outcome of childhood acute lymphoblastic leukemia with a near-haploid or hypodiploid < 45 line. Blood 1990;75:1170–7.

91. Miller DR, Leikin SL, Albo V, et al. Use of prognostic factors in improving the design and efficiency of clinical trials in childhood leukemia: Children's Cancer Study Group Report. Cancer Treat Rep 1980;64:381.

92. Robinson LL, Sather HN, Coccia PF, Nesbit ME, Hammond GD. Assessment of the interrelationship of prognostic factors in childhood acute lymphoblastic leukemia: a report from children's cancer study group. Am J Pediatr Hematol Oncol 1980;2:5.

93. Shaw MT. Monocytic leukemias. Hum Pathol 1980;11:215.

94. Sultan C, Heilmen-Gouault M, Tulliez M. Relationship between blast cell morphology and occurrence of a syndrome of disseminated intravascular coagulation. Br J Haematol 1973;24:255.

95. Gralnick HR, Abrell E. Studies of the procoagulant and fibrinolytic activity of promyelocytes in acute promyelocytic leukemia. Br J Haematol 1973;24:89.

96. Scott RB, Ellison RR, Ley AB. A clinical study of twenty cases of erythroleukemia (Di Guglielmo's syndrome). Am J Med 1964;37:162.

97. Hetzel P, Gee TS. A new observation in the clinical spectrums of erythroleukemia. Am J Med 1978;64:765.

98. Dameshek W. Acute monocytic (histiocytic) leukemia. Ann Intern Med 1960;52:1343.

99. Strau DJ, Mertelsmann R, Koziner B, et al. The acute monocytic leukemias: multidisciplinary studies in 45 patients. Medicine 1980;59:409.

100. Wiernik PH, Serpick AA. Granulocytic sarcoma (chloroma). Blood 1970;35:361.

101. Nieman RS, Barcos M, Costan B, et al. Granulocytic sarcoma: a clinicopathologic study of 61 biopsied cases. Cancer 1981;48:1426.

102. Dutcher JP, Schiffer CA, Wiernik PH. Hyperleukocytosis in adult acute nonlymphocytic leukemia: impact on remission rate and duration and survival. J Clin Oncol 1987;5:1364–72.

103. Wiernik PH. Diagnosis and treatment of acute nonlymphocytic leukemia. In: Wiernik PH, Canellos GP, Kyle RA, Schiffer CA, eds. Neoplastic Diseases of the Blood, Second Edition. New York: Churchill Livingstone, 1991;285–302.

104. Gralnick H, Marchesi S, Givelbar H. Intravascular coagulation in acute leukemia: clinical and subclinical abnormalities. Blood 1972;40:709.

105. Wiernik PH, Serpick AA. Clinical significance of serum and urinary muramidase activity in leukemia and other hematologic malignancies. Am J Med 1969;46:330.

106. Osserman EF, Lawlor DP. Serum and urinary lysozyme (muramidase) in monocytic and myelomonocytic leukemia. J Exp Med 1966;124:921.

107. Brown RK, Read JT, Wiseman BK, Frank WG. The electrophoretic analysis of serum proteins of the blood dyscrasias. J Lab Clin Med 1948;33:1523.

108. Schwarzinger I, Valent P, Koller U, et al. Prognostic significance of surface marker expression on blasts of patients with de novo myeloblastic leukemia. J Clin Oncol 1990;8:423.

109. Fourth International Workshop on Chromosomes in Leukemia: a prospective study of acute nonlymphocytic leukemia. Cancer Genet Cytogenet 1984;11:249.

110. Hallman D, Testa JR. Cytogenetics of acute leukemia. In: Wiernik PH, Canellos GP, Kyle RA, Schiffer CA, eds. Neoplastic Diseases of the Blood, Second Edition. New York: Churchill Livingstone, 1991;215–29.

111. Testa JR, Rowley JD. Cytogenetic patterns in acute nonlymphocytic leukemia. Virchows Arch (Cell Pathol) 1978;29:65.

112. Breitman TR, Selonick SE, Collins SJ. Induction of differentiation of the human promyelocytic leukemia cell line (HL-60) by retinoic acid. Proc Natl Acad Sci U S A 1980;77:2936.

113. Breitman TR, Collins SJ, Keene BR. Terminal differentiation of human promyelocytic leukemic cells in primary culture in response to retinoic acid. Blood 1981;57:1000.

114. Huang M, Ye YC, Chen SR, et al. Use of all-trans retinoic acid in the treatment of acute promyelocytic leukemia. Blood 1988;72:567.

115. Castaigne S, Chomienne C, Daniel MT, et al. All-trans retinoic acid as a differentiation therapy for acute promyelocytic leukemia. I. Clinical results. Blood 1990;76:1704.

116. Chen ZX, Xue Y-Q, Zhang R, et al. A clinical and experimental study on all-trans retinoic acid-treated acute promyeloytic leukemia patients. Blood 1991;78:1413–9.

117. Warrell RP, Frankel SR, Miller WH Jr, et al. Differentiation therapy of acute promyelocytic leukemia with tretinoin (all trans retinoic acid). N Engl J Med 1991;324:1385–93.

118. De The H, Chomienne C, Lanotte M, Degos L, Dejean A. The t(15;17) translocation of acute promyelocytic leukaemia fuses the retinoic acid receptor gene to a novel transcribed locus. Nature 1990;347:558.

119. Leavell BS, Twomey J. Possible leukemoid reaction in disseminated tuberculosis: report of a case with Auer rods. Trans Am Clin Climatol Assoc 1964;75:166.

120. Skarberg KO, Lagerlof B, Reizenstein P. Leukemia, leukemoid reaction and tuberculosis. Acta Med Scand 1967;182:427.

121. Dameshek W. Editorial. The Di Guglielmo syndrome revisited. Blood 1969;34:567.

122. Cohen JR, Creger WP, Greenberg PL, Schrier SL. Subacute myeloid leukemia: a clinical review. Am J Med 1979;66:959.

123. Koeffler HP, Golde DW. Human preleukemia. Ann Intern Med 1980;93:347.

124. Linman JW, Bagby GC. The preleukemic syndrome (hemopoietic dysplasia). Cancer 1978;42:854.

125. Nowell P, Finan J. Chromosome studies in preleukemic states. IV. Myeloproliferative versus cytopenic disorders. Cancer 1978;42:2254.

126. Greenberg PL, Mara E. The preleukemic syndrome: correlation of in vitro parameters of granulopoiesis with clinical features. Am J Med 1969;66:951.

127. Mahmood T, Robinson WA, Hamstra RD, Wallner SF. Macrocytic anemia, thrombocytosis and nonlobulated megakaryocytes. The 5q- syndrome, a distinct entity. Am J Med 1979;66:946.

128. Pedersen-Bjergaard J, Philip P. Cytogenetic characteristics of therapy-related acute nonlymphocytic leukaemia, preleukaemia and acute myeloproliferative syndrome: correlation with clinical data for 61 consecutive cases. Br J Haematol 1978;66:199.

129. Howe RB, Bloomfield CD, McKenna RW. Hypocellular acute leukemia. Am J Med 1982;72:391.

130. Yam LT, Li CY, Necheles TF, Katayama I. Pseudoeosinophilia, eosinophilic endocarditis and eosinophilic leukemia. Am J Med 1972;53:193.

131. Flaum MA, Schooley RT, Fauci AS, Gralnick HR. A clinicopathologic correlation of the idiopathic hypereosinophilic syndrome. I. Hematologic manifestations. Blood 1981;58:1012.

132. Schooley RT, Flaum MA, Gralnick HR, Fauci AS. A clinicopathologic correlation of the idiopathic hypereosinophilic syndrome. II. Clinical manifestations. Blood 1981;58:1021.

133. Parrillo JE, Fauci AS, Wolff SM. Therapy of the hypereosinophilic syndrome. Ann Intern Med 1978;89:167.

134. Parillo JE, Borer JS, Henry WL, Wolff SM, Fauci AS. The cardiovascular manifestations of the hypereosinophilic syndrome: prospective study of 26 patients with review of the literature. Am J Med 1979;67:572.

135. Caplan RM. Urticaria pigmentosa and mastocytosis. JAMA 1965;194:1077.

136. Van Kemmen E. Generalized masteocytosis. Acta Haematol 1974;52:129.

137. Kyle RA, Pease GL. Basophilic leukemia. Arch Intern Med 1966;118:205.

138. Efrati P, Nir E, Yaari A, Berrebi A, Kaplan H, Dvilanski A. Myeloproliferative disorders terminating in acute micromegakaryoblastic leukaemia. Br J Haematol 179;43:79.

139. Pollack A, Rachmelewitz D, Zlotnick D. Plasma cell leukemia. Arch Intern Med 1974;134:131.

140. Pruzanski W, Platts ME, Orgryzlo MA. Leukemic form of immunocytic dyscrasia (plasma cell leukemia). Am J Med 1969;47:60.

141. Kyle RA, Maldonado JE, Bayrd ED. Plasma cell leukemia: report on 17 cases. Arch Intern Med 1974;133:813.

142. Toma VA, Retief FP, Potgieter GM, Anderson JD. Plasma cell leukaemia. Acta Haematol 1980;63:136.

143. Smyth AC, Wiernik PH. Combination chemotherapy of adult acute lymphocytic leukemia. Clin Pharmacol Ther 1976;19:240.

144. Lister TA, Whitehouse JMA, Beard MEJ, et al. Combination chemotherapy for acute lymphoblastic leukaemia in adults. BMJ 1978;1:199.

145. Shaw MT, Raab SO. Adriamycin in combination chemotherapy of adult acute lymphoblastic leukemia. A Southwest Oncology Group Study. Med Pediatr Oncol 1977;3:261.

146. Henderson ES, Scharlau C, Cooper MR, et al. Combination chemotherapy and radiotherapy for acute lymphocytic leukemia in adults: results of CALGB protocol 7113. Leuk Res 1979;3:395.

147. Hoelzer D, Thiel E, Loffler H, et al. Intensified therapy in acute lymphoblastic and acute undifferentiated leukemia in adults. Blood 1984;64:38–47.

148. Radford JE Jr, Burns CP, Jones MP, et al. Adult acute lymphoblastic leukemia: results of the Iowa HOP-L protocol. J Clin Oncol 1989;7:58–66.

149. Hussein KK, Dahlberg S, Head D, et al. Treatment of acute lymphoblastic leukemia in adults with intensive induction, consolidation, and maintenance chemotherapy. Blood 1989;73:57–63.

150. Riehm H, Gadner H, Henze G, Langermann HJ, Odenwald E. The Berlin Childhood Acute Lymphoblastic Leukemia Therapy Study, 1970–1976. Am J Pediatr Hematol Oncol 1980;2:299.

151. Esterhay RJ, Wiernik PH, Groove PH, Markus SD, Wesley MN. Moderate dose methotrexate, vincristine, asparaginase, and dexamethasone for treatment of adult acute lymphocytic leukemia. Blood 1982;59:334.

152. Wiernik PH, Dutcher JP, Gucalp R, et al. MOAD therapy for adult acute lymphocytic leukemia. Proc Am Soc Clin Oncol 1990;9:205.

153. Muriel FS, Pavlovsky S, Penalver JA, et al. Evaluation of induction of remission, intensification, and central nervous system prophylactic treatment in acute lymphoblastic leukemia. Cancer 1974;34:418.

154. Hustu HO, Aur RJA, Verzosa MS, Simone JV, Pinkel D. Prevention of central nervous system leukemia by irradiation. Cancer 1973;32:585.

155. Simone JV, Aur RJA, Hustu HO, Verzosa M. Trends in the treatment of childhood leukemia. In: Neth R, Gallow RC, Mannweiler K, Moloney WC, eds. Modern Trends in Human Leukemia II. Munich: Lehmann, 1976:263–70.

156. Haghbin M, Tan CTC, Clarkson BD. Treatment of acute lymphoblastic leukemia in children with "prophylactic" intrathecal methotrexate and intensive systemic chemotherapy. Cancer Res 1975;35:807.

157. Pavlovsky S, Muriel FS, Garay G, et al. Chemoimmunotherapy with levamisole in acute lymphoblastic leukemia. Cancer 1981;48:1500.

158. Horowitz MM, Messerer D, Hoelzer D, et al. Chemotherapy compared with bone marrow transplantation for adults with acute lymphoblastic leukemia in first remission. Ann Intern Med 1991;115:13–8.

159. Yates JW, Wallace HJ, Ellison RR, Holland JF. Cytosine arabinoside and daunorubicin therapy in acute nonlymphocytic leukemia. Cancer Chemother Rep 1973;57:845.

160. Rai KR, Holland JF, Glidewell OJ, et al. Treatment of acute myelocytic leukemia: a study by Cancer and Leukemia Group B. Blood 1981;58:1203.

161. Rees JKM, Sandler RM, Challener J, Hayhoe FGJ. Treatment of acute myeloid leukemia with a triple cytotoxic regimen. Br J Cancer 1977;36:770.

162. Gale RP, Foon KA, Cline MJ, Zighelboim J. The UCLA Acute Leukemia Study Group: intensive chemotherapy for acute myelogenous leukemia. Ann Intern Med 1981;94:753.

163. Paciucci PA, Ohhuma T, Cuttner J, Silver RT, Holland JF. Mitoxantrone in patients with acute leukemia in relapse. Cancer Res 1983;43:3919.

164. Paciucci PA, Dutcher JP, Cuttner J, Strauman JJ, Wiernik PH, Holland JF. Mitoxantrone and ara-C in previously treated patients with acute myelogenous leukemia. Leukemia 1987;1:565.

165. Berman E, Heller G, Santorsa J, et al. Results of a randomized trial comparing idarubicin and cytosine arabinoside with daunorubicin and cytosine arabinoside in adult patients with newly diagnosed acute myelogenous leukemia. Blood 1991;77:1666.

166. Wiernik PH, Banks PLC, Case J, et al. Cytarabine plus idarubicin or daunorubicin as induction and consolidation therapy for previously untreated adult patients with acute myeloid leukemia. Blood 1992;79:313.

167. Hiddemann W, Kruetzmann H, Straif K, et al. High dose cytosine arabinoside and mitoxantrone: a highly effective regimen in refractory acute myeloid leukemia. Blood 1987;69:744.

168. Cassileth PA, Harrington DP, Hines JD, et al. Maintenance

chemotherapy prolongs remission duration in adult acute non-lymphocytic leukemia. J Clin Oncol 1988;6:583–7.

169. Weinstein HJ, Mayer RJ, Rosenthal DS, et al. Treatment of acute myelogenous leukemia in children and adults. N Engl J Med 1979;303:473.

170. Dutcher JP, Wiernik PH, Markus S, Weinberg V, Schiffer CA, Harwood KV. Intensive maintenance therapy improves survival in adult acute nonlymphocytic leukemia: an eight-year follow-up. Leukemia 1988;2:413.

171. Buchner TH, Urbanitz D, Hiddemann W, et al. Intensified induction and consolidation with or without maintenance chemotherapy for acute myeloid leukemia (AML): two multicenter studies of the German AML Cooperative Group. J Clin Oncol 1985;3:1583.

172. Bodey GP, Freireich EJ, McCredie KB, et al. Prolonged remissions in adults with acute leukemia following late intensification chemotherapy and immunotherapy. Cancer 1981;47:1937.

173. Wolff SN, Herzig RH, Fay JW, et al. High-dose cytarabine and daunorubicin as consolidation therapy for acute myeloid leukemia in first remission: long-term follow-up results. J Clin Oncol 1989;7:1260.

174. Tallman MS, Appelbaum FR, Amos D, et al. Evaluation of intensive postremission chemotherapy for adults with acute nonlymphocytic leukemia using high-dose cytosine arabinoside with L-asparaginase and amscarine with etoposide. J Clin Oncol 1987;5:918.

175. Tallman MS, Kopecky KJ, Amos D, et al. Analysis of prognostic factors for the outcome of marrow transplantation or further chemotherapy for patients with acute nonlymphocytic leukemia in first remission. J Clin Oncol 1989;7:326.

176. Ho DHW. Potential advances in the clinical use of arabinosyl cytosine. Cancer Treat Rep 1977;61:717.

177. Forsthoff CA, Dutcher JP, Wiernik PH. Incidence of central nervous system leukemia in acute nonlymphocytic leukemia. Proc Am Soc Clin Oncol 1983;2:177.

178. Sullivan KM, Shulman HM, Storb R, et al. Chronic graft-versus-host disease in 52 patients: adverse natural course and successful treatment with combination immunosuppression. Blood 1981;57:267.

179. Fritz RD, Forkner CE Jr, Freireich EJ. The association of fatal intracranial hemorrhage and "blastic crisis" in patients with acute leukemia. N Engl J Med 1959;262:59.

180. Wiernik PH, Serpick AA. Factors affecting remission and survival in adult leukemia. Medicine 1970;49:505.

181. Roy AJ, Jaffe N, Djerassi I. Prophylactic platelet transfusions in children with acute leukemia. Transfusion 1973;13:283.

182. Schiffer CA, Aisner J, Wiernik PH. Platelet transfusion therapy for patients with leukemia. In: Greenwalt TJ, Jamieson GA, eds. The Blood Platelet in Transfusion Therapy. New York: Alan R. Liss, 1978:267–79.

183. Dutcher JP, Schiffer CA, Aisner J, Wiernik PH. Alloimmunization following platelet transfusion: the absence of a dose-response relationship. Blood 1981;57:395.

184. Dutcher JP. Platelet transfusion therapy in patients with malignancy. In: Dutcher JP, ed. Modern Transfusion Therapy. Boca Raton, FL: CRC Press, Inc., 1990:25–50.

185. Lohrmann HP, Bull MI, Decter JA. Platelet transfusions from HL-A-compatible correlated donors to alloimmunized patients. Ann Intern Med 1974;80:9.

186. Duquesnoy RJ. Donor selection in platelet transfusion therapy of alloimmunized thrombocytopenic patients. In: Greenwalt TS, Jamieson GA, eds. The Blood Platelet in Transfusion Therapy. New York: Alan R. Liss, 1978:229–43.

187. Schiffer CS, Buchholtz DH, Aisner J. Frozen autologous plate-lets in the supportive care of patients with leukemia. Transfusion 1976;16:321.

188. Schiffer CA, Aisner J, Dutcher JP, Wiernik PH. A clinical program of platelet cryopreservation. In: Vogler WR, ed. Cytapheresis and Plasma Exchange: Clinical Indications. New York: Alan R. Liss, 1982:165–80.

189. Gralnick HR, Bagley J, Abrell E. Heparin treatment for the hemorrhagic diathesis of acute promyelocytic leukemia. Am J Med 1972;52:167.

190. Daly PA, Schiffer CA, Wiernik PH. Acute promyelocytic leukemia: clinical management of 15 patients. Am J Hematol 1980;8:347.

191. The EORTC International Antimicrobial Therapy Project Group. Three antibiotic regimens in the treatment of infection in febrile granulocytopenic patients with cancer. J Infect Dis 1978;137:14.

192. Sugar AM. Empiric treatment of fungal infections in the neutropenic host: review of the literature and guidelines for use. Arch Intern Med 1990;150:2258–64.

193. Hughes WT, Armstrong D, Bodey GP, et al. Guidelines for the use of antimicrobial agents in neutropenic patients with unexplained fever. J Infect Dis 1990;161:381–96.

194. Dutcher JP. Granulocyte transfusion therapy in patients with malignancy. In: Dutcher JP, ed. Modern Transfusion Therapy. Boca Raton, FL: CRC Press, Inc., 1990:135–56.

195. Winston DJ, Ho WG, Gale RP. Prophylactic granulocyte transfusions during chemotherapy of acute nonlymphocytic leukemia. Ann Intern Med 1981;94:616.

196. Strauss RG, Connett JE, Gale RP, et al. A controlled trial of prophylactic granulocyte transfusions during initial induction chemotherapy for acute myelogenous leukemia. N Engl J Med 1981;305:597.

197. Bodey GP, Gehan EA, Freireich EJ. Protected environment-prophylactic antibiotic program in the chemotherapy of acute leukema. Am J Med Sci 1971;262:138.

198. Schimpff SC. Laminar air flow room reverse isolation and microbial suppression to prevent infection in patients with cancer. Cancer Chemother Rep 1975;59:1055.

199. Sullivan MP, Vietti TJ, Haggard ME, Donaldson MH, Krall JM, Gehan EA. Remission maintenance therapy for meningeal leukemia. Blood 1971;38:680.

200. Band PR. Treatment of CNS leukemia with intrathecal cytosine arabinoside. Cancer 1973;32:744.

201. Wang JJ, Pratt CB. Intrathecal arabinosyl cytosine in meningeal leukemia. Cancer 1970;25:531.

202. Moloney WC. Chronic myelogenous leukemia. Cancer 1978;42:865.

203. Pedersen-Bjergaard J, Worm AM, Hainan B. Blastic transformation of chronic myelocytic leukemia, clinical manifestations, prognostic factors and results of therapy. Scand J Haematol 1977;18:292.

204. Rosenthal S, Canellos GP, DeVita VT, Gralnick HR. Characteristics of blast crisis in chronic granulocytic leukemia. Blood 1977;49:705.

205. Barton JC, Conrad ME. Current status of blastic transformation in chronic myelogenous leukemia. Am J Hematol 1978;4:281.

206. Rosner F, Schreiber ZR, Parise F. Leukocyte alkaline phosphatase. Arch Intern Med 1972;130:892.

207. Schiffer CA, Aisner J, Daly PA, Wiernik PH. Increased leukocyte alkaline phosphatase activity following transfusion of leukocytes from a patient with chronic myelogenous leukemia. Am J Med 1979;66:519.

208. Rowley JD. A new consistent chromosomal abnormality in chronic myelogenous leukemia identified by quinacrine fluorescence and Giemsa staining. Nature 1973;243:290.

209. Groffen J, Stephenson JR, Heisterkamp N de Klein A, Bartram CR, Grosveld G. Philadelphia chromosomal breakpoints are clustered within a limited region, *bcr*, on chromosome 22. Cell 1984;36:93–9.

210. Croce CM, Huebner K, Isobe M, et al. Mapping of four distinct BCR-related loci to chromosome region 22q11: order of BCR loci relative to chronic myelogenous leukemia and acute lymphoblastic leukemia. Proc Natl Acad Sci U S A 1987;84:7174–8.

211. Ezdinli EZ, Sokal JE, Crosswhite BS, Sanberg AA. Philadelphia-chromosome positive and negative chronic myelocytic leukemia. Ann Intern Med 1970;72:175.

212. Whang-Peng J, Canellos GP, Carbone PP, Tjio JH. Clinical implications of cytogenetic variants in chronic myelocytic leukemia. Blood 1968;32:755.

213. Kennedy BJ. Hydroxyurea therapy to chronic myelogenous leukemia. Cancer 1972;29:1052.

214. Schwartz JH, Cannellos GP. Hydroxyurea in the management of the hematologic complications of chronic granulocytic leukemia. Blood 1975;46:11.

215. Gralnick HR, Harbor J, Vogel C. Myelofibrosis in chronic granulocytic leukemia. Blood 1971;37:152.

216. Yoffe G, Blick M, Kantarjian H, Spitzer G, Gutterman J, Talpaz M: Molecular analysis of interferon-induced suppression of Philadelphia chromosome in patients with chronic myeloid leukemia. Blood 1987;69:961–3.

217. Talpaz M, Kantarjian H, Kurzrock R, Trujillo JM, Gutterman JU. Interferon-alpha produces sustained cytogenetic responses in chronic myelogenous leukemia: Philadelphia chromosome-positive patients. Ann Intern Med 1991;114:532–8.

218. Rowley JD. Chromosome abnormalities in the acute phase of chronic myelogenous leukemia (CML). Virchows Arch (Cell Pathol) 1978;29:57.

219. Cunningham I, Gee T, Dowling M, et al. Results of treatment of Ph+ chronic myelogenous leukemia with an intensive treatment regimen (L-5 Protocol). Blood 1979;53:375.

220. Fefer A, Cheever MA, Thomas ED, et al. Disappearance of Ph[1]-positive cells in four patients with chronic granulocytic leukemia after chemotherapy, irradiation and marrow transplantation from an identical twin. N Engl J Med 1979;300:333.

221. Oken MM, Sarin PS, Gallo RC, et al. Terminal transferase levels in chronic myelogenous leukemia in blast crisis and in remission. Leuk Res 1978;2:173.

222. Marks SM, Baltimore D, McCaffrey R. Terminal transferase as a predictor of initial responsiveness to vincristine and prednisone in blastic chronic myelogenous leukemia. A co-operative study. N Engl J Med 1978;298:812.

223. Ross DD, Wiernik PH, Sarin PS, Whang-Peng J. Loss of terminal deoxynucleotidyl transferase (TdT) activity as a predictor of emergence of resistance to chemotherapy in a case of chronic myelogenous leukemia in blast crisis. Cancer 1979;44:1566.

224. Schiffer CA, DeBeillis R, Kasdorf H, Wiernik PH. Treatment of the blast crisis of chronic myelogenous leukemia with 5-azacytidine and VP-16-213. Cancer Treat Rep 1982;66:267–71.

225. Dutcher JP, Wiernik PH, Strauman JJ, Spielvogel A, Dukart G. Mitoxantrone and cytosine arabinoside in acute non-lymphocytic leukemia and blast crisis of chronic myelogenous leukemia. Proc Am Soc Clin Oncol 1985;4:170.

226. Dutcher JP, Wiernik PH, Paietta E, Rowe J, Kellermeyer R, Andersen J. Mitoxantrone and 5-azacytidine for patients with accelerated or blast crisis Ph[1] + chronic myelogenous leukemia. Proc Am Soc Clin Oncol 1989;8:205.

227. Boggs DR, Sofferman SA, Winthrobe MM, Cartwright GE. Factors influencing the duration of survival of patients with chronic lymphocytic leukemia. Am J Med 1966;40:243.

228. Rai KR, Sawitsky A. Diagnosis and treatment of chronic lymphocytic leukemia. In: Wiernik PH, Canellos GP, Kyle RA, Schiffer CA, eds. Neoplastic Diseases of the Blood, Second Edition. New York: Churchill Livingstone, 1991;97–110.

229. Rozman C, Montserrat JM, Rodriquez-Fernandez R, et al. Bone marrow histologic pattern—the best single prognostic parameter in chronic lymphocytic leukemia: a multivariate survival analysis in 329 cases. Blood 1984;64:642.

230. Rai KR, Sawitsky A, Cronkite EP, Chanana AD, Levy RN, Pasternack BS. Clinical staging of chronic lymphocytic leukemia. Blood 1975;46:219.

231. Zimmerman TS, Godwin HA, Perry S. Studies of leukocyte kinetics in chronic lymphocytic leukemia. Blood 1968;31:277.

232. Aisenberg AC, Bloch KC, Long JC. Cell surface immunoglobulins in chronic lymphatic leukemia and allied disorders. Am J Med 1973;55:184.

233. Shevach EM. Receptors for complement and immunoglobulin in human leukemic cells and human lymphoblastoid cell lines. J Clin Invest 1972;51:1933.

234. Foa R, Catovsky D, Brozovic M, et al. Clinical staging and immunological findings in chronic lymphocytic leukemia. Cancer 1979;44:483.

235. Binet JL, Auquier A, Dighiero G, et al. A new prognostic classification of chronic lymphocytic leukemia derived from multivariate survival analysis. Cancer 1981;48:198.

236. Knospe WH, Loeb B, Huguley CM. Bi-weekly chlorambucil treatment of chronic lymphocytic leukemia. Cancer 1974;33:555.

237. Sawitsky A, Rai KR, Glidewell O, Silver RT, Participating Members of CALGB (Cancer and Leukemia Group B). Comparison of daily versus intermittent chlorambucil and prednisone therapy in the treatment of patients with chronic lymphocytic leukemia. Blood 1977;50:1049.

238. Han T, Ezdinli EZ, Shimoaka K. Desai DV. Chlorambucil vs. combined chlorambucil-corticosteroid therapy in chronic lymphocytic leukemia. Cancer 1973;31:502.

239. Liepman M, Votaw ML. The treatment of chronic lymphocytic leukemia with COP chemotherapy. Cancer 1978;41:1664.

240. Kempin S, Yagoda A, Crossband E, et al. Complete remission in chronic lymphocytic leukemia (CLL). Proc Am Soc Clin Oncol 1978;19:353.

241. Raphael B, Andersen JW, Silber R, et al. Comparison of chlorambucil and prednisone versus cyclophosphamide, vincristine, and prednisone as initial treatment for chronic lymphocytic leukemia: long-term follow-up of an Eastern Cooperative Oncology Group randomized clinical trial. J Clin Oncol 1991;9:770–6.

242. Richards F II, Spurr CL, Pajak TF, Blake DD, Rabin M. Thymic irradiation: an approach to chronic lymphocytic leukemia. Am J Med 1974;57:862.

243. Byhardt RW, Brace KC, Wiernik PH. The role of splenic irradiation in chronic lymphocytic leukemia. Cancer 1975;35:1621.

244. Johnson RE. Total body irradiation of chronic lymphocytic leukemia. Cancer 1976;37:2691.

245. Sawitsky A, Rai KR, Aral I, et al. Mediastinal irradiation for chronic lymphocytic leukemia. Am J Med 1976;61:892.

246. Piro LD, Carrera CJ, Beutler E, et al. 2-chlorodeoxyadenosine: an effective new agent for the treatment of chronic lymphocytic leukemia. Blood 1988;72:1069.

247. Dillman RO, Mick R, McIntyre OR, et al. Pentostatin in chronic lymphocytic leukemia: a phase II trial of Cancer and Leukemia Group B. J Clin Oncol 1989;7:433.

248. Grever MR, Leiby JM, Kraut EH, et al. Low dose deoxyco-formycin in lymphoid malignancy. J Clin Oncol 1985;3:1196.
249. Keating MJ, Kantarjian H, Talpaz M, et al. Fludarabine: a new agent with major activity against chronic lymphocytic leukemia. Blood 1989;74:19–25.
250. Grever MR, Kopecky KJ, Coltman CA, et al. Fludarabine monophosphate: a potentially useful agent in chronic lymphocytic leukemia. Nouv Rev Fr Hematol 1988;30:457.
251. Cooperative Group for the Study of Immunoglobulin in Chronic Lymphocytic Leukemia. Intravenous immunoglobulin for the prevention of infection in chronic lymphocytic leukemia. A randomized, controlled clinical trial. N Engl J Med 1988;319:902.

14

Non-Hodgkin Lymphoma

*Richard J. Jones, M.D., Richard F. Ambinder, M.D., Ph.D., and
Eric J. Seifter, M.D.*

The term *non-Hodgkin lymphoma* refers to a heterogeneous group of malignancies of the lymphoreticular system. The non-Hodgkin lymphomas encompass more than 10 distinct diseases, each with markedly different biologies and prognoses, ranging from some of the slowest- to the fastest-growing cancers in humans and from incurable to curable. Lymphoid tumors were described first by Hodgkin in 1832;[1] in 1863, Virchow[2] used the term *lymphosarcoma* to distinguish these neoplasms affecting solid organs from leukemias.[2] At the turn of the century, Reed[3] and Sternberg[4] described the giant cells that differentiate Hodgkin disease from non-Hodgkin lymphomas. However, despite the long recognition of these diseases, substantial advances in the understanding of their biology, pathogenesis, and treatment have been made only recently.

Although non-Hodgkin lymphomas are relatively uncommon malignancies, representing less than 5% of new cases of cancer, there are over 20,000 new cases per year, and non-Hodgkin lymphomas are the seventh leading cause of cancer deaths.[5] Furthermore, these statistics underestimate the societal impact of these diseases; the non-Hodgkin lymphomas disproportionately affect relatively young patients compared with the more common cancers.[5] The median age of patients with non-Hodgkin lymphoma is 42 years, and the non-Hodgkin lymphomas are the third most common malignancy in children.

The non-Hodgkin lymphomas also serve as a model for treatment of the more common malignancies. A number of cancer treatment fundamentals have been tested first in patients with non-Hodgkin lymphoma, and this has contributed greatly to our understanding of cancer biology and has provided the framework for our treatment strategies in other cancers. However, although a substantial number of patients with non-Hodgkin lymphoma are cured, the majority of those with non-Hodgkin lymphoma still eventually die of their disease. Thus, considerable progress is still needed both in the area of disease characterization to better predict prognosis and into the mechanisms of treatment resistance to improve the outcome of these patients. This progress can be achieved only through a better understanding of the biology of these important diseases.

ETIOLOGY AND PATHOGENESIS

The cause of lymphomas is unknown; moreover, it is likely that the cause of most lymphomas is multifactorial. Nonetheless, lymphomas and lymphoproliferative diseases provide some of the best-studied examples of the role of viral infection and chromosomal translocation in tumorigenesis. Three examples illustrate the probable role that viral infection plays as a proliferative stimulus to infected lymphocytes, the special character of chromosomal translocations in cells with genes undergoing rearrangement, and the complexity of the interactions involved in tumorigenesis. These examples are Burkitt lymphoma, adult T-cell leukemia/lymphoma, and follicular lymphoma.

Burkitt Lymphoma

In 1958, Burkitt called attention to the lymphoma that now bears his name and is recognized as the most common tumor of children in tropical Africa.[6] Burkitt noted its characteristic and unusual anatomic distribution, particularly involving the jaw. The geographic distribution of the malignancy, restricted to certain climates in equatorial Africa, led to the expectation that a simple causal relationship between an infectious agent and the malignancy might be defined. The study of Burkitt lymphoma tissue ultimately led to discovery of a new virus, Epstein-Barr virus (EBV), present in virtually all cases of African Burkitt lymphoma.[7] EBV is a double-stranded DNA virus capable of infecting B lymphocytes that express the EBV/complement receptor, CD21. B lymphocytes infected by EBV in vitro and in vivo may be transformed into a state of continuous nonmalignant proliferation, known as "immortalization," and at least two EBV genes have been implicated in this process of growth transformation and immortalization.[8]

When first discovered in tumor tissue, it appeared that EBV might be the sole and direct cause of Burkitt lymphoma; however, the distribution of EBV does not explain the Burkitt lymphoma distribution. In fact, quite the reverse appears to be the case, as EBV is ubiquitous, infecting 95% of the world's adult population. EBV typically is acquired in early childhood through salivary transmission, and primary infection in childhood usually is asymptomatic or minimally symptomatic. In Western countries with affluent populations, where exposure generally is delayed until adolescence or young adulthood, primary infection commonly is associated with the syndrome of infectious mononucleosis; atypical lymphocytosis is the normal immune response (mainly $CD8^+$ T cells) to the benign EBV-induced B-cell proliferation of infectious mononucleosis. The geographic distribution of African Burkitt lymphoma more closely corresponds to the distribution of holoendemic malaria than of EBV, and it is generally believed that the relevant consequence of malaria is benign EBV-infected B-cell proliferation. Young children at greatest risk for developing Burkitt lymphoma suffer multiple bouts of clinical malaria per year, and their T-cell control of EBV-induced B-cell proliferation becomes demonstrably impaired.

In settings where there is failure of immune surveillance, EBV-induced B-cell lymphoproliferative disease (and lymphoma) results. The best-studied examples are those following bone marrow and organ transplantation. The incidence of EBV lymphoproliferative disease in allograft recipients ranges from less than 1% to as high as 10%, and preliminary reports suggest that EBV

growth-transforming and immortalizing genes are expressed in the lymphomas associated with immunocompromise.[9] A number of congenital immunodeficiency states, such as ataxia-telangiectasia, Wiskott-Aldrich syndrome, and severe combined immunodeficiency, also are associated with an increased incidence of lymphoma. To the contrary, however, African Burkitt lymphoma is not a direct consequence of EBV-infected B-cell proliferation in the setting of immunosuppression. In contrast to lymphomas associated with immunocompromise, the EBV growth genes seem to be "turned off" in Burkitt lymphoma tissue, and a cellular gene associated with growth regulation (*myc*) is overexpressed by virtue of a family of chromosomal translocations. These translocations juxtapose the *myc* locus on chromosome 8 with the immunoglobulin regulatory loci on chromosomes 14, 2, or 22.[10,11]

The Burkitt family of translocations were the first to be recognized, and they are the best-studied examples of a unique feature of lymphoid malignancies. Immunoglobulin genes responsible for individual antibody production in B cells, as well as T-cell receptor genes, are organized as discontinuous DNA segments in their germline forms.[12] With normal lymphoid development, the DNA segments of the immunoglobulin and T-cell receptor genes rearrange, and this is a major means of providing both antibody and T-cell receptor diversity. This complex process of gene rearrangement can go awry, however, leading to illegitimate recombination between nonhomologous chromosomes and juxtaposing genes that normally are actively transcribed in the involved lymphoid tissue with a proto-oncogene. Following the faulty rearrangement, a cellular proto-oncogene such as *myc* comes under the regulatory control of the rearranged gene locus. In the case of Burkitt lymphoma, the malignant cells are B cells, i.e., cells differentiated toward the production of immunoglobulin; thus, the immunoglobulin regulatory loci in these cells are turned on, and genes (such as *myc*) that are translocated near these loci are also turned on. Presumably, this same translocation would be much less likely to occur in another tissue type (in which immunoglobulin genes were not undergoing spontaneous, developmental rearrangements), and if it did occur, this translocation would not be associated with up-regulation of the *myc* gene because the immunoglobulin regulatory loci would be turned off. It is of interest that the Burkitt family of translocations also is associated with nonendemic Burkitt lymphoma, which has the same diffuse, small, noncleaved cell histology but without the predilection for mandibular involvement, narrow age range, and association with EBV of African (or endemic) Burkitt lymphoma.

In contrast to endemic and nonendemic Burkitt lymphoma, posttransplant lymphomas are not associated with consistent chromosomal translocations; thus, it has been suggested that in the setting of severe immunosuppression, EBV growth genes alone may be sufficient to bring about malignant lymphoproliferation. In other settings, such as malaria, EBV-induced proliferation alone may not be sufficient to produce malignant transformation, perhaps because suppression of T-cell function is not severe enough to allow EBV growth genes to effect malignant transformation. In endemic Burkitt lymphoma, *myc* gene translocation may be the next step as a random consequence of the poorly controlled, EBV-induced B-cell proliferation associated with malaria. After *myc* gene translocation, EBV gene expression may no longer be necessary to sustain growth of the lymphoid clone, and in the context of a functional immune system, expression of these genes actually may be a liability in that they serve to target cells for destruction by cytotoxic T cells. The absence of EBV in nonendemic Burkitt lymphoma suggests that EBV infection is not a prerequisite for the development of this malignancy; other factors may substitute for EBV in the process.

Human T-Cell Leukemia Virus

Another virus also has been identified in lymphoid malignancies: the human T-cell leukemia virus (HTLV-I). As with Burkitt lymphoma, the geographic distribution of the malignancy led to the expectation that a simple causal relationship might be defined. Although the two viruses are very different from each another, there are a number of similarities in their relationships to malignancy.[13] HTLV-I is endemic in some regions of Japan, Africa, and the Caribbean basin,[14] and in some areas, the seropositivity rate increases linearly with age and may reach 20%. Transmission, which may require passage of infected cells, is thought to occur in the perinatal period, but clinical manifestations generally do not develop until midlife. As with EBV, primary infection with HTLV-I may be entirely asymptomatic; fewer than 1% of infected individuals develop malignancy. There is a spectrum of lymphoproliferative disease associated with HTLV-I infection from subclinical disease to adult acute T-cell leukemia/lymphoma, and manifestations of the latter are leukemia, lymphadenopathy sparing the mediastinum, hepatosplenomegaly, skin infiltration, and hypercalcemia.

In contrast to animal models of retroviral oncogenesis, but again similar to EBV, HTLV-I does not contain an oncogene homologous with a cellular gene, nor is there a consistent site of chromosomal integration that might suggest insertional mutagenesis. It has been suggested that early T-cell proliferation may be a function of the HTLV-I tax protein, which may activate cellular genes required for T-cell growth in an autocrine or paracrine fashion involving the interleukin-2 receptor and interleukin-2 gene.[15] However, viral gene expression has not been detected in fully malignant tissue.[16] Perhaps there are further molecular changes on the road to malignancy that render expression of viral genes superfluous, as appears to be the case in Burkitt lymphoma, but it should be noted that in contrast to Burkitt lymphoma, cytogenetic analyses have failed to find a consistent karyotypic abnormality.

Follicular Lymphomas

Most lymphomas do not have any recognized viral cofactors. Follicular lymphomas, which account for approximately half of all lymphomas, are well-studied examples. They are recognized by their characteristic follicular (or nodular) pattern and are invariably B-cell tumors; these tumors usually occur in the middle-aged and elderly and usually are associated with a t(14;18) chromosomal translocation. Molecular characterization of this chromosomal translocation involving recombination between the immunoglobulin heavy-chain locus and another locus of presumed oncogenic potential led to the identification of the *bcl*-2 gene. As with the t(8;14) chromosomal translocation in Burkitt lymphoma, the most important result of this translocation appears to be overexpression of the normal *bcl*-2 gene[17,18] caused by juxtaposing the *bcl*-2 gene of chromosome 18 with the immunoglobulin regulatory loci on chromosome 14. The translocations in both Burkitt and follicular lymphoma are very different from translocations resulting in chimeric proteins, such as the t(9;21) chromosomal translocation of chronic myelogenous leukemia. The t(9;21) translocation results in the synthesis of a novel chimeric protein with growth-transforming properties, but the *bcl*-2 gene, which (in contrast to the *myc* gene) has no retroviral counterpart, promotes the growth and blocks programmed cell death of B lymphocytes.[19] Transgenic mice with an activated *bcl*-2 gene show an abnormal expansion of the B-lymphoid compartment, and lymphocytes from this compartment had an abnormally extended lifespan in tissue culture although they were not malignant per se.[20] As with Burkitt lymphoma and adult T-cell leukemia/lymphoma, one hit, i.e., the t(14;18) chromosomal translocation, appears to be insufficient for full malignant transformation.

In summary, a common theme in lymphomagenesis is lymphocyte-specific proliferative stimuli. These stimuli may be viral (i.e., EBV or HTLV-I, which selectively

**TABLE 14.1.   A Functional Classification of
Non-Hodgkin Lymphoma**

Indolent (low-grade) lymphomas
    Follicular small-cleaved
    Follicular mixed small-cleaved and large cell
    Diffuse small lymphocytic
    Diffuse intermediately differentiated lymphocytic
    Follicular large cell*
    Diffuse small-cleaved cell*
Aggressive (high-grade) lymphomas
    Diffuse mixed small-cleaved and large cell*
    Diffuse large cell*
    Diffuse large cell (immunoblastic)
    Diffuse small noncleaved cell (Burkitt lymphoma)
    Lymphoblastic lymphoma

---

*Officially classified as an intermediate-grade lymphoma by the Working Formulation.

**TABLE 14.2.   A Comparison of Features Typical of Indolent
and Aggressive Lymphomas**

Indolent	Aggressive
Slow growth	Fast growth
Lack of symptoms	"B" symptoms
Strictly nodal and lymphoid organs	Extranodal
Incurable	Curable
Watchful waiting or therapy	Aggressive therapy

target and immortalize B and T cells, respectively), or they may be the consequence of chromosomal translocations that juxtapose a genetic regulatory region turned on in lymphocytes (i.e., the immunoglobulin heavy-chain locus) and a growth gene (*myc* or *bcl-2*). In no case does a single genetic or infectious event appear to be sufficient to transform a lymphocyte to malignancy.

HISTOPATHOLOGIC CLASSIFICATION

The non-Hodgkin lymphomas encompass at least 10 distinct histopathologic entities. The Rappaport classification system was in general use through the 1970s, but this has been supplanted by the International Working Formulation in the United States and the Kiel system in some major European groups.[21,22] We employ the Working Formulation nomenclature in this chapter, but we also present the older Rappaport terminology to allow historical comparisons. The Working Formulation divides the non-Hodgkin lymphomas into three groups based on the extant information about the clinical behavior of the particular histologies: low-grade, intermediate-grade, or high-grade; however, new clinical information about the behavior and curability of certain histologies, as well as recognition of new histologic entities, has called into question many of these Working Formulation divisions. It now appears that all lymphomas can be functionally divided into two groups: indolent and aggressive (Table 14.1). The indolent lymphomas include those classified as low-grade in the Working Formulation and some classified as intermediate-grade, while aggressive lymphomas include those classified as high-grade as well as some classified as intermediate-grade. This grouping facilitates common approaches to staging and therapy; therefore, for the rest

of the chapter, we approach lymphomas based on their clinical behavior as either indolent or aggressive.

The indolent lymphomas share the characteristics of slow growth, long median survivals (ranging from 8 to 12 years), and responsiveness to gentler forms of treatment such as oral chemotherapy (Table 14.2). However, indolent lymphomas also are essentially incurable, with inevitable relapses, declining durations of response, and inexorable progression. The aggressive lymphomas are characterized by fast and explosive growth, frequent constitutional symptoms (fever, night sweats, or weight loss), rapid progression when unresponsive, and the requirement for aggressive forms of therapy. Nevertheless, in contrast to indolent lymphoma, approximately half the patients with aggressive lymphomas are curable using first-line therapy; while short-term prospects appear better for patients with indolent lymphomas, long-term prospects clearly favor those with durable remissions from aggressive lymphomas.

An excisional lymph node biopsy is crucial for proper histopathologic classification. Architectural features defining a follicular or diffuse process are much more difficult to discern by needle biopsy, extranodal sampling, or organ biopsy, and both the size and conformation of lymphocytes can be altered during processing of the bone marrow biopsy. Histopathologic diagnosis by light microscopy remains the bulwark of clinical decision-making; however, controversies in pathologic diagnosis, particularly in distinguishing the non-Hodgkin lymphomas from Hodgkin disease, benign lymphoproliferation, or from undifferentiated carcinoma, sometimes can require more specialized techniques such as cell surface marker or immunoglobulin/T-cell receptor gene rearrangement analyses. Lymphomas present with a follicular or a diffuse pattern in the lymph node. The follicular pattern also is known as nodular in the older Rappaport classification, and the terms are interchangeable. Any mixture of follicular and diffuse patterns is designated by convention as the follicular subtype with associated diffuse elements. Follicular lymphomas tend to behave indolently and be incurable, while diffuse lymphomas may be either indolent or aggressive. The lymphoma classification schemes juxtapose the follicular or diffuse nodal pattern with lymphocyte morphology, judged by size and nuclear shape (Table 14.1).

Indolent Lymphomas

The prototypic indolent lymphoma is follicular small-cleaved cell lymphoma, also known as nodular poorly differentiated lymphocytic lymphoma in the Rappaport system. As with all follicular histologies, these lymphomas are always of B-cell phenotype; the cell type is a small lymphocyte with an indented, folded, or irregular nucleus, also referred to as a "buttock cell." It is unfortunate this cell was designated as "poorly differentiated" in older schemes, because this term implies a poor prognosis or aggressive phenotype to the uninitiated. In fact, just the opposite is true. The small-cleaved cell is associated with indolent behavior and prolonged median survivals characteristic of low-grade lymphomas.

In a less common form of indolent lymphoma, the lymph node pattern is follicular, but the cells reflect a mixture of small-cleaved and large cells. This is termed *follicular mixed lymphoma*, or *nodular mixed lymphoma* in the Rappaport system. The presence of large lymphocytes comprising more than 25% of the total number of lymphocytes and/or the identification of more than five large lymphocytes per high-powered field have been used as criteria to distinguish follicular mixed from follicular small-cleaved cell lymphoma. The large cell was called a histiocyte in the older nomenclature because of its appearance; however, we now know this large cell to be an activated lymphocyte by immunophenotypic analysis.

The third low-grade lymphoma in the Working Formulation is diffuse small lymphocytic or diffuse well-differentiated lymphocytic lymphoma. The cells are small, uniform, mature-appearing lymphocytes, and the presentation is the lymphomatous manifestation of chronic lymphocytic leukemia (CLL). The natural history parallels that expected for CLL, and both diseases can be viewed as a single entity with a full spectrum of presentation, usually between adenopathy alone and a strictly leukemic form. Problems with leukemia, cytopenias, splenomegaly, and autoimmune hemolytic anemia or thrombocytopenia occur in diffuse small lymphocytic lymphoma as they would in CLL.

Follicular large cell lymphoma and diffuse small cleaved-cell lymphoma are classified as intermediate-grade in the Working Formulation, and there has been some controversy historically about the behavior and curability of these two lymphomas, at least partly because of their rarity. However, most data now demonstrate these tumors behave as indolent lymphomas in both their clinical aggressiveness and curability.

This last type of indolent lymphoma is not included in the Working Formulation. This category has been termed diffuse intermediate differentiated lymphocytic lymphoma or mantle zone lymphoma.[23] Small immature follicles are surrounded by a sea of abnormal lymphocytes in the "mantle" zone, and mantle zone or diffuse intermediate differentiated lymphocytic lymphoma type follows a natural history congruent with other indolent lymphomas.

Aggressive Lymphomas

The prototypic aggressive lymphoma is diffuse large cell in the Working Formulation or diffuse histiocytic lymphoma in the Rappaport system. The large cells can be cleaved or noncleaved, with no difference in clinical outcome; in addition, there appears to be no reproducible clinical difference between a so-called immunoblastic large cell versus the standard large cell. The Working Formulation splits diffuse large cell lymphoma into immunoblastic (high-grade) and nonimmunoblastic (intermediate-grade) subtypes. We favor regarding all diffuse large cell types as a functional aggressive lymphoma, which implies rapid growth and potential curability; when viewed this way, diffuse large cell lymphoma is the most common type of aggressive lymphoma in adults and the most frequent among all the lymphoma categories (approximately 40% of all new patients with lymphoma). Another lymphoma classified as intermediate-grade by the Working Formulation, diffuse mixed small-cleaved and large cell lymphoma or diffuse mixed lymphoma also is functionally an aggressive lymphoma, and this lymphoma has relatively fast growth and is curable with the same regimens used for the other aggressive lymphomas. Diffuse large cell lymphoma and diffuse mixed small-cleaved and large cell lymphoma mark as B-cells only 60% to 70% of the time, with the remainder marking as T cells.

The remaining two types of high-grade lymphomas in the Working Formulation are even more explosive in growth, yet still curable, as are all types in this grouping. Burkitt lymphoma presents as a diffuse pattern of small to intermediate-sized lymphocytes with frequent mitoses and a B-cell phenotype. In the older Rappaport system, Burkitt lymphoma also is referred to as diffuse undifferentiated lymphocytic lymphoma; the Working Formulation designates this type as diffuse small noncleaved cell lymphoma. It is important not to confuse diffuse small *noncleaved* cell with diffuse small lymphocytic or diffuse small-cleaved cell, both indolent lymphomas. Lymphoblastic lymphoma is the lymphomatous manifestation of acute lymphocytic leukemia, and a spectrum of presentations occurs between these two entities. The lymphocytes are characteristically T cells with terminal deoxynucleotidyl transferase staining, and both Burkitt lymphoma and lymphoblastic lymphoma are common in childhood.

CLINICAL MANIFESTATIONS

The most common complaint of patients presenting with non-Hodgkin lymphomas is enlarged lymph nodes. The majority of these patients are asymptomatic, and because many other, more common disorders also cause lymphadenopathy, a careful search for benign etiologies should be undertaken. However, there are no features that reliably distinguish benign from neoplastic lymphadenopathy or one type of lymphoma from another. Furthermore, histopathologic examination of the involved tissue is the only definitive way to diagnose lymphoma. Thus, lymph node or other organ biopsy is required to either diagnose or rule out lymphoma; lymph nodes that remain enlarged for more than 3 weeks or are rapidly enlarging should be biopsied.

Unlike patients with Hodgkin disease, "B" symptoms (fevers, night sweats, weight loss) or mediastinal involvement only occur in approximately 20% of patients who present with non-Hodgkin lymphoma. Whereas indolent non-Hodgkin lymphomas usually involve only lymphoid organs (lymph nodes, spleen, and bone marrow), aggressive lymphomas arise from extralymphatic sites in at least one third of cases, and they involve these sites during the course of the illness in the majority of patients. Any organ can be involved by aggressive non-Hodgkin lymphoma; however, organs in the gastrointestinal tract,[24,25] representing approximately 40% of all primary extranodal lymphomas, skin, and bone, are the most common extralymphatic sites.[26]

Most patients with non-Hodgkin lymphoma present with advanced-stage disease. As with Hodgkin disease, the stage of patients with non-Hodgkin disease is classified according to the Ann Arbor Conference[27] (Table 14.3), but this staging system has not been as useful for non-Hodgkin lymphoma as for Hodgkin disease. Less than 10% of patients with indolent lymphomas have pathologically proven stage I or stage II disease, and only about one third of patients with aggressive lymphomas have localized disease.[28]

INDOLENT LYMPHOMAS

The indolent lymphomas (Table 14.1) present almost exclusively in nodal sites and the lymphoid organs. Bone marrow involvement occurs in 50% to 80% of patients, while spleen and liver involvement occur in 40% to 60%. Consequently, most patients have stage IV

TABLE 14.3. The Staging of Lymphomas

Stage	Criteria
I	Involvement of a single lymph node region or single extralymphatic site
II	Involvement of two or more lymph node regions (including a single localized extralymphatic site) on the same side of the diaphragm
III	Involvement of lymph node regions (including localized involvement of one extralymphatic site and/or spleen involvement) on both sides of the diaphragm
IV	Diffuse involvement of one or more extralymphatic organs (i.e., bone marrow, liver, lungs)

disease, but only 10% to 20% present with constitutional "B" symptoms. These lymphomas usually grow slowly, often waxing and waning in size for months or years, and it is not unusual to elicit a several-year history of adenopathy that was ignored because of its indolent behavior.[29] Most of the follicular subtypes, including follicular large cell, have the associated chromosomal abnormality t(14;18) involving the *bcl*-2 gene.

Patients with indolent lymphomas have a slow but inexorable drop in overall survival, with a median survival of 8 to 12 years. In contrast to the more aggressive lymphomas, patients do not have sustained complete remissions and probably are incurable. For older patients, many may die with their disease rather than from it. Indolent lymphomas are unheard of in childhood and are rare in young adults, the incidence of indolent lymphomas gradually increasing with age. The indolent lymphomas are characterized by documented spontaneous regressions that may last from a few months to several years. The median duration of spontaneous regression is about 1 year and the incidence by histology is 30% for follicular small-cleaved cell lymphoma, 17% for follicular mixed lymphoma, and 14% for diffuse small lymphocytic lymphoma (based on Stanford data).[29] The indolent lymphomas also may show histologic progression on subsequent biopsies to more aggressive histologies. This transformation usually is heralded by "B" symptoms and rapid tumor growth, sometimes in extranodal sites not favored by the indolent histologies. The transformation from CLL to diffuse large cell lymphoma has been called Richter syndrome, and patients with any of these histologic progressions have particularly poor survival, with only 20% still alive 2 years after conventional therapy. Approximately one third of patients will show histologic progression by 10 years after diagnosis.

Staging

After confirmation of the histologic diagnosis, staging involves distinguishing between localized disease (stage I or contiguous stage II) or more widespread involvement as this may have therapeutic implications. Physical examination should focus on all nodal sites, including Waldeyer tonsillar ring (pharyngeal) and the epitrochlear nodes. Computed tomographic scans of the neck, chest, abdomen, and pelvis as well as bone marrow biopsy complete the basic staging. Less than 10% of patients with indolent lymphoma have truly localized disease. The more invasive the procedure (i.e., liver biopsy, staging laparotomy), the more likely one will upstage the patient; after computed tomographic scans and bone marrow biopsies alone, 50% of all patients designated as localized disease actually will have more generalized involvement found without more invasive testing. Most patients can be managed with basic staging only because overt generalized disease usually is apparent. When crucial therapeutic decisions are at stake, however, more invasive testing may be warranted.

Therapy

Treatments that have been evaluated extensively for indolent lymphomas include single-agent chemotherapy, combination chemotherapy without doxorubicin (i.e., CVP [vincristine 1.4 mg/m^2 intravenously, prednisone 100 mg orally each day for 5 days, and cyclophosphamide at either 200 to 400 mg/m^2 orally each day for 5 days or 1 g/m^2 intravenously every 3 to 4 weeks]), combination chemotherapy with doxorubicin (i.e., CHOP [cyclophosphamide 750 mg/m^2 intravenously, vincristine 1.4 mg/m^2 intravenously, doxorubicin 50 mg/m^2 intravenously, and prednisone 100 mg orally each day for 5 days given every 3 to 4 weeks]), involved or extended-field radiotherapy, total-nodal irradiation, whole-body irradiation, and combined-modality therapy. The advantages for single-agent therapy include simplicity, lower toxicity, and response rate and survival equivalent to more complicated regimens; a potential disadvantage of employing a single agent daily would be theoretic induction of resistance and mutation. An example of an oral regimen is oral cyclophosphamide 100 to 150 mg/day for 14 days on a 28-day cycle, or 200 to 300 mg/m^2/day for 5 days with prednisone. These various regimens have been tested both prospectively and retrospectively against each other, radiotherapy, and combined-modality therapy, and the following conclusions can be drawn from analyses of these trials:[29]

1. no difference in complete remission rates (60% to 80%) or objective responses (90%);

2. no difference in remission duration;
3. no difference in median survival (8 to 12 years); and
4. no plateau in the survival curves, suggesting inexorable progression of disease.

In another series at Stanford, 83 asymptomatic patients were selected for a watch-and-wait approach, with therapy starting only when symptoms or laboratory abnormalities supervened.[30] The median time to start of therapy was 3 years, but almost 20% of patients were projected free of treatment at 10 years. The overall survival was identical with patients treated at diagnosis (median, 11 years), and on histologic subgroup analysis, the follicular mixed lymphoma category required the initiation of therapy sooner (median time, <1 year).

At present, standard therapy would involve consideration of a watch-and-wait approach. Factors dictating immediate therapy rather than the initiation of therapy on a "watchful-waiting" policy include:

1. constitutional "B" symptoms,
2. rapid growth of lymph nodes,
3. cytopenias due to marrow infiltration (excluding autoimmune etiologies that could respond to steroids), and
4. imminent renal or hepatic dysfunction.

When therapy is required, the choice of radiotherapy versus oral chemotherapy versus intravenous combination chemotherapy is made based on the extent of systemic disease, toxicities of therapy, and the importance of rapid response. Oral chemotherapy often is tolerated better than intravenous combinations, but responses occur more slowly and would be less appropriate for reversal of severe cytopenias or organ dysfunction.

A number of institutions are currently studying the role of autologous bone marrow transplantation in patients with indolent lymphoma as an investigational approach, and it is hoped that this dose-intensive consolidation will result in durable complete remissions or even cures. This modality may work best at the first complete remission, before induction of refractory drug resistance; this approach holds most promise for the younger patients whose long-term prospects are dimmed by the inevitable recurrence and progression of indolent lymphomas. A desire to proceed to such consolidation immediately would be one reason to initiate immediate therapy at diagnosis. The use of bone marrow transplantation remains investigational, however, and because of the need for long follow-up, no answers will be available until the turn of the century.

Localized indolent lymphomas (stage I or contiguous stage II) may be cured by involved-field or extended-field radiotherapy. An 80% relapse-free survival in laparotomy-staged patients versus 50% to 70% in clinically staged patients simply reflects that the more aggressive the staging, the fewer the patients with localized disease. Younger age is a favorable prognostic factor in localized indolent lymphoma. Also, the use of invasive staging (liver biopsy, peritonoscopy, staging laparotomy) outside clinical trials remains quite controversial. Less invasive staging may suffice if one can accept a 50% relapse-free survival, but in very young patients, aggressive staging may be necessary to choose between radiotherapy and autologous transplant consolidation.

A number of newer modalities also have shown some promise in the treatment of indolent lymphomas. Although none of these agents are likely to be curative, they do extend options for controlling these diseases in patients who need treatment. Interferon-α has a 30% to 60% response rate in previously treated follicular small-cleaved cell lymphoma and follicular mixed lymphoma but less than a 10% response rate for diffuse small lymphocytic lymphoma. Doses of 10 million units/m^2 subcutaneously three times a week are employed, and other agents such as 2-chlorodeoxyadenosine and fludarabine also are under investigation. Monoclonal antibodies have been raised against clonal cell surface antigens as a therapeutic approach as well.[31]

In summary, most patients with indolent lymphomas present with advanced disease but enjoy relatively long median survival. Long-term complete remissions are rare, and the disease tends to relapse in the previous nodal sites of involvement, sometimes with altered histology. Spontaneous remissions may occur, and many patients can safely undergo a watchful-waiting approach. The role of intensive consolidation therapy with bone marrow transplantation presently is under investigation.

AGGRESSIVE LYMPHOMAS

Aggressive lymphomas (Table 14.1) represent approximately 50% of the new cases of non-Hodgkin lymphomas. Diffuse large cell lymphoma is the prototype and the most common lymphoma in this group, comprising approximately 40% of the non-Hodgkin lymphomas. With few exceptions, the clinical presentations, diagnostic and therapeutic approaches, and prognoses are similar for all the lymphomas in this category, and virtually all non-Hodgkin lymphomas that arise in children are aggressive non-Hodgkin lymphomas.

Staging

Staging evaluation consists of studies that can distinguish between the 15% to 20% of patients with very localized disease (stage I) and those with more advanced disease (stages II through IV). This differentiation has definite prognostic and possible therapeutic implications. Patients with stage I aggressive non-Hodgkin lymphoma have a better event-free survival than those with more advanced disease (including stage II),[32,33] and patients with stages II through IV disease require aggressive combination chemotherapy while those with truly localized disease can be cured with radiotherapy alone. A complete history and physical examination should pay special attention to all nodal areas and other sites of frequent involvement. Computed tomography or magnetic resonance imaging are the foundation of staging for aggressive non-Hodgkin lymphoma, and because approximately 20% of patients with aggressive non-Hodgkin lymphoma have bone marrow involvement,[34,35] bone marrow examination is necessary to establish the extent of the disease. Lymphangiography and staging laparotomy, still generally considered important staging procedures in Hodgkin disease, have been replaced largely by computed tomography or magnetic resonance imaging scans. The one possible remaining role for these procedures is to rule out more extensive disease (that would require chemotherapy) in patients with clinical stage I disease where radiotherapy as a single modality is planned.

Other than routine blood tests (hematologies, electrolytes, liver functions), few serum tests are helpful in the workup of patients with aggressive lymphomas. Serum levels of calcium and uric acid occasionally are elevated in these patients, and a serum protein electrophoresis may be helpful for following the disease in the uncommon patient whose lymphoma produces a monoclonal immunoglobulin. Serum lactate dehydrogenase also should be checked, as this may be the single most important prognostic variable[36] and also can be used as a disease marker to follow the disease's course.

Therapy

Although patients with stage I disease have an excellent prognosis and expected cure rate of over 80%, the optimal therapy for these patients is somewhat controversial. Radiotherapy yields long-term disease-free survival for approximately 70% of patients with pathologic stage I disease.[32,33,37] The results with radiotherapy will be somewhat worse in those only staged clinically, and radiotherapy alone has not been adequate treatment for patients with stage II disease.[32,33,37] Whether chemotherapy can salvage effectively patients with localized, aggressive lymphomas who fail radiotherapy, as is the case with Hodgkin disease, is unknown. Combination chemotherapy also is effective for these patients,[38,39] and others have used a combination of radiotherapy and chemotherapy.[40,41] There is no firm evidence that any of these approaches are superior, however, and the relative rarity of this disease as well as the excellent outcome regardless of therapeutic approach will make it difficult to determine if one approach is best.

Aggressive combination chemotherapy is required for the treatment of patients with stages II through IV aggressive non-Hodgkin lymphoma. CHOP given every 3 weeks for six to 8 cycles is the prototype of intensive therapy for aggressive non-Hodgkin lymphoma. The largest experience with this regimen was reported by the Southwest Oncology Group; with the longest follow-up being 12 years, they found a complete response rate of over 50% and an actuarial disease-free survival of 30%.[42] Age was the most important factor determining outcome, with approximately 55% disease-free survival of patients under 40 years of age and less than a 20% disease-free survival in those over 65 years. A major reason for the poorer outcomes in older patients was that these patients were less likely to receive full-dose, intensive therapy,[42,43] and failure to maintain dose-intensity has been shown to be an important cause of chemotherapy failure for aggressive non-Hodgkin lymphoma.[44]

In addition to age, other factors have been found to influence the outcome of patients with aggressive lymphomas. Patients presenting with large tumor masses, "B" symptoms, bone marrow involvement, high serum lactate dehydrogenase levels, and poor performance status have been found to have poorer outcomes.[36,45,46] These factors tend not to be independent; most are measures of large tumor burdens. As previously mentioned, serum lactate dehydrogenase may be the single most useful prognostic factor, and the immunophenotype (T cell vs. B cell) also has been reported to be an important prognostic variable for some subgroups of patients with aggressive lymphomas.[47] However, most reports show that when other prognostic factors are taken into account, immunophenotype is not an independent prognostic factor.[48–51]

In the early 1980s, a number of new ("second" and "third" generation) chemotherapy regimens were reported to produce substantially improved results in patients with aggressive lymphomas.[52–55] These regimens tested whether the addition of other drugs (bleomycin, methotrexate, etoposide, cytosine arabinoside) to CHOP and scheduling could overcome drug resistance. Despite the initial enthusiasm associated with these regimens, however, they have not been shown to be superior to CHOP in subsequent trials,[44,56] and it is probable that the apparent improvement over CHOP initially seen with these regimens resulted from patient selection and maintenance of dose intensity. Most of these regimens did not permit the extensive reduction in drug doses that frequently occurred in the early CHOP trials. Currently, there is no evidence that any of the newer regimens are superior to CHOP given intensively, but randomized trials now underway should elucidate the relative effectiveness of the newer regimens versus CHOP.

Very few patients who fail the initial combination chemotherapy for the aggressive lymphomas can be cured with conventional-dose salvage therapy. Thousands of patients worldwide have been treated with dose-intensified cytotoxic therapy followed by bone marrow rescue (bone marrow transplantation) for refractory lymphomas, and the disease-free survival for these patients ranges from 20% to 50%.[57–59] For this reason, bone marrow transplantation has become the treatment of choice for relapsed aggressive lymphoma. The status of lymphoma at the time of transplant is the most important determinant of outcome following bone marrow transplantation; The disease-free survival is less than 10% when transplantation is performed in patients during resistant relapse (patients whose lymphoma no longer responds to conventional salvage therapy).[57,59] In contrast, the disease-free survival is approximately 50% after bone marrow transplantation for relapsed lymphomas that are still sensitive to conventional therapy. Even though bone marrow transplantation is the most effective antilymphoma treatment, it currently cannot be recommended earlier in the natural history (i.e., first remission) of patients with aggressive lymphomas; this is because of its substantial toxicity (transplant-related mortality of approximately 10%) as well as the lack of factors that reliably predict for relapse in a group of patients having a 50% chance of cure with conventional-dose therapy.

Special Considerations

In general, stage for stage, extranodal presentations of aggressive non-Hodgkin lymphomas can be treated the same as the more common nodal presentations. Although surgery has been recommended for patients with gastrointestinal lymphomas to prevent treatment-related perforation and hemorrhage and also decrease relapse,[60] other studies suggest that surgery does not improve outcome over chemotherapy alone.[61] It is likely that surgery is not truly therapeutic for gastrointestinal lymphomas but rather that the results of surgery are simply a prognostic indicator for the extent of the disease. However, certain extranodal presentations do warrant special considerations. Testicular lymphoma seems to have a high rate of early systemic spread especially to the central nervous system (CNS);[62,63] it probably requires chemotherapy and CNS prophylaxis regardless of stage. Patients with aggressive lymphomas that involve the epidural space[64] or paranasal sinuses as well as patients with lymphoblastic or diffuse undifferentiated lymphoma[65] also appear to be at high risk for CNS relapse and probably should receive CNS prophylaxis. The optimal CNS prophylaxis is unknown, but it probably should involve at least six intrathecal injections of methotrexate or cytarabine.[53]

Primary CNS lymphoma is a previously rare tumor that now is becoming increasingly more common, both as a result of (and also unrelated to) the acquired immunodeficiency syndrome (AIDS). Despite being localized initially, primary CNS lymphoma has had a dismal prognosis. However, preliminary studies with combined-modality therapy using chemotherapy, brain irradiation, and intrathecal therapy look promising.[66]

The treatment of virally related lymphomas has not been particularly successful. EBV-related lymphoproliferative diseases in immunocompromised hosts may respond to prompt reduction of immunosuppression (if possible), but if this fails, cytotoxic therapy generally has not been effective.[67] AIDS-related malignant lymphomas generally have had a poor prognosis, largely related to the inability to deliver intensive therapy because of underlying immunocompromise; however, AIDS-related lymphomas may have a similar prognosis to non-AIDS-related lymphomas in the subset of patients with good performance status.[68,69] These patients should receive intensive therapy with curative intent. No therapy, however, has been shown to be curative in HTLV-I T-cell lymphoma.[70]

REFERENCES

1. Hodgkin T. On some of the morbid appearances of the absorbent glands and spleen. Trans Med Chir Soc Lond 1832;17:68–114.
2. Virchow R. Die Krankhoften Geschwulste. Berlin: A. Hirschwald, 1863.
3. Reed DM. On the pathological changes in Hodgkin's disease with especial reference to its relation to tuberculosis. Johns Hopkins Hosp Rep 1902;10:133–96.
4. Sternberg C. Uber eine eigenartige unter dem bilde der pseudoleukamie varlaufende tuberculose des lymphatischen apparates. Ztschr f Heilk 1898;19:21–90.
5. Devita VT, Jaffe ES, Mauch P, Longo DL. Lymphocytic lymphomas. In: DeVita VT, Hellman S, Rosenberg SA, eds. Cancer: Principal and Practice of Oncology. Philadelphia: J.B. Lippincott, 1989:174–98.
6. Burkitt D. A sarcoma involving the jaws in African children. Br J Surg 1958;46:218–223.
7. Miller G. Epstein-Barr virus. Biology, pathogenesis, and medical aspects. In: Fields BN, Knipe DM, eds. Virology. New York: Raven Press, Ltd., 1990:1921–58.
8. Kieff E, Liebowitz D. Epstein-Barr virus and its replication. In: Fields BN, Knipe DM, eds. Virology. New York: Raven Press, 1990:1889–920.
9. Young L, Alfieri C, Hennessy K, et al. Expression of Epstein-Barr virus transformation-associated genes in tissues of patients with EBV lymphoproliferative disease. N Engl J Med 1989; 321:1080–5.
10. Erikson J, ar-Rushdi A, Drwinga HL, Nowell PC, Croce CM. Transcriptional activation of the translocated c-myc oncogene in Burkitt lymphoma. Proc Natl Acad Sci U S A 1983;80:820–4.
11. Dalla-Favera R, Bregni M, Erikson J, Patterson D, Gallo RC, Croce CM. Human c-myc oncogene is located on the region of chromosome 8 that is translocated in Burkitt lymphoma. Proc Natl Acad Sci U S A 1982;79:7824.
12. Waldmann TA, Korsmeyer SJ, Bakhshi A, Arnold A, Kirsch IR. Molecular genetic analysis of human lymphoid neoplasms. Ann Intern Med 1985;102:497–510.
13. Ambinder RF. Human lymphotropic viruses associated with lymphoid malignancy: Epstein-Barr and HTLV-I. Hematol Oncol Clin North Am 1990;4:821–33.
14. Ratner L, Poisez BJ. Leukemias associated with human T cell lymphotropic virus type I in a non endemic region. Medicine 1988;67:401–19.
15. Murphy E, Blattner WA. HTLV-I associated leukemia: a model for chronic retroviral disease. Ann Neurol 1988;23:174–80.
16. Ratner L, Griffiths RC, Marselle L, Hoh M, Wong-Staal R, Saxinger C. A lymphoproliferative disorder caused by human T-lymphotropic virus type I: Demonstration of a continuum between acute and chronic adult T-cell leukemia/lymphoma. Am J Med 1987;83:953–8.
17. Ngan B-Y, Chen-Levy Z, Weiss LM, Warnke RA, Cleary ML. Expression in non-Hodgkin's lymphoma of the bcl-2 protein associated with the t(14;18) chromosomal translocation. N Engl J Med 1988;318:1638–44.
18. Weiss LM, Warnke RA, Sklar J, Cleary ML. Molecular analysis of the t(14;18) chromosomal translocation in malignant lymphomas. N Engl J Med 1987;317:1185–9.
19. Hockenberry D, Nunez G, Milliman C, Schreiber RD, Korsmeyer SJ. Bcl-2 is an inner mitochondrial membrane protein that blocks programmed cell death. Nature 1990;348:334–6.
20. McDonnell T, Deane N, Platt FM, et al. Bcl-2-immunoglobulin transgenic mice demonstrate extended B cell survival and follicular lymphoproliferation. Cell 1989;57:79–88.
21. The Non-Hodgkins Lymphoma Pathologic Classification Project. National Cancer Institute sponsored study of classification of non-Hodgkin's lymphomas: summary and description of a working formulation for clinical usage. Cancer 1982;49:2112–35.
22. Lennert K, Stein H, Kaiserling E. Cytologic and functional criteria for the classification of malignant lymphomas. Br J Cancer 1990;31:29–43.
23. Weisenburger DD, Kim H, Rappaport H. Mantle-zone lymphoma: a follicular variant of intermediate lymphocytic lymphoma. Cancer 1982;49:1429–38.
24. Rosenfelt F, Rosenberg SA. Diffuse histiocytic lymphoma presenting with gastrointestinal tract lesions. Cancer 1980;45:2188–93.
25. Shepherd FA, Evans WK, Kutas G, et al. Chemotherapy following surgery for stages IE and IIE non-Hodgkin's lymphoma of the gastrointestinal tract. J Clin Oncol 1988;6:253–60.
26. Rosenberg SA, Diamond HD, Jaslowitz B, Craver LF. Lymphosarcoma: a review of 1269 cases. Medicine 1961;40:31–84.
27. Carbone PP, Kaplan HS, Mushoff K, Smithers DW, Tubiana M. Report of the Committee on Hodgkin's Disease Staging Classification. Cancer Res 1971;3:1860–1.
28. Sweet DL, Kinzie J, Gaeke ME, Golomb HM, Ferguson DL, Ultmann JE. Survival of patients with localized diffuse histiocytic lymphoma. Blood 1981;58:1218–23.
29. Rosenberg SA. The low-grade non-Hodgkin's lymphomas: challenges and opportunities. J Clin Oncol 1985;3:299–310.
30. Horning SJ, Rosenberg SA. The natural history of initially untreated low-grade non-Hodgkin's lymphomas. N Engl J Med 1984;311:1471–5.
31. Meeker TC, Lowder J, Cleary M, et al. Emergence of idiotype variants during treatment of B-cell lymphoma with antiidiotype antibodies. N Engl J Med 1985;312:1658–65.

32. Nissen NI, Ersboll J, Hansen HS, et al. A randomized study of radiotherapy versus radiotherapy plus chemotherapy in stage I–II non-Hodgkin's lymphomas. Cancer 1983;52:1–7.

33. Vokes EE, Ultmann JE, Golomb HM, et al. Long-term survival of patients with localized diffuse histiocytic lymphoma. J Clin Oncol 1985;3:1309–17.

34. Bennett JM, Cain KC, Glick JH, Johnson GJ, Ezdinli E, O'Connell MJ. The significance of bone marrow involvement in non-Hodgkin's lymphoma: the Eastern Cooperative Oncology Group Experience. J Clin Oncol 1986;4:1462–9.

35. Conlan MG, Bast M, Armitage JO, Weisenburger DD. Bone marrow involvement by non-Hodgkin's lymphoma: the clinical significance of morphologic discordance between the lymph node and bone marrow. J Clin Oncol 1990;8:1163–72.

36. Jagannath S, Velasquez WS, Tucker SL, et al. Tumor burden assessment and its implication for a prognostic model in advanced diffuse large-cell lymphoma. J Clin Oncol 1986;4:859–65.

37. Kaminski MS, Coleman CN, Colby TV, Cox RS, Rosenberg SA. Factors predicting survival in adults with stage I and II large-cell lymphoma treated with primary radiation therapy. Ann Intern Med 1986;104:747–56.

38. Jones SE, Miller TP, Connors JM. Long-term follow-up and analysis for prognostic factors for patients with limited-stage diffuse large-cell lymphoma treated with initial chemotherapy with or without adjuvant radiotherapy. J Clin Oncol 1989;7:1186–91.

39. Link MP, Donaldson SS, Berard CW, Shuster JJ, Murphy SB. Results of treatment of childhood localized non-Hodgkin's lymphoma with combination chemotherapy with or without radiotherapy. N Engl J Med 1990;322:1169–74.

40. Connors JM, Klimo P, Fairey RN, Voss N. Brief chemotherapy and involved field radiation therapy for limited-stage, histologically aggressive lymphoma. Ann Intern Med 1987;107:25–30.

41. Longo DL, Glatstein E, Duffey PL, et al. Treatment of localized aggressive lymphomas with combination chemotherapy followed by involved-field radiation therapy. J Clin Oncol 1989;7:1295–302.

42. Dixon DO, Neilan B, Jones SE, et al. Effect of age on therapeutic outcome in advanced diffuse histiocytic lymphoma: the Southwest Oncology Group Experience. J Clin Oncol 1986;4295–305.

43. Vose JM, Armitage JO, Weisenburger DD, et al. The importance of age in survival of patients treated with chemotherapy for aggressive non-Hodgkin's lymphoma. J Clin Oncol 1988;6:1838–44.

44. Kwak LW, Halpern J, Oshen RA, Horning SJ. Prognostic significance of actual dose intensity in diffuse large-cell lymphoma: results of a tree-structured survival analysis. J Clin Oncol 1990;8:963–77.

45. Shipp MA, Harrington DP, Klatt MM, et al. Identification of major prognostic subgroups of patients with large-cell lymphoma treated with m-BACOD or M-BACOD. Ann Intern Med 1986;104:757–65.

46. Fisher RI, DeVita VT Jr, Johnson BL, Simon R, Young RC. Prognostic factors for advanced diffuse histiocytic lymphoma following treatment with combination chemotherapy. Am J Med 1977;63:177–82.

47. Armitage JO, Vose JM, Linder J, et al. Clinical significance of immunophenotype in diffuse aggressive non-Hodgkin's lymphoma. J Clin Oncol 1989;7:1783–90.

48. Cossman J, Jaffe ES, Fisher RI. Immunologic phenotypes of diffuse, aggressive, non-Hodgkin's lymphomas. Cancer 1984;54:1310–17.

49. Cheng A-L, Chen Y-C, Wang C-H, et al. Direct comparisons of peripheral T-cell lymphoma with diffuse B-cell lymphoma of comparable histological grades: should peripheral T-cell lymphoma be considered separately? J Clin Oncol 1989;7:725–31.

50. Horning SJ, Doggett RS, Warnke RA, Dorfman RF, Cox RS, Levy R. Clinical relevance of immunologic phenotype in diffuse large cell lymphoma. Blood 1984;63:1209–15.

51. Lippman SM, Miller TP, Spier CM, Slymen DJ, Grogan TM. The prognostic significance of the immunotype in diffuse large-cell lymphoma: a comparative study of the T-cell and B-cell phenotype. Blood 1988;72:436–41.

52. Skarin AT, Canellos GP, Rosenthal DS, et al. Improved prognosis of diffuse histiocytic and undifferentiated lymphoma by use of high dose methotrexate alternating with standard agents (M-BACOD). J Clin Oncol 1983;1:91–8.

53. Klimo P, Connors JM. MACOP-B chemotherapy for the treatment of diffuse large-cell lymphoma. Ann Intern Med 1985;102:596–602.

54. Fisher RA, Devita VT Jr, Longo DL, Young RI. In: Skarin AT, ed. Update on Treatment for Diffuse Large Cell Lymphoma. New York: Park Row Publishers, Inc., 1991:31–5.

55. Boyd DB, Coleman M, Papish SW, et al. COPBLAM III: Infusional combination chemotherapy for diffuse large-cell lymphoma. J Clin Oncol 1988;6:425–33.

56. Dana BW, Dahlberg S, Miller TP, et al. m-BACOD treatment for intermediate- and high-grade malignant lymphomas: a Southwest Oncology Group Phase II Trial. J Clin Oncol 1990;8:1155–62.

57. Philip T, Armitage JO, Spitzer G, et al. High-dose therapy and autologous bone marrow transplantation after failure of conventional chemotherapy in adults with intermediate-grade or high-grade non-Hodgkin's lymphoma. N Engl J Med 1987;316:1493–98.

58. Takvorian T, Canellos GP, Ritz J, et al. Prolonged disease-free survival after autologous bone marrow transplantation in patients with non-Hodgkin's lymphoma with a poor prognosis. N Engl J Med 1987;316:1499–505.

59. Jones RJ, Ambinder RF, Piantadosi S, Santos GW. Evidence of a graft-versus-lymphoma effect associated with allogeneic bone marrow transplantation. Blood 1991;77:649–53.

60. List AF, Greer JP, Cousar JC, et al. Non-Hodgkin's lymphoma of the gastrointestinal tract: an analysis of clinical and pathologic features affecting outcome. J Clin Oncol 1988;6:1125–33.

61. Maor MH, Baddux B, Osborne BM, et al. Stages IE and IIE non-Hodgkin's lymphomas of the stomach. Cancer 1984;54:2330–7.

62. Doll DC, Weiss RB. Malignant lymphoma of the testis. Am J Med 1986;81:515–24.

63. Martenson JA Jr, Buskirk SJ, Ilstrup DM, et al. Patterns of failure in primary testicular non-Hodgkin's lymphoma. J Clin Oncol 1988;6:297–302.

64. Mackintosh FR, Colby TV, Podolsky WJ, et al. Central nervous system involvement in non-Hodgkin's lymphoma: an analysis of 105 cases. Cancer 1982;49:586–95.

65. Johnson GJ, Oken MM, Anderson JR, O'Connell MJ, Glick JH. Central nervouse system relapse in unfavourable-histology non-Hodgkin's lymphoma: is prophylaxis indicated? Lancet 1984;ii:685–7.

66. Loeffler JS, Ervin TJ, Mauch P, et al. Primary lymphomas of the central nervous system: patterns of failure and factors that influence survival. J Clin Oncol 1985;3:490–4.

67. List AF, Greco FA, Vogler LB. Lymphoproliferative diseases in immunocompromised hosts: the role of Epstein-Barr virus. J Clin Oncol 1987;5:1673–89.

68. Ziegler JL, Beckstead JA, Volberding PA, et al. Non-Hodgkin's lymphoma in 90 homosexual men. N Engl J Med 1984;311:565–70.

69. Gill PS, Levine AM, Krailo M, et al. AIDS-related malignant lymphoma: results of prospective treatment trials. J Clin Oncol 1987;5:1322–8.

70. Broder S, Bunn PA Jr, Jaffe ES, et al. T-cell lymphoproliferative syndrome associated with human T-cell leukemia/lymphoma virus. Ann Intern Med 1984;100:543–57.

15

Hodgkin Disease

Janice P. Dutcher, M.D., and Peter H. Wiernik, M.D.

Hodgkin disease is a malignant lymphoma with a characteristic histopathologic pattern that includes variable numbers of unique, multinucleate giant cells (Reed-Sternberg cells).

HISTORY

In 1832, Hodgkin read a paper to the Medical-Chirurgical Society in London in which he described the clinical and postmortem findings in six patients with an entity not previously defined. Wilks reported 15 such cases 33 years later; he called the entity *Hodgkin disease*. The histopathology of Hodgkin disease was described by Langhans in 1872 and Greenfield in 1878, and both independently characterized the multinucleate giant cell that has become accepted as the histologic hallmark of the disease. This cell was described in more detail by Sternberg in 1878 and Reed in 1902. Both workers felt that its presence was evidence of an infectious or inflammatory etiology, and failed to recognize the malignant nature of the disease. Between 1937 and 1944, Jackson and Parker provided the first histopathologic classification of Hodgkin disease that related prognosis to microscopic features of pathologic lymph nodes, although Greenfield discovered the nodular sclerosing variety of this entity in 1878, Lukes more clearly described it in 1963 and demonstrated its association with a very favorable prognosis. The histopathologic classification in use today was devised by Lukes and Butler between 1963 and 1966.

The first observation of cutaneous anergy in Hodgkin disease was made by Reed in 1902, and in 1962, Aisen-berg demonstrated that cutaneous anergy was directly related to disease activity. Peters developed the first useful clinical staging system for the disease in 1950, but the introduction of lymphangiography of Kimmonth in 1952 and of exploratory laparotomy by both Glatstein et al. and Serpick et al. in 1969 substantially enhanced staging precision.

Pusey first demonstrated that radiation therapy could produce objective remissions in Hodgkin disease in 1902, and early evidence that such therapy could be curative was developed by Gilbert in 1939, Craft in 1940, and Peters in 1950. With the introduction of megavoltage radiotherapy equipment in the 1950s as well as the refinement in technique made possible by such equipment, the curative potential of radiotherapy became more widely appreciated. The improved efficacy of megavoltage extended-field radiotherapy for the treatment of Hodgkin disease was first demonstrated by Kaplan in 1972,[1] and Eason and Russel reported in 1963 that 15- and 20-year survival rates were identical to 10-year survival rates after radiation therapy.[2]

The favorable effect of systemically administered drugs on Hodgkin disease was first observed in the mid-1940s, with nitrogen mustard; since that time, a number of active chemotherapeutic agents have been discovered. In 1970, DeVita et al.[3] demonstrated that significant numbers of patients with far-advanced Hodgkin disease could obtain a complete remission with combination chemotherapy. They and others subsequently demonstrated cure in a high percentage of complete responders.[4] Thus, almost 150 years elapsed from the first description of the disease to the time when therapeutic intervention resulted in the cure of most patients.

ETIOLOGY

The etiology of Hodgkin disease is unknown. Research on this has been hampered greatly by the fact that no generally accepted animal model for the disease exists, but numerous infectious etiologies proposed in the past have been disproved. A small minority of patients taking phenytoin or related drugs develop lymphadenopathy with a histologic picture resembling Hodgkin disease, but in almost all instances, the lymphadenopathy regresses on discontinuation of the drug.[5] Rarely, however, the patients go on to develop classic Hodgkin disease; in such cases, it is not known whether the drug was etiologic or the patients would have developed Hodgkin disease at the same time without the drug. Some studies have detected a higher incidence of Hodgkin disease in patients with infectious mononucleosis, suggesting that infection with Epstein-Barr virus may lead to neoplasia. However, the association between Hodgkin disease and infectious mononucleosis must be considered unproved. Reed-Sternberg–like cells have been observed in patients with Burkitt lymphoma, a disease also associated with the Epstein-Barr virus, and more recently, the presence of Epstein-Barr (EB) virus has been detected using molecular biologic techniques in involved tissues and the Reed-Sternberg cells in rare patients with Hodgkin disease.[6–8] Nevertheless, no cause-and-effect relationship has been proved.

Reed-Sternberg–like cells recently have been cultured in vitro, thus providing a first step in learning more about the biology of Hodgkin disease.[9,10] Recent studies also have identified a surface lectin on Hodgkin cells that functions as a lymphocyte agglutinin and thus may mediate immunomodulatory effects.[11] Active investigation into the origin and biology of the Reed-Sternberg cell and its relationship to lymphocytes and other tissues is underway,[12,13] but cytogenetic studies have not proved helpful to date.[14]

EPIDEMIOLOGY

The incidence of Hodgkin disease in the United States' white population is approximately 35 and 26 per million males and females, respectively, and the age-specific mortality rates are approximately half the incidence rates for each sex. The mortality from Hodgkin disease in those under the age of 40 years is approximately one third that in those aged 40 or more.

Unlike the other lymphomas, the age-specific incidence curve for Hodgkin disease has two peaks. The first is from the ages of 15 to 40 years and the second from ages 60 to 70. The same-age specific incidence is seen in most countries where it has been studied; however, for unknown reasons, the first peak in the age-specific incidence curve is remarkably less prominent in Japan and the southern United States than elsewhere. One recent evaluation of the occurrence of Hodgkin disease in the United States suggests a decline in incidence in the older age group (> age 40) and an increase in occurrence among young adults (ages 15 to 39).[15]

In the United States, Hodgkin disease is somewhat more prevalent in whites than in nonwhites and in higher socioeconomic than less-fortunate groups. Some data suggest that among those older than age 50, Hodgkin disease may be more prevalent in Jews, and numerous anecdotal reports and small studies suggest that "time and space" clustering of Hodgkin disease cases may exist.[16] Such data support the view that environmental and/or genetic factors may play an etiologic role in this disease, but this view is the subject of much controversy. No proof exists that Hodgkin disease can be transmitted either from the environment to people or among people,[17] and no studies have identified any association between an occupation or other illness and Hodgkin disease.

Recently, the epidemic of human immunodeficiency virus (HIV) appears to have altered the appearance of Hodgkin disease among some patient groups. Despite a general trend toward younger age and nodular sclerosis subtype in the general population, Hodgkin disease among patients infected with HIV is more aggressive.[18–20] This has been noted in reports from both the United States and Europe,[18–20] and these studies report advanced stage at diagnosis, primarily stages III and IV, with more aggressive histology such as mixed cellularity despite the young age of the patients. Both of these disease features previously were more common among the older patient group with Hodgkin disease, and the poorer outcome reported may be related to the advanced stage of the disease at diagnosis or to the complications of treating patients with immunodeficiency. With the current use of antiviral agents, perhaps the outcome of Hodgkin disease in patients infected with HIV will improve.

Several recent reports also have indicated a three- to seven-fold increase in the risk of Hodgkin disease for family members of patients with Hodgkin disease.[21] Most reports describe concurrent occurrence among siblings, suggesting either common genetic or environmental factors.[21–23] In one report of four siblings, a common HLA antigen (DR5) was noted and EB viral titers were within the normal range;[21] in a second report, both siblings had advanced-stage disease of the same histologic type (lymphocyte depleted),[22] and both were diagnosed within 1 month of each other. In our own report, there was a distinct time lag between sibling diagnoses, and the later sibling had more advanced

Hodgkin disease in three families.[23] Our family study also has demonstrated a pattern of increased chromosome fragility among family members developing Hodgkin disease.

CLINICAL FINDINGS

Most patients with Hodgkin disease initially present to a physician with the complaint of a painless, nontender lump in the neck (Fig. 15.1). The enlarged node or nodes often are discovered while bathing or shaving; occasionally, a tight collar leads to the discovery of lymphadenopathy. Self-discovered lymphadenopathy often is the only manifestation of Hodgkin disease at the time of diagnosis. Only a minority of patients, one quarter to one third, will have systemic manifestations of disease such as fever, night sweats, or weight loss, which carry a poor prognosis. Fever usually is low grade, although the temperature may be 104°F (40°C) or more and debilitating. Rarely, fever may be of the Pel-Ebstein type; this type of fever lasts for several days, with afebrile periods of days or weeks separating febrile periods. It is associated with extensive disease and was seen more commonly in the past when diagnosis was not accomplished as quickly as it is today. Constitutional signs of Hodgkin disease are more common in older patients, especially men, and they are indicative of central lymphadenopathy either in the mediastinum, abdomen, or in both. Their cause is unknown.

Other systemic signs of Hodgkin disease do not affect prognosis. Many patients with nodular-sclerosis histol-

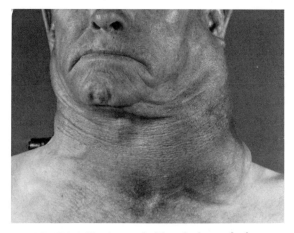

FIGURE 15.1. Massive cervical lymphadenopathy in a man with Hodgkin disease. The patient refused medical attention for at least 1 year after he noticed that his collar size was increasing.

ogy (discussed later) have generalized pruritus that may be severe and lead to excoriation. Rarely, and for unknown reasons, patients may experience pain among involved lymph nodes after the ingestion of alcohol. Alcohol-induced pain is not peculiar to Hodgkin disease, and it may occur in patients with other lymphomas and tumors such as cervical carcinoma as well. However, it still may be helpful in directing the physician's attention to involved node-bearing areas not otherwise suspected.

DIAGNOSIS AND LABORATORY FINDINGS

Hodgkin disease is diagnosed by biopsy of an involved lymph node. Usually, a node in the anterior cervical triangle is chosen for biopsy because of its accessibility. Care must be taken to choose the largest node in a given group of nodes to ensure the best chance of obtaining diagnostic material. Nodes in the posterior neck almost never should be biopsied because of the danger of harming the eleventh cranial nerve. Frequently, a supra-clavicular, axillary, or inguinal node is chosen for biopsy if such a node clinically appears most likely to be pathologic.

The routine laboratory evaluation of a newly diagnosed patient with Hodgkin disease may be unrevealing. In patients with extensive disease, a moderate normochromic and normocytic anemia may be present, and the anemia occasionally may be associated with a positive Coombs test. Rarely, a positive Coombs test may precede the diagnosis of Hodgkin disease by months or years.[24] There may be a peripheral granulocytosis or thrombocytosis, and a significant eosinophilia may be present in patients with pruritus. Lymphopenia may rarely be present, especially if the patient has extensive disease. Lymphopenia is said to confer a poor prognosis, but it is unclear whether the lymphopenia per se or the extensive disease associated with it is responsible for this. The erythrocyte sedimentation rate is abnormal in patients with active disease, and although nonspecific, it is as useful a measure of disease activity as are more elaborate measurements such as serum copper and α_2-globulin levels. Higher erythrocyte sedimentation rates may predict prognosis.

Most patients with early, localized Hodgkin disease have normal reactions to intradermally administered recall antigens, and these patients normally can be sensitized to new ones. Patients with far-advanced disease, especially those with significant systemic signs and symptoms, often are anergic. When these patients respond to therapy, they regain the ability to respond normally to intradermal antigen. Anergy at diagnosis has little prognostic significance considering modern treatment methods.[25]

PATHOLOGY

There are four major histologic types of Hodgkin disease, and the normal lymph node architecture usually is completely destroyed in all of them. In addition, the pathologic assessment of the concentration of malignant Reed-Sternberg cells appears to be of prognostic importance.[26]

Lymphocyte Predominant

In this type of Hodgkin disease, the predominant cell in the lymph node is the mature lymphocyte, which diffusely infiltrates the node. In addition, a Reed-Sternberg cell is seen occasionally. Patients with this type usually have localized disease involving only one or two node-bearing areas, and these patients almost always can be cured with proper treatment and are often young men.

Mixed Cellularity

In this type, the node infiltrate is more pleomorphic, with plasma cells, eosinophils, neutrophils, mature lymphocytes, and many Reed-Sternberg cells readily identified. Such patients often have generalized disease confined to lymph nodes or involving extranodal sites including parenchymal organs. The mixed-cellularity type occurs in patients who tend to be middle-aged or older, and this type has a poorer prognosis than lymphocyte-predominant disease. These patients not infrequently have systemic signs and symptoms of Hodgkin disease, and patients with lymphocyte-predominant disease who relapse often have a mixed-cellularity histology in the nodes bearing recurrent disease.

Lymphocyte Depleted

Patients with this histology characteristically are older and have extensive disease. These patients have the poorest prognosis of all those with Hodgkin disease. The histologic picture may be confused with that of diffuse histiocytic lymphoma, and some patients with lymphocyte-predominant as well as many with mixed-cellularity histology who relapse have a recurrent disease with lymphocyte-depleted histology. The lymph node in lymphocyte-depleted Hodgkin disease is infiltrated by large numbers of Reed-Sternberg cells and little else.

Nodular Sclerosis

It is obvious that a histologic continuum exists from lymphocyte-predominant to mixed-cellularity to lym-

phocyte-depleted histology; in that sequence, prognosis varies directly with the number of mature lymphocytes present and indirectly with the number of Reed-Sternberg cells. In the nodular-sclerosis type, any of these histologies may be seen in the lymph node, but the node itself is divided into multiple nodules by bands of collagen. Often, these nodules can be appreciated by holding the microscopic slide of the biopsy up to the light and viewing it with the naked eye; under the microscope, atypical Reed-Sternberg cells surrounded by clear spaces are seen. These are the so-called *lacunar Hodgkin cells* that probably are caused by artifact of fixation. The presence of these nodules of lymphoid tissue surrounded by collagenous bands confers an excellent prognosis on the patient; only lymphocyte-predominant disease has a better one. Nodular sclerosis is the most common histologic type of Hodgkin disease, and patients with this type usually have disease in multiple node-bearing areas, are often young women, and characteristically have prominent mediastinal lymph node involvement that is appreciated readily on a chest radiograph (Fig. 15.2). Some patients with this type have pruritus, which is not seen with others. Patients with nodular-sclerosis histology who relapse do so with the same histology.

PATTERNS OF SPREAD

In general, Hodgkin disease tends to involve node-bearing areas contiguous to the nodes initially involved. It is useful in planning treatment to think of Hodgkin disease as a unifocal disease, beginning in one node-bearing area and spreading via lymphatics to the next. Thus, if a patient has involvement of the left supraclavicular nodes, there is a reasonable chance that periaortic abdominal lymph nodes are involved; if the right supraclavicular nodes are involved, it is likely that mediastinal nodes are involved as well. Patients with only unilateral high anterior cervical node disease are likely to have no other disease, but if the spleen is involved, it is possible for the liver also to become involved as these organs are connected by lymphatic channels. Lymphatic channels from the spleen connect with subcapsular lymphatics of the liver, and most hepatic Hodgkin disease (which is subcapsular) probably comes to the liver via those lymphatics.[27] Both spleen and liver involvement with Hodgkin disease is nodular rather than diffuse.

Enlarged nodes involved with Hodgkin disease may encroach on normal nonnodal structures and involve them with the disease as well. Thus, a large mediastinal mass may facilitate the spread of Hodgkin disease to compressed lung around its periphery by direct exten-

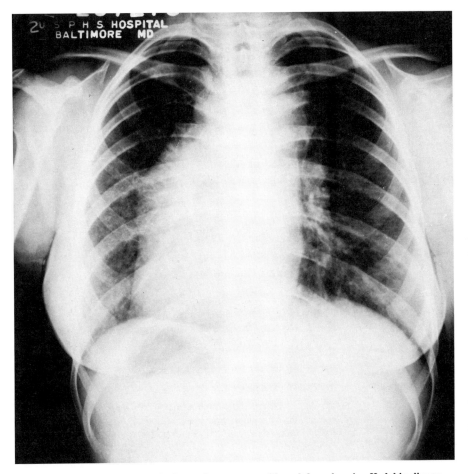

FIGURE 15.2. A large mediastinal mass in a woman with nodular sclerosing Hodgkin disease.

sion (Fig. 15.3). Likewise, a vertebral body may become involved after erosion by a large pathologic periaortic node.

Parenchymal organ involvement other than by direct extension usually occurs only in patients with extensive, generalized nodal disease; therefore, it is unlikely for a patient with disease involving only one or two node-bearing areas on the same side of the diaphragm to have liver, bone marrow, or extensive pulmonary involvement. Rarely, however, the only evidence of Hodgkin disease may be isolated extranodal disease, for example, involving the stomach, testis, or thyroid.

Patients with large, bulky nodes bearing Hodgkin disease are likely to have relatively localized disease confined to one or two node-bearing areas. Patients with palpable but small, shotty nodes are likely to have extensive and widely disseminated disease.

Although unusual in adults, involvement of mesenteric lymph nodes is common in children and patients of all ages with other lymphomas. Hodgkin disease rarely involves lymph nodes in the distal limbs; therefore, epitrochlear or popliteal nodes almost never are involved.

Rarely, Hodgkin disease involves the thymus and no other lymphoid or extranodal tissue; such lesions have been inappropriately termed *granulomatous thymoma* in the past.[28] It is important to recognize this entity, because it essentially always remains localized and often may be cured with local irradiation alone.

STAGING

The rationale for developing a staging system in any malignant disease is to define guidelines for treatment and management and to provide prognostic information. Additionally, in Hodgkin disease, accurate staging has allowed us to limit the therapy given, because the proper

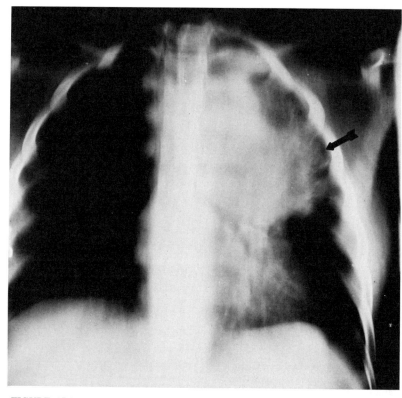

FIGURE 15.3. A tomographic chest radiograph of a man with stage II$_E$A Hodgkin disease. The *arrow* points to limited extranodal disease of the lung proved to be contiguous to the mediastinal mass.

treatment with a localized modality such as radiotherapy requires accurate pretreatment identification of all disease-bearing anatomic sites in the body so that treatment can be delivered accurately.

The staging process that has evolved in the management of Hodgkin disease began with this same premise. To utilize radiotherapy as a therapeutic modality for early stage Hodgkin disease, it is of paramount importance that each anatomic site be investigated by all available diagnostic procedures, whether or not there is clinical evidence of disease. Once all the pretreatment evaluation data are collected, the patient's disease is assigned a Roman numeral stage according to the criteria in Table 15.1. The disease also is assigned a letter stage depending on the presence or absence of significant systemic signs, also as described in Table 15.1. Finally, the substage E is assigned to the patient's disease if there is limited extranodal disease because of direct extension from a nodal mass. Thus, a patient with stage IIIA disease has Hodgkin disease confined to lymph nodes but with nodal involvement on both sides

TABLE 15.1. The Staging of Hodgkin Disease

Stage	Criteria
I	Involvement of only a single node-bearing area (I) or a single extralymphatic site (I$_E$)
II	Involvement of two or more node-bearing areas on the same side of the diaphragm (II) or localized involvement of a single extralymphatic site in addition to two or more node-bearing areas on the same side of the diaphragm (II$_E$)
III	Involvement of node-bearing areas on both sides of the diaphragm (III). The spleen is considered a lymph node; in addition, there may be localized involvement of a single extralymphatic site (III$_E$)
IV	Diffuse, disseminated involvement of one or more extralymphatic organs or tissues by multiple lesions, with or without lymph node disease.

Note: A letter stage assigned to all of the above, either A (no fever, night sweats, or significant loss of body weight) or B (either fever [temperature > 100°F (37.8°C)], significant loss of body weight [at least 10% of usual weight], night sweats, or any combination of the three within 6 months of diagnosis).

of the diaphragm, and this patient has no systemic manifestations of disease (Fig. 15.4). If this patient had direct extension from cervical nodes to the thyroid gland, the disease would be staged III$_E$A. However, some direct extension, such as from a large mediastinal mass into parenchymal lung tissue, has a much poorer prognosis.[29]

There is a direct correlation between stage and prognosis. This previously was much more prominent, when treatment was less effective than it is today; it is still true, however, that patients with stage I disease are much less likely to relapse than patients with stage III disease. More importantly, the prognosis for any patient with A disease is much better than for a patient with B disease, irrespective of the accompanying Roman numeral stage. It also has become clear that patients with stage III disease who have splenic involvement as the only intra-abdominal disease have a much better prognosis than do patients with stage III and splenic as well as upper and lower periaortic nodal disease.[30]

Procedures

Table 15.2 outlines a standard and extended staging evaluation for Hodgkin disease. Computed tomography largely has replaced other radiologic techniques such as chest tomography and the intravenous pyelogram; however, in the abdomen, computed tomographic scans may be deceptively unrevealing in young patients. Lymphangiography still provides one of the best means of adequately examining the lower retroperitoneal and iliac nodes and can demonstrate abnormalities in lymph nodes of normal size. A negative lymphangiogram is approximately 98% accurate, but a positive or "suspicious" study may be only 85% to 90% accurate.[31]

Liver function tests and liver–spleen nuclide scans, or even computed tomographic scans, often provide an inaccurate assessment of these organs. However, if hepatomegaly is present on physical examination, the serum alkaline phosphatase level is elevated, and the liver scan shows both hepatomegaly and focal defects, then the patient almost certainly has Hodgkin disease of the liver.[32] Also, a whole-body gallium citrate scan may be useful in delineating occult disease in the chest or elsewhere, because the isotope is concentrated in certain tumors including those of Hodgkin disease.[33]

Staging Laparotomy

This staging technique continues to be advocated by many as the only method for assessing intra-abdominal

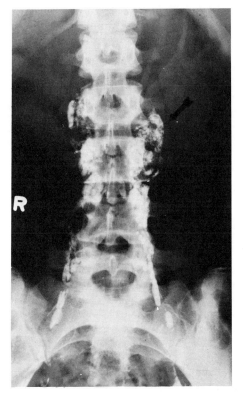

FIGURE 15.4. A positive lymphangiogram in a man with stage IIIA Hodgkin disease. The *arrow* indicates a large, foamy lymph node with filling defects, which is abnormal.

TABLE 15.2. Staging Evaluation for Hodgkin Disease

Surgical biopsy
History and physical examination
  Symptoms (i.e., fever, weight loss, night sweats)
  Adenopathy, organomegaly
Routine laboratory procedures
  Complete blood count
  Serum alkaline phosphatase
  Liver function tests, including lactase dehydrogenase
  Uric acid
  Erythrocyte sedimentation rate
Chest radiograph
Chest computed tomographic scan if mediastinal mass
Abdominal computed tomographic scan
Lymphangiography
Marrow biopsy if:
  Elevated alkaline phosphatase
  Unexplained anemia
  Evidence of bone disease
  Clinical stage III or IV
Bone scan if:
  Elevated alkaline phosphatase
Laparotomy

sites of disease inaccessible to routine radiologic tests. Several series have demonstrated that the use of this technique will upgrade or downstage as many as 80% of patients with Hodgkin disease.[34,35] This is particularly important when radiotherapy is the planned treatment modality. Although certain specific clinical situations may not warrant laparotomy (i.e., stage IIIB, stage IV, and when chemotherapy has been decided as the treatment modality), the majority of patients are likely to benefit from the additional information provided to help direct their treatment.

Certain prelaparotomy evaluations should guide the surgeon's hand at laparotomy. For instance, many lymphangiograms are not uniformly positive but may only show one or two nodes on one side to be suspicious or positive; the surgeon must take the lymphangiogram to the operating room and identify at laparotomy the nodes in question. When the nodes are removed for histologic examination, radiopaque clips should be placed at the biopsy site and an intraoperative abdominal radiograph taken. This radiograph should be compared with the lymphangiogram to ensure that the nodes in question are indeed the nodes biopsied. If the lymphangiogram is negative, random biopsies of both periaortic node chains must be performed. Some intra-abdominal nodes are not visualized on the lymphangiogram (porta hepatis, mesenteric, and splenic hilar nodes), and these must be biopsied as well. The high periaortic nodes are not seen well on a lymphangiogram and also need to be biopsied if possible. The surface of the liver should be examined, and any suspicious lesions must be biopsied. Random wedge biopsies of both lobes should be done if no gross lesions are noted. Splenectomy should be performed and the spleen cut in 3-mm sections, then rotated 90° and cut in 3-mm sections again by the pathologist; each splenic section must be examined carefully for Hodgkin disease. Virtually all splenic Hodgkin lesions can be seen with the unaided eye and vary from the size of a pinhead to several centimeters or more; any suspicious lesion should be examined histologically. If the spleen is examined carefully in this manner, approximately one third of patients not thought to have Hodgkin disease of the spleen before laparotomy will have such disease demonstrated.

When staging laparotomy is performed in the careful manner just described, approximately 30% of patients thought clinically to have stage I or stage II disease will be reclassified as stage III after the procedure. In addition, approximately 10% of all patients undergoing laparotomy will have intra-abdominal disease demonstrated that lies outside the usual radiotherapy port (i.e., disease that would remain untreated after radiation therapy to a standard field). Equally important is the fact that a significant number of patients thought to have liver involvement will be shown to have benign lesions of the liver or none at all, findings that reduce the classification from stage IV to stage III or lower.[36]

Other benefits from staging laparotomy also accrue to the patient. If radiotherapy is administered with curative intent to a splenectomized patient with Hodgkin disease, less normal tissue is irradiated than if the spleen were in place; normal tissue such as the lower left lung and upper pole of the left kidney is spared irradiation. In addition, a histologically proved negative spleen is of paramount prognostic significance, because such patients essentially never have hepatic Hodgkin disease at presentation or later.[37] This observation is important because hepatic involvement is a major cause of death in patients with Hodgkin disease. Also, in women, the ovaries can be removed from their normal location and sutured to the midline behind the uterus,[38] and this maneuver minimizes ovarian exposure to pelvic-node irradiation if it should be necessary either for initial treatment or in the future.

Several long-term studies recently have suggested equivalent efficacy of chemotherapy in early stage Hodgkin's disease.[39–41] These data will be discussed later; suffice it to say that as chemotherapy becomes used more frequently as the primary therapy for early stage Hodgkin disease, an argument can be made to avoid laparotomy. The points against this, however, are the unavailability of knowledge regarding liver involvement in stage III disease and the potential for bulky disease existing in the spleen that would be treated inadequately by a single modality. Thus, even with a lessening of the need for the exact delineation of disease sites, certain patients, particularly those with clinical stage II and stage III disease, may have their treatment enhanced by utilizing information gained from a staging laparotomy.

TREATMENT

Radiotherapy

The accepted primary treatment for Hodgkin disease confined to lymph nodes is extended-field radiotherapy, utilizing megavoltage sources such as cobaltous chloride or a linear accelerator.[42] Such radiation, delivered to a total dose of 40 Gy at a rate of approximately 10 Gy/week, results in a recurrence rate within the irradiated field of 1% to 2%.

Radiotherapy is based on the pathologic stage after all staging procedures described previously have been completed. For stage I disease of the neck, the radiation port includes all neck, supraclavicular, infraclavicular axillary, and upper mediastinal nodes. In stage II disease above the diaphragm, all neck, supraclavicular, infraclavicular axillary, and mediastinal nodes are included, as well as the high periaortic nodes and splenic pedicle nodes. Stage II disease below the diaphragm is irradiated through an inverted-Y port that includes all inguinal, iliac, periaortic, and splenic pedicle nodes. For stage IIIA disease, total-nodal irradiation is administered, to include all of the nodes previously mentioned. Stage IIIB and stage IV disease are treated primarily with chemotherapy (described later), and for stages IB (rare) and IIB (uncommon) disease or for patients with advanced histology (mixed cellularity or lymphocyte depleted), some therapists advise total-nodal radiotherapy, others advise extensive radiotherapy followed by combination chemotherapy, and some advise combination chemotherapy alone.

Bulky mediastinal disease greater than one third of the chest diameter on a posterior-anterior radiograph, even if only stage II, cannot be treated adequately with a single modality, either radiotherapy or chemotherapy. The optimal treatment in this case is involved-field, full-dose radiotherapy with appropriate chemotherapy (six cycles).[29,43–46] In addition, patients with stage IIIA disease and extensive upper and lower abdominal lymph node disease have better disease-free and overall survival after combined-modality treatment than after total-nodal radiotherapy alone.

Chemotherapy

Combination chemotherapy is the modality of choice in patients with advanced Hodgkin disease, stages $IIIA_2$, IIIB, IV (Table 15.3). The regimen of choice has changed over time in an attempt to improve outcome for these patients, because 20% to 40% of patients with advanced or stage B disease eventually will die of Hodgkin disease.

The original curative regimen, MOPP (nitrogen mustard, vincristine [Oncovin], prednisone, and procarbazine), remains an active regimen,[3,4,44] but owing to concerns regarding long-term toxicity and efficacy, MOPP largely has been replaced in cases of advanced Hodgkin disease by a regimen known as ABVD (doxorubicin [Adriamycrin], bleomycin, vinblastine and dacarbazine).[47,48] This regimen, either alone or alternating with MOPP, is highly active and has led to improved relapse-free survival.[48,49] The key to this and other similar approaches (SCAB or MOPP/SCAB) appears to be the addition of doxorubicin to the therapy of advanced disease,[50,51] but whether it is the doxorubicin addition or the alternating noncross-resistant approach that is improving the outcome will require direct comparison.[49] Modifications of the alternating regimen known as the MOPP/ABV hybrid also have been evaluated for reduced toxicity, enhanced delivery of drug, and efficacy;[52,53] the long-term results are promising.[53]

As for early stage disease, the goal is cure with minimization of toxicity whether radiotherapy or chemotherapy is used. The optimal chemotherapeutic regimen to achieve this goal has not been fully determined.

TABLE 15.3. Active Chemotherapeutic Agents and Regimens in Hodgkin Disease

Active Agents	
Nitrogen mustard, Cyclophosphamide, Chlorambucil, Dacarbazine	
Vincristine, Vinblastine, Doxorubicin, Mitoxantrone	
BCNU, CCNU, Streptozotocin	
Procarbazine, Prednisone, Bleomycin	
Regimens	
MOPP	
Nitrogen mustard 6 mg/m^2	Days 1 and 8
Vincristine 1.4 mg/m^2	Days 1 and 8
(maximum 2.0 mg)	
Predisone 40 mg/m^2 orally	Days 1 to 14
Procarbazine 100 mg/m^2 orally	Days 1 to 14
Rest cycle	Days 15 to 28
ABVD	
Doxorubicin 20 mg/m^2	Day 1
Bleomycin 10 mg/m^2	Day 1
Vinblastine 6 mg/m^2	Days 1 and 15
Dacarbazine 375 mg/m^2	Day 1
Rest cycle	Days 16 to 28
SCAB	
Streptozotocin 500 mg/m^2	Days 1 to 5
CCNU 100 mg/m^2 orally	Day 1
Doxorubicin 45 mg/m^2	Day 1
Bleomycin 15 μ/m^2	Days 1 and 8
intramuscular	
MOPP/ABV hybrid	
Nitrogen mustard 6 mg/m^2	Day 1
Vincristine 1.4 mg/m^2	Day 1
(maximum 2.0 mg)	
Procarbazine 100 mg/m^2 orally	Days 1 to 7
Prednisone 40 mg/m^2 orally	Days 1 to 14
Doxorubicin 35 mg/m^2	Day 8
Bleomycin 10 μ/m^2	Day 8
Vinblastine 6 mg/m^2	Day 8
Rest cycle	Days 15 to 28

PROGNOSIS

When treatment is carried out as previously described, essentially all patients with stage IA disease remain disease-free and apparently cured. The cure rate for stage IIA disease is 85% to 90% and 60% to 70% for stage IIIA disease if irradiation alone is used (Fig. 15.5). If radiotherapy is followed by six monthly cycles of MOPP chemotherapy in patients with stage IIA or IIIA

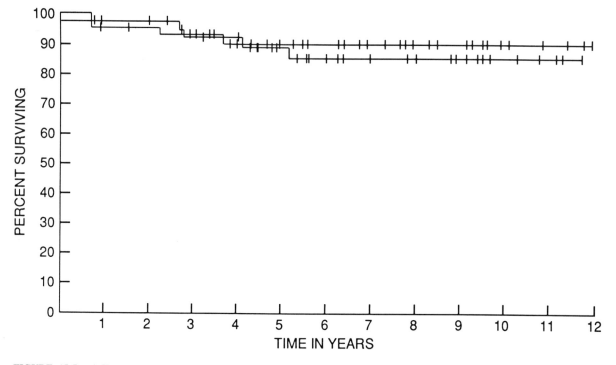

FIGURE 15.5. A Kaplan-Meier plot of the overall survival rate of early-stage patients treated with MOPP; (4 of 44 patients failed) (top) or radiation therapy, (5 of 43 failed) (bottom), excluding those with massive mediastinal disease or stage IIIA disease ($P_2 = 0.68$). (*Source:* Longo et al. 1991[41])

disease, 95% to 100% of patients remain disease-free for 5 years or longer.[4,43,44] Subsets of patients with stage IIA and IIIA disease who particularly benefit from combined modality therapy have been defined; these are patients with bulky disease for whom either modality alone is insufficient.[44,46,54] Long-term follow-up data are encouraging in that relapse appears to have been prevented in a majority of such patients who received combined-modality treatment.[44,54]

The prognosis for patients with stage IB and IIB disease is nearly that of patients with stage IA and IIA disease, especially if combined-modality treatment is employed. Of patients with stage IIIB, IVA, and IVB disease treated with MOPP, 60% to 75% will achieve a complete remission, with median duration of remission in excess of 3.5 years. With ABVD, relapse-free survival at 8 years for patients treated with alternating MOPP/ABVD is 72.6%, compared with 45.1% for MOPP alone,[48] and at least half of the complete responders appear to be cured by such treatment. Patients with bone marrow involvement and stage B systemic signs have a poor prognosis, however, and these patients are rarely cured (Fig. 15.6).

"Salvage" therapy is utilized for patients who relapse after initial therapy. Prognosis at relapse from radiother-apy primarily depends on the extent of the disease at relapse,[55] and prognosis for relapse after chemotherapy depends on response to salvage therapy. A major improvement in therapy with the potential for cure for selected patients who relapse is the use of high-dose chemotherapy with autologous bone marrow support;[56,57] the success of this approach depends on the sensitivity of the disease at relapse to subsequent therapy.

SPECIAL CLINICAL PROBLEMS
Epidural Tumor

Occasionally, a patient with Hodgkin disease presents with back pain and focal neurologic signs, usually in the legs. A myelogram should be performed on an emergency basis, and if a block is demonstrated, the lesion should be treated with radiotherapy as soon as possible to preserve maximal neurologic function.[58] This particular case is a medical emergency.

Skin Disease

Rarely, Hodgkin disease involves the skin, usually an area where lymphatic drainage is blocked by prominent

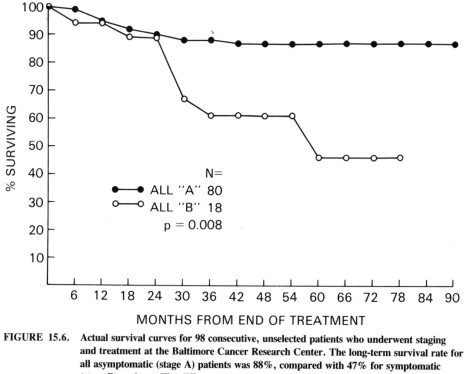

FIGURE 15.6. Actual survival curves for 98 consecutive, unselected patients who underwent staging and treatment at the Baltimore Cancer Research Center. The long-term survival rate for all asymptomatic (stage A) patients was 88%, compared with 47% for symptomatic (stage B) patients. The difference between the curves is statistically highly significant.

lymphadenopathy. Retrograde flow of cells from the pathologic nodes to the skin probably accounts for this lesion and radiation treatment of the involved skin after irradiation to the draining lymph nodes is required.

Stridor

On occasion, a mediastinal mass in a patient with Hodgkin disease will be so massive that it causes airway obstruction by compressing the trachea or smaller air passages. A CT scan can be helpful in delineating the exact site of compression, which should be irradiated immediately to restore normal function and avoid potential catastrophe; no patient should be submitted to laparotomy until such obstruction is irradiated and improving. A single dose of an alkylating agent may allow enough shrinkage to provide time for a tissue diagnosis. Radiotherapy may shrink the tumor so rapidly that exact histologic diagnosis will be impossible.[59]

Infection

Patients with extensive Hodgkin disease who have relapsed or are not responding to initial therapy and have cutaneous anergy also have a propensity to develop fungal, mycobacterial, nocardial, and viral infections, especially if long-term steroid administration has been part of the therapy. The most common fungal infection in such patients is cryptococcal meningitis, and the most common viral infection is herpes zoster. Herpes zoster usually occurs in a localized form and only rarely leads to disseminated viral disease; zoster-immune globulin appears to be of little benefit. The antiviral drug acyclovir may be helpful in reducing the duration of the eruption and is included in the supportive care of this infection. Also, pediatric patients are at greater risk than adults, and those treated with combined-modality therapy are the most likely to develop this complication. The peak occurence is within the first 36 months after beginning treatment.[60,61]

Fever

The fever of Hodgkin disease occasionally will be the most distressing aspect of the illness and can lead to lassitude and uncomfortable night sweats. Often, the fever can be controlled with acetaminophen, but sometimes this is ineffective. In these cases, 25 mg of indomethacin orally three or four times daily may be used. Care must be taken to start the drug when the patient is relatively afebrile; if the drug is begun during a high fever, the temperature may suddenly drop to subnormal levels.

Pregnancy

Approximately two thirds of women who have undergone ovariopexy during staging laparotomy retain normal ovarian function and have normal menses.[17] Those patients who have conceived have delivered apparently normal children, but it is not clear whether fertility is decreased or normal in patients who continue to menstruate. After combination chemotherapy, amenorrhea and aspermia are common, but in some patients, normal function is restored several years posttherapy. It also is clear that many men with Hodgkin disease have oligospermia before therapy.[62,63] All known post-MOPP conceptions that have resulted in delivery have been apparently normal children;[64,65] it is unknown whether the incidence of spontaneous abortion after such therapy is increased.

Renal Manifestations

Except for an occasional instance of a patient with ureteral obstruction secondary to intra-abdominal lymphadenopathy, patients with Hodgkin disease rarely manifest renal complications. On occasion, a nephrotic syndrome is evident at diagnosis that is thought to be caused by a humoral substance elaborated by the tumor that causes glomerular damage, but the syndrome resolves when the Hodgkin disease is treated.[66]

Long-Term Complications of Radiotherapy

RADIATION-RELATED HEART DISEASE. Approximately 30% of patients with Hodgkin disease who receive radiation therapy to the mediastinum will develop radiographic or other evidence of pericardial effusion; the vast majority will regress without therapy and will not recur. Almost all effusions will occur in the first year after treatment is completed, but some patients may have the initial manifestation of pericardial problems 2 years or more after therapy. Almost 20% of patients with radiation-related pericardial injury will develop signs and symptoms of pericardial tamponade, and some will require pericardectomy. In addition, laboratory evidence of myocardial injury can be obtained more frequently than previously appreciated, particularly in patients treated with anteriorly weighted radiation fields.[67–69] The differential diagnosis between radiation-related pericardial disease and recurrent

Hodgkin disease involving the pericardium at times may be difficult, and pericardial biopsy may be required to define the problem.[70] Within the last 10 years, radiation fields have been weighted more equally between anterior and posterior, and this may reduce, but does not eliminate, cardiac injury.[71]

PULMONARY FIBROSIS. Most patients receiving mediastinal irradiation develop some mild pulmonary fibrosis that is of little or no clinical importance in the lung tissue adjacent to the mediastinum. Occasionally, and for unexplained reasons, a patient may develop severe fibrosis even in lung tissue well away from the radiotherapy treatment field that significantly compromises pulmonary function. Again, the differential diagnosis between this complication and recurrent Hodgkin disease may require biopsy.

HYPOTHYROIDISM. Although the larynx is shielded during irradiation of the neck, as many as one fourth to one third of irradiated patients will develop laboratory evidence of thyroid hypofunction associated with elevated thyroid-stimulating hormone levels in the decade following treatment. Thyroid hormone must be administered to such patients to return thyroid-stimulating hormone levels to normal. The combination of elevated thyroid-stimulating hormone levels and hypofunction of the thyroid may lead to carcinoma, and therefore, it can be expected that if thyroid hormone is not administered, an increased incidence of thyroid carcinoma may develop in such patients.[72,73]

SECOND MALIGNANCIES. Radiation therapy is known to be leukemogenic in humans, and there have been many case reports of acute nonlymphocytic leukemia developing in patients with Hodgkin disease treated by radiation therapy or chemotherapy.[74] The incidence of leukemia may even be greater in patients who have received extended courses of treatment or combined-modality therapy;[75] this is especially true when one modality was used initially and then another for the treatment of relapsed Hodgkin disease. Nonhematologic second malignancies also occur at a frequency greater than expected in patients who receive combined-modality therapy; these tumors may occur years after the initial treatment for Hodgkin disease and often are located either within or at the margin of a radiation treatment field.[75–78] Interestingly, there so far appears to be no increased incidence of second malignancies in patients treated with ABVD chemotherapy, while patients treated with MOPP experience an increased incidence of leukemia.

SUMMARY

In the almost 150 years since the original description of Hodgkin disease, it has been transformed by modern therapeutics from a uniformly fatal illness to one that can be cured most of the time. Most of the advances that led to this accomplishment have occurred during the past 25 years. However, despite this fantastic improvement, many patients with Hodgkin disease still die of recurrent disease, but results from studies at several centers indicate that many of these deaths can be avoided by proper staging and careful design of a treatment plan appropriate for the stage and extent of disease. Most significant is the improved disease-free survival among subsets of patients with bulky disease by use of an initial combined-modality treatment approach. In addition, long-term follow-up data have shown that advanced, widely disseminated Hodgkin disease usually responds very favorably to combination chemotherapy and that of patients with stage IIIA disease treated with MOPP chemotherapy, virtually all respond completely and remain disease-free after 10 years of follow-up.[79]

A new concept now being tested is the use of combination chemotherapy in early stage Hodgkin disease. A small study of MOPP chemotherapy in early stage Hodgkin disease in Africa has given results equal to the best radiotherapy treatment studies,[80] and similar results have been obtained by other investigators with long-term follow-up.[39–41,81] Radiotherapy with combination chemotherapy offers superior results over radiotherapy alone in many patients with bulky disease, and in several studies currently being evaluated, combination chemotherapy appears equal in remission-inducing capability and long-term disease-free survival to radiotherapy or combined-modality treatment for early stage disease.

The question must be asked, therefore, whether combination chemotherapy alone might be the optimal treatment for the majority of patients with Hodgkin disease. If the results in years to come indicate that combination chemotherapy is the optimal treatment for most stages, the management of Hodgkin disease will become simpler and more economical. Thus, with the results of treatment improving, management is being directed toward reducing toxicity, and it will then be possible to eliminate most staging procedures, including laparotomy, and to transfer the management of this disease to the office of qualified oncologist or hematologist. The late, serious complications of radiotherapy may be avoided in the majority of patients; most of the serious side effects of MOPP chemotherapy observed are short-term reversible complications that may be more acceptable in the long run. Male sterility is a serious complication in many MOPP-treated patients, however, and methods of avoiding this consequence of therapy will need to be developed if this treatment is to replace radiotherapy. The newer chemotherapy regimens also must be tested against those that have provided long-term disease-free survival and may lead to less short-term and long-term toxicity.

REFERENCES

1. Kaplan HS. Hodgkin's Disease. Cambridge: Harvard University Press, 1972.
2. Eason EC, Russel MH. The cure of Hodgkin's disease. BMJ 1963;1:1704.
3. DeVita VT Jr, Serpick AA, Carbone PP. Combination chemotherapy in the treatment of advanced Hodgkin's disease. Ann Intern Med 1970;73:881.
4. Longo DL, Young RC, Wesley M, et al. Twenty years of MOPP therapy for Hodgkin's disease. J Clin Oncol 1986;4:1295.
5. Choovivathanavanich P, Wallace EM, Scaglione PR. Pseudolymphoma induced by diphenylhydantoin. J Pediatr 1970; 76:621.
6. Mueller N, Evans A, Harris NL, et al. Hodgkin's disease and Epstein-Barr virus. N Engl J Med 1989;320:689.
7. Bignon YT, Bernard D, Cure H, et al. Detection of Epstein-Barr viral genomes in lymph nodes of Hodgkin's disease patients. Mol Carcinog 1990;3:9.
8. Weiss LM, Movahed LA, Warnke RA, Sklar J. Detection of Epstein-Barr viral genomes in Reed-Sternberg cells of Hodgkin's disease. N Engl J Med 1989;320:502.
9. Diehl V, Kirchner HH, Burrichter H, et al. Characteristics of Hodgkin's disease-derived cell lines. Cancer Treat Rep 1982; 66:615.
10. Paietta E, Racevskis J, Stanley ER, et al. Expression of the macrophage growth factor, CSF-1, and its receptor *c-fms* by a Hodgkin's disease-derived cell line and its variants. Cancer Res 1990;50:2049.
11. Paietta E, Hubbard AL, Wiernik PH, et al. Hodgkin's cell lectin: an ectosialyltransferase and lymphocyte agglutinant related to the hepatic asialoglycoprotein receptor. Cancer Res 1987;47:2461.
12. Agnarsson BA, Kadin ME. The immunophenotype of Reed-Sternberg cells. Cancer 1989;63:2083.
13. Casey TT, Olson SJ, Cousar JB, Collins RD. Immunophenotype of Reed-Sternberg cells: a study of 19 cases of Hodgkin's disease in plastic-embedded sections. Blood 1989;74:2624.
14. Tilly H, Bastard C, Delastre T, et al. Cytogenetic studies in untreated Hodgkin's disease. Blood 1991;77:1298.
15. Glacer SL, Swartz WG. Time trends in Hodgkin's disease incidence: the role of diagnostic accuracy. Cancer 1990;66:2196.
16. Vianna NJ, Polan A. Epidemiologic evidence for transmission of Hodgkin's disease. N Engl J Med 1973;289:499.
17. Davis S. Case aggregation in young adult Hodgkin's disease: etiologic evidence from a population experience. Cancer 1986;57:1602.
18. Tirelli U, Vacchar E, Gravosto F, et al. HIV-associated Hodgkin's disease: a report of 53 patients from the European Working Party on HIV-associated neoplasia. Proc Am Soc Clin Oncol 1988;7:2.
19. Gold JE, Altarac D, Ree HJ. HIV-associated Hodgkin disease: a clinical study of 18 cases and review of the literature. Am J Hematol 1991;36:93.
20. Pelstring RJ, Zellmer RB, Sulak LE, et al. Hodgkin's disease in association with human immunodeficiency virus infection. Cancer 1991;67:1865.
21. Robertson SJ, Lowman JT, Grufferman S, et al. Familial Hodgkin's disease. Cancer 1987;59:1314.

22. Durosinmi MA, Nwosu SO, Ogunniyi JO, et al. Hodgkin's disease in siblings: a case report. Afr J Med, Sci 1989;18:219.

23. Wiernik PH, Albertini RJ, Fotino M, Paietta E. Increased peripheral blood T-cell mutant frequencies in healthy mothers of children with familial Hodgkin's disease. Proc Am Soc Clin Oncol 1991;10:287.

24. Cazenave JP, Gagnon JAE, Girouard E, et al. Autoimmune hemolytic anemia terminating 7 years later in Hodgkin's disease. Can Med Assoc J 1973;109:748.

25. Young RC, Corder MP, Haynes HA, et al. Delayed hypersensitivity in Hodgkin's disease. Am J Med 1972;52:63.

26. Specht L, Lauritzen AF, Nordentoft AM, et al. Tumor cell concentration and tumor burden in relation to histopathologic subtype and other prognostic factors in early stage Hodgkin's disease. Cancer 1990;65:2594.

27. Belliveau RE, Wiernik PH, Abt AB. Liver enzymes and pathology in Hodgkin's disease. Cancer 1974;34:300.

28. Fechner RE. Hodgkin's disease of the thymus. Cancer 1969;23:16.

29. Wiernik PH, Slawson RG. Hodgkin's disease with direct extension into pulmonary parenchyma from a mediastinal mass: a presentation requiring special therapeutic considerations. Cancer Treat Rep 1982;66:711.

30. Stein RS, Golomb HM, Wienik PH, et al. Anatomic substages of Stage IIIA Hodgkin's disease: follow-up of a collaborative study. Cancer Treat Rep 1982;66:733.

31. Abt AB, Murphy WL, O'Connell MJ, et al. False positive lymphography in Hodgkin's disease: a histologic-lymphadenographic correlation. Med Pediatr Oncol 1977;3:253.

32. Milder MS, Larson SM, Bagley CM, et al: Liver-spleen scan in Hodgkin's disease. Cancer 1973;31:826.

33. Johnston G, Benua RS, Teates CS. ^{67}Ga-citrate imaging in untreated Hodgkin's disease: preliminary report of cooperative group. J Nucl Med 1974;15:399.

34. Leibenhaut MH, Hoppe RT, Efron B, et al. Prognostic indicators of laparotomy findings in clinical stage I-II supradiaphragmatic Hodgkin's disease. J Clin Oncol 1989;7:81.

35. Mauch P, Larson D, Osteen R, et al. Prognostic factors for positive surgical staging in patients with Hodgkin's disease. J Clin Oncol 1990;8:257.

36. O'Connell MJ, Wiernik PH, Sklansky BD, et al. Staging laparotomy in Hodgkin's disease. Am J Med 1974;57:86.

37. Aisenberg AC, Goldman JM, Raker JW, et al. Spleen involvement at the onset of Hodgkin's disease. Ann Intern Med 1971;74:544.

38. LeFlouch O, Donaldson SS, Kaplan HS. Pregnancy following oophoropexy and total nodal irradiation in women with Hodgkin's disease. Cancer 1976;38:2263.

39. O'Dwyer PJ, Wiernik PH, Stewart MB, Slawson RG. Treatment of early stage Hodgkin's disease: a randomized trial of radiotherapy plus chemotherapy versus chemotherapy alone. In: Cavalli F, Bonadonna G, Rozencweig M, eds. Malignant Lymphomas and Hodgkin's Disease: Experimental and Therapeutic Advances. Amsterdam: Martinus Nijhoff Publishing, 1985:329–36.

40. Pavlovsky S, Dupont J, Jimenez E, et al. Randomized study of chemotherapy alone vs chemotherapy plus radiotherapy in clinical stages IA-IIA Hodgkin's disease. In: Cavalli F, Bonadonna G, Rozencweig M, eds. Malignant Lymphomas and Hodgkin's Disease: Experimental and Therapeutic Advances. Amsterdam: Martinus Nijhoff Publishing, 1985:337–43.

41. Longo DL, Glatstein E, Duffey PL, et al. Radiation therapy versus combination chemotherapy in the treatment of early stage Hodgkin's disease: seven year results of a prospective randomized trial. J Clin Oncol 1991;9:906.

42. Glatstein E. Hodgkin's disease: radiation therapy. In: Coon MF, ed. Current Therapy. Philadelphia: W. B. Saunders, 1977.

43. Wiernik PH, Gustafson J, Schimpff SC, et al. Combined modality treatment of Hodgkin's disease confined to lymph nodes. Am J Med 1979;67:183.

44. Dutcher JP, Wiernik PH. Combined modality treatment of Hodgkin's disease confined to lymph nodes: results 14 years later. In: Cavalli F, Bonadonna G, Rozencweig M, eds. Malignant Lymphomas and Hodgkin's Disease: Experimental and Therapeutic Advances. Amsterdam: Martinus Nijhoff Publishing, 1985;317–33.

45. Proznitz LR, Curtis AM, Knowlton AH, et al. Supradiaphragmatic Hodgkin's disease: significance of large mediastinal masses. Int J Radiat Oncol Biol Phys 1980;6:809.

46. Leopold KA, Canellos GP, Rosenthal D, et al. Stage IA-IIB Hodgkin's disease: staging and treatment of patients with large mediastinal adenopathy. J Clin Oncol 1989;7:1059.

47. Bonadonna G, Zucali R, Monfardini S, et al. Combination chemotherapy of Hodgkin's disease with adriamycin, bleomycin, vinblastine and imidazole carboxamide versus MOPP. Cancer 1975;36:252.

48. Bonadonna G, Valagussa P, Santoro A. Alternating non-cross resistant combination chemotherapy or MOPP in Stage II Hodgkin's disease: a report of 8-year results. Ann Intern Med 1986;104:739.

49. Canellos GP, Propert K, Cooper R, et al. MOPP vs ABVD vs MOPP alternating with ABVD in advanced Hodgkin's disease: a prospective randomized CALGB trial. Proc Am Soc Clin Oncol 1988;7:230a.

50. Wiernik PH, Schiffer CA. Long-term follow-up of advanced Hodgkin's disease patients treated with a combination of streptozotocin, lomustine (CCNU), doxorubicin and bleomycin (SCAB). J Cancer Res Clin Oncol 1988;114:105.

51. Longo DL, Duffey PL, DeVita VT, et al. Treatment of advanced stage Hodgkin's disease: alternating non-cross resistant MOPP/CABS is not superior to MOPP. J Clin Oncol 1991;9:1409.

52. Connors JM, Klimo P. MOPP/ABV hybrid chemotherapy for advanced Hodgkin's disease. Semin Hematol 1987;24(suppl 1):35.

53. Klimo P, Connors JM. An update on the Vancouver experience in the management of advanced Hodgkin's disease treated with the MOPP/ABV hybrid program. Semin Hematol 1988;25(suppl 2):34.

54. Mauch P, Goffman T, Rosenthal DS, et al. Stage III Hodgkin's disease: improved survival with combined modality therapy as compared with radiation therapy alone. J Clin Oncol 1985; 3:1166.

55. Roach M, Brophy F, Cox R, et al. Prognostic factors for patients relapsing after radiotherapy for early stage Hodgkin's disease. J Clin Oncol 1990;8:623.

56. Jagannath S, Dicke KA, Armitage JO, et al. High dose cyclophosphamide, carmustine and etoposide and autologous bone marrow transplantation for relapsed Hodgkin's disease. Ann Intern Med 1986;104:163.

57. Carella AM, Congiu AM, Gaozza E, et al. High-dose chemotherapy with autologous bone marrow transplantation in 50 advanced resistant Hodgkin's disease patients: an Italian study group report. J Clin Oncol 1988;6:1411.

58. Mullins GM, Flynn JPG, El-Mahdi AM, et al. Malignant lymphoma of the spinal epidural space. Ann Intern Med 1971;74:416.

59. Loeffler JS, Leopold KA, Recht A, et al. Emergency prebiopsy radiation for mediastinal masses: impact on subsequent pathologic diagnosis and outcome. J Clin Oncol 1986;4:716.

60. Schimpff SC, O'Connell MJ, Greene WH, et al. Infections in 92 splenectomized patients with Hodgkin's disease. Am J Med 1975;59:695.

61. Guinee VF, Guido JJ, Pfalzgraf KA, et al. The incidence of herpes zoster in patients with Hodgkin's disease. Cancer 1985;56:642.

62. Chapman RM, Sutcliffe SB, Malpas JS. Male gonadal dysfunction in Hodgkin's disease. JAMA 1981;245:1323.

63. Redman JR, Bajorunas DR, Goldstein MC, et al. Semen cryopreservation and artificial insemination for Hodgkin's disease. J Clin Oncol 1987;5:233.

64. Horning SJ, Hoppe RT, Kaplan HS, Rosenberg SA. Female reproductive potential after treatment for Hodgkin's disease. N Engl J Med 1981;304:1377.

65. Andrieu JM, Ochoa-Molina ME. Menstrual cycle, pregnancies and offspring before and after MOPP therapy for Hodgkin's disease. Cancer 1983;52:435.

66. Plager J, Stutzman L. Acute nephrotic syndrome as a manifestation of active Hodgkin's disease. Am J Med 1971;50:56.

67. Brosius FC III, Waller BF, Roberts WC. Radiation heart disease. Am J Med 1981;70:519.

68. Applefeld MM, Slawson RG, Spicer KM, et al. Long-term cardiovascular evaluation of patients with Hodgkin's disease treated by thoracic mantle radiation therapy. Cancer Treat Rep 1982;66:1003.

69. Gomez GA, Park JJ, Panahon AM, et al. Heart size and function after radiation therapy to the mediastinum in patients with Hodgkin's disease. Cancer Treat Rep 1983;67:1099.

70. Serpick A. Clinical case records in chemotherapy: possible radiation pericarditis in Hodgkin's disease. Cancer Chemother Rep 1970;54:199.

71. Green DM, Gingell RL, Pearce J, et al. The effect of mediastinal irradiation on cardiac function of patients treated during childhood and adolescence for Hodgkin's disease. J Clin Oncol 1987;5:239.

72. Schimpff SC, Diggs CH, Wiswell JG, et al. Radiation-related thyroid dysfunction: implications for the treatment of Hodgkin's disease. Ann Intern Med 1980;92:91.

73. Hancock SL, Cox RS, McDougall IR. Thyroid diseases after treatment of Hodgkin's disease. N Engl J Med 1991;325:599.

74. Toland DM, Coltman CA Jr, Moon TE. Second malignancy complicating Hodgkin's disease: the Southwest Oncology Group Experience. Cancer Clin Trials 1978;1:27.

75. Blaney DW, Longo DL, Young RC, et al. Decreasing risk of leukemia with prolonged follow-up after chemotherapy and radiotherapy for Hodgkin's disease. N Engl J Med 1987;316:710.

76. Arseneau JC, Sponzo RW, Levin DO, et al. Nonlymphomatous malignant tumors complicating Hodgkin's disease. N Engl J Med 1972;287:1119.

77. Tucker MA, Coleman CN, Cox RS, et al. Risk of second cancers after treatment for Hodgkin's disease. N Engl J Med 1988; 318:76.

78. Kushner BH, Zauber A, Tan CTC. Second malignancies after childhood Hodgkin's disease. Cancer 1988;62:1364.

79. DeVita VT Jr, Simon RM, Hubbard SM, et al. Curability of advanced Hodgkin's disease with chemotherapy. Ann Intern Med 1980;92:586.

80. Ziegler JL, Bluming AZ, Fass L, et al. Chemotherapy of childhood Hodgkin's disease in Uganda. Lancet 1972;ii:679.

81. Wiernik PH. Combined modality treatment of early stage Hodgkin's disease. In: Wiernik PH, ed. Controversies in Oncology. New York: John Wiley & Sons, 1982:13–5.

16

Plasma Cell Dyscrasias

Robert A. Kyle, M.D.

The monoclonal gammopathies (plasma cell dyscrasias) are a group of disorders characterized by proliferation of a single clone of plasma cells that produce a homogeneous monoclonal (M) protein. Each monoclonal protein consists of two heavy polypeptide chains of the same class and subclass as well as two light polypeptide chains of the same type (Table 16.1). In contrast, each polyclonal immunoglobulin increase consists of one or more heavy-chain classes and both light-chain types.

The different types of monoclonal immunoglobulins (Ig) are designated by capital letters that correspond to the class of their heavy chains, which are designated by Greek letters: γ in IgG, α in IgA, μ in IgM, δ in IgD, and ϵ in IgE. Their subclasses are IgG1, IgG2, IgG3, and IgG4, or IgA1 and IgA2, and their light-chain types are kappa (κ) and lambda (λ).

The monoclonal gammopathies may be classified as follows:

I. Malignant monoclonal gammopathies
   A. Multiple myeloma (IgG, IgA, IgD, IgE, and free light chains)
      1. Overt multiple myeloma
      2. Smoldering multiple myeloma
      3. Plasma cell leukemia
      4. Nonsecretory myeloma
   B. Plasmacytoma
      1. Solitary plasmacytoma of bone
      2. Extramedullary plasmacytoma
   C. Malignant lymphoproliferative diseases
      1. Waldenström macroglobulinemia, or primary macroglobulinemia (IgM)
      2. Malignant lymphoma
   D. Heavy-chain diseases (HCD)
      1. γ (gamma) HCD
      2. α (alpha) HCD
      3. μ (mu) HCD
   E. Amyloidosis (AL)
      1. Primary (AL)
      2. With myeloma (AL)
         (Secondary, localized, and familial amyloidosis have no monoclonal protein)
II. Monoclonal gammopathies of undetermined significance
   A. Benign (IgG, IgA, IgD, IgM, and, rarely, free light chains)
   B. Associated with neoplasms of cell types not known to produce monoclonal proteins
   C. Biclonal gammopathies

This chapter reviews the structure of immunoglobulins and the relationship of normal immunoglobulins to myeloma proteins and macroglobulins, and it presents a brief account of laboratory methods used for the detection and study of monoclonal proteins. The individual monoclonal gammopathies are then discussed.

NORMAL IMMUNOGLOBULINS

Before 1960, the term *gamma globulin* was used to designate those proteins that migrated in the γ mobility region (toward the cathode) of the electrophoretic pattern, but it has long been recognized that they also migrate in the β and α_2 mobility regions. These proteins

TABLE 16.1.   The Classification of Immunoglobulins of Normal Human Serum

	Immunoglobulin				
	IgG	**IgA**	**IgM**	**IgD**	**IgE**
Heavy chain					
Classes	Gamma, γ	Alpha, α	Mu, μ	Delta, δ	Epsilon, ϵ
Subclasses	IgG1, IgG2, IgG3, IgG4	IgA1, IgA2	—	—	—
Light-chain types	Kappa, κ	κ	κ	κ	κ
	Lambda, λ	λ	λ	λ	λ
Molecular formula	$\gamma_2 \kappa_2$	$\alpha_2 \kappa_2$*	$(\mu_2 \kappa_2)5$	$\delta_2 \kappa_2$	$\epsilon_2 \kappa_2$
	$\gamma_2 \lambda_2$	$\alpha_2 \lambda_2$*	$(\mu_2 \lambda_2)5$	$\delta_2 \lambda_2$	$\epsilon_2 \lambda_2$
Designation	IgG-κ	IgA-κ	IgM-κ	IgD-κ	IgE-κ
	IgG-λ	IgA-λ	IgM-λ	IgD-λ	IgE-λ

Source: Kyle and Bayrd 1976[338] Courtesy of Charles C Thomas, Publisher, Springfield, Ill.
*May form polymers.

now are referred to as *immunoglobulins*, and the five groups presently recognized and their properties are listed in Table 16.2.

IgG

Three fourths of the immunoglobulin in normal serum is of the IgG type. It has a molecular weight of 150,000 and a sedimentation coefficient of 6.7S. Its electrophoretic mobility ranges from slow γ (cathodal area) to α_2. Many antibodies to both bacteria and viruses are of the IgG class. A reducing agent such as mercaptoethanol disrupts the disulfide bonds that link the polypeptide chains of the IgG molecule. If the reduced protein is alkylated with iodoacetamide and fractionated in the

presence of a solvent capable of dissociating noncovalent bonds (such as guanidine or urea), two kinds of polypeptide chains can be recovered: heavy and light chains (Fig. 16.1).

HEAVY CHAINS. Both heavy chains of the IgG molecule are of the γ class, and the two light chains are alike, both κ or both λ. Each γ heavy chain has a molecular weight of approximately 55,000 and consists of 440 to 450 amino acids. Each has a variable (V_H) region, in which many amino acid substitutes make each chain different from the next, as well as a constant (C_H) region, in which there are very few amino acid differences from one γ chain to the next. The variable region of the γ chain consists of approximately 110 amino acid

TABLE 16.2.   Properties of Immunoglobulins of Normal Human Serum

	Immunoglobulin				
	IgG	**IgA**	**IgM**	**IgD**	**IgE**
Electrophoretic mobility	γ to α_2	γ to β	γ to β	γ to β	γ to β
Sedimentation coefficient, S	6.7	7.0–15.0	19.0	7.0	8.0
Molecular weight	150,000	160,000–400,000*	900,000	180,000	200,000
Carbohydrate, %	2.6	5.0–10.0	9.8	10.0–12.0	11.0
Biologic half-life (T½), *days*	23.0	5.8	5.1	2.8	2.3
Serum concentration (mean), *mg/ml*	11.4000	1.8000	1.0000	0.0300	0.0003
Total serum immunoglobulin, %	74	21	5	0.200	0.002
Total body pool in intravascular space, %	45	42	76	75	51
Intravascular pool catabolized per day, % (*normal*)	6.7	25.0	18.0	37.0	89.0
Normal synthetic rate, *mg/kg/day*	33.00	24.00	6.70	0.40	0.02
Fixes complement	IgG1 and IgG3; IgG2 is variable	Alternate pathway	Yes	No	—
Crosses placenta	Yes	No	No	No	No

Source: Kyle et al. 1970[339]
*Tends to form polymers of the monomer form.

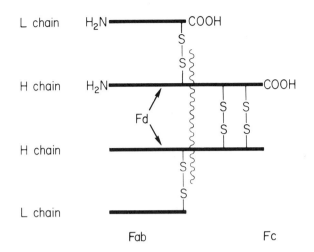

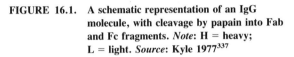

FIGURE 16.1. A schematic representation of an IgG molecule, with cleavage by papain into Fab and Fc fragments. *Note*: H = heavy; L = light. *Source*: Kyle 1977[337]

residues beginning at the amino (NH_2) terminal of the chain. The constant region of the γ chain consists of 310 to 330 amino acids and contains three "homology regions," or "domains," designated $C_\gamma 1$, $C_\gamma 2$, and $C_\gamma 3$. The homology region $C_\gamma 1$ is in the Fd fragment (Fig. 16.1) and runs from approximately amino acid 110 to 220; $C_\gamma 2$ is in the Fc fragment (Fig. 16.1) and extends from approximately amino acid 220 up to 330; and $C_\gamma 3$ extends to the carboxyl terminus.

Immunologic analysis of myeloma proteins has disclosed four distinct subclasses of γ heavy chains, designated IgG1, IgG2, IgG3, and IgG4 (Table 16.3). The average biologic half-life of IgG1, IgG2, and IgG4 myeloma proteins injected into patients with malignancies is 21 days, whereas IgG3 has a half-life of 7 to 8 days.

Although many antigens evoke antibody response within the IgG subclasses that is proportional to their distribution in normal serum, others produce antibodies mainly within one subclass. For example, almost all antibodies to factor VIII (found in hemophiliacs, postpartum women, and elderly patients) are of the IgG4 subclass, while without predilection, only 3% to 4% of the antibodies would be of this subclass.[1]

A high proportion of antibodies to dextran, levan, and teichoic acids is limited to the IgG2 subclass. Antibodies developed against polysaccharide antigens also are found primarily in IgG2.[2]

Among a group of patients with selective IgA deficiency, those with a reduction of IgG2 had frequent respiratory infections, but those with normal IgG2 levels

did not.[3] Of four other patients with no IgG4 (as determined by sensitive radioimmunoassay), all had severe recurrent sinopulmonary infections,[4] and patients with an M protein of different IgG subclasses have greatly different patterns of suppression. For example, patients with IgG2 monoclonal proteins are more likely to have depressed residual IgG than are patients with IgG1, IgG3, or IgG4.[5] IgG classes play an important role in recurrent infections.[6]

We have found that the distribution of IgG subclasses in patients with multiple myeloma did not differ from that in patients with monoclonal gammopathy of undetermined significance.[7] There also was no relationship between clinical and laboratory features in multiple myeloma of different subclass types.

Radial immunodiffusion in agar with appropriate antisera commonly is used for semiquantitative concentrations of IgG subclasses in sera. Subclass typing of IgG may be accomplished with isoelectric focusing in a minigel, followed by passive blotting and capillary diffusion onto nitrocellulose.[8]

LIGHT CHAINS. The light chains were encountered first in 1845, when Macintyre and Henry Bence Jones noted that the urine of a patient with multiple myeloma precipitated when heated, cleared when boiled, and reprecipitated when cooled.[9,10] In 1962, Edelman and Gally demonstrated that the light chains prepared from a serum IgG myeloma protein had the same properties as the Bence Jones protein from the same patient's urine.[11] Thus, it was determined the urinary proteins that evoked such interest from Macintyre and Bence Jones were the light-chain components of the immunoglobulin molecule.

The light chains have a molecular weight of 22,500 and contain from 210 to 220 amino acids. Two distinct groups of Bence Jones proteins (groups I and II) were recognized by Bayne-Jones and Wilson in 1922.[12] The two major classes are now designated κ and λ.[13] Approximately 70% of serum IgG monoclonal proteins are of the κ type and 30% of the λ type. In patients who have Waldenström macroglobulinemia, 80% are κ; the opposite occurs in those who have IgD myeloma, in which 60% are λ.

Analyses of amino acid sequence in individual light chains have disclosed both constant and variable regions. The region of the chain from amino acid 107 to the carboxyl terminus at position 210 to 220 is very similar in chains of the same type (κ or λ) and has been designated as the constant region (C_L) although amino acid substitutions have been found at a dozen different positions in the constant region of human λ chains.[14] The region from the amino terminus (position 1) to approximately position 107 has been different in every

TABLE 16.3. Properties of IgG Subclasses

	Subclass			
	IgG1	IgG2	IgG3	IgG4
Normal				
% IgG	70	20	6	4
mg/dl	5.40	2.10	0.58	0.60
Molecular weight of γ-chain	51,600	51,600	59,500	51,600
Isoelectric point	8.30–9.50	7.00–7.30	8.45–8.95	—
Inter-heavy-chain disulfide bonds, N	2	4	5–13	2
Papain digestion	Sensitive	Resistant	Very sensitive	Resistant
Pepsin digestion	Resistant	Resistant	Sensitive	Sensitive
Biologic half-life (T½), *days*	21	21	7	21
Human monocyte receptors	Yes	No	Yes	No
Fixation of complement	Yes	Variable	Yes	No
Reaction with staphylococcal A protein	Yes	Yes	No	Yes

Source: Schur 1987[6]; Reynolds 1988[2]

light chain analyzed thus far and is called the variable region (V_L); the variable half of the light chain contains the unique thermal solubility characteristics of Bence Jones proteins.[15]

The amino acid differences in the constant regions of the light chains can be related to certain allotypic markers. In the κ chains, if the amino acid leucine is at position 191, the protein is Inv(1) or Inv(2), whereas if valine is at this position, it is Inv(3). However, no genetic factors have been identified in human λ chains. The isotypic markers in λ chains include Oz(+) if lysine is at position 193 and Oz(−) if arginine is present. Another marker in λ chains has been designated as Kern(+) when glycine is present at position 156 and Kern(−) when serine is there. Still another variant, Mcg, has threonine instead of glycine at position 103 (Table 16.4).[16,17]

The human λ-chain gene is in chromosome 22,[18] that for κ on chromosome 2, and that for heavy chain on chromosome 14.[19] The molecular genetics of light chains and their structural diversity, necessary for antibody function, have been discussed elsewhere.[20]

Results of amino acid sequence studies have revealed four basic groups of κ light chains, designated κI, κII, κIII, and κIV.[21] Their frequency of occurrence is approximately 60%, 10%, 28%, and 2%, respectively, and as would be expected these figures reflect the proportion of κI, κII, κIII, and κIV light chains in immunoglobulins of normal serum.[17]

Six subclasses of λ have been reported and have the following distribution: λI, 26%; λII, 38%; λIII, 22%; λIV, 3%, λV, 38%; and λVI, 11%.[22] There is preferential association of λVI subclass with primary systemic amyloidosis,[22] and in fact, all patients with λVI subclass have amyloidosis.

Ordinarily κ chains are in the monomeric form (22,500 mw), but they may exist as noncovalently linked dimers or as a mixture of monomers and dimers,

TABLE 16.4. Properties of IgG Light and Heavy Chains

Property	Light	Heavy
Molecular weight	22,500	55,000
Carbohydrate	None	Present
Classes	κ, λ	IgG1, IgG2, IgG3, IgG4
Allotypes		
Km (1), Km (2), Km (3) [InV]	Cκ	Absent
Isotypes		
Mcg (22%)	CλI	Absent
Kern (18%)	CλII	Absent
Oz (25%)	CλIII	Absent
Gm markers	Absent	Present
Relation to Bence Jones protein	Same	Not related

Source: Kyle and Garton 1991[342]

whereas λ proteins occur as dimers (45,000 mw) linked covalently by their penultimate cysteinyl residues.[17] In addition, κ light chains precipitate maximally over a narrower range of pH than do λ light chains.[23] Recognition of light chains as κ or λ by monospecific antisera depends on the variable and constant domains as well as on the interdomain "switch" region between the variable and constant regions.[24] Bence Jones proteins are synthesized *de novo* and are not degradation products of the complete immunoglobulin in the serum; light chains clearly are catabolized by the renal tubular cells.

Fab AND Fc FRAGMENTS. Treatment of IgG with a proteolytic enzyme, papain, cleaves it into three pieces: two Fab fragments, so named because they possess antigen-combining activity; and an Fc fragment, so named because in certain species it can be crystallized (Figs. 16.1 and 16.2). Each Fab fragment (52,000 mw) consists of the amino terminal region of a heavy chain and a complete light chain. The hinge region, consisting of 15 amino acid residues between $C_{\gamma 1}$ and $C_{\gamma 2}$, is a flexible junction between Fab and Fc fragments, and this hinge permits the angle between the Fab fragments to range from a few degrees to almost 180°.

Three regions of "hypervariability" have been identified in V_L: positions 24 to 34, 50 to 56, and 89 to 97.[25] This hypervariability and the existence of similar hypervariable regions in the variable region of the heavy chain (V_H) in positions 30 to 37, 51 to 68, 84 to 91, and 101 to 110 permit the formation of many different antigen-combining sites, each consisting of fewer than 20 amino acid residues.[26]

The Fc fragment (48,000 mw) consists of the C-terminal region of both heavy chains, which are linked to each other by disulfide bonds. Biologic activities of the Fc fragment include fixation of complement, passive cutaneous anaphylaxis, binding with rheumatoid factors, binding with receptors on macrophages and lymphocytes, reaction with staphylococcal A protein, and transfer across the placenta. Isotypic specificity—specificity for γ, α, μ, δ, or ε—resides in the Fc fragment, and the Fc piece is devoid of antibody activity.

Gm FACTORS. The genetic factors associated with IgG are present on the C region of γ chains and are termed *Gm factors*, or *determinants*.[27] If an Rh-positive red cell is coated with an incomplete Rh antibody, the addition of rheumatoid serum (anti-gamma-globulin) produces agglutination. Serum that prevents agglutination is called Gm+. By alteration of the red cell coating and the agglutinating serum, more than 20 Gm factors can be distinguished. Individual Gm factors are associated with individual subclasses of IgG; there are numerous Gm determinants on IgG1 and IgG3, but few on the other two subclasses.

IgA

Two heavy α-chains and two light chains, both κ or both λ, form IgA (Fig. 16.3).[28] IgA has a molecular weight of 160,000 and a sedimentation coefficient of 7S but also a propensity to form polymers with sedimentation coefficients of 9S to 15S. Its catabolic rate of 5.8 days (T½) is greater than that of IgG. Aggregated IgA can fix the late components of complement, beginning with C3 (alternate pathway). There are two subgroups of the α-chain, α_1 and α_2, resulting in IgA1 and IgA2 proteins; approximately 90% of monoclonal IgA proteins are of the IgA1 class. IgA2 molecules are unique among the immunoglobulins in that the light chains are

IgG – Papain Digestion

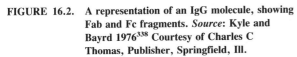

Cleavage by papain

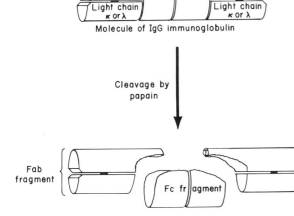

Fab fragment

Fc fragment

FIGURE 16.2. A representation of an IgG molecule, showing Fab and Fc fragments. *Source*: Kyle and Bayrd 1976[338] Courtesy of Charles C Thomas, Publisher, Springfield, Ill.

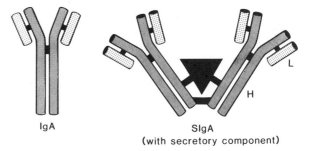

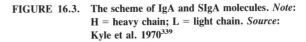

IgA

SIgA
(with secretory component)

FIGURE 16.3. The scheme of IgA and SIgA molecules. *Note*: H = heavy chain; L = light chain. *Source*: Kyle et al. 1970[339]

bound to the α_2-chains by noncovalent forces instead of by disulfide bonds. In a series of 20 healthy persons,[29] 1.37% of all bone marrow plasma cells stained with IgA; the mean percentage of cells staining for IgA1 was 1.19% and that for IgA2 was 0.19%. The cells containing IgA1 constituted 85.7% of all cells that stained for total IgA.

IgA2 has been found in the glomerular deposits of primary IgA nephropathy, in glomerulonephritis accompanying alcoholic cirrhosis, as well as in nephritis from Schönlein-Henoch purpura, whereas lupus nephritis is associated with a preponderance of IgA1.[30] IgA deficiency occurs in two thirds of patients with ataxia-telangiectasia, mainly from a reduction of IgA2.[31]

The daily production of IgA is approximately that of IgG because of the greater catabolism of IgA.[32] Monomeric serum IgA may protect endogenous antigens expressed on various cells and tissues by preventing their interaction with humoral and cellular immune mechanisms that may lead to tissue damage.[33]

Production of IgA begins at 4 weeks after birth, and it approaches the adult level at 1 year of age. No significant changes in concentration occur during adulthood. The major source of monomeric IgA is the bone marrow; spleen cells also produce predominantly monomeric IgA.

SECRETORY IgA. Secretory IgA, or SIgA (Fig. 16.3), is found in high concentration in the secretions of many glands that line the respiratory and gastrointestinal tracts as well as in tears, colostrum, and urine. SIgA has a sedimentation coefficient of 11S and a molecular weight of 390,000. It is composed of two IgA molecules attached by disulfide bonds to a glycoprotein (60,000 to 80,000 mw) called the *secretory component*. The secretory component is synthesized in mucosal epithelial cells, and it increases the resistance of the molecules against digestion by trypsin and pepsin.

In both the gastrointestinal and respiratory tracts, dimeric IgA with J chain (described in the following section) is synthesized in plasma cells and secreted, after which it combines with secretory component on the epithelial cell surface. SIgA then is transported through the cytoplasm in endocytic vesicles to the luminal surface.[34]

In contrast to that in serum IgA, approximately 50% of secretory IgA is of the IgA2 subclass. Approximately 95% of IgA in secretions is polymeric, whereas 90% of serum IgA is monomeric. The intestinal lamina propria cells produce the largest amount of polymeric IgA,[35] and serum IgA does not make a significant contribution to IgA in gastrointestinal fluids.[36]

Secretory IgA exhibits antibacterial and antiviral activity, and evidence indicates that SIgA antibodies are stimulated preferentially by upper respiratory tract infections. SIgA also has a neutralizing effect on viral replication.[37]

In secretions, IgA prevents microorganisms and foreign proteins from adhering to and penetrating the mucosal surfaces.[36] Secretory IgA provides the most potent immunoglobulin signal for the degranulation of eosinophils, and it may be the principal immunoglobulin that mediates eosinophil effector function at mucosal surfaces.[38]

JOINING (J) CHAINS. The J chain is a nonimmunoglobulin with a molecular weight of approximately 15,000.[39] It is bound by disulfide bridges to the Fc portion of the heavy chain and thus forms the dimers or polymers of IgA and the pentamer structure of IgM. It is never found in IgG or in monomers of IgA proteins, yet J chain has been detected in cells secreting IgG. Only one J chain is present in each polymer of IgA or pentamer of IgM; the J chain of IgM and IgA is identical.

IgM

A third immunoglobulin, IgM, is composed of subunits linked by disulfide bonds (Fig. 16.4).[40,41] The heavy chain (μ) of IgM has a molecular weight of approximately 70,000; the subunits, composed of two heavy chains and two light chains, each have a molecular weight of approximately 180,000 to 190,000. Be-

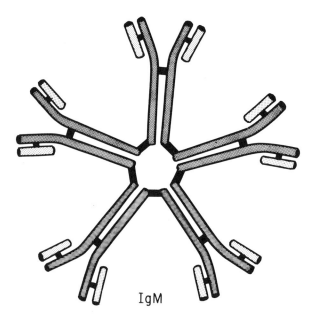

FIGURE 16.4.   An IgM molecule. *Source*: Kyle et al. 1970[339]

cause the molecular weight of IgM is approximately 900,000, it evidently comprises five subunits. The pentamer is assembled in the rough endoplasmic reticulum of plasma cells.[42] The μ-chain consists of one variable (V_H) and four constant (C_μ 1, 2, 3, 4) domains. V_H and $C_\mu 1$ are in the Fd piece, $C_\mu 2$ is in the hinge region, and $C_\mu 3$ and $C_\mu 4$ are in the Fc fragment.[43] Although IgM has a sedimentation coefficient of 19S, more rapidly sedimenting molecules of 22S (composed of dimers of the 19S molecule) and 35S may be seen. Low-molecular-weight IgM (sedimentation coefficient 7S) has been found in patients with various pathologic conditions, including lupus erythematosus, macroglobulinemia, other lymphoproliferative processes, and cirrhosis. Low-molecular-weight IgM (7S) may be detected by nephelometry or immunoblotting.[44]

J chains identical to those associated with IgA polymers also have been isolated from IgM; these aid in initiating or maintaining the tertiary structure of the molecule. Electron microscopy of IgM has shown figures resembling spiders, each with a central ring in which the Fc portions join together and with legs consisting of the Fab fragments. Subclasses of μ-chains have been reported from three laboratories, but they do not correspond. At present, specific subclasses of IgM are not recognized. IgM antibodies are the first produced in a primary immune response, and they avidly fix complement. Cold agglutinins, isoagglutinins, rheumatoid factor, and heterophil and Wasserman antibodies, as well as antibodies to various bacteria, are of the IgM class. Rapid IgM synthesis begins in the first few days of neonatal life, and adult serum levels are attained at 1 year of age. IgM concentrations have been reported to decrease by the sixth decade of life. Also, laser nephelometry frequently overestimates the amount of IgM when compared with densitometry of serum protein electrophoretograms.[45] Consequently, the amount of the IgM monoclonal protein should be followed with either densitometry or nephelometry, but the two methods should not be alternated.

Approximately 80% of IgM monoclonal proteins are of the κ type. This is in contrast to two thirds of IgG and IgA monoclonal proteins.

IgD

In 1965, Rowe and Fahey found a myeloma protein containing a heavy chain unlike those of the other immunoglobulins.[46] This class, IgD, is present in a trimodal distribution, with modes at approximately 0.25, 5, and 35 IU/ml. This distribution suggests that levels of IgD in normal subjects are influenced strongly by inheritance through a monogenic mechanism.[47] IgD is rapidly catabolized and has a serum half-life of 2.8 days. The molecules are relatively heat labile and sensitive to proteases, and they readily break down to Fab and Fc fragments. δ Heavy chains contain three constant domains and a long hinge consisting of 64 amino acid residues. Human IgD has been sequenced,[48] and approximately 75% of IgD is intravascular, a distribution that may be due to irregularities in the shape of the molecule.

Antigen-combining activity associated with IgD has been reported with thyroglobulin, nuclear antigens, and insulin. Most circulating B lymphocytes bear IgD,[49] together with IgM, on their surface as membrane-bound immunoglobulin; however, the function of serum and B-cell membrane-bound IgD is unknown.[50]

IgE

The fifth class of immunoglobulins, IgE, has been purified from the serum of allergic patients.[51] More than 20 cases of IgE myeloma or monoclonal gammopathy have been reported. IgE has a molecular weight of 190,000 and a sedimentation coefficient of 8S. The combination of a short half-life (2.3 days) and a very low rate of synthesis results in an extremely low serum concentration in normal subjects.

IgE mediates the wheal-and-flare reaction associated with reaginic allergies, and it binds to basophils. IgE is fixed on normal human target cells, and histamine is released when the cell-fixed IgE reacts with the allergen. IgE often is increased in patients with extrinsic asthma and hay fever.[52]

The discovery of IgE has not made any significant changes in the treatment of allergic diseases.[53] The physiologic contribution of IgE to the maintenance of health remains speculative.[54]

MONOCLONAL PROTEINS

Relation to Normal Immunoglobulins

Although monoclonal proteins have long been thought of as abnormal, results of studies over the past several years have suggested strongly that they are only excessive quantities of immunoglobulins that occur normally. The striking feature of monoclonal proteins that led investigators to consider them as abnormal is their homogeneity. Whereas normal IgG in human serum is electrophoretically heterogeneous and distributed from the α_2- to the slow γ-regions, IgG monoclonal proteins are localized sharply in their electrophoretic migration.

Kunkel showed that each light-chain type and heavy-chain subclass in monoclonal proteins has its counterpart among normal immunoglobulins and also among antibodies.[55] Even the antigenic determinants (also termed *individual antigenic specificities* or *idiotypic specificities*) thought to be associated uniquely with myeloma proteins have been shown to occur among antibodies.[56] Conversely, studies of highly purified antibodies have revealed a homogeneity approaching that seen in monoclonal proteins, and in some instances, after primary immunization with a carbohydrate antigen, monoclonal immunoglobulins consisting of a single light-chain type and single IgG heavy-chain subclass have been seen.[57]

The possibility expressed by Kunkel that myeloma proteins are individual antibodies and products of the individual plasma cells arising from a single clone of malignant cells has been supported by their antigen-combining activity.[55,58] Monoclonal antibody activity in humans has been associated with cold agglutinin disease as well as with a wide variety of bacterial antigens, including streptolysin O, staphylococcal protein, *Klebsiella polysaccharides*, and brucella.[59] It is almost certain that more monoclonal human proteins will be found to have antibody activity; indeed, it has been postulated that all myeloma proteins may have antibody activity.[60]

In this view, as illustrated in Figure 16.5, the normal collection of IgG molecules comprises minute amounts of homogeneous proteins from many diverse single clones of plasma cells; thus, it is polyclonal. If a single clone escapes the normal controls over its multiplication, it reproduces excessively and synthesizes an excess of protein with a single heavy-chain class and subclass and light-chain type. This monoclonal protein often is associated with a neoplastic process. Support for the single-cell, single-immunoglobulin concept comes from the results of studies of the cellular localization of these proteins; results of experiments performed with antisera to light chains have shown that nearly all individual plasma cells contain κ or λ light chains but not both.

Patterns of Overproduction

Normally, plasma cells produce heavy chains and a slight excess of light chains that spill over into the urine. In IgG myeloma, about three fourths of patients have an excess of light chains that may be excreted into the urine (Bence Jones proteinuria) or catabolized.[61] This small excess of light-chain production could be caused by imbalance in translation or transcription within occasional clones or by a possible suppression of heavy-chain synthesis in such clones. In other instances, no heavy chain is produced by the plasma cell, and only

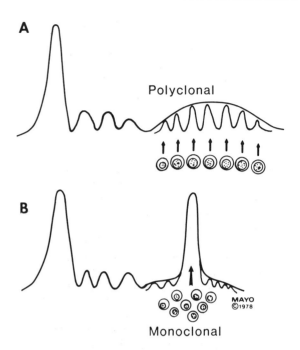

FIGURE 16.5. **Polyclonal and monoclonal electrophoretic patterns. *A*, A broad outline comprising small peaks of many different homogeneous proteins (each represented in normal amount, related by an *arrow* to its peak) that have been produced by many different plasma cell clones (polyclonal). *B*, A tall, narrow peak of homogeneous protein (single heavy-chain class and subclass and single light-chain type) that is excessive output of a single clone (monoclonal). *Source*: Kyle and Greipp 1978[63] Reprinted with permission of the Mayo Foundation**

excessive quantities of light chains are detected (light-chain disease).[62] Finally, a small proportion of myeloma cells do not secrete either heavy or light chains to excess, either because of a simple failure of synthesis or by blocking of secretion, and these are termed *nonsecretory myeloma*.

Apart from these patterns, in a very few cases only a fragment of a light or heavy chain is produced by the cells. In cases of so-called heavy-chain disease, portions of the heavy chains of IgG, IgA, or IgM may be present in serum or urine.

Laboratory Analysis

Analysis of the serum or urine for monoclonal proteins requires a sensitive, rapid, dependable screening method to detect the presence of a monoclonal protein and a specific assay to identify it according to its heavy-chain class and light-chain type.[63] Electrophoresis on cellulose acetate membrane is satisfactory for screening. However, high-resolution agarose gel electrophoresis is more sensitive than cellulose acetate electrophoresis for the detection of small monoclonal proteins;[64] in addition, immunoelectrophoresis, immunofixation, or both should be performed to confirm the presence of a monoclonal protein and distinguish the immunoglobulin class and its light-chain type.

ANALYSIS OF SERUM. **Electrophoresis.** Serum protein electrophoresis should be performed when multiple myeloma, macroglobulinemia, or amyloidosis is suspected. In addition, this test is indicated in any case of unexplained weakness or fatigue, anemia, elevation of the erythrocyte sedimentation rate, back pain, osteoporosis or osteolytic lesions or fractures, immunoglobulin deficiency, hypercalcemia, Bence Jones proteinuria, renal insufficency, or recurrent infection. Also, the physician should perform serum protein electrophoresis in cases of peripheral neuropathy, carpal tunnel syndrome, refractory congestive heart failure, nephrotic syndrome, orthostatic hypotension, or malabsorption, because a localized band or spike would strongly suggest primary amyloidosis.

Interpretation of Results. The first peak at the anodal (positive) end of the serum electrophoretic pattern is albumin and the next peak is α_1-globulin, which contains α_1-antitrypsin, α_1-lipoprotein, and α_1-acid glycoprotein (orosomucoid). The third peak, α_2-globulin, is composed mainly of α_2-macroglobulin, α_2-lipoprotein, haptoglobin, ceruloplasmin, and erythropoietin. The major components of the β-globulin peak are β-lipoprotein, transferrin, plasminogen, complement, and hemopexin. Fibrinogen (in plasma) appears as a discrete band between the β and γ peaks. Addition of thrombin to the sample will produce a clot and disappearance of the band when electrophoresis is repeated. Immunoglobulins (IgG, IgA, IgM, IgD, and IgE) make up the γ-component, but it must be emphasized that immunoglobulins also are found in the β-region and that IgG extends to the α_2-area.

A decrease in albumin and increases in α_1- and α_2-globulins and occasionally in γ-globulin are nonspecific findings seen in inflammatory processes (tissue inflammation and destruction), such as infections or metastatic malignancy. Broad-based γ-globulin peaks or wide bands with fuzzy borders blending into the background are seen in chronic infections, connective tissue diseases, and liver disease. Rarely, two albumin bands (bisalbuminemia) may be found; this is a genetic

abnormality and produces no symptoms. Hypogammaglobulinemia (< 0.6 g/dl) is characterized by a definite decrease in the gamma component, and the diagnosis should be confirmed by quantitative determination of the immunoglobulin levels. Hypogammaglobulinemia is seen in approximately 15% of multiple myeloma patients, and most of these have a large monoclonal protein (Bence Jones) in the urine.

After electrophoresis, a monoclonal protein (a single heavy-chain class and single light-chain type) usually appears as a narrow peak, similar to a church spire, in the γ-, β-, or α_2-region of the densitometer tracing or as a dense, discrete band on the cellulose membrane (Fig. 16.6). In contrast, an excess of polyclonal immunoglobulins (having one or more heavy-chain types with both κ and λ light chains) makes a broad-based peak or broad band (Fig. 16.7) and usually is limited to the γ-region. An occasional serum contains two monoclonal proteins of different immunoglobulin classes, a situation designated as *biclonal gammopathy.*

A tall, narrow, homogeneous peak or a discrete band is most suggestive of monoclonal gammopathy of undetermined significance, myeloma, or Waldenström macroglobulinemia. However, monoclonal peaks also may occur in amyloidosis and lymphoma.

Other Electrophoretic Patterns. It is appropriate at this point to consider the electrophoretic patterns of certain other conditions. The nephrotic syndrome is distinguished by a distinctive serum pattern featuring decreased albumin and γ-globulin and increased α_2- and β-globulins (Fig. 16.8). The increased α_2- or β-globulin may resemble a monoclonal peak of rapid mobility and could be mistaken for myeloma protein. The urinary pattern consists mainly of albumin (Fig. 16.8). Chronic infections, connective tissue diseases, and chronic liver diseases may be characterized by large, broad-based polyclonal patterns. This is true particularly in chronic active hepatitis, in which the γ-component may be 4 or 5 g/dl. Occasionally, a monoclonal protein appears as a broad band on cellulose acetate and is mistaken for a polyclonal increase in immunoglobulins. Presumably, this is caused by the presence of aggregates or polymers, and immunoelectrophoresis is required for identification.

It must be emphasized that a patient can have a monoclonal protein when the total protein concentration, β- and γ-globulin levels, and quantitative immunoglobulin values are all within normal limits. A small monoclonal peak may be concealed among the β- or γ-components and may therefore be missed. A serum monoclonal light chain (Bence Jones proteinemia) rarely is seen in the cellulose acetate tracing. In a number of cases of IgD myeloma, the monoclonal

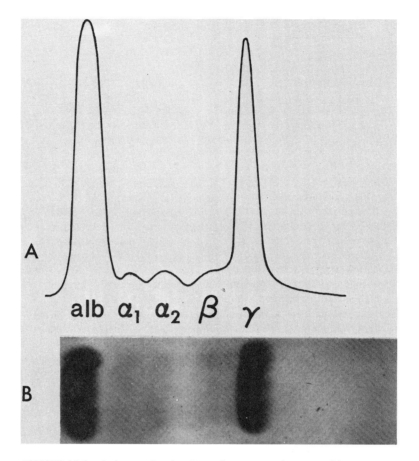

FIGURE 16.6. *A*, A monoclonal pattern of serum protein as traced by densitometer after electrophoresis on cellulose with tall, narrow-based peak of γ mobility. *B*, Monoclonal pattern from electrophoresis of serum on cellulose acetate (anode on left); a dense, localized band representing monoclonal protein is at right. *Source*: Kyle and Greipp 1978[63] Reprinted with permission of the Mayo Foundation

protein appears small or is not evident at all, and often in heavy-chain diseases, the excess of a monoclonal protein is not apparent on the cellulose acetate tracing. Consequently, immunoelectrophoresis is critical.

Immunoelectrophoresis. Immunoelectrophoresis is necessary for identification of the monoclonal protein and for determination of its heavy-chain class and light-chain type. One must perform this test in all cases where a sharp peak or band is found in the cellulose acetate tracing or in which myeloma, macroglobulinemia, amyloidosis, or a related disorder is suspected.

In multiple myeloma, monospecific antisera to IgG, IgA, IgD, or IgE or to κ or λ produce a localized thickening or bowing of the precipitin arc over a narrow mobility range. The immunoelectrophoretic patterns of an IgG-κ monoclonal protein are shown in Figure 16.9.

In Waldenström's macroglobulinemia, IgM antiserum and κ or λ produce a dense localized arc. Sometimes the monoclonal IgM protein does not show an accompanying light-chain abnormality and thus suggests μ heavy-chain disease. However, the addition of a reducing agent such as dithiothreitol to the serum makes IgM-κ or IgM-λ monoclonal protein usually identifiable (Fig. 16.10). We also have found immunofixation to be helpful in this situation (Fig. 16.11).[65,66]

In immunoelectrophoresis of a monoclonal IgG protein, the abnormality in the precipitin arc may occur anywhere from the slow γ- to the α$_2$-regions. Polyclonal increase of a specific immunoglobulin often produces a rather localized thickening of the heavy chain, but there is no corresponding localized thickness of a single light chain because both κ and λ light chains are increased.

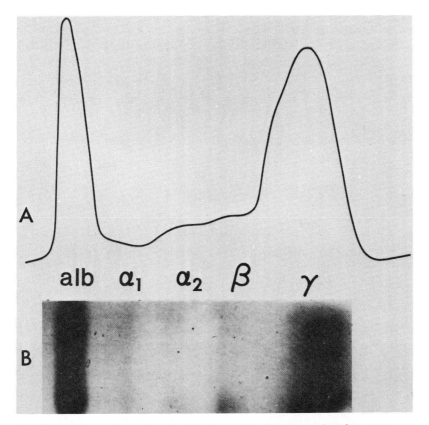

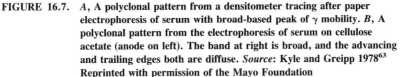

FIGURE 16.7. *A*, A polyclonal pattern from a densitometer tracing after paper electrophoresis of serum with broad-based peak of γ mobility. *B*, A polyclonal pattern from the electrophoresis of serum on cellulose acetate (anode on left). The band at right is broad, and the advancing and trailing edges both are diffuse. *Source*: Kyle and Greipp 1978[63] Reprinted with permission of the Mayo Foundation

All sera must be screened for the presence of IgD or IgE myeloma proteins. This is absolutely essential when bowing of the κ or λ arcs of precipitation is seen without an accompanying abnormality of the IgG, IgA, or IgM arcs. We find it economical to screen the sera of our patients by Ouchterlony immunodiffusion, using antisera to IgD and IgE against each patient's serum. If a precipitin band results, the serum is studied further by immunoelectrophoresis with monospecific antisera to IgD, IgE, κ, and λ.

Immunofixation. This is useful when results of immunoelectrophoresis are equivocal (Fig. 16.12).[65–67] A sharp, well-defined band of a single heavy-chain class and light-chain type is seen in a monoclonal protein, whereas broad, diffuse, heavily stained bands with heavy- and light-chain antisera are characteristic of a polyclonal gammopathy. Technical and interpretive expertise is necessary, because overdilution of a serum

sample will result in loss of the monoclonal band and inadequate dilution may produce a dense polyclonal band that could be misinterpreted as a monoclonal protein.

Immunofixation also is helpful for detecting a small monoclonal protein in the presence of normal background immunoglobulins or a polyclonal increase in immunoglobulins. It is particularly advantageous for the detection of a small monoclonal immunoglobulin or monoclonal light chain in suspected amyloidosis or in apparently solitary or extramedullary plasmacytoma after treatment with radiation. It also is helpful for recognition of a biclonal gammopathy (Fig. 16.13).

In one report, immunofixation detected monoclonal proteins in 15 cases when immunoelectrophoresis failed to recognize them.[68] Despite the advantages of immunofixation, however, immunoelectrophoresis is useful as the initial procedure; it is technically easier, and the results generally are satisfactory. In addition, interpre-

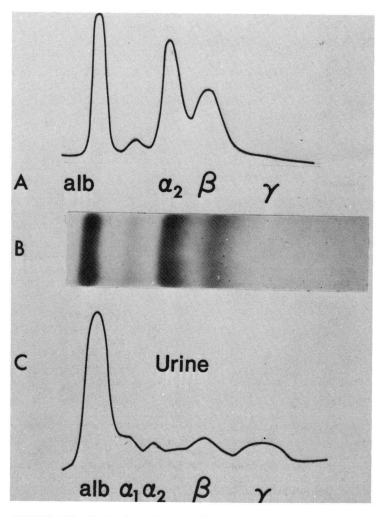

FIGURE 16.8.   **Nephrotic syndrome.** *A*, **The serum electrophoretic pattern (densitometer tracing) showing decreased albumin (*narrow peak*), increased α₂- and β-peaks, and hypogammaglobulinemia. *B*, A cellulose acetate tracing from the same patient. *C*, Urine electrophoretic pattern; most of the protein is albumin.**
Source: **Kyle and Greipp 1978[63] Reprinted with permission of the Mayo Foundation**

tation of immunofixation may be misleading; one can overdiagnose or underdiagnose monoclonal proteins because dilution of the specimen is crucial.

A rate nephelometer using monoclonal specific anti-κ and anti-λ antisera to identify the light-chain component may be used to detect the light-chain type of large monoclonal gammopathies. However, small monoclonal proteins will have a normal κ:λ ratio and consequently will not be recognized.[69] In a series of 336 serum samples, the diagnosis was made in 88% with high-resolution electrophoresis, quantitation of immu-

noglobulins, and the κ:λ ratio, and only 12% required immunofixation for identification.[70]

Immunoblotting. Immunoblotting in combination with high-resolution electrophoresis on agarose may detect monoclonal components in concentrations as low as 0.5 mg/L. In one report, immunoblotting detected a monoclonal protein in 76% of patients older than 95 years and in 79% of those with a kidney transplant; agar electrophoresis and immunofixation had failed to find a definite monoclonal protein in all sera.[71] Norden et al.[72] per-

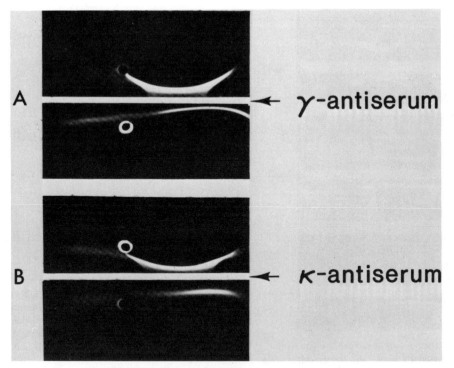

FIGURE 16.9. **Immunoelectrophoretic patterns obtained in myeloma. *A*, Antisera to IgG (γ) shows a thickened arc from the patient's serum in the *top well*; for comparison, a normal arc from normal serum is shown in the *bottom well*. *B*, Antiserum to κ-chains shows a thickened arc similar to the IgG arc (*top well*); for comparison, a normal arc from normal serum is shown in the *bottom well*. Therefore, the patient's serum contains IgG-κ. *Source*: Kyle and Greipp 1978[63] Reprinted with permission of the Mayo Foundation**

formed immunoblotting by using horse-radish peroxidase conjugated antisera to both heavy and light chains; they found that immunoblotting required repeat analysis less frequently than did immunofixation.

Quantitation of Immunoglobulins. This is more useful than immunoelectrophoresis or immunofixation for the detection of hypogammaglobulinemia. Quantitation may be performed by radial immunodiffusion.[73] However, low-molecular-weight (7S) IgM produces a spuriously elevated level, because its rate of diffusion is greater than that of the 19S IgM used as a standard. In contrast, polymeric IgA will produce spuriously low values because the standards consist of 7S IgA. Consequently, radial immunodiffusion is not recommended.

The use of a rate nephelometer is practical for identification of immunoglobulins. In this system, the degree of turbidity produced by antigen–antibody interaction is measured by nephelometry in the near-ultraviolet regions. Because the method is not affected by the molecular size of the antigen, the nephelometric technique measures 7S IgM, polymers of IgA, or aggregates of IgG accurately.

Serum Viscometry. This should be performed when the IgM level is greater than 3 g/dl, the IgA or IgG protein value is more than 4 g/dl, and in any patient with oronasal bleeding, blurred vision, or neurologic symptoms suggestive of a hyperviscosity syndrome. An Ostwald-100 viscometer is a satisfactory instrument for this purpose; however, a Wells-Brookfield viscometer is preferred because it is more accurate, requires less serum, and can perform at different shear rates and different temperatures. In addition, determinations can be made much more rapidly, especially if the viscosity of the serum sample is high. A normal viscosity value is 1.8 centipoises (cP) or less, but symptoms of hyperviscosity are rare unless the value is greater than 4 cP. Indeed, some patients with a value of 10 cP or more do not have symptoms of hyperviscosity.

ANALYSIS OF URINE. In studying patients with gammopathies, urine analysis is essential. Sulfosali

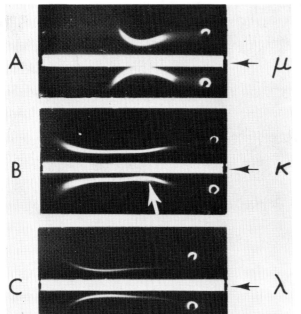

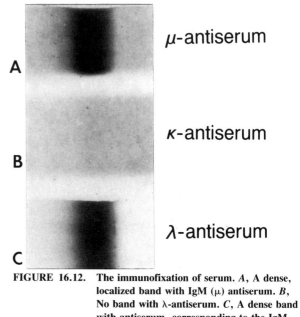

FIGURE 16.10. The *top well* of each slide contains the patient's serum; the *bottom well* contains the same patient's serum exposed to dithiothreitol. *A*, μ-Antiserum in trough, localized IgM arc. *B*, κ-Antiserum in trough. Note the bowing of the κ-arc in the bottom portion of the slide and the normal κ-arc in the top. *C*, λ-Antiserum, normal arcs. *Source*: Kyle and Greipp 1978[63] Reprinted with permission of the Mayo Foundation

FIGURE 16.12. The immunofixation of serum. *A*, A dense, localized band with IgM (μ) antiserum. *B*, No band with λ-antiserum. *C*, A dense band with antiserum, corresponding to the IgM band; the patient has IgM-λ monoclonal protein. *Source*: Kyle and Garton 1986[340]

cylic acid is best for the detection of protein; dipsticks may not detect Bence Jones protein and should not be used as a routine screening test for Bence Jones proteinuria.[74] Most but not all monoclonal light chains in the urine behave as Bence Jones protein: precipitating at

40°C to 60°C, dissolving at 100°C, and reprecipitating on cooling to 40°C to 60°C. Occasionally, the heat test is positive even though the patient has no evidence of myeloma or macroglobulinemia and the urine reveals no sharp peak in the electrophoretic pattern or evidence of a monoclonal light chain on immunoelectrophoresis; such false positive results occur most often in cases of renal insufficiency, malignancy, or connective tissue disease.[75] Conversely, in some cases of myeloma, urine containing large amounts of monoclonal light chains has given negative results with the heat test. Therefore, the heat test for Bence Jones protein cannot be recommended, and the recognition of Bence Jones proteinuria depends on the demonstration of a monoclonal light chain by electrophoresis and immunoelectrophoresis or immunofixation of an adequately concentrated urine specimen.

Electrophoresis and immunoelectrophoresis of urine should be performed in all cases of definite or suspected multiple myeloma, macroglobulinemia, amyloidosis, monoclonal gammopathy of undetermined significance, or heavy-chain disease. For electrophoresis of urine, an aliquot of the 24-hour urine specimen first must be concentrated 200-fold (Minicon-B15 concentrator); rarely, one specimen may be contaminated by another in the concentrator. A urinary monoclonal protein appears as a dense, localized band on the cellulose acetate strip or as a tall, narrow, homogeneous peak on the densitometer tracing (Fig. 16.14). Generally, a monoclonal

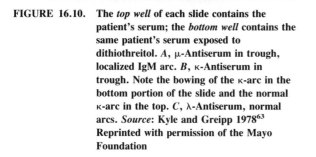

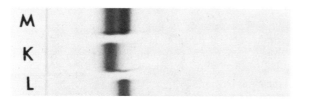

FIGURE 16.11. Immunofixation. Localized IgM bands are seen in the *top portion*. One band corresponds to κ (*middle portion*), and the other band corresponds to λ (*lower portion*). This patient has a biclonal gammopathy (IgM-κ and IgM-λ).

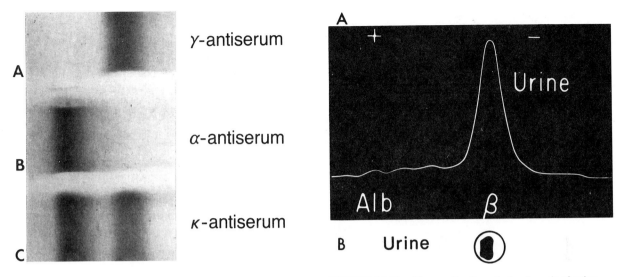

FIGURE 16.13. The immunofixation of serum. *A*, A dense band with IgG (γ) antiserum. *B*, A dense band with IgA (α) antiserum. *C*, Two dense bands with κ-antiserum. The patient has biclonal gammopathy (IgG-κ and IgA-κ). *Source*: Kyle and Garton 1986[340]

FIGURE 16.14. The results of an electrophoresis of urine from a patient with monoclonal protein. *A*, A densitometer tracing with a tall, narrow-based monoclonal peak of β mobility. *B*, A cellulose acetate electrophoretic pattern; the dense band of β mobility represents a monoclonal light chain. *Source*: Kyle and Greipp 1978[63] Reprinted with permission of the Mayo Foundation

protein in urine produces a wider band than a monoclonal protein in serum. A polyclonal increase of light chains is seen as a very broad band extending through most of the γ-area and having fuzzy, indistinct advancing and trailing edges. The densitometer tracing is broad-based, and immunoelectrophoresis shows both κ and λ arcs (Fig. 16.15).

Immunolectrophoresis of concentrated urine is performed with antisera to κ and λ and the appropriate heavy chain. Theoretically, it would be best to use antisera that recognize only free κ- or λ-immunoglobulins rather than light-chain antisera that recognize light chains, which are either free or in an intact immunoglobulin. However, such antisera are not readily available; most are either nonspecific or are not potent enough. In addition, an occasional patient has a heavy-chain fragment that free κ- or λ-antisera would not detect in the urine. Consequently, we use κ- and λ-antisera that are monospecific, potent, and recognize both free and combined light chains. If the monoclonal protein concentration is high, the precipitin arc may overwhelm the antisera or form soluble antigen–antibody complexes (not producing a visible arc), and when this occurs, the physician should repeat immunoelectrophoresis with unconcentrated urine.

Immunoelectrophoresis should be performed on a concentrated urine specimen from a patient with suspected monoclonal gammopathy even if the sulfosali-

cylic acid test is negative for protein. We have seen a number of cases in which the urine osmolality was normal or elevated and the reaction for protein was negative, but electrophoresis of a 160-fold concentrated urine sample revealed a small, localized globulin band and immunoelectrophoresis demonstrated a monoclonal light chain. This finding may be the first clue to amyloidosis.

Immunoelectrophoresis should be performed with monospecific antisera on the urine of all adults with nephrotic syndrome for which the cause is unknown. In a number of our cases, electrophoresis of urine has shown a large amount of albumin and insignificant amounts of globulin, but a small monoclonal light chain actually was found. Many of these patients had primary amyloidosis, although a few had multiple myeloma or light-chain deposition disease. Immunofixation may be helpful in the detection of monoclonal light chains and is more sensitive than immunoelectrophoresis. Immunofixation is most helpful when a monoclonal light chain occurs in the presence of a polyclonal increase in light chains; it also is useful in detecting monoclonal heavy-chain fragments in the urine (Fig. 16.16).

The need for collection of a 24-hour urine specimen cannot be overemphasized. This specimen allows the

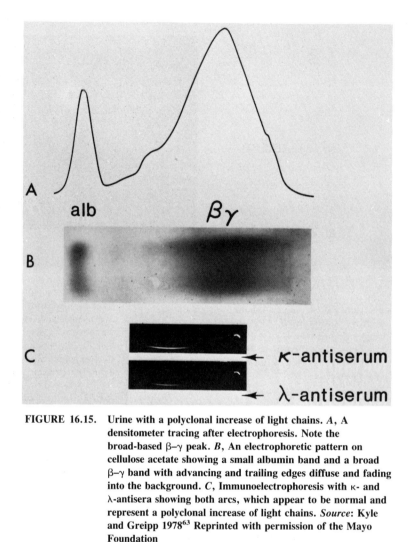

FIGURE 16.15.   Urine with a polyclonal increase of light chains. *A*, A densitometer tracing after electrophoresis. Note the broad-based β–γ peak. *B*, An electrophoretic pattern on cellulose acetate showing a small albumin band and a broad β–γ band with advancing and trailing edges diffuse and fading into the background. *C*, Immunoelectrophoresis with κ- and λ-antisera showing both arcs, which appear to be normal and represent a polyclonal increase of light chains. *Source*: Kyle and Greipp 1978[63] Reprinted with permission of the Mayo Foundation

amount of monoclonal protein excreted in the urine to be measured, and this is an excellent indication of the progress of the disease or the effect of chemotherapy. It also is very useful in following the course of a patient with amyloidosis and the nephrotic syndrome.

MULTIPLE MYELOMA

Multiple myeloma (plasma cell myeloma, myelomatosis, or Kahler disease) is a malignant disease of plasma cells typically involving the bone marrow but often other tissue as well. The "myeloma cell" is an immature and atypical neoplastic plasma cell; myeloma may be regarded as a neoplastic proliferation of a single line of plasma cells engaged in the production of a specific protein as if under constant stimulation. This protein is

monoclonal—one class of heavy chains (γ, α, δ, or ε) and one type of light chain (κ or λ)—and often is referred to as *M* or *myeloma* protein.

Etiology

The cause of multiple myeloma is unknown. Radiation may be a factor in some cases, and five instances of multiple myeloma were found when only 1.8 would be expected 20 years after exposure to more than 50 rads from the atomic bomb among patients 20 to 59 years of age.[76] Also, eight cases of multiple myeloma were found when 4.7 were expected in a long-term follow-up of 14,106 patients with ankylosing spondylitis who were given a single course of radiation therapy.[77]

There is little direct evidence that chemicals cause myeloma in humans, but reports have linked multiple

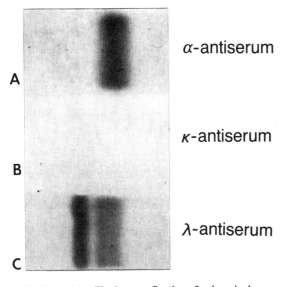

FIGURE 16.16. **The immunofixation of urine.** *A*, **A narrow, localized band with IgA (α) antiserum.** *B*, **No reaction with κ-antiserum.** *C*, **Two discrete bands with λ-antiserum. The patient has a monoclonal λ-protein and an IgG fragment.** *Source*: **Kyle and Garton 1986**[340]

myeloma with asbestos[78] or benzene.[79] An increased risk of multiple myeloma has been recognized in farmers, grain and rubber workers, cosmetologists, furniture workers, and people exposed to pesticides or carbon monoxide.[80] More data are necessary, because the number of cases is small. An occupational risk factor may be responsible for the apparent increased incidence of myeloma in industrialized regions.[81]

Repeated antigenic stimulation of the reticuloendothelial system may contribute to the development of multiple myeloma. In one case-control study, the incidence of chronic infections, connective tissue diseases, allergies, cholecystitis, diverticulitis, or other immune-stimulating conditions was actually less than in the control population.[82]

The likelihood of a genetic factor in some cases is supported by well-documented reports of 23 familial clusters of two or more first-degree relatives (siblings, parents, and children) who had multiple myeloma.[83] In a case-control study of 439 patients with multiple myeloma and 1317 controls, only 3 patients and 4 controls had multiple myeloma in their families.[84]

The possibility of a viral cause also has been suggested in a subset of patients by the finding of Epstein-Barr virus nuclear antigen in 13 (38%) of 34 bone marrow smears from individuals with multiple myeloma.[85] Voelkerding et al.[86] described an IgM-λ nonsecretory plasma-cell malignancy in a 31-year-old man

who was HIV-antibody positive, but further studies are needed to determine whether viruses play a pathogenic role in myeloma.

Approximately half of patients with multiple myeloma are thought to have an abnormal karyotype, with structural changes in chromosomes 1, 11, and 14, as well as trisomy 3, 5, 9, 15, and monosomy 13 and 16. Translocations also have been observed in myeloma and appear to occur predominantly in patients with IgA monoclonal gammopathies.[87]

Incidence and Epidemiology

Multiple myeloma accounts for approximately 1% of all types of malignant disease and slightly more than 10% of hematologic malignancies. In the United States, the death rate for multiple myeloma increased from 0.8 per 100,000 in 1949 to 2.0 per 100,000 in 1969; Sweden and England have reported rates of approximately 3 per 100,000. Data from Olmsted County, Minnesota, revealed a rate of 3 per 100,000 from 1945 to 1954 and a similar rate during the following two decades.[88] The incidence of myeloma increased nearly threefold from 1943 to 1962 in Denmark, but it has remained virtually stable since that time.[89] It seems probable that the death rate for multiple myeloma has not changed; more likely, the apparent increase in recent years is related to the increased availability and use of medical facilities as well as to improved diagnostic techniques rather than a truly increased incidence.

Multiple myeloma occurs in all races and all geographic locations, and its incidence in blacks is twice that in whites. Approximately 60% of all patients are male.

A community cluster of myeloma comprising six cases diagnosed in 1 year (rate, 84 per 100,000) has been reported,[90] and sera were collected from 1200 residents of this community who were 50 years of age or older. Monoclonal serum proteins were found in 1.25% of these residents, a percentage that is not significantly different from that expected in a population of this age, and the cause and significance of this cluster remain unknown. Also, although multiple myeloma has been found in married couples, there is no compelling evidence that direct contact influences transmission of this disease.

Clinical Manifestations

ONSET. Multiple myeloma usually has its onset between the ages of 40 and 70 years, with a peak incidence in the seventh decade of life. It is uncommon before the age of 40 years (2% of our patients were less than 40 years old),[91] and multiple myeloma rarely has been well documented in young adults.[92] Multiple myeloma in children has been reported, but serum and urinary proteins typical of the disease were not always found, and these cases may not actually represent myeloma. It must be emphasized that a diagnosis of myeloma before the age of 30 years is to be accepted only after critical evaluation of all data.

SYMPTOMS. Multiple myeloma is predominantly a disease of the bone marrow, with secondary osteolysis. Bone pain, typically in the back or chest and less often in the extremities, is present at the time of diagnosis in more than two thirds of cases. The pain usually is induced by movement, and it does not occur at night except with change of position. This contrasts with the pain of metastatic carcinoma, which frequently is worse at night. The pain from myeloma may be gradual or sudden in onset, but it often becomes intense and may be protracted or transient, moving from one location to another without apparent reason. Bone tenderness and deformity are common, and persistent localized pain of sudden onset usually indicates a pathologic fracture that often occurs with only minimal trauma. The patient's height also may be reduced by several inches because of vertebral collapse and kyphosis.

Weakness and fatigue are common and often are associated with anemia. Weight loss and night sweats are not prominent until the disease is advanced. Fever from the disease itself occurs much less frequently than in cases of lymphoma or acute leukemia; only 1% of our patients had fever attributed to their myeloma. Most myeloma patients with fever have an infection. Abnormal bleeding, most often as epistaxis or purpura, may be a prominent feature.

In some cases, the major symptoms result from acute infection, renal insufficiency, hypercalcemia, or amyloidosis. Hypercalcemia may be manifested by nausea, vomiting, apathy, weakness, polydipsia, polyuria, and constipation. Congestive heart failure, nephrotic syndrome, joint pains, the carpal tunnel syndrome, or steatorrhea may reflect associated amyloidosis, which occurs in approximately 10% of patients with myeloma. Cryoglobulinemia may produce symptoms on exposure to cold. Rarely, extramedullary tumors in the upper respiratory tract, or elsewhere produce local symptoms.

PHYSICAL FINDINGS. Pallor is the most common physical finding. Bone deformity, pathologic fracture, bone tenderness, and tumor formation also may be seen. The liver is palpable in approximately 20% of patients and the spleen in 5%. Usually, hepatosplenomegaly is of modest degree. Lymphadenopathy is uncommon. Skin involvement is unusual except for petechiae and purpura, and involvement of the sternum may present as a painless, progressive swelling with subsequent defor-mity or fracture. Extramedullary plasmacytomas are uncommon but present as large, exceedingly vascular, subcutaneous masses, often having a purplish hue. Findings caused by local lesions depend, of course, on their location; for example, extradural compression may result in paraplegia. Extramedullary plasmacytomas have been found in almost all tissues. Amyloidosis may produce such diverse abnormalities as defects of cardiac conduction, congestive heart failure, macroglossia, swelling of the joints, and peripheral neuropathy.

Hematologic Data

A normocytic and normochromic anemia occurs eventually in nearly every case of multiple myeloma; anemia is present at the time of diagnosis in about two thirds of cases. The anemia of myeloma is caused mainly by inadequate production of red cells, but a mild shortening of red cell survival as well as iron deficiency and extravascular blood loss also may have an influence. Increased plasma volume, which probably arises from the osmotic effect of the large amount of monoclonal protein, commonly produces hypervolemia in myeloma and decreases the hemoglobin and hematocrit concentrations; thus, significant anemia may be suggested by the hemoglobin or hematocrit value when the red cell mass is only slightly reduced. Overt hemolytic anemia has been reported in myeloma, but the incidence of this is low.

Typically, the erythrocyte sedimentation rate is increased; it was more than 50 mm in 1 hour (Westergren) in three fourths of our patients yet less than 20 mm in another 10%, so a normal sedimentation rate does not exclude the diagnosis of myeloma. Rouleaux are common. Blue-gray staining of the background of the peripheral blood film often is present and is attributed to the increased protein content of the serum.

Ordinarily, the initial leukocyte and platelet counts are normal, but modest decreases are not uncommon. Greater degrees of leukopenia and thrombocytopenia often occur late in the disease after extensive marrow replacement, radiation, or chemotherapy. Fairly often, there are a few immature granulocytes in the peripheral blood, and plasma cells or myeloma cells are seen in the peripheral blood of about 15% of patients. There rarely is clear-cut plasma cell leukemia with leukocyte counts above 50,000 cells/mm^3 and large numbers of myeloma cells in the peripheral blood.

In the absence of fracture with callus formation, serum alkaline phosphatase values are usually normal. Elevated values have been reported, but careful evaluation often shows another cause, such as liver disease, Paget disease, or healing bone fractures. The serum acid phosphatase value may be elevated in myeloma even in the absence of prostatic carcinoma.

Electrophoretic and Immunoelectrophoretic Data

SERUM FINDINGS. A tall, sharp peak on the densitometer tracing or a dense localized band on the cellulose acetate strip (Fig. 16.6) is seen in 80% of myeloma cases. Hypogammaglobulinemia is present in 10% of cases, and a large monoclonal globulin peak in the urine (Bence Jones proteinuria) is usually associated. In 10% of cases, the serum electrophoretic pattern appears normal or contains only a very small peak or band; in our experience, it is unusual to see a band on the cellulose acetate tracing in the presence of Bence Jones proteinemia. These monoclonal light chains presumably are buried in the β- or γ-regions.

Immunoelectrophoresis and immunofixation of the serum reveal a monoclonal protein in slightly more than 90% of patients. In our experience at the Mayo Clinic from 1982 to 1989 with 846 patients who had multiple myeloma, the following M proteins were found: IgG, 52%; IgA, 21%, κ only, 10%; λ only, 7%; IgD, 2%; biclonal, 1%; and no M protein, 7%.

Proteinuria, detected on routine urinalysis, is present initially in about 65% of patients. Immunoelectrophoresis or immunofixation reveals a urinary monoclonal light chain in 75%. The κ:λ ratio is 2:1, and 99% of patients with multiple myeloma have a monoclonal protein in the serum or urine at the time of diagnosis.

Organ Involvement

RENAL. Renal insufficiency is common in myeloma, and elevation of serum creatinine levels was found initially in about 55% of our series. The possibility of myeloma must be considered when any older patient has renal failure of obscure cause.

Hypercalcemia, which was present initially in 30% of our patients, is one of the most common causes of renal insufficiency. If diagnosis is early and therapy prompt, the results are more satisfactory; renal function is frequently improved. Another major cause of renal insufficiency is the so-called myeloma kidney, in which the distal and occasionally the proximal convoluted tubules and collecting tubules become obstructed by large, laminated casts. These casts are composed mainly of precipitated monoclonal light chains. Multinucleated syncytial epithelial cells (giant cells) often are seen at the periphery of the cast. Dilation and atrophy of the renal tubules occur, and eventually, the entire nephron becomes markedly distorted and nonfunctional.[93] Interstitial fibrosis and nephrocalcinosis may occur.[94] Blood pressure is usually normal, even in the presence of marked renal insufficiency.

The degree of renal insufficiency correlates best with tubular atrophy and degeneration and with the magnitude of Bence Jones proteinuria.[95] Eight of 11 patients

who excreted more than 1 g of Bence Jones protein daily had severe renal impairment, but all 9 without Bence Jones proteinuria had a creatinine clearance rate greater than 50 ml/minute. Most of those in the former group had severe derangement of renal histology, manifested mainly by tubular atrophy.[95] However, we have seen several patients producing from 1 to more than 10 g of Bence Jones proteinuria daily for 5 to 20 years without developing significant renal insufficiency; apparently, some Bence Jones proteins have a nephrotoxic effect and others do not.

The mechanism of nephrotoxicity of Bence Jones proteins is unknown. Clyne et al.[96] suggested that Bence Jones proteins with an isoelectric point above 5.5 become positively charged when the urine pH is below 5.5 and coprecipitate with negatively charged Tamm-Horsfall mucoprotein that normally coats the tubule, thus forming tubular casts. However, the role of the isoelectric point in Bence Jones protein is controversial. In a study of 23 patients with multiple myeloma, Coward et al.[97] found no relationship between urinary light-chain excretion and the level of creatinine clearance; Rota et al.[98] also found that the isoelectric point did not have a crucial role in renal failure.

Hyperuricemia, acute and chronic pyelonephritis, infiltration of the kidney by plasma cells, and increased blood viscosity may all contribute to renal insufficiency. Antibiotics such as aminoglycosides may produce an asymptomatic increase in serum creatinine levels or be responsible for acute renal failure. Nonsteroidal anti-inflammatory agents also may promote renal failure.[98]

Amyloid deposition also may produce the nephrotic syndrome, renal insufficiency, or both. Histologic documentation of amyloidosis was found in 7% of our patients with myeloma; the actual incidence is higher because of number of cases in which amyloidosis was suspected but histologic proof was not sought as it would not have altered the course of therapy.[91]

Acute renal failure has followed intravenous urography, but it appears that the risk is slight if dehydration from water deprivation and laxatives is minimized and abdominal compression and hypotension are avoided during the procedure. Occasionally, acute renal failure may occur in the absence of prior urography. Hypercalcemia may be a significant factor in its precipitation.[99]

Multiple myeloma may be associated with Fanconi syndrome. In these cases, Bence Jones proteinuria is almost always of the κ type. Plasmacytosis or frank myeloma is seen in the bone marrow, and crystalline cytoplasmic inclusions commonly are seen in the plasma cells of the bone marrow and in the renal tubular cells. Eventually, amyloidosis or multiple myeloma may occur.[100] Improvement of some manifestations of Fanconi syndrome has been reported when Bence Jones proteinuria has decreased because of chemotherapy for the underlying multiple myeloma.[101]

Myeloma cells have been found in the urinary sediment of patients with myeloma. However, there has been no correlation found between the presence of plasma cells in the urine, the light-chain type, and the presence of renal insufficiency.[102]

Monoclonal light chains may be deposited in the renal glomerulus and manifested by renal insufficiency. This has been designated as *light-chain deposition disease*. The patient may present with nephrotic syndrome or renal failure, and the clinical spectrum ranges from patients with overt multiple myeloma, Waldenström macroglobulinemia, or other lymphoproliferative disease to patients without evidence of a malignant lymphoplasmacytic disorder.[103,104] Typically, nodular glomerulosclerosis is present. The deposits consist of monoclonal κ or, rarely, λ light chains. Approximately half of the patients have a circulating free serum or urine monoclonal light chain.[105]

NEUROLOGIC FINDINGS. Involvement of the nervous system is not uncommon in myeloma. Radiculopathy is the single most frequent neurologic complication, and it usually is lumbosacral. Root pain results from compression of the nerve by the vertebral lesion or by the collapsed bone itself.

Compression of the spinal cord or cauda equina, usually produced by myeloma arising in the marrow cavity of the vertebra and extending to the extradural space, has been reported in 5% to 10% of patients with myeloma. The usual manifestation is back pain with radicular features, weakness or paralysis of the lower extremities, or bowel and bladder paralysis. This may be the initial sign of multiple myeloma, or it may occur during the course of the disease. Treatment of extradural plasmacytoma consists of irradiation or surgical decompression followed by irradiation of the site.[106] The ultimate prognosis should not influence unduly the decision to operate; survival for only a year as an ambulatory patient is to be preferred to paraplegia for the duration of the disease.

Peripheral neuropathy involving the motor or sensory modality or both may occur in multiple myeloma. It may precede the diagnosis of multiple myeloma and may dominate the clinical picture. It usually is associated with amyloidosis. In a review, Kelly et al.[107] described 10 patients with typical multiple myeloma and peripheral neuropathy; eight exhibited a mixed sensorimotor neuropathy that was symmetric and slowly progressive. Four of these 8 were found to have amyloid deposits in the sural nerve, and their neuropathy was painful and did not respond to chemotherapy. In the 4 patients without amyloid deposits, pain and weakness were not promi-

nent features, but the neuropathy still did not improve with chemotherapy. A ninth patient had a purely sensory neuropathy, and the tenth had a predominantly motor neuropathy.

Intracranial plasmacytomas usually are extensions of myelomatous lesions of the skull; infrequently, plasmacytoma of the dura mater (independent of skull lesions) has been seen. Plasmacytomas may involve the hypothalamus, temporal cortex, corpus callosum, and posterior fossa. Destruction of the sella has been reported, with involvement of the third, fourth, and sixth cranial nerves. Slager et al.[108] described a patient with ataxia, stiff neck, and lethargy who had plasma cells in the cerebrospinal fluid. At autopsy, the leptomeninges were infiltrated by plasma cells, but the dura and adjacent brain parenchyma were not involved. A combination of radiation therapy and intrathecal chemotherapy may be of some benefit.[109]

Patients with IgG or IgA monoclonal proteins in the serum usually have monoclonal proteins in the cerebrospinal fluid, but this does not seem to elevate the total protein concentration in the cerebrospinal fluid. There is no correlation between the concentration of monoclonal protein or total protein in the serum or cerebrospinal fluid and the presence of polyneuropathy or severity of electroencephalographic abnormality. Occasionally, myeloma cells may be seen in the cerebrospinal fluid.

Amyloid deposits in cases of myeloma may compress the median nerve, producing the carpal tunnel syndrome, or may involve the autonomic nervous system, contributing to orthostatic hypotension. Rarely, amyloid deposits may be found in the nerves of patients with myeloma and peripheral neuropathy, and multiple myeloma may be associated with progressive multifocal leukoencephalopathy.

GASTROINTESTINAL FINDINGS. Multiple myeloma may involve the stomach and present as a prominence of the rugal folds. Among 900 reviewed cases of myeloma, the gastrointestinal tract was affected in only 16. Hepatomegaly from plasma cell infiltration occurs in about 5% of patients, but this is not of major prognostic significance.[110] At autopsy, hepatomegaly and plasma cell infiltration of the liver are common, and jaundice and ascites sometimes are seen as well.[111] Hemorrhagic ascites has been reported, and multiple myeloma may involve the head of the pancreas and produce obstructive jaundice.[112]

RESPIRATORY FINDINGS. Thoracic skeletal involvement was seen in 28% of our cases.[113] The most frequent abnormality was osteolytic lesions, which were seen in over half the positive chest roentgenograms. Plasmacytomas appeared radiographically as either expanding bony lesions or as soft tissue masses, with or without associated bone destruction, in 12% of our cases of multiple myeloma. Plasmacytomas arise most frequently from the ribs but can originate from the vertebrae, subcutaneous tissue, or mediastinum. Pleural effusions were found in 6% of our patients. Most commonly, this was from congestive heart failure caused by amyloidosis, but in 1% of the patients, it was caused by multiple myeloma involving the pleura. The pleural fluid contained a monoclonal protein and in several cases myeloma cells.[113] Myeloma may cause pulmonary infiltration, but this is not roentgenographically distinguishable from infiltration caused by infections.

CARDIAC FINDINGS. Myeloma involving the pericardium may produce cardiac tamponade, and plasma cells have been identified in the pericardial fluid. Rarely, a plasmacytoma may involve the atria or the sinoatrial node and cause atrial fibrillation.

SKELETAL FINDINGS. Conventional roentgenograms showed abnormalities in 79% of our patients with multiple myeloma.[91] This proportion undoubtedly would have been higher if roentgenography had been performed more frequently throughout each patient's illness. More than half of our patients had a combination of osteoporosis, lytic lesions, and fractures. Generalized osteoporosis may be the only skeletal manifestation of myeloma, and the characteristic lesions are the so-called punched-out lytic areas without associated osteoblastic reaction. The lesions may be sharply circumscribed or, when superimposed on diffuse demineralization, poorly defined. To decide whether or not a poorly defined refraction is abnormal may be difficult, particularly in distinguishing venous lakes from lytic lesions in the skull. Also, multiple lytic lesions are not diagnostic of myeloma and cannot be distinguished roentgenographically from those caused by metastatic carcinoma.

The vertebrae, skull, thoracic cage, pelvis, and proximal humeri and femurs are the usual sites of involvement. Lesions infrequently appear in distal portions of the extremities, but involvement of the mandible is not infrequent (several of our patients have suffered pathologic fractures while eating). Pathologic or compression fractures, especially vertebral, are common and always should suggest the possibility of myeloma. In contrast to the frequency with which they are the site of metastatic carcinoma, the vertebral pedicles are seldom involved by myeloma. Lesions frequently extend into the soft tissues, particularly from the ribs and vertebral column, and this feature should suggest myeloma.

Technetium-99m bone scans generally are inferior to conventional roentgenograms for detecting lesions in myeloma. On the other hand, bone metastases from prostate carcinoma are much more likely to be detected by bone scans than by roentgenograms.[114] Computed tomography may be helpful when skeletal pain is atypical and radiographs show no abnormality; in this setting, computed tomography often reveals lytic lesions. Computed tomography also has been useful in distinguishing overt multiple myeloma producing skeletal pain from smoldering multiple myeloma or monoclonal gammopathy of undetermined significance associated with a large monoclonal protein and osteoporosis with compression fractures.[115] Magnetic resonance imaging also is more sensitive than roentgenograms or radionucleotide bone scans.[116]

The mechanism of bone resorption in myeloma is mainly osteoclastic. Osteoclast-activating factor represents a family of bone-resorbing factors produced by lymphocytes and monocytes. Durie et al.[117] demonstrated a close relationship between the production of osteoclast-activating factor by bone marrow cells and the extent of skeletal destruction. Measurement of serum bone gla-protein levels is a promising marker for bone turnover and response to chemotherapy in myeloma as well.[118]

MISCELLANEOUS FINDINGS. Orbital involvement has been reported in 35 cases of multiple myeloma, manifested as proptosis in most of them.[119] Myeloma may involve the skin and may produce large reddish-purple, subcutaneous nodules. Many of these resemble reticulum cell sarcoma histologically. Breast masses have been reported as the initial finding in myeloma, and hypopituitarism has been caused by a myelomatous sellar lesion destroying the pituitary gland.

In addition to these extraosseous sites of myeloma, lesions may occur in the lungs, spleen, liver, lymph nodes, adrenal glands, and retroperitoneal regions. It is said that most patients with extramedullary involvement have IgA myeloma proteins, but there are some with IgG and IgD myeloma.

System Involvement

IMMUNOLOGIC ASPECTS. The plasma cell is a B lymphocyte that has undergone differentiation and transformation. It can synthesize and secrete immunoglobulin, but in the process of differentiation, it loses certain surface markers, such as surface immunoglobulin, Ia antigen, and receptors for the Fc portion of IgG, C3b, and C3d.

T cells play an important role in normal B-cell differentiation. Although characteristic changes in various T-cell populations can be demonstrated in patients with multiple myeloma, it is unclear whether these alterations are reactive to the monoclonal gammopathy or are causally related. In general, patients with multiple myeloma have reduced percentages of CD4 cells, increased percentages of CD8 cells, and reduced T-helper:T-suppressor ratios.[120,121]

Fifty-five percent of bone marrow aneuploid myeloma cells express the pre-B common acute lymphoblastic leukemia antigen (CALLA).[122] A coexpression of CALLA and monoclonal cytoplasmic immunoglobulin by the same aneuploid myeloma cell suggests a new tumor cell phenotype, without a known counterpart in normal B-cell differentiation. It has been postulated that subpopulations expressing CALLA and containing cytoplasmic immunoglobulins may represent maturation stages of myeloma and that the diploid cells may be the precursors of the aneuploid plasma cells.[123]

A myeloma pre-B-like malignant hybrid with coexpression of cytoplasmic μ, CALLA, terminal deoxynucleotidyl transferase (pre-B phenotype), and plasma cell antigens (PCA-1 and PC-1) has been found in both direct and cultured bone marrow.[124] Heavy- and light-chain immunoglobulin gene rearrangements demonstrated monoclonality of these cells, and double-labelling experiments (immunophenotype and labelling index) have demonstrated that the cultured pre-B-like myeloma hybrid has a proliferative component exceeding that of myeloma; these pre-B myeloma cells were postulated to be the stem cell population of myeloma.

Plasma cell precursors of myeloma probably circulate in the peripheral blood, and several investigators have demonstrated that a subpopulation of peripheral blood lymphocytes express the same idiotype found in the myeloma cells.[125,126] In addition, clonal gene rearrangements in the peripheral blood of patients with myeloma are identical to those seen in marrow cells.[127]

Several lymphoid growth factors are involved in the differentiation of normal B cells. Resting B cells enter into DNA synthesis by interleukin (IL)-4, proliferate with IL-5, and differentiate into plasma cells via IL-6. When cultured in vitro in the presence of IL-3 and IL-6, peripheral blood mononuclear cells from patients with myeloma generate a population of morphologically evident plasma cells after 6 days; in one study, these cells expressed the same light and heavy chain produced by the bone marrow malignant plasma cells.[128] Those authors concluded that circulating malignant plasma cells precursors exist and that their growth and terminal differentiation are under the synergistic control of IL-3 and IL-6.

Multiple myeloma is associated with the overproduction of cytokines, which may be responsible for the osteolytic bone lesions and polyclonal hypogammaglobulinemia associated with myeloma. Recombinant IL-6

in vitro produces plasma cell proliferation, which is directly correlated with the labelling index of the myeloma cells in vivo.[129] Kawano et al.[130] proposed that IL-6 was an autocrine growth factor for myeloma cells; in contrast, Klein et al.[131] showed that the increased production of IL-6 in the bone marrow of patients with progressive multiple myeloma was confined to the adherent cells of the bone marrow environment and not the myeloma cells. This suggests a paracrine rather than an autocrine effect on myeloma cell growth by IL-6. Kishimoto[132] postulated that IL-6 induces a polyclonal proliferation of plasma cells and that a second event, such as altered oncogene expression, may transform cells into a monoclonal process. Significant serum IL-6 levels were detected in only 3% of patients with monoclonal gammopathy of undetermined significance but were found in 35% of those with overt multiple myeloma and 100% of patients with plasma cell leukemia.[133] The use of anti-IL-6 antibodies may be beneficial for the treatment of aggressive multiple myeloma. There is no question that IL-6 is a potent growth factor for myeloma, and its altered expression may be involved in multiple myeloma.

Although increase of total serum γ-globulin is characteristic of multiple myeloma, patients with this disorder actually have a deficiency of functional immunoglobulins and low serum titers of antibodies to various antigens. This may be caused by suppressor T lymphocytes or macrophages.[134] In some patients with myeloma, macrophages suppress the primary antibody response by secreting a low-molecular-weight immunosuppressor; induction of secretion of macrophage immunosuppressor is caused in turn by secretion of a high-molecular-weight suppressor by the malignant plasma cells.[135] The role of immunosuppression in myeloma has been reviewed elsewhere.[136]

INFECTIONS. The incidence of infections increases in multiple myeloma.[137] The pathogens seen most frequently have been *Diplococcus pneumoniae* and *Staphylococcus aureus* in pulmonary infections and *Escherichia coli* in urinary infections; subsequently, gram-negative organisms have been reported to account for more than half of all infections.[138] The greatest risk of infection in multiple myeloma is during the first 2 months after the initiation of chemotherapy, and elevated serum creatinine levels and decreased polyclonal serum immunoglobulins also were associated with a higher incidence of infection in one study.[139]

The impairment of antibody response, deficiency of normal immunoglobulins, reduction of delayed hypersensitivity, and in some instances, depression of reticuloendothelial function and impairment of neutrophil activity may contribute to the increased susceptibility to infections among patients with myeloma. The propensity to infection is increased further by chemotherapeutic depression of the immune response and production of neutropenia.

Herpes zoster is not uncommon in multiple myeloma. Acquired immunodeficiency syndrome also has been associated with multiple myeloma.[140]

COAGULATION ABNORMALITIES. Bleeding may be a prominent feature in multiple myeloma. Qualitative platelet abnormalities may result from the coating of platelets by myeloma protein.[141] Inhibitors of coagulation factors and thrombocytopenia from marrow involvement or chemotherapy also may contribute, and the M protein may possess a heparin-like anticoagulant activity and produce bleeding.[142] Abnormal clot retraction, leaving the clot bulky and gelatinous, may result from binding of the Fab fragment of the myeloma protein to fibrin. Intravascular coagulation, amyloid deposition, and hepatic or renal insufficiency may produce bleeding, and functional deficiency of protein C, presumably from the presence of the monoclonal protein, in a patient with myeloma has produced fulminant necrosis of the skin and subcutaneous tissues.[143]

A tendency to thrombosis manifested by a shortened coagulation time, increased fibrinogen concentration, decreased antiplasmin concentration, and increased levels of factor VIII has been detected. Because patients with myeloma are in the older age groups and may be debilitated and bedridden, circumstances that contribute to thrombosis, the significance of these findings is debatable.

Diagnosis

Bone pain, anemia, and an excessive erythrocyte sedimentation rate or increased rouleaux constitute a triad that strongly suggests multiple myeloma. A number of other findings are suggestive by themselves, such as multiple osteolytic lesions, pathologic fractures, bone tumors, osteoporosis, hypercalcemia, uremia, cryoglobulinemia, pyroglobulinemia, hyperglobulinemia. Bence Jones proteinuria, and protein electrophoretic abnormalities. Blood typing and erythrocyte counting may prove difficult; indeed, the inability to type or crossmatch blood for transfusion may be an initial clue to the diagnosis of myeloma.

If the diagnosis of multiple myeloma is suspected, the physician should obtain, in addition to a complete history and physical examination, determinations of hemoglobin or hematocrit levels; leukocyte, differential, and platelet counts; measurements of serum creatinine, calcium, phosphorus, alkaline phosphatase, and uric acid; a radiographic survey of bones, including humeri and femurs; serum protein electrophoresis; measurement of serum immunoglobulins; serum immunoelectrophoresis or immunofixation (or both); tests for cryoglobulins and viscosity if the M spike is large or if symptoms suggesting hyperviscosity are present; bone marrow aspirate and biopsy; routine urinalysis; and electrophoresis, immunolectrophoresis, and immunofixation of an adequately concentrated aliquot from a 24-hour urine specimen.

The diagnosis depends on demonstration of increased numbers of atypical, immature plasma cells (Fig. 16.17). These plasma cells vary from small and relatively mature to large and anaplastic. The morphology varies greatly among patients, and although asynchronism (cytoplasmic maturity disproportionate to the degree of nuclear differentiation) is common in the plasma cells of patients with multiple myeloma,[144] we have found that plasma cell asynchrony, nucleolar size, nuclear chromatin pattern, and nuclear size do not reliably distinguish multiple myeloma from monoclonal gammopathy of undetermined significance. A monoclonal immunoglobulin in the plasma cells of patients with multiple myeloma can be identified by the immunoperoxidase method.[145] This is helpful for differentiating plasma cell proliferation in multiple myeloma or monoclonal gammopathy of undetermined significance from benign reactive plasmacytosis due to carcinoma, connective tissue disease, liver disease, hypersensitivity states, and infections; this approach also is helpful for recognizing neoplastic plasma cells with unusual morphologic characteristics.

Although plasma cells generally compose 10% or more of all nucleated cells in myeloma, they may be less than 5% or almost 100% of the marrow cells. They may present diffusely, in small clumps, in syncytia, or in large sheets. Marrow involvement often is focal rather than diffuse, and consequently, specimens may vary strikingly. In the same case, one marrow aspirate may consist of nothing but myeloma cells, whereas the next, obtained from another site, may be normal or nearly so. Repeated bone marrow examination may be necessary for the diagnosis; the presence of large homogeneous nodules or infiltrates of plasma cells in bone marrow sections is a reliable morphologic criterion for the diagnosis of multiple myeloma. These nodules are not always present, however, nor are they always diagnostic of multiple myeloma. Buss et al.[146] reported that 2% of patients with reactive plasmacytosis had large homogeneous nodules or infiltrates of plasma cells, whereas 26% of patients with well-documented multiple myeloma did not.

Electron microscopy of the plasma cell demonstrates a prominent, well-developed endoplasmic reticulum

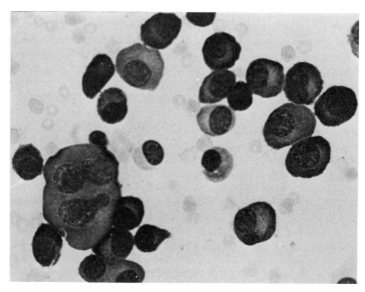

FIGURE 16.17.   The typical condition of marrow in multiple myeloma. Replacement is extensive, nucleoli are common, and polyploidy is evident (Wright stain; × 470). *Source*: Kyle and Bayrd 1976[338] Courtesy of Charles C Thomas, Publisher, Springfield, Ill.

(ergastoplasm) and a prominent, well-organized Golgi complex. The endoplasmic reticulum is the primary site of protein synthesis and may be dilated from protein storage. Protein also may be stored in the Golgi complex prior to secretion.

Minimal criteria for the diagnosis of multiple myeloma include the presence of at least 10% abnormal plasma cells in the bone marrow or histologic proof of a plasmacytoma, the usual clinical features of myeloma, and at least one of the following abnormalities: monoclonal protein in the serum (usually > 3 g/dl), monoclonal protein in the urine, or osteolytic lesions. Connective tissue diseases, chronic infections, carcinoma, lymphoma, and leukemia should be excluded unless other features enable the diagnosis of multiple myeloma to be clearly made.

Distinguishing multiple myeloma from monoclonal gammopathy of undetermined significance may be very difficult. The presence of a serum M protein of more than 3 g/dl is suggestive of multiple myeloma rather than monoclonal gammopathy of undetermined significance, but some exceptions, such as smoldering multiple myeloma, exist. Levels of the immunoglobulin class not associated with the M protein are reduced in multiple myeloma, but these also may be decreased in patients with benign monoclonal gammopathy. The presence of a monoclonal light chain (Bence Jones proteinuria) is

suggestive of a neoplastic process, but small amounts of monoclonal light chain may occur in benign monoclonal gammopathy as well.

The plasma cell labelling index may be useful in differentiating multiple myeloma from monoclonal gammopathy of undetermined significance or smoldering multiple myeloma. A monoclonal antibody (BU-1) reactive with 5-bromo-2-deoxyuridine recognizes cells that synthesize DNA. The BU-1 monoclonal antibody does not require denaturation, and consequently, fluorescein-conjugated immunoglobulin antisera (κ and λ) identify monoclonal plasma cells. The labelling index can be performed in 4 to 5 hours and is a practical aid for assisting in therapeutic decisions.[147] An elevated plasma cell labelling index is strong evidence for overt multiple myeloma, but many patients with symptomatic myeloma have a normal plasma cell labelling index.

Elevated levels of β_2-microglobulin, the presence of J chains, elevated plasma cell acid phosphatase levels, reduced numbers of CD-4 lymphocytes, and increased numbers of monoclonal-idiotype peripheral blood lymphocytes or immunoglobulin-secreting cells in the peripheral blood do not differentiate multiple myeloma reliably from monoclonal gammopathy of undetermined significance. Also, no single technique differentiates benign from malignant plasma cell proliferation. The most dependable means is serial measurement of the M protein in the serum and urine as well as periodic re-evaluation of clinical and laboratory features to determine whether multiple myeloma, systemic amyloidosis, macroglobulinemia, or other malignant lymphoplasma cell proliferative disease has developed.

Association with Other Diseases

RHEUMATOID ARTHRITIS. The association of rheumatoid arthritis has been reported with benign monoclonal gammopathy, multiple myeloma, Waldenström macroglobulinemia, and γ heavy-chain disease. The onset of rheumatoid arthritis usually antedates detection of the protein abnormality, but in our experience, the incidence of multiple myeloma among 279 consecutive patients with rheumatoid arthritis did not appear significantly greater than that in a control group. The association of systemic lupus erythematosus and multiple myeloma also has been noted, but this relationship may be fortuitous.[148]

SERUM LIPIDS AND XANTHOMATOSIS. The serum cholesterol concentration is lower than normal in many cases of multiple myeloma. On the other hand, myeloma and hyperlipidemia have been reported in 19 cases, usually in conjunction with xanthomas,[149] and plane xanthomatosis, a rare entity characterized by diffuse and tannish or yellowish areas of varied shape and size, has been reported in 15 cases of multiple myeloma.[150] Plane xanthomatosis usually precedes the discovery of myeloma, but it occasionally occurs during the course of myeloma.

NEOPLASMS. Myeloma and carcinoma of the colon have been associated.[151] However, in view of the prevalence of carcinoma of the colon, it seems probable that this association is only coincidental. The association of chronic lymphocytic leukemia and multiple myeloma also has been described,[152] but in most instances, two distinct clonal proliferations are present. However, in one case, the finding of shared idiotypes between the IgG-κ molecule synthesized by the chronic lymphocytic leukemia cells and the IgA-κ molecule secreted by the plasma cell proliferation was strong evidence that a single clonal event occurred.[153]

In a study of 628 patients with multiple myeloma who survived at least 2 months, the prevalence and types of solid tumors were no different from those in normal patients of the same age and duration of risk.[154] Thus, long-term chemotherapy does not appear to contribute to the incidence of second solid tumors in patients with multiple myeloma.

Cutaneous T-cell lymphoma (Sézary syndrome and mycosis fungoides) has been reported with multiple myeloma,[155,156] and the simultaneous presentation of typical hairy-cell leukemia and multiple myeloma has been well documented.[157] More than a dozen cases of Kaposi sarcoma and multiple myeloma have been published as well.[158]

MISCELLANEOUS DISEASES. Vandermolen et al.[159] describe four patients with fibrosis of the bone marrow and plasma cell dyscrasia. Severe anemia, leukopenia, and thrombocytopenia were present, but the patients did not have the typical features of agnogenic myeloid metaplasia, such as poikilocytosis, splenomegaly, and leukoerythroblastosis. The size of the M spike was modest, and osteolytic lesions were found infrequently.

The association of multiple myeloma with pernicious anemia, polycythemia vera, myelofibrosis with myeloid metaplasia, red-cell aplasia and thymoma, aplastic anemia, Paget disease, refractory sideroblastic anemia, Gaucher disease, sarcoidosis, erythema elevatum diutinum, bullous pyoderma gangrenosum, hyperparathyroidism, hypereosinophilic syndrome, progressive muscular dystrophy, Bowen disease, and idiopathic thrombocytopenic purpura has been reported,[160] but adequately controlled studies are necessary to make certain there is truly increased frequency of myeloma with these entities rather than mere coincidence. In most cases, mere coincidence seems likely, because unusual concurrences of these diseases are most likely to be reported in the literature.

Course and Prognosis

Multiple myeloma runs a progressive course. Formerly, median survival ranged from 3.5 to 8.5 months, but chemotherapy now has extended it to between 2 and 3 years; almost 20% of our patients survived for 5 years or longer. The major causes of death are infection and renal insufficiency.

To determine myeloma cell mass, Salmon and Smith[161] measured immunoglobulin production per plasma cell in vitro. They calculated the rate of M protein production from the serum concentration of monoclonal protein, plasma volume, and M protein fractional catabolic rate, and immunoglobulin production per plasma cell was measured in vitro. From these two determinations, the total number of myeloma cells present was measured as follows:

myeloma cell number equals

$$\frac{\text{total body M-component synthesis rate}}{\text{cellular M-component synthesis rate}}$$

Durie and Salmon[162] then devised a clinical staging system based on a combination of factors that correlated with the myeloma cell mass. Those patients with high cell mass ($> 1.2 \times 10^{12}/m^2$)—stage III—had at least one of the following: hemoglobin of less than 8.5 g/dl, serum calcium concentration of more than 12 mg/dl, serum IgG monoclonal component of more than 7 g/dl, IgA of more than 5 g/dl, Bence Jones proteinuria of more than 12 g/day, or advanced lytic bone lesions. Those with low cell mass ($< 0.6 \times 10^{12}/m^2$)—stage I—had all of the following characteristics: hemoglobin of more than 10.0 g/dl, normal serum calcium concentration, serum IgG monoclonal component of less than 5 g/dl or IgA of less than 3 g/dl or Bence Jones proteinuria of less than 4 g/day, and no generalized lytic lesions detectable by skeletal survey. Those patients whose cell mass was between the limits specified were designated as intermediate—stage II.

Patients were subclassified by their serum creatinine values as either A (< 2 mg/dl) or B (≥ 2 mg/dl). Median survival was 61.2 months for stage IA patients and 40.1 months for stage IIIA patients. Renal insufficiency was associated dramatically with poorer survival; patients with stage IIIB disease had a median survival of 14.7 months.[163] In patients with Bence Jones λ myeloma, the measured myeloma cell mass was twofold higher than that predicted from clinical staging,[164] and this may contribute to the shorter survival in patients with λ light-chain myeloma. Other investigators have attempted to improve on the accuracy of this clinical staging system, but no system has proved superior to that of Durie and Salmon. We believe that the major benefit of the clinical staging system is to allow comparison of therapy results in clinical trials.

The serum β_2-microglobulin level is the single most powerful prognostic factor in previously untreated multiple myeloma;[165] the bone marrow plasma cell labelling index and the age of the patient also are additional prognostic factors.[166] Plasmablastic morphology is associated with a shorter survival (10 months) than that in patients with other types of morphology (35 months) ($P < 0.05$). There were no significant differences in survival among patients with mature, intermediate, and immature types, or among patients with different morphologic grades or asynchrony scores.[167] Bartl et al.[168] recognized six histologic types and developed three prognostic grades in 674 patients with multiple myeloma. In this study, all patients with high-grade malignancy (20 patients, 3%) had plasmablastic proliferation, and the median survival was 8 months.

Multiple myeloma is a slowly proliferating tumor that in many cases seems to pause after a year or two of presumably rapid subclinical growth. In general, patients with high tumor cell mass have a lower labelling index than those with low tumor cell mass, although a high labelling index may be found in some cases with a large tumor. This latter combination indicates a poor prognosis.[163] Latreille et al.[169] also reported that the labelling index is a highly significant prognostic factor. The response rate does not differ significantly between patients with high [H3]-thymidine labelling indexes and those with low labelling index levels, but the survival is longer in patients with low labelling indexes. Also, the median response is shorter in patients with elevated labelling indexes than in those with normal values.[170] We also determine the plasma cell labelling index of peripheral blood with our BU-1 monoclonal antibody; we found that an elevated peripheral blood labelling index recognized 63% of patients with untreated symptomatic multiple myeloma. The peripheral blood labelling index was elevated in 4 of 29 patients with an apparent smoldering multiple myeloma or monoclonal gammopathy of undetermined significance, and all four patients developed symptomatic multiple myeloma requiring chemotherapy within 6 months. The peripheral blood labelling index also correlated well with the bone marrow labelling index.[171]

After a clinical response to therapy, the plasma cell labelling index is very low and the tumor burden remains in a plateau phase in almost one half of myeloma patients.[172] These very slowly proliferating cells are resistant to agents affecting the cell cycle, such as melphalan, cyclophosphamide, and carmustine. During relapse, the growth fraction of malignant plasma cells increases, and the reinstitution of cell-cycle drugs may be effective again.[173]

OTHER PROGNOSTIC FACTORS. The presence of chromosomal abnormalities indicates a poor prognosis; in one series of 32 patients with untreated multiple myeloma, survival was 6 months for those with chromosomal abnormalities.[174] Lewis and MacKenzie[175] also noted chromosomal abnormalities in 30 patients with multiple myeloma.

A high RNA content in the tumor cell was associated with better response rates to both initial therapy and salvage therapy in 77 previously untreated patients with myeloma.[176] Patients with hypodiploid DNA levels and low RNA content usually do not respond to chemotherapy and also have a shortened survival.[177]

The presence of CALLA positivity has been reported to correlate with aggressive clinical disease. The median survival was 6 months for patients with CALLA positivity in contrast to 56 months for those with CALLA negativity.[178] However, others have reported that CALLA positivity is not associated with more aggressive disease. Myeloma colony growth in culture also is indicative of poor prognosis, and large myeloma colonies were identified in the cultures of 14 patients with multiple myeloma. The median survival of these patients was 3.5 months, compared with 38.5 months for those without large myeloma colonies.[179]

LONG-TERM SURVIVAL. In one report, 19 of 870 patients (2.2%) with multiple myeloma survived for 10 years or longer.[180] All 19 patients had symptoms that required chemotherapy at the time of diagnosis, and the major difference between the long-term survivors and the other 851 patients was their response to therapy. Renal insufficiency and hypercalcemia were more common in the larger group. Also, Alexanian[181] reported that 13 of 305 patients (4%) lived for more than 10 years; most of the long-term survivors in this study were younger than 65 years and responded well to chemotherapy.

An aggressive preterminal phase may occur in patients who have multiple myeloma. This is characterized by the sudden appearance and rapid growth of soft tissue masses, fever without demonstrable infection, pancytopenia unrelated to chemotherapy, and a median survival of approximately 3 months. Biopsy of the soft tissue masses shows primitive plasma cells that are easily confused with those of histiocytic lymphoma, and multiple myeloma in this phase generally is resistant to chemotherapy.[182]

Treatment

Most patients with multiple myeloma have symptoms or laboratory evidence of significant disease at the time of diagnosis and clearly need to be treated. However, some patients have no symptoms, and their laboratory abnormalities are stable. In these cases, it may be difficult to distinguish multiple myeloma from monoclonal gammopathy of undetermined significance. We believe that such patients should not be treated but should be re-examined at 3- to 6-month intervals. If clinical and laboratory examinations show no progression, continued observation with repeated evaluation is indicated. We also have observed a number of patients with smoldering myeloma for more than 5 years without treatment.

IRRADIATION. Because it is generalized at the time of diagnosis, radiation therapy should not be used in multiple myeloma unless pain is severe and localized. Palliative irradiation in a dose of 2000 to 3000 rads usually is effective. Although radiation therapy effectively relieves pain in most instances, the patient frequently returns in a short time with pain at another site. Radiation therapy may be repeated, but it ultimately is limited by the development of leukopenia or thrombocytopenia, which in turn restricts the use of chemotherapy. If patients with multiple myeloma are to be treated with radiation, it is best to complete the palliative therapy 3 weeks before starting chemotherapy and to repeat leukocyte and platelet counts before the start of chemotherapy, because the myelosuppressive effects of both radiation and chemotherapy are cumulative. Thus, irradiation in multiple myeloma is adjunctive and limited, and it should be used only for "focal lesions."

CHEMOTHERAPY. Chemotherapy is the best initial treatment for generalized myeloma unless there is disabling pain that is clearly the result of a well-defined focal process. If analgesics together with chemotherapy can control the pain, chemotherapy is preferred to repeated local irradiation, because the bone marrow reserve of many patients is limited and local irradiation does not benefit systemic disease.

The major controversy in chemotherapy is whether melphalan and prednisone or a combination of alkylating agents should be used. The oral administration of melphalan (L-phenylalanine mustard, Alkeran, Burroughs Wellcome Co., Research Triangle Park, NC) and prednisone is a standard form of therapy, and it produces objective response in 50% to 60% of patients. Melphalan may be given orally in a daily dosage of 0.15 mg/kg for 7 days (amounting to between 8 and 10 mg daily for an average-sized person and between 56 and 70 mg per course) with 20 mg of prednisone given 3 times daily for the same period. The dose of melphalan should be calculated on the basis of the patient's ideal body weight. The melphalan and prednisone regimen should be repeated every 6 weeks, and the patient should avoid alcohol- and caffeine-containing products and take antacids while receiving the prednisone. Leukocyte and platelet counts must be determined at 3-week intervals after the start of chemotherapy, and the dose of melphalan should be altered until modest midcycle cytopenia occurs. Melphalan should be given while the patient is fasting, because absorption is delayed and reduced to approximately 50% after food is eaten.[183] Absorption of melphalan may be poor in some patients, and the oral dosage must be increased appropriately.

If the leukocyte and platelet counts are low at 6 weeks, chemotherapy should be delayed and the counts redetermined at weekly intervals until they increase. If the leukocyte and platelet values remain low, or if the counts obtained at 3 weeks are unduly low, the melphalan dose in the next 7-day course should be reduced accordingly. At least three courses of melphalan and prednisone should be given before this treatment is discontinued unless there are significant toxic reactions or the disease progresses despite adequate therapy.

Objective evidence of response may not be achieved for several months, and one should not change to another therapeutic regimen unless there is evidence of progressive disease or intolerable side effects.

Many combinations of chemotherapeutic agents have been used because of the obvious shortcomings of melphalan and prednisone. The best known combination, the M-2 protocol, includes melphalan, cyclophosphamide, carmustine, vincristine, and prednisone. This regimen produced objective response in 78% of 81 previously untreated patients and a median survival of 38 months.[184]

Harley et al.[185] reported that myeloma patients who were considered poor risks because of high tumor cell load or other findings survived longer if treated with melphalan, cyclophosphamide, carmustine, and prednisone than if treated with only melphalan and prednisone. Conversely, good-risk patients generally did better with only melphalan and prednisone than with the four-drug combination. However, Bergsagel et al.[186] concluded from a prospective study that melphalan, cyclophosphamide, carmustine, and prednisone in alternating or concurrent schedules were not more effective than a combination of only melphalan and prednisone. Also, they found no difference between the reponse of good-risk and poor-risk patients. In a group of 132 azotemic patients with multiple myeloma, a Medical Research Council therapeutic trial that compared the effectiveness of intravenous cyclophosphamide with a combination of cyclophosphamide, melphalan, prednisone, and lomustine revealed poor results with both regimens.[187]

In a prospective study, courses of a combination of vincristine, melphalan, cyclophosphamide, and prednisone were alternated with either the combination of vincristine, cyclophosphamide, doxorubicin, and prednisone or the combination of vincristine, carmustine, doxorubicin, and prednisone. The median survival was 48 months in patients receiving the combinations of chemotherapy and 23 months in those receiving melphalan and prednisone.[188] In another report[189] using the same combinations of alternating alkylating agents with only a minimal difference in dosage, the response rates were virtually the same for melphalan and prednisone (53% and 60%); the slightly longer survival of patients treated with melphalan and prednisone (38 vs. 28 months) was attributed to a higher frequency of favorable prognostic factors and the use of vincristine and doxorubicin combinations when the myeloma became resistant.

In a randomized trial comparing the M-2 protocol (vincristine, carmustine, melphalan, cyclophosphamide, and prednisone) with a combination of melphalan and prednisone, objective response was noted in 72% of patients receiving the combination and in 51% of those receiving melphalan and prednisone. The median survivals of 31 and 30 months, respectively, were not significantly different, and there was greater toxicity associated with the combination of alkylating agents.[190]

The controversy of a single versus a combination of alkylating agents has not been resolved. Ten prospective, randomized studies of melphalan and prednisone versus a drug combination failed to show clearly that drug combinations were better than melphalan and prednisone for the treatment of multiple myeloma.[191] Sporn and McIntyre[192] presented an analysis of therapy in patients with previously untreated multiple myeloma, and it is obvious that new agents with greater specificity and effectiveness must be found before the treatment of multiple myeloma can be improved. In short, we do not have adequate chemotherapy for this disease.

Also, the ideal duration of chemotherapy is unknown. Cessation of chemotherapy after 1 to 2 years usually results in relapse, and response to resumed therapy may be of both lesser frequency and degree than response to the initial chemotherapy. However, no difference in survival was found in a prospective study that compared patients randomized to continuing melphalan and prednisone with those on no-maintenance therapy.[193]

Since the first report suggesting the possible role of alkylating agents in the development of acute leukemia in multiple myeloma,[194] many cases have been recognized.[195,196] In the Medical Research Council's first two trials, 12 of 648 patients with myeloma developed myelodysplasia or acute leukemia; the 5-year actuarial prevalance was 3% and the 8-year prevalance 10%.[197] The peak incidence of acute leukemia occurs 3.5 to 5 years after the initiation of therapy, and in one series, the actuarial risk of developing acute leukemia within 50 months was 19.6%.[198] Melphalan appears to be a more potent leukemogenic agent than cyclophosphamide.[199]

The most important risk factor in one study was the total amount of melphalan given during the most recent 3-year period.[197] Multiple myeloma and acute leukemia have been recognized simultaneously or within months of each other in several instances when patients have not received radiation or chemotherapy, but this simultaneous occurrence probably is fortuitous.[195] Also, second malignancy after chemotherapy recently has been reviewed elsewhere.[200]

Chemotherapy often produces cytopenia and usually is the cause of low leukocyte and platelet values obtained during its use; however, progressive invasion of bone marrow by plasma cells or the development of myelodysplasia or acute leukemia also may be responsible. Performance of a bone marrow aspiration and biopsy with chromosome studies readily makes the correct diagnosis apparent. The presence of ringed sideroblasts in the bone marrow and missing chromosomes 5 or 7 are characteristic of myelodysplasia or acute leukemia. Le Beau et al.[201] found a clonal chromosomal abnormality in 97% of 63 patients with a therapy-related myelodysplastic syndrome or acute non-lymphocytic leukemia after chemotherapy or radiotherapy. Fifty-five of these 63 patients (87%) had a clonal abnormality of chromosomes 5 or 7 or both. Also, antileukemic therapy is disappointing, and survival is short.[202]

In conclusion, it seems reasonable to continue chemotherapy for 1 to 2 years and then stop if the M protein levels in the serum and urine have been stable for at least 6 months and the patient has no other evidence of active disease. The patient should be followed closely, however, and chemotherapy reinstituted when relapse occurs.

The role of interferon-α_2 in the prolongation of remission in patients with multiple myeloma is of great interest. In one recent report, 101 patients who had obtained an objective response or stable disease after chemotherapy either with single or multiple alkylating agents were randomized to receive interferon-α_2 or no treatment for maintenance. The relapse rate was 40% for patients given interferon-α_2 for maintenance and 67% for those randomized to no-maintenance therapy, and the median duration of response was 25.8 months for those receiving interferon-α_2 and 14.2 months for the control group. The median survival from the time of randomization was 38.3 months in the control group, but this had not been reached in those receiving interferon-α_2.[203]

TREATMENT OF REFRACTORY MULTIPLE MYELOMA. Almost all patients with multiple myeloma who respond to chemotherapy eventually will relapse if they do not die of another disease. Further, approximately one third of patients initially treated with chemotherapy will not obtain an objective response. The highest response rates reported for patients with multiple myeloma resistant to alkylating agents have been with VAD (vincristine, Adriamycin [doxorubicin], and dexamethasone). VAD has induced remission in two thirds of patients who had relapsed, whereas dexamethasone alone produced remission in only 21%.[204] VBAP—a combination of vincristine (2 mg), carmustine (30 mg/m^2), and doxorubicin (30 mg/m^2) on day 1 and prednisone (60 mg daily) for 5 days—every 3 to 4 weeks has produced some benefit in approximately 40% of patients. Interferon has been disappointing in the therapy of patients with multiple myeloma refractory to alkylating agents,[205] and results from combinations of chemotherapeutic agents as well as newer single agents for

patients with previously treated myeloma have been summarized elsewhere.[206]

NEWER THERAPEUTIC APPROACHES. The use of high-dose melphalan therapy (140 mg/m^2 as a single intravenous dose) produced a complete response in 27% of 41 previously untreated patients age 63 years or younger.[207] However, the median duration of remission was a disappointing 19 months.

The combination of VBMCP (vincristine, carmustine, melphalan, cyclophosphamide, and prednisone) with alternating cycles of interferon-α_2 has produced an objective response in 80% of previously untreated patients with myeloma; 40% in one study had a complete or near-complete response.[208] This experience has resulted in a prospective randomized study currently under way by the Eastern Cooperative Oncology Group, in which patients are randomized to VBMCP, VBMCP plus interferon-α_2 in alternating cycles, or VBMCP with high-dose cyclophosphamide in cycles 3 and 5. To obtain more biologic data to develop better therapeutic approaches, the plasma cell labelling index, β_2-microglobulin level, ploidy determination, presence of circulating myeloma cells, phenotyping, T and B lymphocyte subsets, morphologic review, and clonal DNA analysis are being analyzed at regular intervals.

Bone marrow transplantation from an identical twin (syngeneic) has been reported in five cases, and one of these five died at 1 month from cytomegalovirus-associated interstitial pneumonitis. Three had relapse of myeloma at 6, 17, and 18 months, and the fifth was alive and well after 5.5 years but with a small, persistent M protein.[209]

Allogeneic bone marrow transplantations have been performed utilizing HLA-compatible donors. Gahrton et al.[210] reported that 10 of 14 patients with multiple myeloma survived for a median of 12 months. Five had no signs of active myeloma, whereas 4 had minimal persistent disease and one was in relapse. Barlogie et al.[211] used melphalan (140 mg/m^2) and total-body irradiation (850 cGy) followed by autologous or allogeneic bone marrow transplantation; survival ranged from 2 to 14 months.

Autologous bone marrow transplantation potentially is applicable to more patients, but two major problems exist: the eradication of multiple myeloma from the patient, and the removal of myeloma cells and their precursors from the autologous marrow. Purging of the marrow with monoclonal antibodies or chemotherapy is being investigated at several laboratories. The use of stem cells from autologous peripheral blood has reconstituted successfully the marrow of patients with multiple myeloma treated by high-dose chemotherapy and total-body irradiation.[212]

Multidrug resistance to chemotherapy is another major problem in the treatment of multiple myeloma. The use of verapamil to reduce resistance to doxorubicin is an interesting approach.[213]

MONITORING OF RESPONSE. The effect of chemotherapy should be assessed at regular intervals by determination of the hemoglobin as well as serum and urine M-protein concentrations, examination of the bone marrow, and evaluation of skeletal roentgenograms. Objective response consists of the following: at least 50% reduction of M protein in the serum and at least 50% reduction of M protein in urine. Secondary signs of response include increase of hemoglobin by 2.0 g/dl, decrease of plasma cells in the bone marrow by 50%, and increase of performance as well as decrease of pain by two or more grades.

THERAPY FOR SPECIAL PROBLEMS. Hypercalcemia occurs in at least one third of patients with multiple myeloma. It first must be considered to be recognized, and investigation for it is required by the presence of anorexia, nausea, vomiting, polyuria, increased constipation, weakness, confusion, stupor, or coma. When hypercalcemia is symptomatic, treatment is urgent. Hypercalcemia often leads to renal insufficiency, but prompt treatment improves renal function.

Because dehydration often accompanies hypercalcemia, hydrate the patient. Saline solution is the agent of choice, because sodium promotes renal excretion of calcium. The addition of furosemide (Lasix, Hoechst-Roussel Pharmaceuticals, Inc., Somerville, NJ), 40 mg every 4 hours, may be beneficial; during diuretic therapy, electrolyte levels must be closely monitored. In addition to hydration and diuresis, we use prednisone in an initial dose of 100 mg daily; this must be reduced after a few days and discontinued as quickly as possible. If these measures fail, mithramycin may be given intravenously in a dose of 25 μg/kg body weight. It produces its effect within 24 to 48 hours, but hypercalcemia often recurs after 2 to 3 days. Calcitonin has been used with some success as well, but in a prospective study, gallium nitrate was more effective than calcitonin for treatment of calcium-related hypercalcemia.[214] Aminohydroxypropylidene bisphosphonate also is effective in the treatment of hypercalcemia,[215,216] and hemodialysis using a low-calcium dialysate may be useful. Because prolonged bed rest often contributes to hypercalcemia, encourage patients with myeloma to be as active as possible.

One of the major causes of death in multiple myeloma is renal insufficiency. Hypercalcemia is one of the most treatable of the factors producing uremia, and if hyperuricemia occurs, allopurinol provides effective therapy.

If the patient is allergic to this agent, sodium bicarbonate, 0.6 to 0.9 g three or four times daily, and acetazolamide (Diamox), 250 mg at bedtime, should alkalize the urine. Polycitra also may be used.

The development of acute renal failure also is a serious complication in multiple myeloma. Prompt correction of dehydration is of utmost importance, and because metabolic acidosis usually is present, sodium bicarbonate should be administered either orally or intravenously. Furosemide should be given to maintain a high urine flow rate (100 ml/hour), and hemodialysis is necessary for renal failure. Plasmapheresis has been reported to be of benefit as well.[217] In a prospective study, we randomized patients to a regimen of forced diuresis and chemotherapy or to forced diuresis, chemotherapy, and plasmapheresis; we found that patients with severe myeloma cast formation or other irreversible changes were unlikely to benefit from plasmapheresis.[218] Also, renal transplantation for myeloma kidney has resulted in prolonged survival. Obviously, the multiple myeloma must be kept under control.

Bacterial infections are frequent in myeloma and often are fatal. Significant fever is an indication for appropriate cultures, roentgenography, and consideration of antibiotic therapy; the selection of antibiotics can be made more specific once the results of the cultures are known. Occasionally, in cases of multiple, recurrent, and severe bacterial infections, we have used penicillin prophylactically with good results. Intravenously administered γ-globulin is helpful but expensive, and pneumococcal vaccine and influenza immunization should be given to all patients with multiple myeloma despite their impairment of antibody response.

Among the major problems of patients with myeloma are skeletal lesions, with pain and fracture. Although bone lesions are reported to heal with chemotherapy, we have been disappointed in this regard. Frequently, a brace or supporting garment is helpful, but avoidance of trauma is more important as even mild stress may result in multiple fractures. Nevertheless, encourage the patient to be as active as possible, because confinement to bed increases demineralization of the skeleton. Give analgesics to control pain so the patient can be ambulatory, and physical therapy also may be beneficial. Fixation of a long-bone fracture with an intramedullary rod and methacrylate has given very satisfactory results in our experience. Oral diphosphonates, which reduce osteoblastic activity, may be helpful as well, and the use of fluoride, which stimulates osteoblastic activity, and calcium, which produces calcification of the osteoid tissue, may be of benefit.

Symptomatic hyperviscosity, which may include oronasal bleeding, blurred vision, neurologic symptoms, and congestive heart failure, should be treated with plasma exchange. Most patients have symptoms when the relative serum viscosity reaches 6 or 7 cP (normal, <1.8 cP), but the relationship between serum viscosity and clinical manifestations is not precise.

An extradural plasmacytoma pressing the spinal cord must be considered in every patient with multiple myeloma who develops weakness of the lower extremities or difficulty in voiding or defecating. The sudden onset of severe thoracic pain or the presence of a paraspinal mass also raises the possibility of spinal cord compression. In the event of any of these symptoms, magnetic resonance imaging, computed tomography, or myelography is essential. Radiation therapy in a dose of approximately 3000 rads (30 Gy) is helpful, but dexamethasone must be administered daily during radiation therapy to reduce edema. If the neurologic deficit worsens during irradiation, surgical decompression must be done and radiotherapy then resumed.

In nearly every case of myeloma, anemia eventually develops, and transfusion of packed red cells remains the cornerstone of therapy. A hemoglobin concentration of 8 to 10 g/dl is adequate in most cases unless there is significant coronary artery disease or cerebrovascular insufficiency. Successful treatment for the primary disease with alkylating agents and corticosteroids may restore erythropoiesis. Androgens also may raise the hemoglobin level in some patients, but in our experience, the results generally have been disappointing. Erythropoietin has been reported to increase hemoglobin levels in patients with multiple myeloma, and this may be a useful therapeutic approach in patients during a plateau state who have symptoms of anemia.[219]

Any patient with a serious disease such as multiple myeloma has psychologic problems as well and needs substantial and continuing emotional support. The approach must be positive. The physician must have confidence in his or her ability to cope with the patient's problems, and the patient should be able to sense this confidence. Potential benefits of therapy should be emphasized; it reassures the patient to know that some persons survive for 10 or more years while receiving treatment. It is vital that the physician caring for the patient with myeloma has both the interest and the capacity to deal with incurable disease over a span of months to years with assurance, sympathy, and resourcefulness.

VARIANT FORMS OF MYELOMA

Smoldering Multiple Myeloma

The diagnosis of smoldering multiple myeloma depends on the presence of an M protein greater than 3 g/dl in the serum and more than 10% atypical plasma cells in the bone marrow but no anemia, renal insufficiency, or skeletal lesions.[220] Often, a small amount of M protein is found in the urine, and the concentration of uninvolved or normal immunoglobulins in the serum is decreased. Clusters or aggregates of plasma cells often are seen in the biopsy specimen of the bone marrow, and the plasma cell labelling index is low. In some patients, symptomatic multiple myeloma does not develop for years. It is important to recognize these patients, because they should not be treated unless progression occurs. One must realize that most patients who satisfy the criteria for the diagnosis of multiple myeloma have symptomatic disease and require therapy. Patients with smoldering multiple myeloma also constitute less than 5% of patients with multiple myeloma. Biologically, patients with smoldering multiple myeloma have a "benign" monoclonal gammopathy (monoclonal gammopathy of undetermined significance), but it is difficult to accept that diagnosis initially when the M protein is more than 3 g/dl and the bone marrow contains more than 10% plasma cells.

Plasma Cell Leukemia

Patients with plasma cell leukemia have more than 20% plasma cells in the peripheral blood and an absolute plasma cell content of at least 2000 cells/µl. Plasma cell leukemia may be classified as primary when it is diagnosed in the leukemic phase, or as secondary when there is leukemic transformation of a previously recognized multiple myeloma. Approximately 60% of patients have the primary form. Patients with primary plasma cell leukemia are younger (median age, 53 vs. 62 years), have a greater incidence of hepatosplenomegaly (50% vs. 17%) and lymphadenopathy (12% vs. 6%), a higher platelet count (94,000 vs. 26,000 cells/µl), fewer lytic bone lesions (44% vs. 72%), a small serum M-protein component (median, 1.6 vs. 4.4 g/dl), and a longer survival (median, 6.8 vs. 1.3 months) than patients with secondary plasma cell leukemia.

Treatment of primary plasma cell leukemia is unsatisfactory at present. Melphalan and prednisone may produce remission,[221] and while the response rate is higher with combination chemotherapy than with a single alkylating agent, unfortunately, the survival is still short.

Secondary plasma cell leukemia rarely responds to chemotherapy, because affected patients already have received alkylating agents and are resistant to them. In our series, the median survival was 1.3 months.[222]

Nonsecretory Myeloma

Patients with nonsecretory myeloma have no M protein in either their serum or urine; in our experience, this occurs in less than 1% of patients with multiple myeloma. From January 1, 1982, to December 31, 1986, we saw 462 patients with multiple myeloma, including 14 who had no M protein in the serum and urine; however, 10 of these 14 had had an M protein at the time of diagnosis elsewhere and had been treated when we first saw them. Only 4 patients had no M protein in their serum or urine at the time of diagnosis. Thus, approximately 1% of our patients with multiple myeloma had the nonsecretory form. For certainty of diagnosis, a monoclonal protein must be identified in the plasma cells by immunoperoxidase or immunofluorescence methods. In some patients, evidence of a monoclonal protein cannot be found within the cell, suggesting that no such protein is present, and more than a dozen such patients have been described.[223]

The more carefully the serum and urine are studied for evidence of a monoclonal protein, the fewer cases of nonsecretory myeloma will be found. In one instance, a small monoclonal IgG-κ protein was found with immunoisoelectric focusing after repeated electrophoreses and immunoelectrophoreses were negative.[224]

Survival similar to that of patients with multiple myeloma[225] or longer[226] has been reported.

IgD Myeloma

IgD myeloma differs enough in a number of respects from IgG and IgA myeloma to warrant discussion as a separate entity, and more than 130 cases have been reported since the discovery of IgD immunoglobulin in 1965.[227] The size of the electrophoretic peak of serum monoclonal protein usually is much less than that seen in IgG and IgA myeloma; indeed, more than 10% of cases have no visible monoclonal component on serum electrophoresis. Monoclonal λ light chains have been reported in 90% of patients, but in our experience, only 55% had a monoclonal λ-protein. Plasma cell leukemia, amyloidosis, and extramedullary plasmacytomas have been reported more frequently with IgD myeloma, and survival generally is believed to be less than with other types. However, IgD myeloma often is not diagnosed until later in its course.[228] We have seen several patients with IgD myeloma who survived longer than 5 years.

Osteosclerotic Myeloma (POEMS Syndrome)

The major clinical feature in osteosclerotic myeloma is a chronic inflammatory-demyelinating polyneuropathy with predominantly motor disability. Single or multiple osteosclerotic bone lesions are characteristic,[229] and the acronym *POEMS* (*p*olyneuropathy, *o*rga-

nomegaly, *e*ndocrinopathy, *M* protein, and *s*kin changes) describes the complete syndrome.[230]

Symptoms of peripheral neuropathy generally precede the diagnosis. Sensory symptoms consisting of tingling and paresthesias are followed by weakness. The symptoms begin in the feet and spread proximally, and severe weakness occurs in most patients. Except for the presence of papilledema, the cranial nerves are not involved; the autonomic nervous system is intact. Hepatomegaly occurs in almost one half of patients, but splenomegaly and lymphadenopathy occur only in a minority. Hyperpigmentation and hypertrichosis may be striking, and gynecomastia and atrophic testes as well as clubbing of the fingers and toes may be seen.

In contrast to multiple myeloma, the hemoglobin level usually is normal, and polycythemia often is present.[231] Thrombocytosis occurs in more than one half of patients, but renal insufficiency and hypercalcemia rarely are found. The bone marrow aspirate and biopsy usually contain less than 5% plasma cells, so myeloma rarely can be diagnosed solely on the basis of the bone marrow examination. A monoclonal protein is found in the serum in most cases, but the size is usually modest (median, 1.1 g/dl) and rarely more than 3 g/dl. Almost all are λ.[232] The presence of a monoclonal light chain in the urine (Bence Jones proteinuria) is infrequent, but when present, it is of modest amount. The protein level in cerebrospinal fluid is elevated, and slowing of conduction velocities in motor nerves is found. Osteosclerotic lesions also are seen in the roentgenograms of all patients; the lesions may be small and misinterpreted as benign bony sclerosis. The diagnosis is confirmed by biopsy of an osteosclerotic lesion and demonstration of a plasmacytoma.

Castleman disease (plasma-cell type) may be found.[233] Osteosclerotic myeloma also may be associated with angiofollicular lymphoid lesions resembling Castleman disease.[234]

In patients with a single lesion or multiple osteolytic lesions in a limited area, radiation will produce substantial improvement of the neuropathy in more than one half. In patients with widespread osteosclerotic lesions, chemotherapy with melphalan and prednisone may be helpful.

Solitary Plasmacytoma (Solitary Myeloma) of Bone

There can be no doubt that some plasmacytomas arise singly and remain solitary, but in most instances, widespread multiple myeloma develops years after the initial lesion. Indeed, some regard solitary plasmacytoma as only the first manifestation of multiple myeloma. The diagnosis of the solitary plasmacytoma is based on histologic proof that the tumor consists of plasma cells identical to those seen in myeloma, and in addition to histologic confirmation of the identity of the lesion, complete skeletal roentgenograms must show no other lesions of myeloma, the bone marrow aspirate must contain no evidence of multiple myeloma, and immuno-electrophoresis of the serum and concentrated urine should show no monoclonal protein. Some exceptions to the last criterion occur, but therapy for the solitary lesion usually results in disappearance of the monoclonal protein.

The most uncertain criterion for the diagnosis of solitary plasmacytoma of bone is the length of observation necessary before being sure that the disease will not become generalized; dissemination or recurrence of plasmacytoma has occurred as late as 21 years after discovery. The potential for multiple myeloma to develop in a patient who has had a solitary plasmacytoma exists for many years, and there can never be absolute certainty that multiple myeloma will not occur at some later date. However, the possibility that a plasmacytoma will remain solitary is supported by a case without evidence of multiple myeloma 35 years after histologic diagnosis of the solitary plasmacytoma. Meyer and Schulz[235] reported that 9 of their 12 patients with solitary myeloma showed dissemination 2 to 10 years after diagnosis (average, 5 years). In a review of 96 published cases and 18 personal cases of solitary myeloma, Bataille and Sany[236] reported that 12% had local recurrence, 15% had new solitary lesions at distant sites, and 58% had developed typical multiple myeloma at the end of 10 years. Disease-free survival at 10 years ranges from 15% to 25%;[236,237] approximately 50% of patients with solitary plasmacytoma of bone survive for 10 years.[237,238] There is some truth in the adage that a solitary plasmacytoma is one that grows slowly enough for the patient to die of some other disease.

Treatment for solitary plasmacytoma consists of supervoltage irradiation in the range of 4000 to 5000 rads. There is no evidence that surgical removal of the plasmacytoma is superior to adequate irradiation; amputation is not indicated for solitary plasmacytoma. Electrophoresis, immunoelectrophoresis, and immunofixation of the serum and urine are helpful in following the course of a solitary plasmacytoma.

Extramedullary Plasmacytoma

Plasma cell tumors that arise outside the bone marrow are extramedullary plasmacytomas. They may behave benignly or may disseminate later to produce widespread disease. They may be single or multiple and may or may not be invasive. The upper respiratory tract, including the nasal cavity and sinuses, nasopharynx, and larynx, is the most frequent location of lesions,[239] and extramedullary plasmacytomas also may involve the esophagus, stomach, small or large bowel, kidney, skin, testes, thyroid, orbit, salivary glands, dura mater, brain, urinary bladder, thyroid, lung, breast, and lymph nodes.[160] Epistaxis, rhinorrhea, and nasal obstruction are the most frequent symptoms. Extramedullary plasmacytomas also may spread locally or develop into widespread multiple myeloma.

Woodruff et al.[240] reported 14 cases of extramedullary plasmacytoma, and after treatment with radiotherapy, only 1 had persistent local disease and 1 subsequently showed evidence of disseminated myeloma. Among another group of 12 patients with extramedullary plasmacytoma, only 2 subsequently developed multiple myeloma during a follow-up period of 14 to 320 months.[241] Knowling et al.[242] reported progression in 5 of 25 patients; 1 developed a single bony lesion, 2 had progression to multiple myeloma, and 2 developed multiple extramedullary plasmacytomas. Predominance of IgA monoclonal proteins in extramedullary plasmacytoma has been noted as well.[243]

The diagnosis depends on the documentation of a plasmacytoma that stains with a single heavy-chain type and single light-chain class. Computed tomography is useful in delineating the extent of the plasmacytoma, and treatment consists of tumoricidal radiation.

WALDENSTRÖM MACROGLOBULINEMIA (PRIMARY MACROGLOBULINEMIA)

In 1944, Waldenström described two patients with oronasal bleeding, severe normocytic and normochromic anemia, excessive erythrocyte sedimentation, lymphadenopathy, and low serum fibrinogen values.[244] Both had an abnormally large amount of a homogeneous γ-globulin with a sedimentation coefficient of 19S to 20S, corresponding to a molecular weight of more than 1,000,000. (The description of a third patient did not permit a definite diagnosis of macroglobulinemia.) Subsequently, the serum globulin was identified as an immunoglobulin and was designated IgM. As an entity, macroglobulinemia bears similarities to multiple myeloma, lymphoma, and chronic lymphocytic leukemia, and it should be considered as a malignant lymphoplasmoproliferative disorder.[245]

Etiology and Pathogenesis

Although the cause of Waldenström macroglobulinemia is unknown, the disease may be more frequent in certain families. In one, two brothers had macroglobulinemia with a very similar clinical pattern and protein abnormality, and serum from their mother also showed a narrow band on electrophoresis and increased IgM on immunoelectrophoresis. Blattner et al.[246] described a father and two children with an IgM monoclonal protein and a lymphoproliferative process and a third child with Waldenström macroglobulinemia. All had HLA haplotype A2, B8, and DRw3, as well as the B-cell alloantigens Ia-172 and 350. Two other family members had thyroiditis. Two studies of relatives of patients with Waldenström macroglobulinemia revealed an increased frequency of IgM monoclonal proteins as well as quantitative abnormalities, suggesting a genetic element in some cases. Macroglobulinemia also has been found in monozygotic twins,[247] and although radiation can cause acute leukemia, there is only one reported case of Waldenström macroglobulinemia occurring after radiotherapy, which was given for ankylosing spondylitis.[248]

Chromosomal abnormalities are frequent, but no specific abnormality has been recognized. In one series, 17 of 19 patients had clonal chromosomal abnormalities most commonly involving chromosomes 10, 11, 12, 15, 20, and 21.[249] Peripheral blood lymphocytes expressed CD9 (BA-2) and CD24 (BA-1) and stained with a single class of light chain. Reduction in CD4 T cells also was common.[250]

The basic abnormality in macroglobulinemia is uncontrolled proliferation of cells with lymphocyte–plasma cell characteristics. They vary morphologically, ranging from small lymphocytes to frank plasma cells, and frequently, their cytoplasm is ragged. Some of the cells contain intranuclear and intracytoplasmic periodic acid-Schiff–positive material that is probably identical to circulating macroglobulin. Electron microscopic features include a well-developed endoplasmic reticulum having rough dilated areas filled with protein. The lymphoplasma cells appear to be the production site of the macroglobulin, which can be demonstrated by immunofluorescence in cells from lymph node imprints, bone marrow, and buffy-coat smears. Idiotypic antibodies have been found on lymphocytes and plasmacytoid cells in the bone marrow and in circulating mature plasma cells in Waldenström macroglobulinemia.[251] All cells with surface idiotypic determinants also had the heavy- and light-chain isotypes of the serum M protein. The lymphocyte immunofluorescent patterns revealed by double staining with antiidiotype and anti–light chain antibodies were identical, firmly supporting the view that this disease is a differentiating B-lymphocyte malignancy.

For the unwary observer, lymph nodes in macroglobulinemia are very difficult to distinguish by light microscopy from nodes in lymphosarcoma or chronic lymphocytic leukemia. Usually, the nodes are normal in size or only slightly enlarged and show capsular, hilar, and trabecular invasion. Retention of a surprisingly normal reticulum pattern, scarcity of peripheral follicles, scantiness of mitotic figures, excess of clearly recognizable plasma cells, presence of periodic acid-Schiff–positive intranuclear inclusions, and increased numbers of mast cells should suggest the diagnosis of macroglobulinemia.

Clinical Manifestations and Related Features

SYMPTOMS AND PHYSICAL SIGNS. Macroglobulinemia of Waldenström has a predilection for older men. In our series of 71 patients, ages ranged from 30 to 89 years (median, 63 years). Only 1% were younger than 40 years, and 62% were male.[252] As a rule, the onset is insidious; weakness, fatigue, and bleeding (especially oozing from the oronasal region) are not uncommon presenting symptoms. Blurring or other impairment of vision affects about one third of patients and may be the major complaint. Recurrent infections, dyspnea, congestive heart failure, weight loss, and neurologic symptoms occur; however, bone pain is virtually nonexistent in contrast to multiple myeloma. Pallor, mild splenomegaly, hepatomegaly, and peripheral lymphadenopathy are the most common physical findings. The liver was palpable in 25% and the spleen in 20% of our patients, and lymphadenopathy was noted in 17%. Retinal lesions, including hemorrhages, exudates, and venous congestion with vascular segmentation (sausage formation) may be the most impressive features, but they can be caused by hyperviscosity from other causes.

NEUROLOGIC MANIFESTATIONS. Some 25% of patients with Waldenström macroglobulinemia have neurologic abnormalities, and these include peripheral neuropathy, a syndrome such as Guillain-Barré, encephalopathy, and subarachnoid hemorrhage. Peripheral neuropathy may be the initial symptom and usually involves both sensory and motor modalities; it appears similar to the peripheral neuropathy of carcinoma or multiple myeloma. Also, IgM has been found in the myelin sheath.[253] Dysfunction of the auditory and vestibular apparatus is not uncommon, and sudden deafness may be the presenting symptom.[254] Progressive spinal muscular atrophy has been reported, as has multifocal leukoencephalopathy. The association of macroglobulinemia and encephalopathy constitutes the Bing-Neel syndrome.

OTHER CLINICAL FEATURES. The incidence of infection is twice that of normal. *Pneumocystis carinii* and cytomegalic inclusion disease have been reported in macroglobulinemia.

A bleeding diathesis in macroglobulinemia is not uncommon. Abnormalities in platelet adhesiveness, prothrombin time, and thromboplastin generation may be seen, and values of factor VIII may be low. Thrombocytopenia or hyperviscosity also may contribute to the bleeding diathesis.

Abnormalities of Other Organs

Renal failure is uncommon. Deposits of IgM on the endothelial aspect of the basement membrane may become large enough to occlude the capillary lumen and resemble thrombi. Lymphocytic or plasma cell infiltration identical to that in the bone marrow has been reported in two thirds of cases. Occasionally, amyloid may be deposited in the glomerulus. Acute renal failure may be precipitated by dehydration. Nephrotic syndrome from deposition of monoclonal IgM with high-titer glomerular autoantibodies to the glomerular basement membrane has been described. The nephrotic syndrome and IgM deposits in the glomerular basement membrane disappeared after chlorambucil and prednisone therapy.[255] Also, approximately 80% of our patients have Bence Jones proteinuria.

Pulmonary involvement is manifested by diffuse pulmonary infiltrates, isolated masses, or pleural effusion. The pulmonary masses consist of plasmacytoid lymphocytes, and the pulmonary lesions often respond to treatment with chlorambucil, cyclophosphamide, or radiation and do not appear to affect prognosis adversely.[256] Pleural effusion also may occur.[257]

Diarrhea and steatorrhea are uncommon complicating features of macroglobulinemia. Deposition of monoclonal IgM or the infiltration of lymphocytes and plasma cells may be responsible;[258] nodular regenerative hyperplasia of the liver has been found in three patients with a monoclonal IgM protein and in a fourth with a polyclonal increase of IgM. Three of the patients had a lymphoproliferative process.[259] Involvement of the orbit and lacrimal glands also has been seen in macroglobulinemia.

Macroglobulinemia has been reported in association with amyloidosis, nonlymphoid malignancies, rheumatoid arthritis, ankylosing spondylitis, Sjögren syndrome, and acute leukemia.

Hyperviscosity Syndrome

Bleeding is the most common symptom, with chronic nasal bleeding and oozing from the gums the most frequent, but the same condition may be manifested as postsurgical hemorrhage or gastrointestinal bleeding. Flame-shaped retinal hemorrhages are common, and papilledema may be seen. The patient may complain of blurring or loss of vision, and neurologic symptoms include dizziness, headache, vertigo, nystagmus, decreased hearing, ataxia, paresthesias, diplopia, somnolence, and coma. Hyperviscosity can precipitate or aggravate congestive heart failure.[260]

In our experience, 15 of 51 patients (29.4%) with Waldenström macroglobulinemia had a serum viscosity of more than 4 cP (normal, ≤ 1.8 cP). Unexpectedly, 5 of the patients had no symptoms related to hyperviscosity. Nine patients had bleeding, and 3 complained of blurred vision.[252] Crawford et al.[261] also reported that six of eight patients with a serum viscosity of more than 5 cP had symptoms, but none of their patients had symptoms of hyperviscosity if the level was less than 3 cP.

Most patients have symptoms when the relative serum viscosity reaches 6 or 7 cP. The relation between serum viscosity and clinical manifestations is not precise, and we have seen a patient with a serum viscosity of 15 cP who had no symptoms of the hyperviscosity syndrome. Although this syndrome is common in macroglobulinemia, it also may be associated with either IgG or IgA myeloma, especially if the IgA myeloma protein is polymerized.[262] Hyperviscosity was present in 4.2% of a series of 234 patients with IgG myeloma,[263] and patients with symptomatic hyperviscosity should be treated with plasmapheresis. Plasma exchange of 3000 to 4000 ml should be performed daily until the patient is asymptomatic; the blood volume should be maintained with albumin rather than plasma.

Laboratory Findings

PERIPHERAL BLOOD AND BONE MARROW. Almost all patients with Waldenström macroglobulinemia have moderate to severe degrees of normocytic and normochromic anemia. Depression of erythropoiesis (presumably caused by the abnormal proliferation of lymphocytes in the marrow) and excessive destruction or loss of red cells are the usual causes. Occasionally, Coombs-positive hemolytic anemia is seen. The plasma volume may be increased greatly, thus lessening the hemoglobin and hematocrit values independently of change in the red cell mass so that the anemia may be more apparent than real. Rouleaux formation is striking, and erythrocyte sedimentation is increased greatly. Occasionally, it may be recorded as 0 because of the excessive gelation of the protein. The leukocyte and platelet counts usually, however, are normal, but mild decreases may be seen. Lymphocytosis or monocytosis is not uncommon. In many cases of macroglobulinemia, the serum cholesterol concentration is low, particularly if the amount of protein is large. Hyperuricemia also may be present.

The bone marrow aspirate usually is hypocellular, but fixed sections are very cellular and extensively infiltrated with lymphoid cells. The lymphocytes tend to be small, often are basophilic, and resemble plasma cells. Naked nuclei are common, and small ragged lymphocytes with so-called cytoplasmic shedding may be evident. The number of plasma cells always is greater than normal, and normal marrow elements are correspondingly decreased. Also, the number of mast cells is increased, which may help to differentiate macroglobulinemia from myeloma or lymphoma.

PROTEIN ABNORMALITIES. The serum protein electrophoretic pattern of Waldenström macroglobulinemia is indistinguishable from that of multiple myeloma; it is a sharp, narrow peak or dense band migrating with γ- or β-globulin mobility. Analysis of serum by immunoelectrophoresis with a specific antiserum to IgM (μ-chain) reveals a localized dense precipitin arc (Fig. 16.18). Approximately 75% of monoclonal IgM proteins are of the κ type. In our series of 71 cases, the M spike ranged from 3 to 7.9 g/dl (median, 4.3 g/dl), and 80% of our patients had a monoclonal light chain in the urine. Frequently, low-molecular-weight (7S) IgM is present, and it may account for as much as 40% of the excess IgM immunoglobulins. About 10% of macroglobulins are cryoprecipitable and are designated as macrocryoglobulins.

ROENTGENOGRAPHIC FEATURES. The bones most often appear normal, but diffuse osteoporosis may be seen. Bone destruction with lytic lesions occurs in less than 10% of cases. Lymphangiography in Waldenström macroglobulinemia often shows enlarged nodes with irregular filling defects and a reticular or "foamy" appearance indistinguishable from lymphosarcoma.

Diagnosis

The combination of typical symptoms and physical findings, usually more than 3 g/dl of monoclonal IgM protein, as well as appropriate abnormalities of the bone marrow provide the diagnosis of Waldenström macroglobulinemia. The major problems in differential diagnosis involve the distinction from multiple myeloma, chronic lymphocytic leukemia, lymphoma, and monoclonal gammopathy of undetermined significance of the IgM type. These diseases are closely related, and some patients actually have characteristics of more than one disorder.

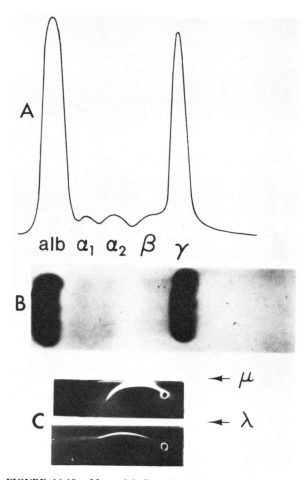

FIGURE 16.18. **Macroglobulinemia.** *A,* **The monoclonal pattern of serum protein as traced by densitometer after electrophoresis on cellulose, showing a tall, narrow-based peak of γ mobility.** *B,* **The monoclonal pattern from electrophoresis of serum on cellulose acetate (anode on left); the dense, localized band at the right represents a monoclonal protein.** *C,* **Immunoelectrophoresis showing a dense μ-arc and a similar λ-arc. The patient has an IgM-λ monoclonal protein.** *Source:* **Kyle and Greipp 1978[63] Reprinted with permission of the Mayo Foundation**

In our review of 430 patients with an IgM monoclonal gammopathy, we defined Waldenström macroglobulinemia as having an IgM serum spike of 3 g/dl or more and an increase in lymphocytes or plasma cells in the bone marrow. We defined a malignant lymphoproliferative process as an increase in lymphocytes and plasma cells in the bone marrow, no evidence of chronic lymphocytic leukemia or lymphoma, and a serum spike of less than 3 g/dl. The patients with malignant lymphoproliferative disease required therapy because of anemia or constitutional symptoms, and their median survival is essentially the same as patients with Waldenström macroglobulinemia (5.5 vs. 5.0 years). There is no reason to separate patients with a malignant lymphoproliferative disease from those with Waldenström macroglobulinemia on the basis of the size of their M spike.[252]

The presence of a monoclonal IgM protein less than 2.0 g/dl, absence of anemia and organomegaly, presence of mild lymphocytosis of the bone marrow, and no constitutional symptoms are suggestive of monoclonal gammopathy of undetermined significance of the IgM type. Long-term follow-up of 242 patients with monoclonal gammopathy of undetermined significance of the IgM type revealed that 40 (17%) developed a serious disease (Waldenström macroglobulinemia in 22, lymphoproliferative disease in 9, lymphoma in 6, chronic lymphocytic leukemia in 1, and amyloidosis in 2); the median duration from recognition of the M protein until development of serious disease ranged from 4 to 9 years. Nineteen additional patients had an increase in the serum M spike, but the diagnosis of macroglobulinemia or other malignant lymphoproliferative disease could not be made. The patient with monoclonal gammopathy of undetermined significance must be observed carefully, because in some patients with apparently benign monoclonal gammopathy, Waldenström macroglobulinemia or related diseases subsequently develop.[252]

We have seen several patients with IgA or IgG multiple myeloma but a large number of lymphocytoid cells in the bone marrow.[264] Levine et al.[265] also have recognized patients with plasmacytoid–lymphocytic morphology but with a monoclonal IgG or IgA protein. We classify such cases as IgG or IgA myeloma. Conversely, we have seen patients with large amounts of monoclonal IgM proteins in the serum, anemia, oronasal bleeding, and blurred vision, but who also had lytic bone lesions and typical immature plasma cells of the bone marrow characteristic of myeloma. We prefer to classify these cases as macroglobulinemia rather than as IgM myeloma.[266,267] Although the problem is insoluble at present, results of future studies, including data on the response to melphalan or chlorambucil, may show how to combine or separate these entities correctly.

IgM may be increased in various disorders, including rheumatoid arthritis, Sjögren syndrome, lupus erythematosus, cirrhosis, recurrent infections, parasitic infestations, and sarcoidosis. In these conditions, the macroglobulins usually are polyclonal and their concentration in the serum generally lower than in Waldenström macroglobulinemia with monoclonal IgM.

Course and Treatment

In our experience, the median survival of patients with Waldenström macroglobulinemia is 5 years. Bartl et al.[268] distinguished three types of macroglobulinemia based on bone marrow involvement: lymphoplasmacytoid (47%), lymphoplasmacytic (42%), and polymorphous (11%) and median survivals of 74, 25, and 12 months, respectively.

Patients with Waldenström macroglobulinemia should not be treated unless they have anemia; constitutional symptoms such as weakness, fatigue, night sweats, weight loss, or hyperviscosity; or significant hepatosplenomegaly or lymphadenopathy. Patients with monoclonal gammopathy of undetermined significance should not be treated but should be followed carefully for the development of symptomatic disease.

Specific therapy should be directed against the abnormal proliferation of lymphocytes and plasma cells. Chlorambucil, in an initial dose of 6 to 8 mg daily, is a useful agent, but the dosage must be altered depending on the leukocyte and platelet counts, which should be determined every 2 weeks. A combination of chlorambucil and prednisone for 1 week every 4 to 6 weeks also is efficacious, and combination chemotherapy with the M-2 protocol (carmustine, cyclophosphamide, vincristine, melphalan, and prednisone) may be helpful.[269] Acute leukemia may develop in patients who have had macroglobulinemia treated with alkylating agents;[270] consequently, chemotherapy should be discontinued if the patient has been treated for 2 years and the disease has reached a plateau. Chemotherapy should be reinstituted when the disease relapses. If hyperviscosity is present, plasma exchange will alleviate the symptoms quickly.

Transfusions of packed red cells should be given for symptomatic anemia. One must be aware of the increased plasma volume in many of these patients, resulting in spuriously low hemoglobin and hematocrit levels; consequently, transfusion therapy should not be based only on a low hemoglobin or hematocrit value.

CRYOGLOBULINEMIA

Cryoglobulins (proteins that precipitate or gel when cooled and dissolve when heated) (Fig. 16.19) may be classified simply in the following categories: type I, monoclonal, consisting of IgG, IgM, IgA, or rarely, monoclonal light chains (Bence Jones proteins); type II, mixed, in which two or more immunoglobulins are found and one is monoclonal; and type III, polyclonal, in which no monoclonal protein is found. Cryoglobulins also are designated as idiopathic or essential when they are not associated with any recognizable disease.

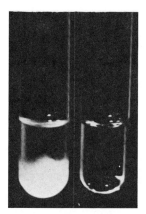

FIGURE 16.19.   Cryoglobulinemia. The *left panel* shows the precipitate formed at exposure to 0°C. The *right panel* shows the disappearance of the precipitate when heated to 37°C. *Source*: Kyle and Greipp 1978[63] Reprinted with permission of the Mayo Foundation

In most cases, monoclonal cryoglobulins (type I) are IgM or IgG, but IgA and Bence Jones cryoglobulins have been reported. Type I cryoglobulins are associated with macroglobulinemia, multiple myeloma, or monoclonal gammopathy of undetermined significance, and the protein itself probably undergoes a temperature-dependent conformational change that results in polymerization at low temperatures.[271]

Patients with monoclonal cryoglobulinemia may have symptoms of cold intolerance such as Raynaud phenomenon, purpura, cold urticaria, neuropathy, leg ulcers, and gangrene of the extremities. Indeed, we have seen severe Raynaud phenomenon as well as skin ulceration and sloughing occur in several patients with only 1 to 2 g/dl of monoclonal IgG protein because their cryoglobulins precipitated at 25°C to 26°C.[272] In contrast, however, we have been impressed with a number of patients who had 4 to 5 g/dl of a monoclonal IgG or IgM cryoprotein but no symptoms whatever on exposure to cold.

Cryoglobulinemia may produce a spurious elevation of the leukocyte count by the model S Coulter counter. It is thought this is caused by particles formed by combination of the cryoglobulin and fibrinogen.

Most commonly, mixed cryoglobulins (type II) consist of IgM–IgG, but IgG–IgG and IgA–IgG have been reported.[273] Usually, the quantity of the cold-precipitating protein is less than 0.2 g/dl and the serum protein electrophoretic pattern indicates normality or diffuse hypergammaglobulinemia.

Clinical Manifestations

Patients with mixed cryoglobulinemia frequently have vasculitis, glomerulonephritis, or lymphoproliferative or chronic infectious processes. Purpura and polyarthralgias are common as well. Involvement of the joints is symmetrical, but deformities rarely develop. Raynaud phenomenon, necrosis of the skin, and neurologic symptoms may occur,[274] and renal involvement also is common. In almost 80% of biopsy specimens, glomerular damage can be seen as a diffuse, proliferative glomerulonephritis, with thickening of the glomerular basement membrane.[275] A nephrotic syndrome may occur,[276] but renal insufficiency is not common. Development of end-stage renal failure also is infrequent. Hepatic dysfunction and serologic evidence of previous infection with hepatitis B virus have been reported in some series as well.[277] Infiltration of liver portal tracts with lymphocytes that stain with the same immunoglobulin type as in the serum was noted in 9 of 12 cases of essential mixed cryoglobulinemia, and the bone marrow biopsy specimens of most of these patients had multiple foci of plasmacytoid cells. The authors postulated that many cases of mixed cryoglobulinemia may have a low-grade lymphomatous process.[278]

Treatment

Orally administered corticosteroids are the most frequently used therapeutic agents. If there is no response, α_2 interferon, cyclophosphamide, chlorambucil, or azathioprine may be useful, and plasmapheresis has been effective in some instances. The physician must be aware that renal manifestations will wax and wane and that spontaneous remissions may occur.

Type III (polyclonal) cryoglobulinemia is not associated with a monoclonal component.[279] Polyclonal cryoglobulinemia is found in many patients with infectious or inflammatory diseases, and it usually is asymptomatic.

PYROGLOBULINEMIA

Pyroglobulins are immunoglobulins that precipitate when heated to 56°C and do not dissolve when cooled.[280] They resemble Bence Jones proteins in that they precipitate when heated from 56°C to 60°C, but they can be distinguished easily by immunoelectrophoresis with appropriate antisera. Pyroglobulins usually are of the IgG class, but IgM and IgA have been reported.[281] In most cases, pyroglobulinemia is associated with multiple myeloma, but it also may occur in macroglobulinemia, lymphoproliferative syndromes, and other neoplastic diseases. Pyroglobulinemia is not associated with any symptoms and may be regarded as a laboratory curiosity.

CRYOFIBRINOGEN

Cryofibrinogen becomes apparent when plasma is cooled to 0°C. Its presence was recognized first in a case of bronchogenic carcinoma. Cryofibrinogens are not uncommon, and they have been associated with metastatic carcinoma, connective tissue diseases, myocardial infarction, pregnancy, and even with normal health.

HEAVY-CHAIN DISEASES

Heavy-chain diseases are characterized by the presence of monoclonal proteins that comprise a portion of the immunoglobulin heavy chain in the serum, urine, or both. In the first report of γ heavy-chain disease, Franklin et al.[282] postulated the existence of two additional heavy-chain diseases, α and μ, a prophecy now fulfilled. These heavy chains are devoid of light chains and represent a lymphoplasma cell proliferative process.

γ Heavy-Chain Disease

The abnormal protein consists of a γ-chain with significant deletions of amino acids, including the deletion of the CH1 domain of the constant (C) region in all instances. The molecular weight of the monomeric chain ranges from 27,000 to 49,000.

Patients with γ heavy-chain disease usually present with a lymphoma-like illness, but the clinical findings are diverse, ranging from an aggressive lymphoproliferative process to an asymptomatic state.[283] The median age is approximately 61 years, but the disease has begun before the age of 20 years in several cases.

Weakness, fatigue, and fever are common, but other features that have been noted include parotid swelling, severe soreness of the tongue, nodular infiltration of the skin, extranodal non-Hodgkin lymphoma, autoimmune hemolytic anemia, idiopathic thrombocytopenic purpura, rapid enlargement of the thyroid, neutropenia from hypersplenism, and an atypical lymphoproliferative process. Hepatosplenomegaly and lymphadenopathy were seen in about 60% of patients in one study.[283]

Laboratory abnormalities included anemia in 79% of patients initially and in nearly all eventually. Five patients had a Coombs-positive autoimmune hemolytic anemia, and the serum protein electrophoretic pattern frequently showed no localized band or spike. In fact, the electrophoretogram often showed a broad-based band more suggestive of a polyclonal than a monoclonal protein (Fig. 16.20). Some patterns revealed hypogammaglobulinemia and a very small increase in the β-band. Other patterns appeared normal, and immunoelectrophoresis was necessary for detection of the monoclonal γ heavy chain. The mobility of the monoclonal protein was most commonly in the β-area but ranged from α_1 to slow γ. The level of the monoclonal serum protein varied from immeasurable to 9 g/dl, and in 76% of cases, it was IgG1 subclass. Proteinuria ranged from a trace to 20 g daily but was less than 1 g in most cases. Increased numbers of plasma cells, lymphocytes, or plasmacytoid lymphocytes were seen in the bone marrow and lymph node biopsies, and the histologic picture was variable. One of our patients had a typical plasmacytoma of the thyroid, while another had an extranodal non-Hodgkin lymphoma. γ Heavy-chain disease has been associated with nodular sclerosing Hodgkin disease[284] and rheumatoid arthritis,[285] and Hodgkin disease was reported in a patient with a serum protein electrophoretic abnormality who subsequently developed symptomatic Hodgkin disease (mixed cellularity). The Hodgkin disease responded to chemotherapy, but the γ heavy chain persisted in both the serum and urine.[286] The presence of the γ heavy-chain protein does not appear to influence the course or prognosis of the underlying disorder.[287]

The clinical course of γ heavy-chain disease varies from a rapid progression downhill, with death in a few weeks, to the asymptomatic presence of a stable monoclonal heavy chain in the serum and urine. In one case, the monoclonal γ heavy chain disappeared without therapy, and in another, it disappeared after recovery from a serious illness. The clinical course may be prolonged; for instance, the diagnosis in one case was preceded 22 years before by cervical lymphadenopathy and 17 years before by hemolytic anemia. The median survival among 49 cases reported in the literature was 12 months, with a range of 1 to 264 months.

Treatment is not indicated for the asymptomatic patient. We have seen responses to cyclophosphamide, vincristine, and prednisone in combination. If there is no response to this regimen, doxorubicin should be added.

Nine additional patients with γ heavy-chain disease differed in that they had a monoclonal complete immunoglobulin in the serum as well as a monoclonal γ heavy chain in the serum or urine. In addition, seven of these patients had Bence Jones proteinuria. The clinical patterns in these cases varied.

α Heavy-Chain Disease

First described in 1968, α heavy-chain disease has become the most frequently reported type, with more

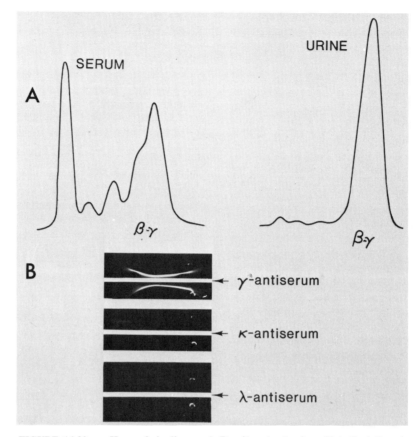

FIGURE 16.20. γ **Heavy-chain disease.** *A,* **Densitometer tracings. Note the tall peak of β–γ mobility in serum and the tall β–γ peak in urine.** *B,* **Immunoelectrophoresis. The** *top well* **in each immunoelectrophoretic pattern represents serum; the** *bottom well* **represents concentrated urine. With γ-antiserum, a dense, thickened, asymmetric arc is seen in both serum and urine. With κ-antiserum, a faint, fuzzy arc is seen in serum; no arc is seen in urine. With λ-antiserum, there is a faint, fuzzy λ-arc in serum and none in urine. This patient has a monoclonal γ-chain in serum and urine (γ heavy-chain disease).** *Source:* **Kyle and Greipp 1978[63] Reprinted with permission of the Mayo Foundation**

than 200 cases recognized.[288–290] α Heavy-chain disease is a proliferative disorder of β-lymphoid cells, usually involving the gastrointestinal tract and producing an internally deleted α-chain devoid of light chains. Typically, a severe malabsorption syndrome is present.

Most patients have come from North Africa or the Middle East, but cases have been reported as well from South America, the Far East, and both Southern and Eastern Europe. It is not restricted to a specific ethnic group. The incidence is slightly greater in males than in females and is highest in the third decade of life; however, α heavy-chain disease has been reported in children.[291] It appears in undernourished populations with poor hygiene and frequent infestation by intestinal pathogens.

Clinical features include diarrhea, steatorrhea, weight loss, abdominal pain, and vomiting; hepatosplenomegaly and peripheral lymphadenopathy are uncommon findings. Clubbing of the fingers as well as retardation of physical growth and secondary sexual characteristics may be seen.

Atypical involvement of the gastrointestinal tract has been reported; for example, Tungekar et al.[292] reported four cases of gastric lymphoma with α heavy-chain disease. Another atypical patient had generalized lymphadenopathy, splenomegaly, and cutaneous infiltration but no involvement of the gastrointestinal or respiratory tract.[293]

Plasma cell infiltration of the jejunal mucosa, either with or without involvement of the mesenteric or para-aortic lymph nodes, is the most common pathologic feature. However, ulcerative and constrictive transmural tumors of the upper intestine have been seen as well.[294]

The serum protein electrophoretic pattern is normal in half the cases; in the remainder, an unimpressive broad band may appear in the α_2- or β-regions. The diagnosis of α heavy-chain disease depends on recognition of a monoclonal α heavy chain that is not associated with a light chain. An antiserum to Fab-α is absorbed with κ- and λ-proteins and is made specific for the Fab portion of the α heavy chain. Immunoselection by immunoelectrophoresis into gel containing the anti-Fab-α antisera provides the most sensitive and specific detection system for α heavy-chain disease.[295] The amount of α-chain in the urine is small, and Bence Jones proteinuria has never been reported. The immunoperoxidase technique also is useful for differentiating α heavy-chain disease from Mediterranean or Middle East lymphoma.[296]

Chromosomal abnormalities have been found in the lymphoid cells of patients with α heavy-chain disease, and Berger et al.[297] reported abnormal karyotypes in three of four patients. In two, a rearrangement of 14q32 was observed. Immunoglobulin heavy- and light-chain gene rearrangements were found as well in three patients with α heavy-chain disease; two of the patients had early-stage disease responsive to antibiotics, suggesting that the disease is neoplastic even in its early stages.[298]

In addition, nonsecretory α heavy-chain disease has been well documented. In one case, α_1-chains had rearrangements of the α-chain gene as well as the κ-chain gene.[299]

Most often, α heavy-chain disease is progressive and fatal, yet remissions in response to melphalan or cyclophosphamide and prednisone—and surprisingly, to antibiotics—have been recorded. In one case, oral tetracycline and intensive nutritional support produced a symptomatic remission, but the patient still had duodenal mucosal abnormalities and free α-chains in the serum.[300] The Tunisian-French Intestinal Lymphoma Study Group reported 21 Tunisian patients with α heavy-chain disease,[301] and 2 of 6 patients with stage A disease obtained a complete remission with antibiotics. The four antibiotic failures received chemotherapy, but they did not respond. Nine of the 15 patients with stage B or C disease obtained a complete remission with a combination of chemotherapeutic agents, and survival for the total group was 90% at 2 years and 67% at 3 years.[301]

μ Heavy-Chain Disease

A case of μ heavy-chain disease associated with chronic lymphocytic leukemia and amyloidosis was reported in 1970. Seven cases were described by Franklin in 1975, and chronic lymphocytic leukemia was associated in all but one.[302] The lack of peripheral lymphadenopathy, the presence of vacuolated plasma cells in the bone marrow, and the large amounts of Bence Jones protein excreted in the urine distinguished these from the usual cases of chronic lymphocytic leukemia. The serum protein electrophoretic pattern usually appears normal, except for hypogammaglobulinemia, and the presence of a dense band is unusual. In fact, an abnormal band has been found in only 4 of the 15 reported cases of μ heavy-chain disease. Bence Jones proteinuria has been reported in two thirds of cases, but μ-chain fragments in the urine are rare.[303] Some cases of μ heavy-chain disease have features resembling lymphoma or multiple myeloma with amyloidosis, and one patient presented with systemic lupus erythematosus and was found to have a free μ heavy chain and a monoclonal IgG-κ protein in the serum.[304] We have seen a patient with a small μ heavy chain who had increased numbers of small lymphocytes and plasmacytoid lymphocytes in the marrow but was asymptomatic; he was stable for 3 years, then developed an aggressive malignant lymphoproliferative disease and died 6 months later. More cases of μ heavy-chain disease will be recognized, and its clinical spectrum will broaden, as has happened with γ heavy-chain disease. The course of μ heavy-chain disease is variable, and survival ranges from a few months to many years. Treatment with corticosteroids and alkylating agents has produced benefit in some patients.

AMYLOIDOSIS

Amyloid, a substance that appears homogeneous and amorphous under the light microscope, stains pink with hematoxylin-and-eosin and metachromatically with methyl violet and crystal violet. Under polarized light, Congo red produces a green birefringence of amyloid, and it is the most specific stain for detection of this substance. Under the electron microscope, amyloid is seen to consist of rigid, nonbranching fibrils 50 to 150 Å in width and of indefinite length.

Amyloid fibrils are arranged in a β-pleated sheet conformation, as revealed by low angle x-ray diffrac-

TABLE 16.5. Types of Amyloidosis

Class	Amyloid Type	Major Protein Component
Primary amyloidosis: no evidence of preceding or coexisting disease except multiple myeloma	AL	κ or λ
Secondary amyloidosis: coexistence of other conditions, such as rheumatoid arthritis or chronic infection	AA	Protein A
Localized amyloidosis: involvement of a single organ without evidence of generalized involvement	AL	κ or λ
Familial amyloidosis		
Neurologic		
Portuguese	AF_p	Transthyretin (prealbumin)
Japanese	AF_j	Transthyretin (prealbumin)
Swedish	AF_s	Transthyretin (prealbumin)
Cardiopathic		Transthyretin (prealbumin)
Nephropathic		
Familial Mediterranean fever		Protein A
Senile cardiac amyloidosis	AS_{cI}	Transthyretin (prealbumin)
Dialysis arthropathy	AB	β_2-Microglobulin

Source: Kyle and Greipp 1983[343]

tion. This feature permits Congo red binding. The fibrils are insoluble, generally resist proteolytic digestion, and are the components of the amyloid deposits that replace and destroy normal cardiac, renal, and other tissues.

The amyloid in primary amyloidosis (AL), in comparison with that in secondary amyloidosis (AA), has been said to stain atypically and to involve the heart, tongue, gastrointestinal tract, nerves, and skin, whereas AA mainly involves the liver, kidney, and spleen. However, it must be emphasized that no consistent differences between AL and AA have been demonstrated by staining characteristics, organ distribution, or even electron microscopy. Amyloid consisting of protein A loses its affinity for Congo red after exposure to potassium permanganate, whereas amyloid in patients with primary or myeloma-associated amyloidosis, senile cardiac amyloid, familial amyloidosis, or nodular pulmonary amyloidosis (AL protein) is resistant to potassium permanganate.[305,306]

Another structure that has been described in all amyloid tissue is the P-component protein (AP).[307] This is a glycoprotein and is not related to immunoglobulins.

Classification

There is no truly satisfactory classification of amyloidosis, but we prefer that shown in Table 16.5. This classification has the advantage of exploiting what is currently known about the biochemistry of the amyloid fibril.

Biochemistry and Pathogenesis

Glenner et al.[308] demonstrated that amyloid fibrils from a patient with AL amyloidosis were virtually identical to the variable portion of a monoclonal light chain (Bence Jones protein); thus, the variable portion of a monoclonal light chain, or in some instances the intact light chain, constitutes the fibril subunit of AL amyloidosis. The light-chain class more frequently is λ than κ (2:1) in AL. In more than half of the cases, λ-chains are of the λ_{VI} subclass,[22] and in fact, all recognized λ_{VI} proteins have been associated with amyloidosis. In 5 of 14 patients with AL, Buxbaum and Hauser[309] demonstrated the synthesis of immunologically identical light chains that were of lower molecular weight than intact light chains. Others also have reported the secretion of free light chains and light-chain fragments in patients with AL.[310] This suggests that patients with AL may have aberrant de novo synthesis of light chains or abnormal proteolytic processing.

The mechanism for the deposition of monoclonal light chains as amyloid is unclear. Amyloid fibrils have been recognized in both plasma cells and macrophages near the plasma cells.

In AA amyloidosis, the major component of the amyloid fibril is protein A. It has a molecular weight of 8500, consists of 76 amino acids, and is unrelated to any known immunoglobulin.[311] With the use of an antiserum to AA (amyloid A), an antigenically related larger molecule (12,500 mw) known as serum SAA-related protein has been found in the sera of normal patients as well as in those with amyloidosis. Protein A is derived by the proteolytic cleavage of SAA-related protein. SAA-related protein levels are greatly increased in AA amyloidosis and modestly elevated in AL, but they are within normal limits in familial amyloidosis. SAA-related protein levels are greatly elevated in rheumatoid arthritis and Crohn disease but only modestly increased in lupus erythematosus and chronic ulcerative colitis; the SAA-related protein level corresponds to the incidence of secondary amyloidosis in these patients.[312]

The catabolism, or breakdown, of amyloid fibrils may be an important factor in the pathogenesis of amyloidosis. Lavie et al.[313] reported that monocytes from patients with amyloidosis did not degrade SAA-related protein, whereas the monocytes from normal patients did so, thus suggesting that macrophage dysfunction may contribute to the development of amyloidosis. It appears that amyloidosis may be the result of an interplay of several factors, including the slow removal and excess formation of amyloid fibrils. More studies are needed to elucidate these mechanisms.

Primary Amyloidosis and Amyloidosis with Myeloma

On the basis of the appearance and number of the plasma cells in the bone marrow, the amount of monoclonal protein in the serum and urine, and the presence or absence of skeletal lesions, a series of patients with systemic amyloidosis was divided into two groups: those with primary amyloidosis, and those having amyloidosis with multiple myeloma.[314] It must be emphasized that these two groups represent the same fundamental disease process and that differentiation is sometimes both difficult and artificial.

CLINICAL FEATURES. Primary amyloidosis and amyloidosis with myeloma occur more often in men than in women. The mean age at diagnosis, approximately 61 years, is virtually identical to that for multiple myeloma.

The most common presenting symptoms are fatigue or weakness, weight loss, ankle edema, dyspnea, paresthesias, and lightheadedness or syncope. Weight loss may be striking, amounting to 20 kg or more in some instances. Hoarseness or change of voice as well as jaw claudication also may occur.

The principal initial physical findings include ankle edema, purpura, and enlargement of the liver and tongue. Macroglossia, which occurs in approximately 10% of cases, may be extremely impressive. Splenomegaly is an initial finding in 5% of cases and, when present, is modest in degree. Purpura is not infrequent and often involves the face, neck, and upper eyelids. Purpura of the eyelids after pinching is a characteristic sign of amyloidosis, and periorbital purpura may be striking after proctoscopy (postproctoscopic palpebral purpura—PPPP). Bleeding may occur because of acquired deficiency of factor X, presumably caused by binding of factor X to amyloid.[315] Edema is common and may be associated with congestive heart failure or the nephrotic syndrome, and orthostatic hypotension may be a prominent feature.

Among our patients with primary amyloidosis, the nephrotic syndrome was present in 32%, congestive heart failure in 26%, carpal tunnel syndrome in 16%, peripheral neuropathy in 17%, and orthostatic hypotension in 16%. In most cases, these abnormalities had existed from 1 to 3 years, reflecting the delay in diagnosis of this disease.

LABORATORY FINDINGS. Anemia is not a prominent feature in AL amyloidosis, and when present, it usually is due to renal insufficiency, multiple myeloma, or gastrointestinal bleeding. Thrombocytosis occurs in 5% to 10% of patients, and proteinuria is present in approximately 80%. Renal insufficiency is present in half the patients at the time of diagnosis. The creatinine level is 2 mg/dl or more in one fourth of patients, and hyperbilirubinemia is an infrequent finding but an ominous sign when present. The thrombin time is prolonged in 60% of patients, but the prothrombin time is increased in approximately 15%. The factor X level is decreased in less than 5% and is rarely the cause of bleeding.

Serum protein electrophoresis reveals a localized band or spike in slightly less than half the cases. Hypogammaglobulinemia is found in nearly one fourth of patients, and immunoelectrophoresis or immunofixation reveals a monoclonal serum protein in two thirds. Bence Jones proteinemia is found in one fifth of patients, and immunoelectrophoresis or immunofixation of the urine shows a monoclonal light chain in approximately two thirds. A monoclonal protein is found in the serum or urine in approximately 90%. In our experience, the median percentage of plasma cells in the bone marrow is 6%, and only 15% of our patients had more than 20% plasma cells in the marrow. Roentgenograms of the bones are normal unless the patient has multiple myeloma.

THE INVOLVEMENT OF INDIVIDUAL ORGAN SYSTEMS

Renal. Nephrotic syndrome is present in one third of patients at the time of diagnosis. The degree of proteinuria does not correlate well with the extent of amyloid deposition in the kidneys, and the severity of proteinuria correlates better with the presence of spicules and podocyte destruction than with the amount of amyloid deposited in the glomerulus.[316] Gross hematuria is rare, but renal vein thrombosis or the adult Fanconi syndrome has been associated with amyloidosis.

Cardiac and Circulatory. Congestive heart failure is present in approximately 25% of patients at the time of diagnosis, and it develops during the course of the disease in an additional 10%. The electrocardiogram frequently shows either low voltage in the limb leads or characteristics consistent with an anteroseptal infarction (loss of anterior forces); however, there is no evidence of myocardial infarction at autopsy.[317] Cardiac arrhythmias and conduction disturbances are common.

Echocardiography is a valuable technique for the evaluation of amyloid heart disease. Increased thickness of the ventricular wall and septum correlates with an increased incidence of congestive heart failure.[318] Early cardiac amyloidosis is characterized by abnormal relaxation. Advanced involvement is characterized by restrictive hemodynamics. Granular sparkling, left atrial enlargement, and reduced systolic function occur later. Constrictive pericarditis or hypertrophic obstructive cardiomyopathy may be difficult to differentiate from amyloid heart disease. Intermittent claudication of the extremities or the jaw may be a prominent feature,[319] and orthostatic hypotension occurs in approximately 15% of all patients.

Neurologic. Sensorimotor peripheral neuropathy, characterized by dysesthesias involving the lower extremities, occurs in one sixth of patients. Autonomic dysfunction may be a prominent feature and often is manifested by orthostatic hypotension, diarrhea, or impotence.[320]

Other Organs. Histologic involvement of the gastrointestinal tract occurs in most patients, but it is usually asymptomatic. Occasionally, pseudo-obstruction of the bowel or malabsorption may be seen. Ascites is not common, but hepatic involvement is. Liver failure is rare.[321]

Histologic involvement of the blood vessels and alveolar septa of the lungs is common, but dyspnea from involvement of alveolar septa is rare. Amyloidosis may involve periarticular structures and may resemble rheumatoid arthritis. Rarely, amyloid deposits produce osteolytic lesions, but extensive deposits of amyloid may cause weakness and pseudohypertrophy of skeletal muscles. Involvement of the skin by amyloidosis may take the form of petechiae, ecchymoses, papules, plaques, nodules, tumors, bullous lesions, and thickening of the skin (resembling scleroderma). Amyloidosis of the lacrimal and parotid glands may produce dryness of the eyes and mouth, and rapid enlargement of the thyroid in

amyloidosis has been reported, as well as panhypopituitarism from destruction of the pituitary by amyloid deposits.

DIAGNOSIS. The possibility of AL amyloidosis must be considered in every patient with an M protein in the serum or urine and who has nephrotic syndrome, refractory congestive heart failure, sensorimotor peripheral neuropathy, carpal tunnel syndrome, giant hepatomegaly, or idiopathic malabsorption. The initial diagnostic procedure should be an abdominal fat aspirate, which is positive in more than 70% of patients.[322] A bone marrow aspiration and biopsy should be performed to determine the degree of plasmacytosis, and stains for amyloid are positive in almost half of patients. A rectal biopsy specimen should be taken if the abdominal fat and bone marrow biopsy results are negative. The specimen must include the submucosa, and it is positive in approximately 80% of patients. If these sites are negative, tissue should be obtained from an organ with suspected involvement.

Renal biopsy produces an even higher incidence of positive findings, but the procedure is more difficult than rectal biopsy and may cause bleeding. Liver biopsy frequently reveals amyloid; however, it may cause bleeding as well. In some instances, rupture of the liver has occurred. Always examine tissue obtained at carpal tunnel decompression for amyloid, because it is positive in more than 90% of patients with amyloidosis. Biopsies of the sural nerve, small intestine, endomyocardium, and skin may be important aids to recognition.

Congo red produces an apple-green birefringence under polarizing light and is the most commonly used stain. Although false-positive and false-negative results may occur, it is more reliable than methyl violet, crystal violet, or thioflavin T. However, electron microscopy also may be necessary for the identification of the typical fibrils.

AA amyloid loses its affinity for Congo red after exposure to potassium permanganate, whereas AL amyloid does not. However, false-positive and false-negative instances do occur. Specific antisera to protein A, transthyretin, and κ and λ correctly identify the type of systemic amyloidosis,[323] and the use of ^{123}I-labelled serum amyloid P component is helpful for localizing amyloid deposits in vivo. Increased uptake of ^{99m}Tc pyrophosphate is not a reliable test for diagnosis.[324]

PROGNOSIS AND THERAPY. Currently, the median survival of patients with AL amyloidosis is almost 2 years. Survival varies greatly depending on the associated syndrome, ranging from 6 months for those with congestive heart failure to more than 5 years when only peripheral neuropathy is present. Cardiac involvement accounts for the death of almost half of all patients.

Therapy of AL amyloidosis is unsatisfactory. Because amyloid fibrils consist of the variable portion of a monoclonal immunoglobulin light chain, treatment with alkylating agents that are known to be effective against plasma cell proliferative processes should be attempted. In one prospective randomized study, the median survival was 25 months for patients receiving melphalan and prednisone and 18 months for those receiving colchicine; when the survival of patients who received only one regimen was analyzed, or when survival was analyzed from study entry until death or progression of disease, a significant survival difference favoring melphalan and prednisone was evident.[325] These results suggest that treatment with melphalan and prednisone is superior to colchicine for AL amyloidosis. However, the development of a myelodysplastic syndrome or acute nonlymphocytic leukemia in AL amyloidosis has been recognized as well.

We also have used dimethylsulfoxide, but the results were not impressive. Also, chronic hemodialysis and renal transplantation have been performed in some cases with renal failure.

One of the major problems in the treatment of amyloidosis is assessing the response. At present, the investigator is limited to the evaluation of organ function and measurement of the monoclonal protein in the serum and urine. A simple measure is needed for measuring the amount of amyloid in a patient. Perhaps ^{123}I-labelled serum amyloid P component may prove to be useful in this regard.

Secondary, localized, and familial amyloidosis are not discussed in this review. For these, the reader is directed to a recently published monograph.[326]

MONOCLONAL GAMMOPATHY OF UNDETERMINED SIGNIFICANCE

The term *monoclonal gammopathy of undetermined significance* denotes the presence of a monoclonal protein in persons with no evidence of myeloma, macroglobulinemia, or other related diseases.[327,328] It is a more satisfactory term than *benign monoclonal gammopathy*, because it cannot be determined whether a monoclonal protein will remain unchanged or is an evolving myeloma or macroglobulinemia. Synonyms include idopathic, asymptomatic, benign, nonmyelomatous, discrete, cryptogenic, and rudimentary dysimmunoglobulinemia, lanthanic monoclonal gammopathy, idiopathic paraproteinemia, and asymptomatic paraimmunoglobulinemia.

The incidence of monoclonal proteins without myeloma or macroglobulinemia is approximately 1% among the population over the age of 50 years and 3% among those over the age of 70 years.

Differentiation from Myeloma and Macroglobulinemia

Those with MGUS have less than 3.0 g/dl of the monoclonal protein in the serum, fewer than 5% plasma cells in bone marrow aspirates, no anemia or osteolytic lesions, normal concentration of serum albumin, no monoclonal protein in the urine (Bence Jones proteinuria), and no evidence of progression for at least 5 years. Monoclonal gammopathy of undetermined significance cannot be differentiated adequately from multiple myeloma by the morphologic abnormalities of the plasma cells, presence or absence of chromosomal abnormalities, concentrations of uninvolved immunoglobulins, presence or absence of small amounts of monoclonal light chain in the urine, levels of serum β_2-microglobulin, the presence of J chains in the plasma cells, or elevated plasma cell acid phosphatase levels. The plasma cell labelling index, reduction of CD4 cells in peripheral blood, increased numbers of monoclonal-idiotype peripheral blood lymphocytes, or immunoglobulin-secreting cells may be of some help, but no single technique exists that reliably differentiates benign from malignant plasma cell proliferation. The most dependable means is the serial measurement of the M-protein level in both the serum and urine and the periodic re-evaluation of clinical and laboratory features to determine whether multiple myeloma, systemic amyloidosis, macroglobulinemia, or other malignant proliferative disease has developed.

We have observed 241 patients with a monoclonal protein in the serum who initially had no evidence of multiple myeloma, macroglobulinemia, amyloidosis, or lymphoma.[327,329,330] Nineteen years after diagnosis of monoclonal gammopathy of undetermined significance, the patients were classified as follows: group 1, patients without significant increase in monoclonal protein (benign) (24%); group 2, patients with an increased M-protein value to more than 3 g/dl but who did not require treatment for myeloma or macroglobulinemia (3%); group 3, patients who had died without developing multiple myeloma or related diseases (51%); and group 4, patients in whom multiple myeloma, macroglobulinemia, or amyloidosis developed (24%).

The interval from the recognition of the M protein to the diagnosis of multiple myeloma ranged from 23 to 251 months (median, 115 months [9.6 years]) in the 36 patients. Macroglobulinemia of Waldenström developed in seven patients, with a median interval of 8.5

years from the recognition of the M protein to the diagnosis of macroglobulinemia. Systemic amyloidosis (AL) was found in 7 patients from 6 to 16.5 years (median, 8 years) after the recognition of the M protein. Two patients developed an aggressive malignant lymphoma 7 and 22 years after the recognition of the monoclonal gammopathy, and one patient developed chronic lymphocytic leukemia 4.5 years later.

Treatment for monoclonal gammopathy of undetermined significance is not indicated. However, frequent re-examination is necessary to ensure that the concentration of the monoclonal protein is stable and that myeloma, macroglobulinemia, or amyloidosis has not developed.

Association with Other Diseases

Although monoclonal gammopathy of undetermined significance frequently exists without any other abnormalities, certain diseases often occur in association with it, as would be expected in an older population. It therefore is essential to have a control group when considering such an association to show if it merely is coincidence. Monoclonal gammopathy frequently has been reported as being increased with carcinoma of the colon; however, in two large studies, the incidence of monoclonal proteins among patients with nonreticu-loendothelial neoplasms was no greater than that expected in a population of similar age.

Surgical removal of the tumors has no effect on the concentration of the monoclonal protein. In no instance has removal of a malignant solid tumor caused the serum monoclonal protein to disappear.

An increased incidence of monoclonal IgM proteins has been noted in cases of chronic lymphocytic leukemia, lymphocytic lymphoma, and histiocytic (reticulum cell) sarcoma. No increased incidence of monoclonal proteins has been recognized in Hodgkin disease or in nodular lymphomas.[331] Although monoclonal proteins have been found in the serum of patients with leukemia, there are not enough data to determine whether the incidence is greater than in a normal population. Monoclonal gammopathies are associated with acquired immunodeficiency syndrome as well as renal, bone marrow, and liver transplants.[332]

Lichen myxedematosus is a rare dermatologic lesion that frequently is associated with a small monoclonal IgG λ-protein migrating toward the cathode. Monoclonal gammopathies have been associated with pernicious anemia, von Willebrand disease, Gaucher disease, liver disease, rheumatoid arthritis, lupus erythematosus, myasthenia gravis, hyperparathyroidism, peripheral neuropathy, acute leukemia, angioedema, red cell aplasia, capillary leak syndrome, Sézary syndrome, pyoderma gangrenosum, hereditary spherocytosis, Sjögren

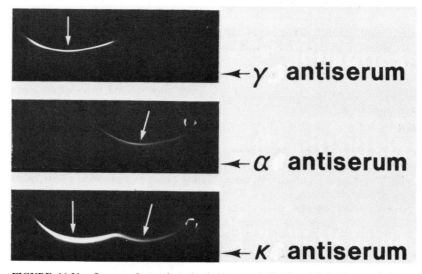

FIGURE 16.21. **Immunoelectrophoresis. Antisera to IgG (γ) and IgA (α) caused the bowing of the arcs that corresponds to the double bowing of the κ-arc. This patient has IgG-κ and IgA-κ biclonal gammopathy.** *Source*: Kyle 1982[341]

syndrome, renal papillary necrosis, and necrobiotic xanthogranuloma. The association of monoclonal proteins with these diseases is very likely coincidental.[332]

In some cases of monoclonal gammopathy of undetermined significance, myeloma, and macroglobulinemia, the immunoglobulin has exhibited unusual specificities to dextran, actin, antistreptolysin O, antinuclear activity, and peripheral nerve myelin (MAG).[333]

BICLONAL GAMMOPATHIES

The biclonal gammopathies are a group of disorders characterized by the production of two distinct monoclonal proteins (Fig. 16.21). They may be caused either by proliferation of two separate clones of plasma cells, each producing an unrelated monoclonal immunoglobulin, or by production of two monoclonal proteins by a single clone of plasma cells with incomplete class switching. In a review of 57 cases of biclonal gammopathy we found that 65% had a biclonal gammopathy of undetermined significance.[334] One patient with biclonal gammopathy of undetermined significance developed symptomatic myeloma after 2 years.

Among the 57 patients, 9 (16%) had multiple myeloma, and 11 (19%) had a lymphoproliferative disorder. The most frequent combinations of proteins were IgG–IgA (53%), IgG–IgM (26%), and IgG–IgG (10%). Of the 115 monoclonal proteins, 70% were κ and 30% λ. The same light-chain class, that is, both κ or both λ, was found in each biclonal pair in 63% of cases.

Nilsson et al.[335] reported that almost half of their 20 patients with biclonal gammopathy had biclonal gammopathy of undetermined significance, and multiple myeloma subsequently developed in two. Also, Riddell et al.[336] reported that 28 of 1135 patients (2.5%) with monoclonal gammopathy actually had biclonal gammopathy.

ACKNOWLEDGMENTS

This investigation was supported in part by Research Grant CA-16835 from the National Institutes of Health, Public Health Service, and the Toor Fund.

REFERENCES

1. Shapiro SS. Characterization of factor VIII antibodies. Ann N Y Acad Sci 1975;240:350.
2. Reynolds HY. Immunoglobulin G and its function in the human respiratory tract. Mayo Clin Proc 1988;63:161.
3. Oxelius V-A, Laurell A-B, Lindquist B, et al. IgG subclasses in selective IgA deficiency: importance of IgG2–IgA deficiency. N Engl J Med 1981;304:1476.
4. Beck CS, Heiner DC. Selective immunoglobulin G_4 deficiency and recurrent infections of the respiratory tract. Am Rev Respir Dis 1981;124:94.
5. Papadea C, Reimer CB, Check IJ. IgG subclass distribution in patients with multiple myeloma or with monoclonal gammopathy of undetermined significance. Ann Clin Lab Sci 1989;19:27.
6. Schur PH. IgG subclasses—a review. Ann Allergy 1987;58:89.
7. Kyle RA, Gleich GJ. IgG subclasses in monoclonal gammopathy of undetermined significance. J Lab Clin Med 1982; 100:806.
8. Fasullo FJ Jr, Fritsche HA Jr, Liu FJ, Hamilton RG. IgG heavy-chain subclass typing of myeloma paraproteins by isoelectric focusing immunoblot analysis. Clin Chem 1989; 35:364.
9. Macintyre W. Case of mollities and fragilitas ossium, accompanied with urine strongly charged with animal matter. R Med Chir Soc Lond Trans 1850;33:211.
10. Bence Jones H. Papers on chemical pathology: prefaced by the Gulstonian lectures, read at the Royal College of Physicians, 1846. Lancet 1847;ii:88.
11. Edelman GM, Gally JA. The nature of Bence Jones proteins: chemical similarities to polypeptide chains of myeloma globulins and normal γ-globulins. J Exp Med 1962;116:207.
12. Bayne-Jones S, Wilson DW. Immunological reactions of Bence Jones proteins. II. Differences between Bence Jones proteins from various sources. Bull Johns Hopkins Hosp 1922;33:119.
13. Korngold L, Lipari R. Multiple-myeloma proteins. III. The antigenic relationship of Bence Jones proteins to normal gamma-globulin and multiple-myeloma serum proteins. Cancer 1956;9:262.
14. Lieu T-S, Deutsch HF, Tischendorf FW. Human λ-chain sequence variations and serologic associations. Immunochemistry 1977;14:429.
15. Solomon A, McLaughlin CL. Bence Jones proteins and light chains of immunoglobulins. I. Formation and characterization of amino-terminal (variant) and carboxyl-terminal (constant) halves. J Biol Chem 1969;244:3393.
16. Fett JW, Deutsch HF. Primary structure of the Mcg λ chain. Biochemistry 1974;13:4102.
17. Solomon A. Bence Jones proteins and light chains of immunoglobulins. N Engl J Med 1976;294:17,91.
18. Erikson J, Martinis J, Croce CM. Assignment of the genes for human λ immunoglobulin chains to chromosome 22. Nature 1981;294:173.
19. Rowley JD. Identification of the constant chromosome regions involved in human hematologic malignant disease. Science 1982;216:749.
20. Solomon A. Light chains of immunoglobulins: structural-genetic correlates. Blood 1986;68:603.
21. Wang AC, Fudenberg HH, Wells JV, Roelcke D. Letter to the editor. A new subgroup of the kappa chain variable region associated with anti-Pr cold agglutinins. Nature [New Biol] 1973;243:126.
22. Solomon A, Kyle RA, Frangione B. Light chain variable region subgroups of monoclonal immunoglobulins in amyloidosis AL. In: Glenner GG, Osserman EF, Benditt EP, Calkins E, Cohen AS, Zucker-Franklin D, eds. Amyloidosis. New York: Plenum Press, 1986:449–62.
23. Putnam FW, Easley CW, Lynn LT, Ritchie AE, Phelps RA. The heat precipitation of Bence Jones proteins. I. Optimum conditions. Arch Biochem Biophys. 1959;83:115.
24. Solomon A. Bence Jones proteins and light chains of immunoglobulins. XIV. Conformational dependency and molecular localization of the kappa (κ) and lambda (λ) antigenic determinants. Scand J Immunol 1976;5:685.

25. Wu TT, Kabat EA. An analysis of the sequences of the variable regions of Bence Jones proteins and myeloma light chains and their implications for antibody complementarity. J Exp Med 1970;132:211.

26. Capra JD, Kehoe JM. Hypervariable regions, idiotypy, and the antibody-combining site. Adv Immunol 1975;20:1.

27. Steinberg AG. Globulin polymorphisms in man. Annu Rev Genet 1969;3:25.

28. Tomasi TB Jr. Human immunoglobulin A. N Engl J Med 1968; 279:1327.

29. Lenormand P, Crocker J. Distribution of IgA$_1$ and IgA$_2$ subclasses in normal bone marrow trephines and in trephines infiltrated by IgA producing multiple myeloma. J Clin Pathol 1987;40:200.

30. André C, Berthoux FC, André F, Gillon J, Genin C, Sabatier J-C. Prevalence of IgA2 deposits in IgA nephropathies: a clue to their pathogenesis. N Engl J Med 1980;303:1343.

31. Rivat-Peran L, Buriot D, Salier J-P, Rivat C, Dumitresco S-M, Griscelli C. Immunoglobulins in ataxia-telangiectasia: evidence for IgG4 and IgA2 subclass deficiencies. Clin Immunol Immunopathol 1981;20:99.

32. Heremans JF. Immunoglobulin A. In: Sela M, ed. The Antigens, Volume 2. New York: Academic Press, 1974:395.

33. Mestecky J, Russell MW, Jackson S, Brown TA. The human IgA system: a reassessment. Clin Immunol Immunopathol 1986;40:105.

34. Goodman MR, Link DW, Brown WR, Nakane PK. Ultrastructural evidence of transport of secretory IgA across bronchial epithelium. Am Rev Respir Dis 1981;123:115.

35. Kutteh WH, Prince SJ, Mestecky J. Tissue origins of human polymeric and monomeric IgA. J Immunol 1982;128:990.

36. Conley ME, Delacroix DL. Intravascular and mucosal immunoglobulin A: two separate but related systems of immune defense? Ann Intern Med 1987;106:892.

37. DeCoteau WE. The role of secretory IgA in defense of the distal lung. Ann N Y Acad Sci 1974;221:214.

38. Abu-Ghazaleh RI, Fujisawa T, Mestecky J, Kyle RA, Gleich GJ. IgA-induced eosinophil degranulation. J Immunol 1989; 142:2393.

39. Koshland ME. Structure and function of the J chain. Adv Immunol 1975;20:41.

40. Metzger H. Structure and function of γM macroglobulins. Adv Immunol 1970;12:57.

41. Hayzer DJ, Jaton J-C. Immunoglobulin M (IgM). Methods Enzymol 1985;116:26.

42. Tartakoff A, Vassalli P. Plasma cell immunoglobulin M molecules: their biosynthesis, assembly, and intracellular transport. J Cell Biol 1979;83:284.

43. Putnam FW, Florent G, Paul C, Shinoda T, Shimizu A. Complete amino acid sequence of the mu heavy chain of a human IgM immunoglobulin. Science 1973;182:287.

44. Harries R, Beckman I, Roberts-Thomson P. Low molecular weight IgM detection using immunoblotting. J Immunol Methods 1986;88:97.

45. Abu-Farsakh FA, Abu-Farsakh HA. M-component overestimated by laser nephelometry in Waldenström's macroglobulinemia. Clin Chem 1988;34:428.

46. Rowe DS, Fahey JL. A new class of human immunoglobulins. I. A unique myeloma protein. II. Normal serum IgD. J Exp Med 1965;121:171.

47. Dunnette SL, Gleich GJ, Miller RD, Kyle RA. Measurement of IgD by a double antibody radioimmunoassay: demonstration of an apparent trimodal distribution of IgD levels in normal human sera. J Immunol 1977;119:1727.

48. Putnam FW, Takahashi N, Tetaert D, Lin L-C, Debuire B. The last of the immunoglobulins: complete amino acid sequence of human IgD. Ann N Y Acad Sci 1982;399:41.

49. Van Boxel JA, Paul WE, Terry WD, Green I. IgD-bearing human lymphocytes. J Immunol 1972;109:648.

50. Spiegelberg HL. Immunoglobulin D (IgD). Methods Enzymol 1985;116:95.

51. Ishizaka K, Ishizaka T, Hornbrook MM. Physicochemical properties of reaginic antibody. V. Correlation of reaginic activity with γE-globulin antibody. J Immunol 1966;97:840.

52. Yunginger JW, Gleich GJ. The impact of the discovery of IgE on the practice of allergy. Pediatr Clin North Am 1975;22:3.

53. Ishizaka K. Twenty years with IgE. From the identification of IgE to regulatory factors for the IgE response (American Association of Immunologists: Presidential Address). J Immunol 1985;135:i.

54. Geha RS. Human IgE. J Allergy Clin Immunol 1984;74:109.

55. Kunkel HG. The "abnormality" of myeloma proteins. Cancer Res 1968;28:1351.

56. Natvig JB, Kunkel HG. Human immunoglobulins: classes, subclasses, genetic variants, and idiotypes. Adv Immunol 1973;16:1.

57. Krause RM. The search for antibodies with molecular uniformity. Adv Immunol 1970;12:1.

58. Potter M. Myeloma proteins (M-components) with antibody-like activity. N Engl J Med 1971;284:831.

59. Seligmann M, Brouet JC. Antibody activity of human myeloma globulins. Semin Hematol 1973;10:163.

60. Osterland CK, Espinoza LR. Biological properties of myeloma proteins. Arch Intern Med 1975;135:32.

61. Buxbaum JN. The biosynthesis, assembly, and secretion of immunoglobulins. Semin Hematol 1973;10:33.

62. Stone MJ, Frenkel EP. The clinical spectrum of light chain myeloma: a study of 35 patients with special reference to the occurrence of amyloidosis. Am J Med 1975;58:601.

63. Kyle RA, Greipp PR. Series on clinical testing. 3. The laboratory investigation of monoclonal gammopathies. Mayo Clin Proc 1978;53:719.

64. Reichert CM, Everett DF Jr, Nadler PI, Papadopoulos NM. High-resolution zone electrophoresis, combined with immunofixation, in the detection of an occult myeloma paraprotein. Clin Chem 1982;28:2312.

65. Cawley LP, Minard BJ, Tourtellotte WW, Ma BI, Chelle C. Immunofixation electrophoretic techniques applied to identification of proteins in serum and cerebrospinal fluid. Clin Chem 1976;22:1262.

66. Ritchie RF, Smith R. Immunofixation. III. Application to the study of monoclonal proteins. Clin Chem 1976;22:1982.

67. Roberts RT. Usefulness of immunofixation electrophoresis in the clinical laboratory. Clin Lab Med 1986;6:601.

68. Duc J, Morel B, Peitrequin R, Frei PC. Identification of monoclonal gammopathies: a comparison of immunofixation, immunoelectrophoresis and measurements of kappa- and lambda-immunoglobulin levels. J Clin Lab Immunol 1988;26:141.

69. Deegan MJ, Perry M, Hayashi H. A rapid method for identifying the light chain component of a monoclonal protein (abstract). Blood 1985;66(suppl 1):186A.

70. Keren DF, Warren JS, Lowe JB. Strategy to diagnose monoclonal gammopathies in serum: high-resolution electrophoresis, immunofixation, and κ/λ quantification. Clin Chem 1988; 34:2196.

71. Radl J, Wels J, Hoogeveen CM. Immunoblotting with (sub)-class-specific antibodies reveals a high frequency of monoclonal gammopathies in persons thought to be immunodeficient. Clin Chem 1988;34:1839.

72. Norden AGW, Fulcher LM, Heys AD. Rapid typing of serum

paraproteins by immunoblotting without antigen-excess artifacts. Clin Chem 1987;33:1433.

73. Fahey JL, McKelvey EM. Quantitative determination of serum immunoglobulins in antibody-agar plates. J Immunol 1965; 94:84.

74. Hinberg IH, Katz L, Waddell L. Sensitivity of in vitro diagnostic dipstick tests to urinary protein. Clin Biochem 1978;11:62.

75. Perry MC, Kyle RA. The clinical significance of Bence Jones proteinuria. Mayo Clin Proc 1975;50:234.

76. Ichimaru M, Ishimaru T, Mikami M, Matsunaga M. Multiple myeloma among atomic bomb survivors in Hiroshima and Nagasaki, 1950–76: relationship to radiation dose absorbed by marrow. J Natl Cancer Inst 1982;69:323.

77. Darby SC, Doll R, Gill SK, Smith PG. Long-term mortality after a single treatment course with x-rays in patients treated for ankylosing spondylitis. Br J Cancer 1987;55:179.

78. Kagan E, Jacobson RJ. Lymphoid and plasma cell malignancies: asbestos-related disorders of long latency. Am J Clin Pathol 1983;80:14.

79. Aksoy M, Erdem Ş, Dinçol G, Kutlar A, Bakioğlu I, Hepyüksel T. Clinical observations showing the role of some factors in the etiology of multiple myeloma: a study in 7 patients. Acta Haematol (Basel) 1984;71:116.

80. Cuzick J, De Stavola B. Multiple myeloma—a case-control study. Br J Cancer 1988;57:516.

81. Cuzick J, Velez R, Doll R. International variations and temporal trends in mortality from multiple myeloma. Int J Cancer 1983;32:13.

82. Cohen HJ, Bernstein RJ, Grufferman S. Role of immune stimulation in the etiology of multiple myeloma: a case control study. Am J Hematol 1987;24:119.

83. Maldonado JE, Kyle RA. Familial myeloma: report of eight families and a study of serum proteins in their relatives. Am J Med 1974;57:875.

84. Bourguet CC, Grufferman S, Delzell E, Delong ER, Cohen HJ. Multiple myeloma and family history of cancer: a case-control study. Cancer 1985;56:2133.

85. Rodriguez MA, Durie BGM, Meltzer PS. Evidence that a subset of human myelomas contain Epstein-Barr virus (abstract). Proc Am Soc Clin Oncol 1985;4:13.

86. Voelkerding KV, Sandhaus LM, Kim HC, et al. Plasma cell malignancy in the acquired immune deficiency syndrome: association with Epstein-Barr virus. Am J Clin Pathol 1989;92:222.

87. Gould J, Alexanian R, Goodacre A, Pathak S, Hecht B, Barlogie B. Plasma cell karyotype in multiple myeloma. Blood 1988;71:453.

88. Linos A, Kyle RA, O'Fallon WM, Kurland LT. Incidence and secular trend of multiple myeloma in Olmsted County, Minnesota: 1965–77. J Natl Cancer Inst 1981;66:17.

89. Hansen NE, Karle H, Olsen JH. Trends in the incidence of multiple myeloma in Denmark 1943–1982: a study of 5500 patients. Eur J Haematol 1989;42:72.

90. Kyle RA, Herber L, Evatt BL, Heath CW Jr. Multiple myeloma: a community cluster. JAMA 1970;213:1339.

91. Kyle RA. Multiple myeloma: review of 869 cases. Mayo Clin Proc 1975;50:29.

92. Lazarus HM, Kellermeyer RW, Aikawa M, Herzig RH. Multiple myeloma in young men: clinical course and electron microscopic studies of bone marrow plasma cells. Cancer 1980; 46:1397.

93. Levi DF, Williams RC Jr, Lindstrom FD. Immunofluorescent studies of the myeloma kidney with special reference to light chain disease. Am J Med 1968;44:922.

94. Kyle RA. Monoclonal gammopathies and the kidney. Annu Rev Med 1989;40:53.

95. DeFronzo RA, Cooke CR, Wright JR, Humphrey RL. Renal function in patients with multiple myeloma. Medicine (Baltimore) 1978;57:151.

96. Clyne DH, Pesce AJ, Thompson RE. Nephrotoxicity of Bence Jones proteins in the rat: importance of protein isoelectric point. Kidney Int 1979;16:345.

97. Coward RA, Delamore IW, Mallick NP, Robinson EL. The importance of urinary immunoglobulin light chain isoelectric point (pI) in nephrotoxicity in multiple myeloma. Clin Sci 1984;66:229.

98. Rota S, Mougenot B, Baudouin B, et al. Multiple myeloma and severe renal failure: a clinicopathologic study of outcome and prognosis in 34 patients. Medicine 1987;66:126.

99. DeFronzo RA, Humphrey RL, Wright JR, Cooke CR. Acute renal failure in multiple myeloma. Medicine (Baltimore) 1975;54:209.

100. Maldonado JE, Velosa JA, Kyle RA, Wagoner RD, Holley KE, Salassa RM. Fanconi syndrome in adults: a manifestation of a latent form of myeloma. Am J Med 1975;58:354.

101. Gailani S, Seon B-K, Henderson ES. κ light chain—myeloma associated with adult Fanconi syndrome: response of the nephropathy to treatment of myeloma. Med Pediatr Oncol 1978;4:141.

102. Pringle JP, Graham RC, Bernier GM. Detection of myeloma cells in the urine sediment. Blood 1974;43:137.

103. Noel LH, Droz D, Ganeval D, Grunfeld JP. Renal granular monoclonal light chain deposits: morphological aspects in 11 cases. Clin Nephrol 1984;21:263.

104. Alpers CE, Tu W-H, Hopper J Jr, Biava CG. Single light chain subclass (kappa chain) immunoglobulin deposition in glomerulonephritis. Hum Pathol 1985;16:294.

105. Tubbs RR, Gephardt GN, McMahon JT, Hall PM, Valenzuela R, Vidt DG. Light chain nephropathy. Am J Med 1981;71:263.

106. Bruckman JE, Bloomer WD. Management of spinal cord compression. Semin Oncol 1978;5:135.

107. Kelly JJ Jr, Kyle RA, Miles JM, O'Brien PC, Dyck PJ. The spectrum of peripheral neuropathy in myeloma. Neurology (NY) 1981;31:24.

108. Slager UT, Taylor WF, Opfell RW, Myers A. Leptomeningeal myeloma. Arch Pathol Lab Med 1979;103:680.

109. Gomez GA, Krishnamsetty RM. Successful treatment of meningeal myeloma with combination of radiation therapy, chemotherapy, and intrathecal therapy. Arch Intern Med 1986;146:194.

110. Perez-Soler R, Esteban R, Allende E, Salomo CT, Julia A, Guardia J. Liver involvement in multiple myeloma. Am J Hematol 1985;20:25.

111. Thomas FB, Clausen KP, Greenberger NJ. Liver disease in multiple myeloma. Arch Intern Med 1973;132:195.

112. Zafaranloo S, Bryk D, Gerard PS. Obstructive jaundice secondary to mulitple myeloma—a case report. Comput Radiol 1986;10:197.

113. Kintzer JS Jr, Rosenow EC III, Kyle RA. Thoracic and pulmonary abnormalities in multiple myeloma: a review of 958 cases. Arch Intern Med 1978;138:727.

114. Wahner HW, Kyle RA, Beabout JW. Scintigraphic evaluation of the skeleton in multiple myeloma. Mayo Clin Proc 1980;55:739.

115. Kyle RA, Schreiman JS, McLeod RA, Beabout JW. Computed tomography in diagnosis and management of multiple myeloma and its variants. Arch Intern Med 1985;145:1451.

116. Daffner RH, Lupetin AR, Dash N, Deeb ZL, Sefczek RJ, Schapiro RL. MRI in the detection of malignant infiltration of bone marrow. AJR Am J Roentgenol 1986;146:353.

117. Durie BGM, Salmon SE, Mundy GR. Relation of osteoclast

activating factor production to extent of bone disease in multiple myeloma. Br J Haematol 1981;47:21.

118. Bataille R, Delmas P, Sany J. Serum bone gla-protein in multiple myeloma. Cancer 1987;59:329.

119. Orellana J, Friedman AH. Ocular manifestations of multiple myeloma, Waldenström's macroglubinemia and benign monoclonal gammopathy. Surv Ophthalmol 1981;26:157.

120. De Rossi G, De Sanctis G, Bottari V, et al. Surface markers and cytotoxic activities of lymphocytes in monoclonal gammopathy of undetermined significance and untreated multiple myeloma: increased phytohemagglutinin-induced cellular cytotoxicity and inverted helper/suppressor cell ratio are features common to both diseases. Cancer Immunol Immunother 1987;25:133.

121. Pilarski LM, Andrews EJ, Serra HM, Ruether BA, Mant MJ. Comparative analysis of immunodeficiency in patients with monoclonal gammopathy of undetermined significance and patients with untreated multiple myeloma. Scand J Immunol 1989;29:217.

122. Epstein J, Barlogie B, Katzmann J, Alexanian R. Phenotypic heterogeneity in aneuploid multiple myeloma indicates pre-B cell involvement. Blood 1988;71:861.

123. Barlogie B, Epstein J, Selvanayagam P, Alexanian R. Plasma cell myeloma—new biological insights and advances in therapy. Blood 1989;73:865.

124. Grogan TM, Durie BGM, Lomen C, et al. Delineation of a novel pre-B cell component in plasma cell myeloma: immunochemical, immunophenotypic, genotypic, cytologic, cell culture, and kinetic features. Blood 1987;70:932.

125. Carmagnola AL, Boccadoro M, Massaia M, Pileri A. The idiotypic specificities of lymphocytes in human monoclonal gammopathies: analysis with the fluorescence activated cell sorter. Clin Exp Immunol 1983;51:173.

126. Sugai S, Takiguchi T, Hirose Y, Konaka Y, Shimizu S, Konda S. B-cell malignancy and monoclonal gammopathy, and idiotype of cell surface and serum immunoglobulin. Jpn J Clin Oncol 1983;13:533.

127. Berenson J, Wong R, Kim K, Brown N, Lichtenstein A. Evidence for peripheral blood B lymphocyte but not T lymphocyte involvement in multiple myeloma. Blood 1987;70:1550.

128. Bergui L, Schena M, Gaidano G, Riva M, Caligaris-Cappio F. Interleukin 3 and interleukin 6 synergistically promote the proliferation and differentiation of malignant plasma cell precursors in multiple myeloma. J Exp Med 1989;170:613.

129. Zhang XG, Klein B, Bataille R. Interleukin-6 is a potent myeloma-cell growth factor in patients with aggressive multiple myeloma. Blood 1989;74:11.

130. Kawano M, Hirano T, Matsuda T, et al. Autocrine generation and requirement of BSF-2/IL-6 for human multiple myeloma. Nature 1988;332:83.

131. Klein B, Zhang X-G, Jourdan M, et al. Paracrine rather than autocrine regulation of myeloma-cell growth and differentiation by interleukin-6. Blood 1989;73:517.

132. Kishimoto T. The biology of interleukin-6. Blood 1989;74:1.

133. Bataille R, Jourdan M, Zhang X-G, Klein B. Serum levels of interleukin 6, a potent myeloma cell growth factor, as a reflect of disease severity in plasma cell dyscrasias. J Clin Invest 1989; 84:2008.

134. Broder S, Waldmann TA. The suppressor-cell network in cancer. N Engl J Med 1978;299:1281.

135. Katzmann JA. Myeloma-induced immunosuppression: a multistep mechanism. J Immunol 1978;121:1405.

136. Jacobson DR, Zolla-Pazner S. Immunosuppression and infection in multiple myeloma. Semin Oncol 1986;13:282.

137. Fahey JL, Scoggins R, Utz JP, Szwed CF. Infection, antibody response and gamma globulin components in multiple myeloma and macroglobulinemia. Am J Med 1963;35:698.

138. Shaikh BS, Lombard RM, Appelbaum PC, Bentz MS. Changing patterns of infections in patients with multiple myeloma. Oncology (Basel) 1982;39:78.

139. Perri RT, Hebbel RP, Oken MM. Influence of treatment and response status on infection risk in multiple myeloma. Am J Med 1981;71:935.

140. Thomas MAB, Isbister JP, Ibels LS, Cooper DA, Wells JV, McMahon C. IgA kappa multiple myeloma and lymphadenopathy syndrome associated with AIDS virus infection. Aust N Z J Med 1986;16:402.

141. McGrath KM, Stuart JJ, Richards F II. Correlation between serum IgG, platelet membrane IgG, and platelet function in hypergammaglobulinaemic states. Br J Haematol 1979;42:585.

142. Chapman GS, George CB, Danley DL. Heparin-like anticoagulant associated with plasma cell myeloma. Am J Clin Pathol 1985;83:764.

143. Gruber A, Blaskó G, Sas G. Functional deficiency of protein C and skin necrosis in multiple myeloma. Thromb Res 1986; 42:579.

144. Graham RC Jr, Bernier GM. The bone marrow in multiple myeloma: correlation of plasma cell ultrastructure and clinical state. Medicine (Baltimore) 1975;54:225.

145. Hitzman JL, Li C-Y, Kyle RA. Immunoperoxidase staining of bone marrow sections. Cancer 1981;48:2438.

146. Buss DH, Prichard RW, Hartz JW, Cooper MR, Feigin GA. Initial bone marrow findings in multiple myeloma: significance of plasma cell nodules. Arch Pathol Lab Med 1986;110:30.

147. Greipp PR, Witzig TE, Gonchoroff NJ, et al. Immunofluorescence labeling indices in myeloma and related monoclonal gammopathies. Mayo Clin Proc 1987;62:969.

148. Butler RC, Thomas SM, Thompson JM, Keat ACS. Anaplastic myeloma in systemic lupus erythematosus. Ann Rheum Dis 1984;43:653.

149. Özer FL, Telatar H, Telatar F, Müftüoğlu E. Monoclonal gammopathy with hyperlipidemia. Am J Med 1970;49:841.

150. Moschella SL. Plane xanthomatosis associated with myelomatosis. Arch Dermatol 1970;101:683.

151. Shanbrom E. Multiple myeloma and coexistent carcinoma of the sigmoid colon: a review of the literature and report of four cases. Am J Clin Pathol 1963;40:67.

152. Brouet JC, Fermand JP, Laurent G, et al. The association of chronic lymphocytic leukaemia and multiple myeloma: a study of eleven patients. Br J Haematol 1985;59:55.

153. Fermand JP, James JM, Herait P, Brouet JC. Associated chronic lymphocytic leukemia and multiple myeloma: origin from a single clone. Blood 1985;66:291.

154. Stegman R, Alexanian R. Solid tumors in multiple myeloma. Ann Intern Med 1979;90:780.

155. Venencie PY, Winkelmann RK, Puissant A, Kyle RA. Monoclonal gammopathy in Sézary syndrome: report of three cases and review of the literature. Arch Dermatol 1984;120:605.

156. Venencie PY, Winkelmann RK, Friedman SJ, Kyle RA, Puissant A. Monoclonal gammopathy and mycosis fungoides: report of four cases and review of the literature. J Am Acad Dermatol 1984;11:576.

157. Lawlor E, Willoughby R, O'Briain DS, Daly PA. Multiple neoplasms in hairy cell leukaemia. Acta Haematol (Basel) 1984;72:57.

158. Geerling S. Kaposi's sarcoma associated with multiple myeloma. South Med J 1984;77:931.

159. Vandermolen L, Rice L, Lynch EC. Plasma cell dyscrasia with marrow fibrosis: clinicopathologic syndrome. Am J Med 1985;79:297.

160. Kyle RA, Greipp PR. Plasma cell dyscrasias: current status. Crit Rev Oncol Hematol 1988;8:93.

161. Salmon SE, Smith BA. Immunoglobulin synthesis and total

body tumor cell number in IgG multiple myeloma. J Clin Invest 1970;49:1114.

162. Durie BGM, Salmon SE. A clinical staging system for multiple myeloma: correlation of measured myeloma cell mass with presenting clinical features, response to treatment, and survival. Cancer 1975;36:842.

163. Durie BGM, Salmon SE, Moon TE. Pretreatment tumor mass, cell kinetics, and prognosis in multiple myeloma. Blood 1980;55:364.

164. Durie BGM, Cole PW, Chen H-SG, Himmelstein KJ, Salmon SE. Synthesis and metabolism of Bence Jones protein and calculation of tumour burden in patients with Bence Jones myeloma. Br J Haematol 1981;47:7.

165. Cuzick J, Cooper EH, MacLennan ICM. The prognostic value of serum β2 microglobulin compared with other presentation features in myelomatosis (a report to the Medical Research Council's Working Party on Leukaemia in Adults). Br J Cancer 1985;52:1.

166. Greipp PR, Katzmann JA, O'Fallon WM, Kyle RA. Value of β_2-microglobulin level and plasma cell labeling indices as prognostic factors in patients with newly diagnosed myeloma. Blood 1988;72:219.

167. Greipp PR, Raymond NM, Kyle RA, O'Fallon WM. Multiple myeloma: significance of plasmablastic subtype in morphological classification. Blood 1985;65:305.

168. Bartl R, Frisch B, Fateh-Moghadam A, Kettner G, Jaeger K, Sommerfeld W. Histologic classification and staging of multiple myeloma: a retrospective and prospective study of 674 cases. Am J Clin Pathol 1987;87:342.

169. Latreille J, Barlogie B, Johnston D, Drewinko B, Alexanian R. Ploidy and proliferative characteristics in monoclonal gammopathies. Blood 1982;59:43.

170. Montecucco C, Riccardi A, Ucci G, et al. Analysis of human myeloma cell population kinetics. Acta Haematol (Basel) 1986;75:153.

171. Witzig TE, Gonchoroff NJ, Katzmann JA, Therneau TM, Kyle RA, Greipp PR. Peripheral blood B cell labeling indices are a measure of disease activity in patients with monoclonal gammopathies. J Clin Oncol 1988;6:1041.

172. Durie BGM, Russell DH, Salmon SE. Reappraisal of plateau phase in myeloma. Lancet 1980;ii:65.

173. Drewinko B, Alexanian R, Boyer H, Barlogie B, Rubinow SI. The growth fraction of human myeloma cells. Blood 1981;57:333.

174. Dewald GW, Kyle RA, Hicks GA, Greipp PR. The clinical significance of cytogenetic studies in 100 patients with multiple myeloma, plasma cell leukemia, or amyloidosis. Blood 1985;66:380.

175. Lewis JP, MacKenzie MR. Non-random chromosomal aberrations associated with multiple myeloma. Hematol Oncol 1984;2:307.

176. Barlogie B, Alexanian R, Gehan EA, Smallwood L, Smith T, Drewinko B. Marrow cytometry and prognosis in myeloma. J Clin Invest 1983;72:853.

177. Smith L, Barlogie B, Alexanian R. Biclonal and hypodiploid multiple myeloma. Am J Med 1986;80:841.

178. Durie BGM, Grogan TM. CALLA-positive myeloma: an aggressive subtype with poor survival. Blood 1985;66:229.

179. Takahashi T, Lim B, Jamal N, et al. Colony growth and self renewal of plasma cell precursors in multiple myeloma. J Clin Oncol 1985;3:1613.

180. Kyle RA. Long-term survival in multiple myeloma. N Engl J Med 1983;308:314.

181. Alexanian R. Ten-year survival in multiple myeloma. Arch Intern Med 1985;145:2073.

182. Suchman AL, Coleman M, Mouradian JA, Wolf DJ, Saletan S. Aggressive plasma cell myeloma: a terminal phase. Arch Intern Med 1981;141:1315.

183. Bosanquet AG, Gilby ED. Comparison of the fed and fasting states on the absorption of melphalan in multiple myeloma. Cancer Chemother Pharmacol 1984;12:183.

184. Lee BJ, Lake-Lewin D, Meyers JE. Intensive treatment of multiple myeloma. In: Wiernik PH, ed. Controversies in Oncology. New York: John Wiley & Sons, 1982:61.

185. Harley JB, Pajak TF, McIntyre OR, et al. Improved survival of increased-risk myeloma patients on combined triple-alkylating-agent therapy: a study of the CALGB. Blood 1979;54:13.

186. Bergsagel DE, Bailey AJ, Langley GR, MacDonald RN, White DF, Miller AB. The chemotherapy of plasma-cell myeloma and the incidence of acute leukemia. N Engl J Med 1979;301:743.

187. Medical Research Council. Treatment comparisons in the third MRC myelomatosis trial. Br J Cancer 1980;42:823.

188. Durie BGM, Dixon DO, Carter S, et al. Improved survival duration with combination chemotherapy induction for multiple myeloma: a Southwest Oncology Group study. J Clin Oncol 1986;4:1227.

189. Alexanian R, Dreicer R. Chemotherapy for multiple myeloma. Cancer 1984;53:583.

190. Oken MM, Tsiatis A, Abramson N, Glick J. Evaluation of intensive (VBMCP) vs standard (MP) therapy for multiple myeloma (abstract). Proc Am Soc Clin Oncol Annu Meet 1987;6:203.

191. Bergsagel DE. Is aggressive chemotherapy more effective in the treatment of plasma cell myeloma? Eur J Cancer Clin Oncol 1989;25:159.

192. Sporn JR, McIntyre OR. Chemotherapy of previously untreated multiple myeloma patients: an analysis of recent treatment results. Semin Oncol 1986;13:318.

193. Belch A, Shelley W, Bergsagel D, et al. A randomized trial of maintenance *versus* no maintenance melphalan and prednisone in responding multiple myeloma patients. Br J Cancer 1988;57:94.

194. Kyle RA, Pierre RV, Bayrd ED. Multiple myeloma and acute myelomonocytic leukemia: report of four cases possibly related to melphalan. N Engl J Med 1970;283:1121.

195. Rosner F, Grünwald HW. Simultaneous occurrence of multiple myeloma and acute myeloblastic leukemia: fact or myth? Am J Med 1984;76:891.

196. Rosner F, Grünwald HW. Multiple myeloma and Waldenström's macroglobulinemia terminating in acute leukemia: review with emphasis on karyotypic and ultrastructural abnormalities. N Y State J Med 1980;80:558.

197. Cuzick J, Erskine S, Edelman D, Galton DAG. A comparison of the incidence of the myelodysplastic syndrome and acute myeloid leukaemia following melphalan and cyclophosphamide treatment for myelomatosis: a report to the Medical Research Council's Working Party on Leukaemia in Adults. Br J Cancer 1987;55:523.

198. Bergsagel DE, Bailey AJ, Langley GR, MacDonald RN, White DF, Miller AB. The incidence of acute leukemia in myeloma patients treated with alkylating agents (abstract). In: Lecture and Symposium Abstracts. Joint Meeting of the 18th Congress of the International Society of Hematology and 16th Congress of the International Society of Blood Transfusion, Montreal, Quebec, Canada, August 16–22, 1980, p 60.

199. Greene MH, Harris EL, Gershenson DM, et al. Melphalan may be a more potent leukemogen than cyclophosphamide. Ann Intern Med 1986;105:360.

200. Kyle RA, Gertz MA. Second malignancies after chemotherapy. In: Perry MC, ed. The Chemotherapy Source Book. Baltimore: Williams & Wilkins, 1992:689.

201. Le Beau MM, Albain KS, Larson RA, et al. Clinical and

cytogenetic correlations in 63 patients with therapy-related myelodysplastic syndromes and acute nonlymphocytic leukemia: further evidence for characteristic abnormalities of chromosomes no. 5 and 7. J Clin Oncol 1986;4:325.

202. Duane SF, Peterson BA, Bloomfield CD, Michels SD, Hurd DD. Response of therapy-associated acute nonlymphocytic leukemia to intensive induction chemotherapy. Med Pediatr Oncol 1985;13:207.

203. Mandelli F, Avvisati G, Amadori S, et al. Maintenance treatment with recombinant interferon alpha-2b in patients with multiple meyloma responding to conventional induction chemotherapy. N Engl J Med 1990;322:1430.

204. Alexanian R, Barlogie B, Dixon D. High-dose glucocorticoid treatment of resistant myeloma. Ann Intern Med 1986;105:8.

205. Quesada JR, Gutterman JU. Annotation: alpha interferons in B-cell neoplasms. Br J Haematol 1986;64:639.

206. Buzaid AC, Durie BGM. Management of refractory myeloma: a review. J Clin Oncol 1988;6:889.

207. Selby PJ, McElwain TJ, Nandi AC, et al. Multiple myeloma treated with high dose intravenous melphalan. Br J Haematol 1987;66:55.

208. Kyle RA, Oken MM, Greipp PR, Kay NE, Tsiotis A, O'Connell MJ. Alternating cycles of VBMCP with interferon (rIFN α_2) in the treatment of multiple myeloma (abstract). Read at the Twenty-Second Congress of the International Society of Hematology, Milan, Italy, August 28 to September 2, 1988.

209. Fefer A, Cheever MA, Greenberg PD: Identical-twin (syngeneic) marrow transplantation for hematologic cancers. J Natl Cancer Inst 1986;76:1269.

210. Gahrton G, Tura S, Flesch M, et al. Bone marrow transplantation in multiple myeloma: report from the European Cooperative Group for Bone Marrow Transplantation. Blood 1987;69:1262.

211. Barlogie B, Alexanian R, Dicke KA, Zagars G. High dose melphalan (HDM) and total body irradiation (TBI) for refractory multiple myeloma. Proc Am Soc Clin Oncol Annu Meet 1987;6:192.

212. Fermand J-P, Levy Y, Gerota J, et al. Treatment of aggressive multiple myeloma by high-dose chemotherapy and total body irradiation followed by blood stem cells autologous graft. Blood 1989;73:20.

213. Dalton WS, Grogan TM, Meltzer PS, et al. Drug-resistance in multiple myeloma and non-Hodgkin's lymphoma: detection of P-glycoprotein and potential circumvention by addition of verapamil to chemotherapy. J Clin Oncol 1989;7:415.

214. Warrell RP Jr, Israel R, Frisone M, Snyder T, Gaynor JJ, Bockman RS. Gallium nitrate for acute treatment of cancer-related hypercalcemia: a randomized, double-blind comparison to calcitonin. Ann Intern Med 1988;108:669.

215. Ralston SH, Alzaid AA, Gallacher SJ, Gardner MD, Cowan RA, Boyle IT. Clinical experience with aminohydroxypropylidene bisphosphonate (APD) in the management of cancer-associated hypercalcaemia. Q J Med 1988;69:825.

216. Thiébaud D, Jaeger Ph, Jacquet AF, Burckhardt P. Dose-response in the treatment of hypercalcemia of malignancy by a single infusion of the biphosphonate AHPrBP. J Clin Oncol 1988;6:762.

217. Pasquali S, Cagnoli L, Rovinetti C, Rigotti A, Zucchelli P. Plasma exchange therapy in rapidly progressive renal failure due to multiple myeloma. Int J Artif Organs 1985;8(suppl 2):27.

218. Johnson WJ, Kyle RA, Pineda AA, O'Brien PC, Holley KE. Treatment of renal failure associated with multiple myeloma: plasmapheresis, hemodialysis, and chemotherapy. Arch Intern Med 1990;150:863.

219. Ludwig H, Fritz E, Kotzmann H, Höcker P, Gisslinger H, Barnas U. Erythropoietin treatment of anemia associated with multiple myeloma. N Engl J Med 1990;322:1693.

220. Kyle RA, Greipp PR. Smoldering multiple myeloma. N Engl J Med 1980;302:1347.

221. Walker JD, Kaczmarski RS. Survival of twenty-two months in a patient with primary plasma cell leukaemia treated with melphalan and prednisolone. Postgrad Med J 1988;64:232.

222. Noel P, Kyle RA. Plasma cell leukemia: an evaluation of response to therapy. Am J Med 1987;83:1062.

223. Franchi F, Seminara P, Teodori L, Adone G, Bianco P. The non-producer plasma cell myeloma: report of a case and review of the literature. Blut 1986;52:281.

224. Sheehan T, Sinclair D, Tansey P, O'Donnell JR. Demonstration of serum monoclonal immunoglobulin in a case of non-secretory myeloma by immunoisoelectric focusing. J Clin Pathol 1985; 38:806.

225. Cavo M, Galieni P, Gobbi M, et al. Nonsecretory multiple myeloma: presenting findings, clinical course and prognosis. Acta Haematol (Basel) 1985;74:27.

226. Dreicer R, Alexanian R. Nonsecretory multiple myeloma. Am J Hematol 1982;13:313.

227. Jancelewicz Z, Takatsuki K, Sugai S, Pruzanski W. IgD multiple myeloma: review of 133 cases. Arch Intern Med 1975; 135:87.

228. Fibbe WE, Jansen J. Prognostic factors in IgD myeloma: a study of 21 cases. Scand J Haematol 1984;33:471.

229. Takatsuki K, Sanada I. Plasma cell dyscrasia with polyneuropathy and endocrine disorder: clinical and laboratory features of 109 reported cases. Jpn J Clin Oncol 1983;13:543.

230. Bardwick PA, Zvaifler NJ, Gill GN, Newman D, Greenway GD, Resnick DL. Plasma cell dyscrasia with polyneuropathy, organomegaly, endocrinopathy, M protein, and skin changes: the POEMS syndrome; report on two cases and a review of the literature. Medicine (Baltimore) 1980;59:311.

231. Delauche MC, Clauvel JP, Seligmann M. Peripheral neuropathy and plasma cell neoplasias: a report of 10 cases. Br J Haematol 1981;48:383.

232. Kelly JJ Jr, Kyle RA, Miles JM, Dyck PJ. Osteosclerotic myeloma and peripheral neuropathy. Neurology 1983;33:202.

233. Case Records of the Massachusetts General Hospital (Case 10-1987). N Engl J Med 1987;316:606.

234. Kobayashi H, Sakaki A, Ii K, Hizawa K, Sano T, Ogushi F. Plasma-cell dyscrasia with polyneuropathy and endocrine disorders associated with dysfunction of salivary glands. Am J Surg Pathol 1985;9:759.

235. Meyer JE, Schulz MD. "Solitary" myeloma of bone: a review of 12 cases. Cancer 1974;34:438.

236. Bataille R, Sany J. Solitary myeloma: clinical and prognostic features of a review of 114 cases. Cancer 1981;48:845.

237. Frassica DA, Frassica FJ, Schray MF, Sim FH, Kyle RA. Solitary plasmacytoma of bone: Mayo Clinic experience. Int J Radiat Oncol Biol Phys 1989;16:43.

238. Chak LY, Cox RS, Bostwick DG, Hoppe RT. Solitary plasmacytoma of bone: treatment, progression, and survival. J Clin Oncol 1987;5:1811.

239. Wiltshaw E. The natural history of extramedullary plasmacytoma and its relation to solitary myeloma of bone and myelomatosis. Medicine (Baltimore) 1976;55:217.

240. Woodruff RK, Whittle JM, Malpas JS. Solitary plasmacytoma. I. Extramedullary soft tissue plasmacytoma. Cancer 1979; 43:2340.

241. Corwin J, Lindberg RD. Solitary plasmacytoma of bone vs. extramedullary plasmacytoma and their relationship to multiple myeloma. Cancer 1979;43:1007.

242. Knowling MA, Harwood AR, Bergsagel DE. Comparison of extramedullary plasmacytomas with solitary and multiple plasma cell tumors of bone. J Clin Oncol 1983;1:255.

243. Papadimitriou CS, Schwarze EW. Extramedullary non-gas-

trointestinal plasmocytoma: an immunohistochemical study of sixteen cases. Pathol Res Pract 1983;176:306.

244. Waldenström J. Incipient myelomatosis or "essential" hyperglobulinemia with fibrinogenopenia: a new syndrome? Acta Med Scand 1944;117:216.

245. McCallister BD, Bayrd ED, Harrison EG Jr, McGuckin WF. Primary macroglobulinemia: review with a report of thirty-one cases and notes on the value of continuous chlorambucil therapy. Am J Med 1967;43:394.

246. Blattner WA, Garber JE, Mann DL, et al. Waldenström's macroglobulinemia and autoimmune disease in a family. Ann Intern Med 1980;93:830.

247. Fine JM, Muller JY, Rochu D, et al. Waldenström's macroglobulinemia in monozygotic twins. Acta Med Scand 1986;220:369.

248. Epenetos AA, Rohatiner A, Slevin M, Woothipoom W. Ankylosing spondylitis and Waldenström's macroglobulinemia: a case report. Clin Oncol 1980;6:83.

249. Palka G, Spadano A, Geraci L, et al. Chromosome changes in 19 patients with Waldenström's macroglobulinemia. Cancer Genet Cytogenet 1987;29:261.

250. Pilarski LM, Andrews EJ, Serra HM, Ledbetter JA, Ruether BA, Mant MJ. Abnormalities in lymphocyte profile and specificity repertoire of patients with Waldenström's macroglobulinemia, multiple myeloma, and IgM monoclonal gammopathy of undetermined significance. Am J Hematol 1989;30:53.

251. Pettersson D, Mellstedt H, Holm G. Characterization of the monoclonal blood and bone marrow B lymphocytes in Waldenström's macroglobulinaemia. Scand J Immunol 1980;11:593.

252. Kyle RA, Garton JP. The spectrum of IgM monoclonal gammopathy in 430 cases. Mayo Clin Proc 1987;62:719.

253. Julien J, Vital C, Vallat J-M. Lagueny A, Deminiere C, Darriet D. Polyneuropathy in Waldenström's macroglobulinemia: deposition of M component on myelin sheaths. Arch Neurol 1978;35:423.

254. Platia EV, Saral R. Deafness and Waldenström's macroglobulinemia. South Med J 1979;72:1495.

255. Lindström FD, Hed J, Eneström S. Renal pathology of Waldenström's macroglobulinaemia with monoclonal antiglomerular antibodies and nephrotic syndrome. Clin Exp Immunol 1980;41:196.

256. Rausch PG, Herion JC. Pulmonary manifestations of Waldenström macroglobulinemia. Am J Hematol 1980;9:201.

257. Monteagudo M, Lima J, Garcia-Bragado F, Alvarez J. Chylous pleural effusion as the initial manifestation of Waldenström's macroglobulinemia. Eur J Respir Dis 1987;70:326.

258. Brandt LJ, Davidoff A, Bernstein LH, Biempica L. Rindfleisch B, Goldstein ML. Small-intestinal involvement in Waldenström's macroglobulinemia: case report and review of the literature. Dig Dis Sci 1981;26:174.

259. Wanless IR, Solt LC, Kortan P, Deck JHN, Gardiner GW, Prokipchuk EJ. Nodular regenerative hyperplasia of the liver associated with macroglobulinemia: a clue to the pathogenesis. Am J Med 1981;70:1203.

260. Bloch KJ, Maki DG. Hyperviscosity syndromes associated with immunoglobulin abnormalities. Semin Hematol 1973;10:113.

261. Crawford J, Cox EB, Cohen HJ. Evaluation of hyperviscosity in monoclonal gammopathies. Am J Med 1985;79:13.

262. Preston FE, Cooke KB, Foster ME, Winfield DA, Lee D. Myelomatosis and the hyperviscosity syndrome. Br J Haematol 1978;38:517.

263. Pruzanski W, Watt JG. Serum viscosity and hyperviscosity syndrome in IgG multiple myeloma: report on 10 patients and a review of the literature. Ann Intern Med 1972;77:853.

264. Maldonado JE, Kyle RA, Brown AL Jr, Bayrd ED. "Intermediate" cell types and mixed cell proliferation in multiple myeloma: electron microscopic observations. Blood 1966;27:212.

265. Levine AM, Lichtenstein A, Gresik MV, Taylor CR, Feinstein DI, Lukes RJ. Clinical and immunologic spectrum of plasmacytoid lymphocytic lymphoma without serum monoclonal IgM. Br J Haematol 1980;46:225.

266. Zarrabi MH, Stark RS, Kane P, Dannaher CL, Chandor S. IgM myeloma, a distinct entity in the spectrum of B-cell neoplasia. Am J Clin Pathol 1981;75:1.

267. Takahashi K, Yamamura F, Motoyama H. IgM myeloma—its distinction from Waldenström's macroglobulinemia. Acta Pathol Jpn 1986;36:1553.

268. Bartl R, Frisch B, Mahl G, et al. Bone marrow histology in Waldenström's macroglobulinaemia: clinical relevance of subtype recognition. Scand J Haematol 1983;31:359.

269. Case DC Jr, Schulman P, Herring WB. Waldenström's macroglobulinemia: combination chemotherapy with the M-2 protocol (BCNU, cyclophosphamide, vincristine, melphalan and prednisone) (abstract). Blood 1985;66(suppl 1):213A.

270. Horsman DE, Card RT, Skinnider LF. Waldenström macroglobulinemia terminating in acute leukemia: a report of three cases. Am J Hematol 1983;15:97.

271. Wang A-C. Molecular basis for cryoprecipitation. Springer Semin Immunopathol 1988;10:21.

272. Letendre L, Kyle RA. Monoclonal cryoglobulinemia with high thermal insolubility. Mayo Clin Proc 1982;57:629.

273. Brouet J-C, Clauvel J-P, Danon F, Klein M, Seligmann M. Biologic and clinical significance of cryoglobulins: a report of 86 cases. Am J Med 1974;57:775.

274. Montagnino G. Reappraisal of the clinical expression of mixed cryoglobulinemia. Springer Semin Immunopathol 1988;10:1.

275. D'Amico G, Colasanti G, Ferrario F, Sinico AR, Bucci A, Fornasier A. Renal involvement in essential mixed cryoglobulinemia: a peculiar type of immune-mediated renal disease. Adv Nephrol 1988;17:219.

276. Tarantino A, De Vecchi A, Montagnino G, et al. Renal disease in essential mixed cryoglobulinaemia: long-term follow-up of 44 patients. Q J Med 1981;50:1.

277. Gorevic PD, Kassab HJ, Levo Y, et al. Mixed cryoglobulinemia: clinical aspects and long-term follow-up of 40 patients. Am J Med 1980;69:287.

278. Monteverde A, Rivano MT, Allegra GC, et al. Essential mixed cryoglobulinemia, type II: a manifestation of a low-grade malignant lymphoma? Clinical-morphological study of 12 cases with special reference to immunohistochemical findings in liver frozen sections. Acta Haematol (Basel) 1988;79:20.

279. Grey HM, Kohler PF. Cryoimmunoglobulins. Semin Hematol 1973;10:87.

280. Dammacco F, Miglietta A, Lobreglio G, Bonomo L. Cryoglobulins and pyroglobulins: an overview. Ric Clin Lab 1986;16:247.

281. Invernizzi F, Cattaneo R, Rosso di San Secondo V, Balestrieri G, Zanussi C. Pyroglobulinemia: a report of eight patients with associated paraproteinemia. Acta Haematol (Basel) 1973;50:65.

282. Franklin EC, Lowenstein J, Bigelow B, Meltzer M. Heavy chain disease—a new disorder of serum γ-globulins: report of the first case. Am J Med 1964;37:332.

283. Kyle RA, Greipp PR, Banks PM. The diverse picture of gamma heavy-chain disease: report of seven cases and review of literature. Mayo Clin Proc 1981;56:439.

284. Roda L, David M-J, Biron P, Souche S, Creyssel R. Gamma heavy chain disease DUB: clinical, immunochemical and pathological studies. Haematologica (Pavia) 1985;70:232.

285. Dickson JR, Harth M, Bell DA, Komar R, Chodirker WB. Gamma heavy chain disease and rheumatoid arthritis. Semin Arthritis Rheum 1989;18:247.

286. Di Benedetto G, Cataldi A, Verde A, Gloghini A, Nicolò G, Pistoia V. Gamma heavy chain disease associated with Hodgkin's disease: clinical, pathologic, and immunologic features of one case. Cancer 1989;63:1804.

287. Fermand J-P, Brouet J-C, Danon F, Seligmann M. Gamma heavy chain "disease": heterogeneity of the clinicopathologic features; report of 16 cases and review of the literature. Medicine (Baltimore) 1989;68:321.

288. Seligmann M. Immunochemical, clinical, and pathological features of α-chain disease. Arch Intern Med 1975;135:78.

289. Rambaud JC, Galian A, Matuchansky C, et al. Natural history of alpha-chain disease and the so-called Mediterranean lymphoma. Recent Results Cancer Res 1978;64:271.

290. Haghighi P, Wolf PL. Alpha-heavy chain disease. Clin Lab Med 1986;6:477.

291. Bowie MD, Hill ID. α-Chain disease in children. J Pediatr 1988;112:46.

292. Tungekar MF, Omar YT, Behbehani K. Gastric alpha heavy chain disease. Oncology 1987;44:360.

293. Takahashi K, Naito M, Matsuoka Y, Takatsuki K. A new form of alpha-chain disease with generalized lymph node involvement. Pathol Res Pract 1988;183:717.

294. Haghighi P, Kharazmi A, Gerami C, et al. Primary upper small-intestinal lymphoma and alpha-chain disease: report of 10 cases emphasizing pathological aspects. Am J Surg Pathol 1978;2:147.

295. Doe WF, Danon F, Seligmann M. Immunodiagnosis of alpha chain disease. Clin Exp Immunol 1979;36:189.

296. Isaacson P. Middle East lymphoma and α-chain disease: an immunohistochemical study. Am J Surg Pathol 1979;3:431.

297. Berger R, Bernheim A, Tsapis A, Brouet J-C, Seligmann M. Cytogenetic studies in four cases of alpha chain disease. Cancer Genet Cytogenet 1986;22:219.

298. Smith WJ, Price SK, Isaacson PG. Immunoglobulin gene rearrangement in immunoproliferative small intestinal disease (IPSID). J Clin Pathol 1987;40:1291.

299. Matuchansky C, Cogné M, Lemaire M, et al. Nonsecretory α-chain disease with immunoproliferative small-intestinal disease. N Engl J Med 1989;320:1534.

300. O'Keefe SJD, Winter TA, Newton KA, Ogden JM, Young GO, Price SK. Severe malnutrition associated with α-heavy chain disease: response to tetracycline and intensive nutritional support. Am J Gastroenterol 1988;83:995.

301. Ben-Ayed F, Halphen M, Najjar T, et al. Treatment of alpha chain disease: results of a prospective study in 21 Tunisian patients by the Tunisian-French Intestinal Lymphoma Study Group. Cancer 1989;63:1251.

302. Franklin EC. μ-Chain disease. Arch Intern Med 1975;135:71.

303. Brouet J-C, Seligmann M, Danon F, Belpomme D, Fine J-M. μ-Chain disease: report of two new cases. Arch Intern Med 1979;139:672.

304. Leach IH, Jenkins JS, Murray-Leslie CF, Powell RJ. Mu-heavy chain and monoclonal IgG κ paraproteinaemia in systemic lupus erythematosus. Br J Rheumatol 1987;26:460.

305. Wright JR, Calkins E, Humphrey RL. Potassium permanganate reaction in amyloidosis: a histologic method to assist in differentiating forms of this disease. Lab Invest 1977;36:274.

306. Smith RRL, Hutchins GM, Moore GW, Humphrey RL. Type and distribution of pulmonary parenchymal and vascular amyloid: correlation with cardiac amyloidosis. Am J Med 1979;66:96.

307. Holck M, Husby G, Sletten K, Natvig JB. The amyloid P-component (protein AP): an integral part of the amyloid substance? Scand J Immunol 1979;10:55.

308. Glenner GG, Terry W, Harada M, Isersky C, Page D. Amyloid fibril proteins: proof of homology with immunoglobulin light chains by sequence analyses. Science 1971;172:1150.

309. Buxbaum J, Hauser D. Aberrant immunoglobulin synthesis in light chain amyloidosis: free light chain and light chain fragment production by human bone marrow cells in short-term tissue culture. J Clin Invest 1986;78:798.

310. Preud'homme JL, Ganeval D, Grünfeld JP, Striker L, Brouet JC. Immunoglobulin synthesis in primary and myeloma amyloidosis. Clin Exp Immunol 1988;73:389.

311. Levin M, Franklin EC, Frangione B, Pras M. The amino acid sequence of a major nonimmunoglobulin component of some amyloid fibrils. J Clin Invest 1972;51:2773.

312. De Beer FC, Mallya RK, Fagan EA, Lanham JG, Hughes GRV, Pepys MB. Serum amyloid-A protein concentration in inflammatory diseases and its relationship to the incidence of reactive systemic amyloidosis. Lancet 1982;ii:231.

313. Lavie G, Zucker-Franklin D, Franklin EC. Degradation of serum amyloid A protein by surface-associated enzymes of human blood monocytes. J Exp Med 1978;148:1020.

314. Kyle RA, Bayrd ED. Amyloidosis: review of 236 cases. Medicine (Baltimore) 1975;54:271.

315. Greipp PR, Kyle RA, Bowie EJW. Factor X deficiency in primary amyloidosis: resolution after splenectomy. N Engl J Med 1979;301:1050.

316. Dikman SH, Churg J, Kahn T. Morphologic and clinical correlates in renal amyloidosis. Hum Pathol 1981;12:160.

317. Smith TJ, Kyle RA, Lie JT. Clinical significance of histopathologic patterns of cardiac amyloidosis. Mayo Clin Proc 1984;59:547.

318. Cueto-Garcia L, Reeder GS, Kyle RA, et al. Echocardiographic findings in systemic amyloidosis: spectrum of cardiac involvement and relation to survival. J Am Coll Cardiol 1985;6:737.

319. Gertz MA, Kyle RA, Griffing WL, Hunder GG. Jaw claudication in primary systemic amyloidosis. Medicine (Baltimore) 1986;65:173.

320. Kelly JJ Jr, Kyle RA, O'Brien PC, Dyck PJ. The natural history of peripheral neuropathy in primary systemic amyloidosis. Ann Neurol 1979;6:1.

321. Gertz MA, Kyle RA. Hepatic amyloidosis (primary [AL], immunoglobulin light chain): the natural history in 80 patients. Am J Med 1988;85:73.

322. Gertz MA, Li C-Y, Shirahama T, Kyle RA. Utility of subcutaneous fat aspiration for the diagnosis of systemic amyloidosis (immunoglobulin light chain). Arch Intern Med 1988;148:929.

323. Linke RP, Nathrath WBJ, Eulitz M. Classification of amyloid syndromes from tissue sections using antibodies against various amyloid fibril proteins: report of 142 cases. In: Glenner GG, Osserman EF, Benditt EP, Calkins E, Cohen AS, Zucker-Franklin D, eds. Amyloidosis. New York: Plenum Press, 1986:599.

324. Gertz MA, Brown ML, Hauser MF, Kyle RA. Utility of technetium Tc 99m pyrophosphate bone scanning in cardiac amyloidosis. Arch Intern Med 1987;147:1039.

325. Kyle RA, Greipp PR, Garton JP, Gertz MA. Primary systemic amyloidosis: comparison of melphalan/prednisone versus colchicine. Am J Med 1985;79:708.

326. Kyle RA, Gertz MA. Systemic amyloidosis. Crit Rev Oncol Hematol 1990;10:49.

327. Kyle RA. Monoclonal gammopathy of undetermined significance: Natural history of 241 cases. Am J Med 1978;64:814.

328. Ritzmann SE, Loukas D, Sakai H, Daniels JC, Levin WC. Idiopathic (asymptomatic) monoclonal gammopathies. Arch Intern Med 1975;135:95.

329. Kyle RA. Monoclonal gammopathy of undetermined significance (MGUS): a review. Clin Haematol 1982;11:123.

330. Kyle RA. 'Benign' monoclonal gammopathy: a misnomer? JAMA 1984;251:1849.

331. Alexanian R. Monoclonal gammopathy in lymphoma. Arch Intern Med 1975;135:62.

332. Kyle RA, Lust JA. Monoclonal gammopathies of undetermined significance. Semin Hematol 1989;26:176.

333. Merlini G, Farhangi M, Osserman EF. Monoclonal immuno-globulins with antibody activity in myeloma, macroglobuline-mia and related plasma cell dyscrasias. Semin Oncol 1986; 13:350.

334. Kyle RA, Robinson RA, Katzmann JA. The clinical aspects of biclonal gammopathies: review of 57 cases. Am J Med 1981;71:999.

335. Nilsson T, Norberg B, Rudolphi O, Jacobsson L. Double gammopathies: incidence and clinical course of 20 patients. Scand J Haematol 1986;36:103.

336. Riddell S, Traczyk Z, Paraskevas F, Israels LG. The double gammopathies: clinical and immunological studies. Medicine (Baltimore) 1986;65:135.

337. Kyle RA. Immunoglobulins and syndromes associated with monoclonal gammopathies. In: Tice's Practice of Medicine, Volume 1. Hagerstown, MD: Harper & Row, 1977;48:3.

338. Kyle RA, Bayrd ED. The Monoclonal Gammopathies: Multiple Myeloma and Related Plasma-cell Disorders. Springfield, IL: Charles C Thomas, 1976:3,10.

339. Kyle RA, Bieger RC, Gleich GJ. Diagnosis of syndromes associated with hyperglobulinemia. Med Clin North Am 1970; 54:917.

340. Kyle RA, Garton JP. Laboratory monitoring of myeloma pro-teins. Semin Oncol 1986;13:310.

341. Kyle RA. The laboratory evaluation of immunosecretory states. Clin Lab Annu 1982;1:383.

342. Kyle RA, Garton JP. Immunoglobulins and laboratory recogni-tion of monoclonal proteins. In: Wiernik PH, Canellos GP, Kyle RA, Schiffer CA, eds. Neoplastic Diseases of the Blood, Second Edition. New York: Churchill Livingstone, 1991.

343. Kyle RA, Greipp PR. Amyloidosis (AL): clinical and laboratory features in 229 cases. Mayo Clin Proc 1983;58:665.

17

Platelets

Scott Murphy, M.D.

Easy bruising, epistaxis, and menorrhagia are three common complaints with which physicians must deal, and in addition to prolonged and excessive bleeding after surgery or dental work, these may be caused by abnormalities of the number and function of platelets. In patients with severe thrombocytopenia, these problems may be associated with the formation of petechiae in the skin or similar capillary bleeding in the mucous membranes of the mouth, retina, and gastrointestinal tract. The term *petechia* is used to refer to a minute, round, red spot that is not raised and does not blanch with pressure. *Purpura* is a more general term, used to refer to coalescent petechiae and ecchymoses that often are described by patients as "black-and-blue marks." In various combinations, these clinical manifestations also may result from a number of diseases where blood vessels and connective tissue are abnormal; patients with platelet disorders rarely have bleeding into the joints, muscles, or viscera as seen in those with deficiencies of plasma coagulation proteins.

Four major categories of disease produce these findings, and the first is *thrombocytopenia*. In general, there are few, if any, clinical manifestations of a decrease in the number of platelets from normal to the 50,000 to 150,000 cells/mm^3 range. In this range, abnormal bleeding suggests the presence of an associated defect in platelet function, and if the platelet count is in the range of 20,000 to 50,000 cells/mm^3, then minor bruising, menorrhagia, and bleeding after surgery may be expected.[1] However, it often is surprising to see how well patients with platelet counts in this range can tolerate

significant surgical stress. At platelet levels below 20,000 cells/mm^3, petechiae and spontaneous ecchymoses become increasingly common, and serious manifestations such as gastrointestinal, urinary tract, and central nervous system bleeding may occur as the platelet count approaches 0 cells/mm^3. However, some patients can tolerate low levels for long periods without serious sequelae.

Disorders of platelet function is the second category. Platelet dysfunction occurs as both an isolated phenomenon and a result of systemic disease. Petechiae are uncommon in this group as long as the platelet count is normal, but the other bleeding manifestations listed previously are common.

Myeloproliferative disease is the third, and this group includes polycythemia vera, chronic granulocytic leukemia, myelofibrosis, and essential thrombocythemia. In some of these patients, bleeding may result from a defect in platelet function, but it appears to be related to thrombocytosis per se in others. In general, however, bleeding from thrombocytosis alone occurs only when the platelet count exceeds 1 million cells/mm^3.

Blood vessel and connective tissue disease is the fourth. In these patients, the type of bleeding seen is that which is characteristic for the particular disease. For example, patients with small-vessel vasculitis predominantly have petechiae and purpura, and patients with hereditary hemorrhagic telangiectasia have epistaxis and gastrointestinal bleeding. In general, patients in this category do not have abnormal bleeding associated with surgery and dental work.

THROMBOCYTOPENIA

The platelet count in normal individuals varies over a rather wide range, from 150,000 to 450,000 cells/mm^3. However, within the normal population, mean platelet volume also varies over a wide range, and there is an inverse relationship between the platelet count and the mean platelet volume. As a result, the concentration of the platelet mass in the blood is more constant in the normal population than might be supposed.[2]

The pathophysiologic classification of diseases producing thrombocytopenia is based primarily on platelet kinetics as assessed by measurements of the recovery and survival of labelled platelets; platelets may be obtained from the patient by serial centrifugation, labelled with either radioactive chromium (^{51}Cr) or indium (^{111}In), and then reinfused. Two measurements are made: immediate isotope recovery in the circulation, and subsequent lifespan. In normal individuals, the total body platelet mass is divided between the circulating blood and a pool of platelets in the spleen that is in excess of what would be predicted based on splenic blood volume.[3] These splenic platelets are freely exchangeable with the circulating pool, and there is approximately one platelet in the splenic pool for every two in the circulation. Thus, when labelled platelets are infused into normal individuals, the isotope recovery in the circulation is only approximately 66% because of the distribution of labelled platelets into the splenic pool; after splenectomy, the isotope recovery approaches 100%. In patients with splenomegaly from any cause, the fraction of the total body platelet mass in the splenic pool increases in rough proportion to the splenic size. Thus, isotope recovery sometimes is reduced to 10% to 20% in patients with splenomegaly. (Figure 17.1 presents this concept graphically.) Therefore, the clinical evaluation of patients with thrombocytopenia should begin during the physical examination with careful palpation for splenic enlargement.

The lifespan of platelets is measured by determining the disappearance rate of platelet-associated isotope from the circulation. In normal individuals, this lifespan of platelet-associated isotope is from 8 to 10 days. Patients with thrombocytopenia can be categorized as having impaired production in which isotope recovery and lifespan are normal or only slightly reduced, disorders of distribution in which isotope recovery is reduced but isotope lifespan is normal or nearly so, or accelerated destruction in which isotope recovery is normal but isotope lifespan is short.

It is important to remember that cell counters used in clinical laboratories will report thrombocytopenia that is spurious in approximately 0.1% of patients.[4] In general,

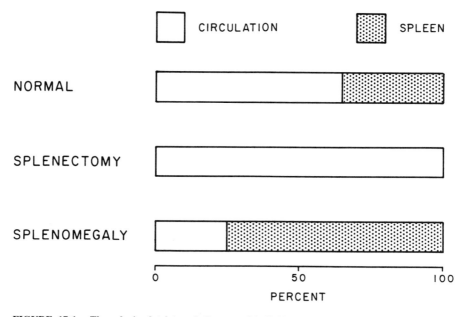

FIGURE 17.1. The splenic platelet pool. In normal individuals, two thirds of the body's platelets are in circulation and one third is in the splenic pool, which is freely exchangeable with circulation. After splenectomy, the body's total platelet mass is in circulation, and the normal physiologic role of the spleen is exaggerated in patients with splenomegaly.

this is due to platelet clumping in vitro after drawing blood into the anticoagulant, ethylenediaminetetraacetic acid. Confirmation of this spurious thrombocytopenia can be obtained by identifying platelet aggregates on blood smears and by obtaining a normal platelet count using citrate as the anticoagulant.

Impaired Platelet Production

Decreased production of platelets implies a defect in the function of megakaryocytes, the precursor cells for platelets in the bone marrow. Although megakaryocytes constitute less than 0.1% of all marrow cells, they are easily recognized because of their large size and lobulated nuclei. Their development from the hematopoietic stem cell results from a series of cell divisions that are not recognizable morphologically, and this development can be modulated, at least in vitro, by cytokines such as interleukin-3, interleukin-6, and granulocyte-macrophage colony-stimulating factor as well as others.[5] By the time that they are recognizable, megakaryocytes have ploidy values of 4N, 8N, 16N, 32N, and so on. The full maturation of recognizable megakaryocytes to the point of platelet production appears to be regulated by yet another cytokine, thrombopoietin.

The complete evaluation of a patient with thrombocytopenia requires marrow aspiration so that smears may be prepared as well as a needle biopsy for the preparation of tissue sections. In most instances of impaired platelet production, there is either a reduced number of megakaryocytes in the marrow or abnormalities in their morphology, and these are appreciated best by examining tissue sections. In addition, there almost invariably are abnormalities of the white and red blood cell series; a deficit in platelet production rarely is seen without abnormalities of the other marrow elements as well.

CAUSES.

Marrow Suppression by Chemotherapy and Radiotherapy. Because of increasingly aggressive therapy of malignant disease, bone marrow suppression by either chemotherapy or radiotherapy has become the most common cause of thrombocytopenia. Radiotherapy and a variety of chemotherapeutic agents predictably suppress marrow proliferation in a dose-related fashion, but for unknown reasons, leukopenia usually appears first and is more severe than thrombocytopenia. Thrombocytopenia rarely is the predominant, dose-limiting problem; however, there are two notable exceptions. The nitrosoureas rather typically produce a late thrombocytopenia 3 to 6 weeks after administration, when the white blood cell count has recovered, and recovery is usually prompt, within 1 to 2 weeks after the nadir. On the other hand, marrow hypoplasia produced by busulfan may be followed by months of severe thrombocytopenia long after the granulocyte count has returned to normal, or at least to levels adequate to protect against infection.

In addition to the predictable marrow hypoplasia produced by these drugs, other drugs also are capable of producing severe marrow failure in an idiosyncratic fashion; most notable among these are chloramphenicol, phenylbutazone, gold compounds, phenytoin, and the sulfonamides. It is extremely rare for these drugs to cause impaired platelet production without serious deficits in granulocyte and erythrocyte production as well.

Malignant Invasion of the Marrow. When malignant tissue invades the marrow, the production of normal blood cells commonly is impaired. The traditional concept of myelophthisic anemia implies that normal cells fail to develop because of inadequate space; however, biopsy specimens from many of these patients demonstrate ample residual fat spaces. Therefore, the mechanisms of the suppression of production must be biochemical and more complex than a mere limitation of space. Also, malignancy may be missed if only smears of marrow aspirates are evaluated, but it will be obvious on sections of a needle biopsy.

The most common malignancy to produce this picture is acute leukemia. The diagnosis is based on the recognition of leukemic blasts in blood and marrow smears and usually is straightforward. One variant, acute promyelocytic leukemia, is associated with particularly severe thrombocytopenia and hemorrhage, because there is an associated, disseminated intravascular coagulation. The latter appears to be provoked by the release from leukemic cells of procoagulant material that leads to a rapid consumption of platelets and coagulation factors; successful treatment requires intensive infusion of platelets and coagulation factors.[6]

Diagnosis may be more difficult in patients with the so-called dysmyelopoietic or myelodysplastic syndromes.[7] Approximately 50% of these more difficult cases will have thrombocytopenia associated with variable degrees of anemia and leukopenia along with a hyperplastic marrow. These patients generally are subclassified according to the French-American-British criteria into refractory anemia, acquired idiopathic sideroblastic anemia, chronic myelomonocytic leukemia, or refractory anemia with excess blasts. Thrombocytopenia is a poor prognostic factor,[8] and in contrast to impaired platelet production produced by chemotherapeutic drugs, normal or even increased numbers of megakaryocytes may be present in the marrow of these patients. Abnormalities of megakaryocyte morphology include a predominance of cells with a single or bilobed nucleus associated with decreased numbers of normal forms with multilobed nuclei. However, this finding is inconstant, and it is difficult to use megakaryocyte morphology to make a diagnosis.

When present, thrombocytopenia undoubtedly reflects a megakaryocytic abnormality, yet platelet kinetics may be complex. It is likely there is ineffective thrombopoiesis similar to the ineffective erythropoiesis that is so typical of these patients; in fact, one report exists of a shortened platelet survival time associated with normal survival of labelled normal platelets.[9] This suggests that platelets are made so badly that they never leave the marrow or, if they do, their intravascular survival is short.

Invasion of the marrow by malignant lymphoma or carcinomas such as lung, breast, stomach, colon, and prostate also may produce severe thrombocytopenia along with anemia and leukopenia. In these patients, it is common to see nucleated red cells and immature granulocytic precursors in the peripheral blood (the so-called leukoerythroblastic blood picture).

Megaloblastic Anemia. Severe thrombocytopenia may be a component of the pancytopenia that is produced by deficiencies in folic acid and vitamin B_{12}, and platelet counts as low as 10,000 cells/mm^3 have been observed. Rarely, thrombocytopenic bleeding may be the most striking clinical finding. The characteristic blood and marrow morphology makes the diagnosis obvious, and the platelet level returns to normal within 1 to 2 weeks after the initiation of replacement therapy.

Aplastic Anemia: Acquired and Congenital. Patients may develop acquired aplastic anemia from drugs (as described earlier), in the aftermath of an episode of infectious hepatitis, as part of the paroxysmal nocturnal hemoglobinuria syndrome, or idiopathically. In addition, Fanconi anemia, which is an aplastic pancytopenia, develops between the ages of 5 and 10 years, apparently on a congenital basis. In both acquired and congenital anemia, there is pancytopenia in the peripheral blood, and the marrow biopsy shows decreased hematopoietic marrow and increased fat spaces. In idiopathic aplastic anemia, there commonly is an infiltrate of lymphocytes and plasma cells within the interstitial spaces of the marrow,[10] and this morphologic finding may correlate with the concept that cytotoxic T cells suppress stem cell proliferation in many of these cases. Thrombocytopenic bleeding, increased incidence of infection, and refractory anemia are the major clinical problems that arise from the failure of blood production; not uncommonly, bleeding is the major problem.

In addition, there is a rare congenital disorder characterized by the marked depletion or total absence of megakaryocytes and with no associated abnormality of the granulocytic or erythrocytic series. Because the radii are commonly absent in these patients, the syndrome has been termed *TAR (thrombocytopenia with absent radius) syndrome.* Twenty percent of families have more than one affected member,[11] and the inheritance appears to be autosomal recessive. All patients have additional skeletal abnormalities, one third have cardiac anomalies, and as a rule, hemorrhagic symptoms begin in the first year of life. If the patient survives this first year, the prognosis is relatively good and survival into adulthood not uncommon.

The major cause of thrombocytopenia in aplastic anemia is certainly failure of platelet production from a decreased number of megakaryocytes; however, the platelet survival time is not necessarily normal. The mean platelet lifespan in one study was 9.6 days in normal controls, 7.0 days in patients with platelet counts in the range of 50,000 to 100,000 cells/mm^3, and 5.1 days in patients with platelet counts less than 50,000 cells/mm^3.[12] These data are consistent with a model in which the maximum platelet lifespan is 10.5 days with a fixed requirement of 7100 cells/mm^3/day to support vascular integrity. This requirement accounts for progressive shortening of the platelet lifespan as the platelet count falls, because an increasing percentage of the platelets produced each day will be required for this function.

Acquired amegakaryocytic thrombocytopenia with minimal or no involvement of other marrow cell lines is rarely seen.[13] Observation over time suggests that many of these patients have variants of aplastic anemia or dysmyelopoietic syndromes, with particularly severe involvement of megakaryocytes, and a favorable response in many cases to therapy that is effective in aplastic anemia supports this view.[14]

THERAPY.

Specific. In many of these patients, there is specific therapy for the underlying condition; for example, megaloblastic anemia can be treated with administration of the appropriate vitamin. In young patients with aplastic anemia, bone marrow transplantation from an HLA-identical sibling may be curative,[15] but with increasing age over 25 years, there is a progressive risk of morbidity and mortality from graft-versus-host disease after marrow transplantation. Both these patients and those without matched donors may be treated with antilymphocyte[16] or antithymocyte[17] globulin with or without high-dose corticosteroids. The mechanism of action is unknown, but this therapy may reverse an abnormal immune-mediated suppression of bone marrow function. Also, with supportive care, a remission commonly can be produced by chemotherapy in acute leukemia and lymphoma and, but more rarely, in metastatic carcinoma.

Supportive Care. Most platelet transfusions are given in the form of platelet concentrates that are harvested from routine donations of units (450 ml) of whole blood. Such a concentrate is termed a *unit* and should contain 6 to 10 $\times 10^{10}$ platelets; in addition, there will be approximately 10^8 contaminating leukocytes. Theoretically, the administration of 1 unit should raise the platelet count of a recipient with 1 m^2 body surface area by 20,000 cells/mm^3, but clinical experience has shown that the average posttransfusion increment in platelet count is usually one half the predicted result because of coexistent infection, fever, bleeding, disseminated intravascular coagulation, splenomegaly, and the presence of alloantibodies stimulated by the previous administration of blood products.[18] Thus, when administering prophylactic transfusions to patients with platelet counts in the range of 0 to 20,000 cells/mm^3, an initial dose of 3 units/m^2 is recommended to raise the platelet count to a protective level of 20,000 to 50,000 cells/mm^3. Clinical experience also has indicated that platelet survival in the days after infusion is considerably shorter than the theoretic 8 to 10 days, even in the recipient with stable thrombocytopenia, and that survival is shortened even further by the complicating factors previously listed; therefore, repeated transfusion (at least twice weekly) is required to maintain a protective level.

The major indication for platelet transfusion is the severe thrombocytopenia that often results from marrow hypoplasia due to cytoreductive therapy of malignancies. The model has been the therapy of acute leukemia, and studies[1] before the availability of platelet transfusion suggested that the risk of life-threatening hemorrhage rose from 3% of days at a platelet count of 15,000 cells/mm^3 to 30% of days at a platelet count of less than 1000 cells/mm^3. Thus, there is a general consensus[19] that these patients should be transfused prophylactically when the platelet count falls below 15,000 cells/mm^3, particularly if there are clinical factors such as fever and sepsis that predispose to bleeding, administration of drugs that interfere with platelet function, gastrointestinal ulceration, coexistent abnormality of coagulation factors, or high leukocyte counts.

The need for prophylactic transfusion is less in other patients with decreased platelet production, such as those with stable aplastic anemia and myelodysplastic syndromes. These patients commonly lack the previously listed complicating clinical factors and tend to be free of serious hemorrhage for months or years, even when the platelet count is in the range of 5000 to 15,000 cells/mm^3. Such patients may be managed with the judicious use of therapeutic transfusion at the time of hemorrhage or invasive procedures, but of course, these situations must be evaluated on an individual basis. Some patients, particularly those with baseline platelet counts below 5000 cells/mm^3 require continuing prophylactic support.

Within 2 weeks to 6 months, with a median of approximately 6 weeks, many patients treated with repeated platelet infusions will become refractory owing to the formation of alloantibodies. The incidence of this complication varies with the underlying diagnosis, but it is seen in approximately one third and two thirds of patients with acute leukemia and aplastic anemia, respectively. In the refractory patient, platelet counts obtained 1 hour after infusion are no different from those obtained before the infusion; thus, a poor 1-hour increment in platelet count is a sensitive and easy measurement that can be used to detect refractoriness. However, this measure is not specific, because nonimmunologic factors in the patient can produce the same poor therapeutic result.[18]

Often, the refractory patient can be managed with platelets from single donors; using a variety of pheresis machines, one can obtain the equivalent of 4 to 6 units of platelets from a single donor in approximately 2 hours. Concepts of how single donors should be selected are based on the fact that most of the alloantibodies responsible for refractoriness are directed against HLA antigens. The vast majority of refractory patients have lymphocytotoxic anti-HLA antibodies in their circulation, and if one can find a donor with no HLA antigens that the patient lacks, then the response generally will be good. There are exceptions, however, and some donors provide excellent support even though they possess an antigen that the recipient lacks but seems not to recognize as foreign. In any event, approximately 50% of refractory patients can be managed for a long period with single-donor platelets. Unfortunately, there is still quite a bit of trial and error in the selection process.

Considerable evidence exists suggesting that HLA immunization requires exposure to both class I antigens that are present on platelets and most leukocytes and class II antigens that are present only on monocytes and some subclasses of B cells.[20] Therefore, providing leukocyte-depleted platelet transfusions may delay or prevent alloimmunization, and this approach is suggested for patients who are initiating a therapeutic program that will require prolonged platelet support.

Certain types of thrombocytopenic bleeding also respond to the administration of ϵ-aminocaproic acid,[21] which blocks the fibrinolytic activity of plasmin that is generated by the action of tissue-type plasminogen activator on plasminogen. Tissue-type plasminogen activator activity is high in secretions from the mucous membranes of the nose, oropharynx, and gastrointestinal tract as well as in the urine. Bleeding in these areas due to defective platelet function may slow if fibrinolysis is inhibited, and a commonly effective dose would be 2 to 4 g by mouth every 6 to 8 hours.

Disorders of Platelet Distribution

The spleen is the only well-documented site in which there is temporary sequestration of platelets capable of returning to the circulation; therefore, the disorders of distribution are those diseases in which normal splenic function is exaggerated by splenomegaly. The size of the splenic platelet pool depends on the splenic blood flow and the intrasplenic platelet transit time. In a wide variety of disease states, splenic blood flow increases as splenic volume increases, whereas platelet transit time does not.[22] Therefore, the percentage of the total body platelet mass pooled in the spleen increases with increased splenic size, and this is the major cause of thrombocytopenia in patients with large spleens. However, this correlation between splenic size and the degree of reduction in the peripheral platelet count is poor if a variety of diseases are examined. Many, such as the myeloproliferative diseases, are complicated by an associated autonomous increase in the rate of platelet production that masks the increased size of the splenic platelet pool. Also, diseases such as the malignant lymphomas may be complicated by decreased platelet production associated with tumor involvement of the marrow or accelerated immune destruction; therefore, the degree of reduction in the peripheral platelet count is greater than would be expected based on the size of the spleen.

The most common clinical situation in which thrombocytopenia results almost entirely from an increase in the size of the splenic platelet pool is hepatic cirrhosis associated with portal hypertension. Many of these patients have platelet counts in the range of 20,000 to 100,000 cells/mm^3, plentiful megakaryocytes in the marrow, normal or nearly normal platelet lifespan, and prominent splenomegaly.[23] In itself, a platelet count in this range is not a major problem; however, it can be when it is associated with an impaired synthesis of clotting factors by the diseased liver and anatomic defects such as esophageal varices. In such cases, splenectomy or portal decompression with a distal splenorenal shunt generally results in an appropriate elevation of the platelet count. In contrast, transfused platelets will be distributed between the circulating and splenic pools in the same fashion as the patient's own platelets, so one expects little elevation of the platelet count and little clinical benefit from platelet transfusions unless massive doses are administered.

Accelerated Platelet Destruction

Accelerated platelet destruction as an isolated clinical phenomenon is seen in idiopathic thrombocytopenic purpura (ITP). Many patients present with a clinical picture resembling ITP, but one must separate true ITP from the many illnesses that mimic it. Therefore, it is useful to think in terms of the ITP clinical picture. This is characterized by thrombocytopenia in the peripheral blood with normal values in the red and white cell series; mean platelet volume is increased, with the degree of increase roughly proportional to the degree of the lowering of the platelet count.[24] The marrow should be normal, although there may be increased numbers of megakaryocytes and perhaps iron deficiency secondary to chronic bleeding, and the only abnormalities on physical examination are related to bleeding. Also, the spleen and lymph nodes are not enlarged. Accelerated platelet destruction leading to the ITP clinical picture can be produced either by immunologic or nonimmunologic mechanisms.

IMMUNOLOGIC DISORDERS.

True Idiopathic Thrombocytopenic Purpura. Idiopathic thrombocytopenic purpura is a relatively common illness; in childhood, it usually presents acutely, most often 1 to 3 weeks following a viral infection. There is no gender predilection in childhood, and the disease generally runs a self-limited course with spontaneous remission occurring in less than 3 months.

This picture may be seen in adults, but the adult form more commonly has a chronic onset with easy bruising, petechiae formation, and menorrhagia. Adult women are affected much more frequently than men, with a peak incidence in the twenties and thirties. The severity of thrombocytopenia may wax and wane, occasionally with striking cycles between severe thrombocytopenia and thrombocytosis.[25] Spontaneous remission in adults is the exception and generally occurs within the first 3 months after thrombocytopenia is first documented.

It has been known for decades that a factor producing thrombocytopenia is present in the IgG fraction of the plasma of these patients, and this was first demonstrated by the administration of ITP plasma to normal volunteers. Using many different types of assays, it has been shown that more than 90% of patients with ITP have increased levels of platelet-associated IgG;[26] thus, these assays are very sensitive for the diagnosis. Unfortunately, they are not specific. Many patients with thrombocytopenia on a nonimmune basis also have increased levels of platelet-associated IgG. A major cause for this problem is that more than 99% of the total platelet-associated IgG is stored within platelet granules and is not, therefore, antibody to platelet surface antigens.[26] The platelet content of granular IgG is increased when there is accelerated platelet destruction, apparently due to changes in thrombopoiesis occurring in response to it; thus, levels of platelet-associated IgG have been reported to be increased in many diseases where platelet survival is short but that conventionally have not been considered to have an immune etiology. Furthermore, even assays that are designed to measure only surface IgG sometimes share this problem. The reasons for this are unknown; however, a new generation of assays that measure antibody specific for platelet surface glycoproteins[27,28] should eventually circumvent this problem of nonspecificity. Using one of these assays, 80% of patients with chronic ITP had autoantibodies against platelets, 65% against glycoprotein IIb/IIIa, and 15% against glycoprotein Ib/IX.[29] Because this new generation of assays is not yet widely available, however, differential diagnosis of ITP still is accomplished by excluding the mimicking diseases described later.

All of these patients have a reduced platelet lifespan, with the degree of shortening roughly proportional to the degree of lowering of the platelet count (Fig. 17.2). In addition, the antiplatelet antibody has activity against megakaryocytes, and platelet production is inhibited in

some cases.[30] The increase in platelet size appears to be related, to some extent, to the accelerated rate of platelet destruction, because on average, young platelets are larger than old ones. However, the major factor is that the marrow responds to peripheral platelet destruction by the production of platelets with increased size.[31] In most patients, the removal of IgG-coated platelets is accomplished primarily in the spleen,[32] and the spleen apparently is far more sensitive to the IgG-mediated membrane defect than other portions of the reticuloendothelial system. In addition, it has been estimated that the spleen produces much of the antiplatelet antibody, so high concentrations are achieved locally. In any event, splenectomy produces a lasting remission in the majority of these patients.

Platelet function in most patients with ITP is normal relative to the circulating platelet mass; however, in a significant minority, hemorrhagic symptoms are present even when the platelet count is greater than 50,000 cells/mm^3.[33] We assume that the antiplatelet antibody alters platelet function in these patients.

The circulating antiplatelet IgG is capable of crossing the placenta and producing thrombocytopenia in newborn babies of women with ITP. This may occur after either splenectomy or drug therapy has produced a

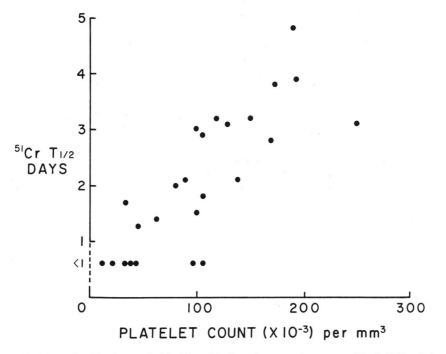

FIGURE 17.2. Platelet survival in idiopathic thrombocytopenic purpura. The half-life of ^{51}Cr-labelled platelets (normally 3 to 5 days) is graphed against the platelet count. There is a correlation between the degree of lowering of the platelet count and the degree of shortening of the platelet lifespan.

remission in the mother. In one series of women with a history of ITP,[34] the incidence of neonatal platelet counts lower than 100,000 and 50,000 cells/mm^3 were 40% and 20%, respectively, and there was no correlation between maternal and neonatal platelet counts. The major risk is bleeding in the central nervous system of the fetus during vaginal delivery, and in this same series, the incidence of intracranial hemorrhage was 12% for babies delivered vaginally and 0% for those delivered by caesarian section. It now is possible to select babies who require caesarian section by determining the fetal platelet count before term by percutaneous umbilical blood sampling.[35] In evaluating pregnant women without a history of ITP, it is important to remember that it is normal for approximately 10% to have a fall in their platelet count to between 80,000 and 150,000 cells/mm^3.[36]

Treatment of ITP. The increased application of blood studies to health-maintenance programs as well as the wider availability of platelet counting have resulted in the increased detection of asymptomatic cases. I have elected to follow such patients if the platelet count consistently is above 30,000 cells/mm^3. Such patients generally remain stable for years, without improvement or deterioration of the platelet level.[37] If the count is lower and the patient has bleeding manifestations, then steroid therapy, 1 mg/kg prednisone daily or the equivalent, should be started; this usually results in a gratifying rise in the platelet count and alleviation of symptoms within a few days. It generally has been assumed that steroids act by inhibiting phagocytosis of IgG-coated platelets by the reticuloendothelial system, but there is recent evidence suggesting that the rate of platelet production may increase as well.[38] As soon as a satisfactory, stable elevation of the platelet count has been obtained, the steroids should be tapered, and if the dose required to control the symptoms is not prohibitively high, patients can be maintained on steroid therapy for 3 months to allow the 10% to 30% who will remit spontaneously to do so.[39] In those who do not, a decision must be made about splenectomy at this point. If the patient can be maintained with prednisone (10 mg daily or less), then splenectomy can be deferred; if higher doses are required or steroid complications are becoming evident, then splenectomy should be performed if there are no contraindications.

After splenectomy, 60% of patients have a complete and permanent remission, predominantly due to normalization of platelet survival. Twenty percent do not have a complete remission but do have an elevation of the platelet count to a level where they are free of symptoms without medical therapy, and 20% continue to have thrombocytopenia and hemorrhagic manifestations re-

quiring therapy. Some of these 20% can be managed by administering low doses of corticosteroids; the goal should be control of symptoms at a platelet level greater than 30,000 cells/mm^3, a level where spontaneous serious hemorrhage is rare.

There are a variety of options for patients who continue to have thrombocytopenic symptoms on low doses of steroids after splenectomy. The most reliable way to produce a short-term rise in the platelet count is to infuse γ-globulin intravenously in doses of 1 to 2 g/kg over 2 to 5 days; approximately two thirds of patients will have an elevation that will persist for 1 to 3 weeks.[40] Maintenance infusions of 0.5 to 1 g/kg then can be given every 1 to 3 weeks. In one series,[41] 40% of patients so treated eventually went into a prolonged remission without treatment. Cyclophosphamide and azathioprine,[42] administered orally in doses of 100 to 150 mg daily, have produced remissions in 30% to 60% of patients; 2 to 4 weeks of therapy are required to obtain an effect. These agents are much better suited for long-term therapy than intravenous γ-globulin, and remissions have been maintained for years with them. However, there is always a concern about the long-term oncogenic effects of these agents. Other therapies described include danazol,[43] vinca alkaloids,[44] and recombinant α interferon.[45]

The role of platelet transfusion in ITP is limited, because the transfused platelets will have a short survival as the patient's own platelets do. Nonetheless, platelet transfusion can raise the platelet count for several hours,[46] and it may be helpful in a patient with active or life-threatening hemorrhage or in anticipation of surgery.

Immune Thrombocytopenia Related to Systemic Illness. Table 17.1 lists systemic illnesses in which immune thrombocytopenia can be a component. Patients with fully developed acquired immunodeficiency syndrome often have pancytopenia related to many causes;[47] however, from the beginning of the AIDS epidemic, it has been recognized that individuals infected with the human immunodeficiency virus com-

TABLE 17.1. Systemic Diseases with Immune Thrombocytopenia

Acquired immunodeficiency syndrome
Systemic lupus erythematosus
Chronic lymphocytic leukemia and lymphoma
Sarcoidosis
Solid tumors
Mononucleosis
Common variable immunodeficiency
Bone marrow transplantation and graft-versus-host disease

monly develop a syndrome indistinguishable from ITP before they develop other manifestations of AIDS and abnormalities in the red and white cell series. Patients with human immunodeficiency virus–related ITP have the same likelihood of going on to full-blown AIDS as do nonthrombocytopenic seropositive individuals.[48] Platelet survival time is reduced in these patients, but there also is a component of decreased production as sometimes exists in true ITP.[49] It was initially proposed that accelerated platelet destruction was caused by non-specific deposition of complement and immune complexes on the platelet surface,[50] but there is more recent evidence for the presence of an antibody directed against platelet antigens analogous to the situation in true ITP.[51,52]

These patients respond to therapy with corticosteroids, intravenous γ-globulin, and splenectomy with the same rate as do patients having true ITP.[53] In addition, there generally is an increase in the platelet count during therapy with azidothymidine;[47] in general, azidothymidine should be the initial treatment used considering the potential immunosuppressive effects of the other treatments, particularly corticosteroids. Most patients will require no therapy if the platelet count is 30,000 cells/mm^3, but there is a significant exception when the syndrome develops in patients with hemophilia in whom the risk of central nervous system hemorrhage increases when the platelet count is below 50,000 cells/mm^3 because of the coexistent plasma clotting defect.[54]

The clinical picture of ITP can be the presenting manifestation of patients with systemic lupus erythematosus,[55,56] Hodgkins disease,[57] non-Hodgkins lymphoma, and sarcoidosis[58] when no other manifestation of these illnesses is apparent. Thus, in a patient with apparent ITP, the presence of a palpable spleen or enlarged lymph nodes should initiate an investigation for these illnesses. On occasion, these diagnoses are made when the spleen is examined microscopically after splenectomy for otherwise typical ITP, but accelerated platelet destruction may become apparent for the first time at any point during the course of these illnesses or in chronic lymphocytic leukemia as well.[59] The mechanisms involved are believed to be immunologic and similar to those of true ITP, and in general, it is best to give these patients treatment for their primary illness. This generally includes steroids. If significant thrombocytopenia persists as steroids are withdrawn, however, splenectomy often will be helpful. More rarely, immune thrombocytopenia has been observed in association with solid tumors,[60] infectious mononucleosis,[61] and common variable immunodeficiency.[62]

Approximately 20% of patients who have received an allogeneic bone marrow transplantation have a chronic thrombocytopenia despite full engraftment leading to adequate production of both red cells and granulocytes.[63,64] Marrow examination shows adequate megakaryocytes, and kinetic studies indicate shortened platelet survival with no evidence for excessive splenic pooling. There is a strong correlation with the presence of graft-versus-host disease, and it also is likely that the thrombocytopenia is an autoimmune phenomenon associated with that syndrome.

Drug-Related Thrombocytopenia. Many drugs have been reported to cause the clinical picture of ITP,[65] and in any large series, quinidine/quinine, the sulfonamides, heparin, and gold compounds are the major offenders. Most of these reports describe the acute onset of thrombocytopenia that, when the drug is withdrawn, remits within a time-frame consistent with that drug's metabolism. It generally has not been considered wise to re-expose the patient to the drug to prove an etiologic connection, and useful in vitro assays to prove the presence of drug-related platelet antibodies are not widely available. In practice, one should stop all drugs that one can in the patient who presents with the ITP picture. Prompt remission suggests involvement of the drug in the etiology of the thrombocytopenia.

The mechanism of quinidine/quinine–related thrombocytopenia has been investigated extensively.[66,67] In a minority of individuals, the administration of the drug elicits formation of an IgG antibody that can participate in a high-affinity antibody-drug-platelet complex, leading to platelet destruction. The affinity of any two of the reactants without the third is low, and when the drug is withdrawn, remission occurs rapidly because the drug is excreted rapidly. The antibody then continues to circulate harmlessly for many months; thrombocytopenia recurs only if the drug is readministered. If the antibody titer falls to low-enough levels, then the drug can be given without causing thrombocytopenia. However, an anamnestic response is to be expected, and thrombocytopenia will recur if the drug is continued.

Many studies suggest that heparin-induced thrombocytopenia,[68] which occurs in approximately 1% of patients treated with the drug, has an immunologic basis and that bovine heparin produces more thrombocytopenia than porcine heparin. An antibody formed against heparin binds to circulating heparin, resulting in an immune complex which then can bind to circulating platelets, and in approximately 10% of affected patients, platelet activation occurs and leads to thrombotic complications, particularly in the peripheral, coronary, and cerebral arterial circulation.[69] Fortunately, remission is prompt once the administration of heparin is stopped.

The thrombocytopenia associated with gold compounds generally persists for 6 to 12 months.[70] Fortunately, the platelet count rises promptly with steroid therapy, and the response can be maintained until remission occurs. Pathophysiologic mechanisms are unclear, because gold and gold-related antibodies cannot be demonstrated in the plasma or associated with circulating platelets during the thrombocytopenic phase. Similarly, the pathophysiologic mechanisms leading to thrombocytopenia for drugs other than quinidine/quinine and heparin are inadequately defined.

Posttransfusion Purpura. Posttransfusion purpura is a rare clinical syndrome consisting of life-threatening thrombocytopenic purpura that occurs approximately 1 week after blood transfusion.[71] Typically, the precipitating transfusion is a routine unit of stored whole blood or packed red cells. Most patients have been exposed to foreign blood in the past, either by pregnancy or previous transfusion, and the majority of patients have been women. Recovery occurs spontaneously within 10 days to 2 months, and on recovery, platelets in the majority of patients have been found to lack the antigen Pl^{A1}, which is carried on the platelet surface glycoprotein IIIa. Also, during the acute phase, the serum of these patients contains an antibody against Pl^{A1}. In thoroughly studied cases, the transfused blood always has contained the antigen to which the antibody is directed. This is not surprising, because 97% of the population have platelets that contain the Pl^{A1} antigen. The unsolved mystery of this disease is how the antibody mediates the destruction of the patient's own platelets that lack the antigen involved; in rare cases, the syndrome results from alloimmunization against the antigens Pl^{A2} or Pen^a carried on glycoprotein IIIa or against Bak^a or Bak^b carried on glycoprotein IIb.[72]

If the clinical picture is characteristic, then the diagnosis can be made with virtual certainty if an anti-Pl^{A1} antibody can be demonstrated in the patient's serum. However, the absence of an anti-Pl^{A1} antibody does not exclude the diagnosis, because a platelet antigen other than Pl^{A1} can be involved. The demonstration of an antibody without Pl^{A1} specificity provides only circumstantial evidence as previously transfused patients often have antiplatelet antibodies without coexistent thrombocytopenia. Recent studies indicate that the treatment of choice is intravenous immunoglobulin, 1 g/kg, given in two doses over 48 hours.[73] This usually results in a prompt response. Plasma exchange may be used in refractory cases, and success with transfusion of antigen-negative platelets also has been reported.[74] However, the accelerated in vivo destruction of the patient's own antigen-negative platelets would argue against the success of the transfusion approach.

Neonatal Thrombocytopenia. The thrombocytopenia that is observed in newborn babies of women with ITP

already has been discussed, but neonatal thrombocytopenia also is seen in the babies of normal women due to the formation of alloantibody against fetal platelets that have crossed the placenta into the maternal circulation during the pregnancy. The alloantibodies cross the placenta into the fetal circulation, causing thrombocytopenia as early as the twentieth week of pregnancy.[75] In many ways, this disease is analogous to antibody-mediated erythroblastosis fetalis. However, a major difference is that this disease typically occurs in the first pregnancy, and this is rare in erythroblastosis fetalis. In several series, the platelets of 50% to 80% of these mothers were found to lack Pl^{A1} while antibody against Pl^{A1} could be detected in their serum; a variety of antigenic discrepancies have been found in other cases as well.[76] Also, the bleeding tendency of the fetus can be so severe that intracranial hemorrhage can occur in the uterus.

The ideal therapy for the first affected child of a woman with this syndrome is transfusion using a unit of the mother's platelets; these platelets, which lack the antigen against which the alloantibody is directed, normally survive in the infant's circulation. When the mother's platelets are collected, it is advisable to resuspend them in normal plasma so that additional alloantibody is not infused into the infant. With this approach, most newborn babies do well if they have not had serious hemorrhage either before or during delivery. The risk of recurrence in subsequent pregnancies is high; therefore, as an experimental approach, it has been recommended[75,77] that periodic percutaneous umbilical blood sampling of fetal blood be done beginning at 20 to 22 weeks of gestation and that infusion of intravenous γ-globulin and/or maternal platelets be given to the affected fetus. Elective caesarian section before the onset of labor should be performed if the fetus is thrombocytopenic.

NONIMMUNOLOGIC DISORDERS. A variety of diseases mimic ITP, but an immunologic mechanism leading directly to platelet destruction is not involved. Of these diseases, one of the most common is the syndrome of disseminated intravascular coagulation, in which there are deficiencies of plasma coagulation proteins as well as elevation in the titer of fibrin and fibrinogen degradation products; these findings are not seen in ITP. In the consumptive coagulopathy seen with viral and bacterial sepsis, the degree of platelet depletion may be far greater than that of the coagulation factors, and in some cases, the discrepancy may be so great that isolated platelet consumption is the only clinical problem.[78]

Five other disease groups are in this category as well. These include thrombotic thrombocytopenic purpura, ethanol-induced thrombocytopenia, thrombocytopenia due to massive bleeding, thrombocytopenia related to toxemia of pregnancy, and hereditary thrombocytopenia.

Thrombotic Thrombocytopenic Purpura. In this disease, the clinical picture is highly variable, but five findings commonly are seen in various combinations: fever, microangiopathic hemolytic anemia, thrombocytopenia with normal or increased numbers of megakaryocytes in the marrow, renal failure, and fluctuating central nervous system deficits. The lactate dehydrogenase usually is very high, reflecting the hemolytic state. This disease typically has a fulminant or subacute onset, but more chronic disease that waxes and wanes also has been observed. In the past, this disease was nearly uniformly fatal, but in the 1980s, it became clear that approximately 80% of patients will survive if treated promptly with daily, intensive plasma exchange.[79] Although there is much speculation, the pathogenesis of the illness is unknown; the success of plasma exchange suggests there is a circulating deleterious factor in plasma that is responsible or that a normally present beneficial factor is absent during active disease. Most patients can be held in remission with plasma exchange until the disease activity subsides gradually and permanently over several weeks. Splenectomy is effective for the minority of patients who respond suboptimally to plasma exchange or who continue to require it beyond 1 month,[80] and both dextran and corticosteroids may be tried in patients who are refractory to plasmapheresis and splenectomy.

Thrombotic thrombocytopenic purpura is a disease of young adults. The hemolytic-uremic syndrome that is seen in children is closely related but with much more prominent renal failure and less prominent thrombocytopenia and neurologic disease. Yet another related process is the hemolytic-uremic syndrome seen in patients with adenocarcinoma.[81] Anemia, thrombocytopenia, and renal failure are prominent, but fever and neurologic disease rare. The vast majority of patients have received treatment with mitomycin, but the mechanism of the drug's effect is unknown.

Ethanol-Induced Thrombocytopenia. The alcoholic who also is a "binge" drinker may present at the hospital with an extremely low platelet count; levels as low as 10,000 cells/mm^3 have been observed. Undoubtedly, the mechanism is multifactorial, but megakaryocytes are present in the marrow and the condition therefore mimics ITP. In the typical case, the platelet count begins to rise as soon as the patient is withdrawn from alcohol, and within 5 to 10 days, the platelet count is normal. In fact, it is highly characteristic for a rebound thrombocytosis to persist for several weeks after recovery.

When these patients are first seen, there is no way to be certain they do not have ITP. Fortunately, the thrombocytopenia usually is not severe enough to require therapy, and the diagnosis is apparent when spontaneous recovery occurs. However, the thrombocytopenia occasionally is severe enough that the physician feels obliged to prescribe corticosteroids because of the concern that the patient has ITP. This should be avoided if possible, because steroid therapy may impair defenses against complicating infection.

Thrombocytopenia Due to Massive Bleeding. Whole blood that has been refrigerated in the blood bank for more than few hours contains few viable platelets. Therefore, if a patient bleeds massively and stored blood is used for replacement, the patient's platelet count is reduced, because the splenic reservoir is too small to keep up with the external losses. In general, this rarely is a significant clinical problem, at least until the number of blood units infused exceeds 10; at this point, platelet levels will be reduced to from 50,000 to 100,000 cells/mm^3. Platelet transfusions should be administered if there is pathologic bleeding, but there is no benefit from administering transfusion simply because the platelet count is low.[82]

Thrombocytopenia Related To Toxemia. Preeclampsia is defined by the presence of hypertension and proteinuria after the twentieth week of gestation. Fifteen percent to 20% of patients will have thrombocytopenia (frequently less than 50,000 cells/mm^3),[83] it has been emphasized that microangiopathic hemolytic anemia as well as elevated liver enzymes may accompany the low platelet count (the HELLP syndrome), overshadowing modest degrees of hypertension.[83,84] It generally is agreed that delivery is the therapy of choice, because the abnormalities subside quickly thereafter.

Hereditary Thrombocytopenia. A few patients who appear to have ITP actually have hereditary thrombocytopenia. It is essential to obtain a family history in all patients with the clinical picture of ITP, and the physician should be particularly suspicious if the thrombocytopenia dates to early childhood without the spontaneous remission that is typical of childhood ITP. One should be even more suspicious if there is a poor response to steroid therapy or splenectomy. If suspicion is strong, platelet counts of family members should be obtained, and platelet survival studies may provide definitive information. In some families, the patient's own platelets may have normal survival; in others, survival may be short. However, platelet survival is normal if labelled normal platelets are infused into the patient, because there are no extracellular factors that lead to premature platelet destruction. This contrasts with ITP, in which normal platelets have short survival. Such studies may be definitive, but they also should be approached with great caution because of the risk of transmitting infectious diseases by cross transfusion.

The hereditary thrombocytopenias are best classified according to the mode of inheritance as well as platelet size.[85] Thrombocytopenia, eczema, and increased susceptibility to infection are inherited as an X-linked, recessive trait in the Wiskott-Aldrich syndrome, and the platelets characteristically are smaller than normal. This may be appreciated on peripheral blood smear. Autologous platelet survival is short, and in some families, thrombocytopenia may be striking, with little or no increase in infection or eczema. Splenectomy improves the thrombocytopenia but also increases the risk of overwhelming bacterial infection; if splenectomy is performed, then continuous, lifelong prophylactic antibiotic coverage should be instituted.[86] In patients with recurrent infections, the mortality in childhood is high, and bone marrow transplantation clearly is warranted.

In two well-defined diseases, the Bernard-Soulier syndrome and the May-Hegglin anomaly, the platelets are massive. As mentioned previously, platelets in ITP commonly are larger than normal, but this enlargement is a relatively subtle finding on a routine blood smear. There is no problem, however, identifying the huge platelets in the Bernard-Soulier syndrome and the May-Hegglin anomaly on casual examination of a smear. The Bernard-Soulier syndrome is discussed in the section on disorders of platelet function; in the May-Hegglin anomaly, modest thrombocytopenia with huge platelets is associated with the presence of pale-blue inclusions, termed as *Döhle bodies,* in the granulocytes.[87] Inheritance is by an autosomal dominant mode. These patients rarely have difficulty with severe hemorrhage, and therapy generally is not required. Autologous platelet survival is normal.

Finally, there is a group of families in which inheritance is autosomal dominant and platelet size is normal.[88] Autologous platelet survival may be normal or short. These patients can be distinguished from those with ITP by family studies and platelet survival measurements. The thrombocytopenia does not respond to the administration of steroids or to splenectomy, but these patients rarely are thrombocytopenic enough to require therapy. Platelet transfusions may be useful in acute bleeding episodes and in preparation for surgery.

DISORDERS OF PLATELET FUNCTION

When number of platelets is normal, hemorrhagic symptoms sometimes arise owing to a defect in platelet function. As mentioned in the introduction, these patients come to the physician's attention because of easy bruising, epistaxis, menorrhagia, and excessive bleeding after surgery or dental work. Petechiae are not common, unlike patients with severe thrombocytopenia.

Before discussing this group of diseases, it is helpful to review how normal platelets carry out their function at a site of vessel injury; of course, this must be a great oversimplification of a very complicated process.[89] When the endothelium is interrupted, von Willebrand factor binds to subendothelial tissues and is altered so that it also binds to the surface membrane glycoprotein Ib-IX complex of nearby platelets.[90] Thus, platelet adherence to subendothelial tissue occurs, and as adherence is occurring, thrombin is being generated through the extrinsic and intrinsic clotting systems. Both adherence to subendothelial tissue and thrombin exposure stimulate platelets to undergo the release reaction. Platelets have dense storage granules that contain adenosine diphosphate (ADP) as well as adenosine triphosphate (ATP), calcium, and serotonin; during the release reaction, these storage granules are secreted into the extracellular space where ADP acts as a primary platelet-aggregating agent. ADP acts by altering the surface membrane glycoprotein IIb-IIIa complex so that it can serve as a binding site for fibrinogen. Bound fibrinogen molecules then can provide molecular bridges between adjacent platelets. Other platelet agonists, such as thrombin, bound von Willebrand factor, and thromboxane A_2 (discussed later), alter the glycoprotein IIb-IIIa complex in a similar fashion; thus, a mass of platelets forms at the site of endothelial disruption, providing initial hemostasis.

The biochemical pathway from agonist binding to the release reaction is complex. When von Willebrand factor or thrombin bind, various phosphorylated inositol species are released from membrane phosphotidyl inositides; in turn, these species release calcium from internal stores, leading to an increase in cytoplasmic calcium that appears to be crucial for cell activation. During activation, arachidonic acid is made available from cellular membranes to be acted on by an intraplatelet enzyme, cyclooxygenase, with the eventual formation of prostaglandins and thromboxanes. Of these, the most important is thromboxane A_2, a potent inducer of the release reaction. Cyclooxygenase is inhibited by aspirin and other nonsteroidal anti-inflammatory agents, such as indomethacin and phenylbutazone.

In the test tube, thrombin, connective tissue, ADP, and epinephrine can induce the release reaction by activating the cyclooxygenase pathway; in addition, strong agonists such as thrombin and high concentrations of connective tissue have the capacity to induce the release reaction even when the cyclooxygenase pathway is completely inhibited by aspirin. However, weak agonists such as ADP and epinephrine as well as low concentrations of collagen require the generation of thromboxane A_2 to produce release. The antibiotic ristocetin is used in laboratory testing, because it mimics the effect of binding to subendothelial tissue on von Willebrand factor; thus, in the test tube, ristocetin alters von Willebrand factor so that it binds to glycoprotein Ib-IX, inducing platelet aggregation.

Patients suspected of having platelet function defects may be evaluated by measuring the bleeding time and studying platelet aggregation. The most widely used technique for measuring the bleeding time is the template version of the original Ivy method. A blood pressure cuff is placed on the upper arm and inflated to 40 mm Hg to produce a consistent intravascular pressure in the capillaries distal to it. Then, with the aid of the template device, an incision is made 1-mm deep and 10-mm long; bleeding normally ceases within 4 to 8 minutes. The measurement is sensitive enough to detect the rather modest defect produced by aspirin ingestion, and the measurement appears to be abnormal in the majority of patients with clinically significant disorders of platelet function. Therefore, this technique has been relied on heavily as a screening test for platelet dysfunction. However, a few patients with platelet dysfunction and von Willebrand disease may have normal bleeding times either occasionally or continuously, and more detailed studies should be pursued if the patient's clinical history is strongly suggestive even if the bleeding time is normal. In addition, there is no convincing evidence for a strong correlation between the degree of prolongation of the bleeding time and the risk of bleeding with surgery.[91] This test is used best as one of a panel designed to detect disease and not as a guide to therapy.

Aggregation studies are performed with blood that has been drawn into sodium citrate and then centrifuged at a slow speed so that a supernatant of platelet-rich plasma forms (Fig. 17.3). Aliquots of the platelet-rich plasma are placed in a cuvette and stirred at a constant rate and temperature, and light transmission through the platelet-rich plasma is recorded continuously. Aggregating agents, usually ADP, epinephrine, connective tissue, arachidonic acid, and ristocetin, are introduced into the cuvette, and aggregation is recorded as an increase in light transmission. ADP and epinephrine produce a primary wave of aggregation that at the appropriate concentration of the aggregating agent is followed by a secondary wave; connective tissue, arachidonic acid, and ristocetin produce only one wave. The secondary waves of aggregation with ADP and epinephrine as well as the single wave with arachidonic acid and low concentrations of connective tissue are all

accompanied by the synthesis of thromboxane A_2 and inhibited by aspirin. Therefore, it is impossible to interpret aggregation studies unless the patient has refrained from using aspirin and other nonsteroidal anti-inflammatory agents. The inhibitory effect of aspirin on aggregation with connective tissue can be overcome by high concentrations, so those concentrations in the range of sensitivity for the aspirin defect should be used. Primary aggregation with ADP and epinephrine is not affected by aspirin, and in addition, an aliquot of PRP may be used to measure the platelet content of both ADP and ATP to look for a deficiency of dense storage granules.

Disorders of platelet function are best described by separating them into intrinsic and extrinsic defects. The intrinsic defects are those found within the platelet itself; the extrinsic defects are those resulting from abnormalities in the environment.

Intrinsic Defects

DEFECTS OF ADHERENCE. The Bernard-Soulier syndrome, when fully expressed, is transmitted as an autosomal recessive defect.[92] On peripheral blood smear, the platelets are giant and completely granulated. The platelet count typically is modestly reduced, but the bleeding tendency is far greater than can be explained by the degree of thrombocytopenia. However, platelet mass per volume of blood actually may be normal. The bleeding time is prolonged, and aggregation with ADP, epinephrine, arachidonic acid, and connective tissue is normal in both the primary and secondary phases. However, there is no aggregation with ristocetin. Aggregation with ristocetin also is lacking in severe von Willebrand disease, but the defect in this situation can be corrected by the addition of normal von Willebrand factor, demonstrating that the defect itself is in the plasma and not in the platelets. In the Bernard-Soulier syndrome, the defect cannot be corrected by the addition of normal von Willebrand factor and is related to a much-reduced concentration of membrane glycoprotein Ib-IX.[90] As would be predicted, platelets in the blood from patients with von Willebrand disease and the Bernard-Soulier syndrome have reduced adherence to subendothelial tissue in in vitro models,[93] and parents of the patients affected have abnormally large platelets and decreased glycoprotein Ib-IX but not thrombocytopenia or a clinically significant defect in platelet function.

Although the aggregation and biochemical defects are relatively constant from patient to patient, the severity of the clinical picture is variable. Some patients do reasonably well, particularly as they progress into adult life. Administration of corticosteroids and splenectomy are

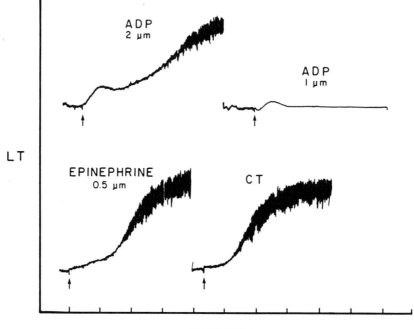

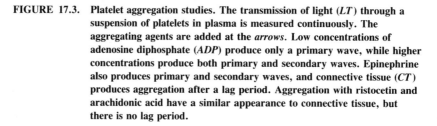

FIGURE 17.3.   Platelet aggregation studies. The transmission of light (*LT*) through a suspension of platelets in plasma is measured continuously. The aggregating agents are added at the *arrows*. Low concentrations of adenosine diphosphate (*ADP*) produce only a primary wave, while higher concentrations produce both primary and secondary waves. Epinephrine also produces primary and secondary waves, and connective tissue (*CT*) produces aggregation after a lag period. Aggregation with ristocetin and arachidonic acid have a similar appearance to connective tissue, but there is no lag period.

not helpful, but platelet transfusions are effective during acute bleeding episodes.

DEFECTS OF RELEASE.

Drug-Induced. As previously mentioned, aspirin and the other nonsteroidal anti-inflammatory agents inhibit the production of thromboxane A_2 from arachidonic acid. One aspirin tablet by mouth suffices to produce complete inhibition that lasts for the lifespan of the platelet, long after the drug itself has disappeared from the circulation; inhibition by the other drugs requires that the drug be present. Thus, the defect produced by the other nonsteroidal anti-inflammatory drugs might be placed more properly under the extrinsic abnormalities of platelet function. Aspirin ingestion is followed by a modest prolongation of the bleeding time, absence of secondary aggregation waves with ADP and epinephrine, and inhibited primary aggregation with arachidonic acid as well as low concentrations of connective tissue. These defects can be detected for at least 48 to 72 hours after ingestion, until the marrow has produced a subpopulation of unaffected platelets, and because one aspirin tablet is innocuous in a normal person, the abnormalities in the laboratory studies clearly are more striking than the clinical consequences. However, several clinical studies have shown that aspirin ingestion increases bleeding to a modest degree during some forms of surgery.[89] In addition, aspirin ingestion can produce a marked prolongation of the bleeding time and a more serious bleeding tendency in patients with decreased concentrations of plasma coagulation factors (e.g., hemophiliacs and patients on oral anticoagulants).[94] Aspirin should be avoided in such patients as well as those with thrombocytopenia or disorders of platelet function.

Primary. Primary release defects represent a group that is probably quite heterogeneous. The common characteristics are easy bruising, increased tendency to bleeding after surgical or dental procedures, and minimal to marked prolongation of the bleeding time. Initially, these patients were described as consistently having abnormalities in the results of platelet aggregation studies, and it was felt that most patients fell into two broad categories: aspirin-like defects, or storage pool disease. In the aspirin-like defect, all defects characteristic of the aspirin effect are seen in a patient who has not been using the drug; patients with storage pool disease were described as having defective aggregation responses to epinephrine, ADP, and collagen, along with (by definition) decreased concentration of platelet ADP, ATP, and serotonin. In typical cases of storage pool disease, the platelets demonstrate a decreased number of the very dense granules that contain these compounds, so when the platelet is stimulated with release inducers, decreased concentrations of ADP and ATP are released. The defect has been seen as a hereditary trait with an autosomal dominant transmission and also in persons with no family history of bleeding. When combined with albinism, this defect has been labelled the Hermansky-Pudlak syndrome.

It now has become apparent that these syndromes are very heterogeneous and only a minority of patients with a bleeding tendency and prolonged bleeding time have one of the two classically defined patterns.[95] In one series,[96] normal aggregation studies, storage pool contents, and studies for von Willebrand disease were found in 27% of patients referred because of prolonged bleeding time, and easily another quarter of such patients have miscellaneous aggregation abnormalities that cannot be categorized clearly. Furthermore, at least one quarter of patients with storage pool disease as defined by prolonged bleeding time and decreased platelet content of ADP and ATP have normal aggregation studies.[97] Figure 17.4 shows my experience with such patients.

Clinically, one should be cautious about labelling these patients as "bleeders," because necessary surgery may be withheld or unnecessary platelet transfusions administered at surgery. Certainly, platelet transfusion makes sense, but the risks of posttransfusion hepatitis

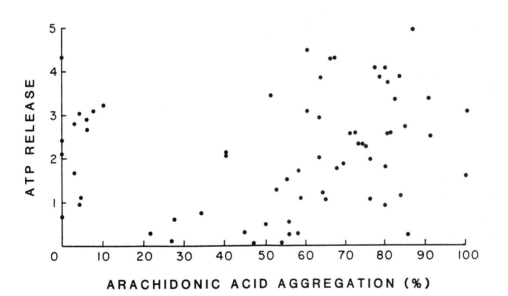

FIGURE 17.4.   The author's experience with platelet function testing in patients referred for suspected platelet dysfunction, generally with a prolonged bleeding time. Adenosine triphosphate (*ATP*) released with a high concentration of thrombin (5 units/ml) reflects the platelet storage pool's contents of adenine nucleotides. Normal values are about 2 μmol/10^{11} platelets. The aggregation of arachidonic acid reflects the activity of the aspirin-inhibitable pathway, and normal values are above 40%. Some patients have an isolated aspirin-like defect (absent aggregation with arachidonic acid) or storage pool disease (decreased release of ATP), but a few have both. Many also have neither. (*Source:* data collected with Dr. Arun Sheth.)

may be greater than the risk of bleeding if a careful surgical technique is employed. Measures described in the section on nonspecific therapy probably are preferable.

DEFECTS OF PRIMARY AGGREGATION. Glanzmann thrombasthenia is an autosomal recessive disorder in which the patient's platelets do not aggregate with any concentration of ADP, epinephrine, connective tissue, or thrombin.[98] This functional abnormality results from the absence, near absence, or malfunction of the membrane glycoprotein IIb-IIIa complex and the consequent inability of the platelet to bind fibrinogen after stimulation. Despite this severe defect in vitro, however, spontaneous hemorrhage is rare, and most patients live a normal lifespan. Pathologic hemorrhage usually is confined to periods of hemostatic stress, such as menses and after surgery, and such episodes commonly require support with platelet transfusion. However, there is marked variability from patient to patient and no correlation with glycoprotein IIb-IIIa levels.

Extrinsic Defects

Platelet function may be abnormal not because the circulating platelets are abnormal but because a necessary plasma cofactor is absent or the external environment inhibits platelet function. The distinction is critical, because appropriate treatment involves altering the environment and not supplying normal platelets by platelet transfusion. The best documented example is von Willebrand disease, in which the appropriate therapy is to raise the level of von Willebrand factor.

UREMIA. It is likely that the bleeding tendency seen in uremic patients is due to an extrinsic defect, although our understanding in this area is quite limited. In uremia, both the platelet count and the levels of plasma coagulation factors are normal; in a minority, a modest thrombocytopenia is seen. However, the bleeding time generally is prolonged very disproportionately to the thrombocytopenia, and there is no consensus in the literature as to the mechanism of the bleeding tendency. Still, most would agree that the defect is produced by metabolites retained in the circulation as a result of renal failure; guanidinosuccinic acid, phenolic acids, and urea have been proposed. The bleeding tendency improves with adequate dialysis and maintenance of the hematocrit at a level greater than 30, either by transfusion or by therapy with erythropoietin. These are the mainstays of therapy, and additional, nonspecific therapies are discussed later. Platelet transfusion is not recommended, because the transfused platelets will be affected in the same way as the patient's own.

DRUG-INDUCED DEFECTS. Aspirin is the only drug whose use has been associated conclusively with clinical bleeding.[89] Drugs other than nonsteroidal anti-inflammatory agents may well inhibit platelet function; however, it is wise to maintain some skepticism in this area. Many drugs alter platelet aggregation when added to a platelet suspension in vitro yet exert no demonstrable effect when administered to humans in clinical doses, either parenterally or by mouth. One at least would like to see a clear-cut increase in the bleeding time or an alteration of the aggregation patterns with standard doses and routes of administration before concluding that a drug inhibits platelet function. Aside from the nonsteroidal antiinflammatory agents, few drugs have been shown by these criteria to have an effect on platelets. Exceptions are the β-lactam antibiotics;[99] they clearly prolong the bleeding time and impair platelet aggregation when given in the massive doses that commonly are used. However, it has never been proven that clinical bleeding is increased with their use. It also is important to realize that sulfinpyrazone and dipyridamole, both drugs commonly prescribed as antiplatelet agents, have not been shown convincingly to affect platelet function in vivo when administered in standard doses; it may be that they exert their antithrombotic actions by an effect on the vasculature and not on the platelets.

PARAPROTEINS. The hemorrhagic diathesis commonly seen in patients with high concentrations of paraproteins, such as those with Waldenström macroglobulinemia and multiple myeloma, also is listed in this category. The mucous membrane and dermal bleeding seen in these patients is very similar to that observed in those with platelet dysfunction and appears to be related, at least in part, to a deleterious effect of the protein on the platelet. As a generalization, patients with pathologic bleeding have a paraprotein level in excess of 5 g/100 ml. The mechanism of this effect is not known, but many patients do have a prolonged bleeding time.[100] In addition, there generally is an increase in plasma viscosity, and some paraproteins also interfere with the polymerization of fibrin. Therefore, there may be several mechanisms leading to a hemorrhagic state. For immediate management, lowering the paraprotein level by plasmapheresis is beneficial; long-term management depends on lowering the paraprotein level with cytotoxic chemotherapy directed against the underlying lymphoproliferative malignancy.

CARDIOPULMONARY BYPASS. During extracorporeal circulation, patients acquire a complex coagulopathy that includes a modest reduction in the platelet count to the range of 50,000 to 100,000 cells/mm^3 and abnormal platelet function.[101] The platelet defect is related to the release of intracellular granules and surface glycoprotein abnormalities that apparently are induced by contact with the extracorporeal apparatus; platelet function returns to normal within several hours after return to normal circulation. Platelet transfusion is unnecessary as a routine and should be reserved for patients who appear to be bleeding pathologically.

NONSPECIFIC THERAPY. Several nonspecific measures have been used to reduce bleeding time and, presumably, bleeding tendency in patients with platelet function disorders.[21] In normal individuals, 1-desamino-8-D-arginine vasopressin (DDAVP) induces the release of von Willebrand factor from endothelial cells, and it has been proposed that the excess circulating von Willebrand factor increases the ability of platelets to adhere to subendothelial tissue, thereby improving a variety of bleeding tendencies. DDAVP has been effective in aspirin-induced defects, storage pool disease, isolated prolongation of the bleeding time, uremia, and cardiopulmonary bypass; patients with thrombocytopenia and Glanzmann thrombasthenia have not responded. The effect is greatest 1 to 2 hours after intravenous infusion and disappears approximately 12 hours later. Infusions may be repeated every 12 to 24 hours, but tachyphylaxis after several doses is common though not universal. Because of its efficacy and safety, DDAVP is the recommended therapy at the time of surgery for patients who have been shown to respond to it with shortening of the bleeding time. DDAVP also allows the risks of platelet transfusion to be avoided. Conjugated estrogens also have been found to be effective in uremia, and if there is no contraindication, ϵ-aminocaproic acid may provide nonspecific benefit in these patients just as it does in those with thrombocytopenia.

MYELOPROLIFERATIVE DISEASE AND DYSMYELOPOIETIC SYNDROMES

The myeloproliferative diseases are characterized by the autonomous overproduction of erythrocytes, granulocytes, and platelets, either singly or in combination. Four syndromes (polycythemia vera, chronic granulocytic leukemia, myelofibrosis, and essential thrombocythemia) have relatively characteristic clinical pictures, but many examples of overlap occur. These patients often must be distinguished from those with reactive thrombocytosis, in whom an elevated platelet count is seen in response to an underlying malignancy, inflammatory condition, or iron deficiency. Patients with myeloproliferative disease may have a hemorrhagic tendency even when they also have an elevated or

normal platelet count or when a minor reduction in platelet count seems insufficient to explain the degree of bleeding. There are three settings in which bleeding is seen: abnormal platelet function, elevated platelet count, and elevated hematocrit.

Abnormal Platelet Function

Because circulating blood cells arise from an abnormal stem cell in these patients, it is not unexpected that platelets will have abnormal function in some cases, and this is reflected in a prolonged bleeding time, which is seen most commonly in myelofibrosis.[102] Although bleeding can occur when the platelet count is normal, it is most important in the late stages of the illness, when the count falls to from 50,000 to 100,000 cells/mm^3, a range where bleeding should not occur from thrombocytopenia per se. The same phenomenon also may be seen in patients with dysmyelopoietic syndromes.

The mechanism of the platelet dysfunction is not known; however, many patients with myeloproliferative disease and dysmyelopoietic syndromes have abnormal aggregation studies. The absence of primary and secondary waves of aggregation with administration of epinephrine are particularly common, yet the majority of patients with abnormal aggregation studies have neither a prolonged bleeding time nor a clinical bleeding tendency. Also, some patients with markedly prolonged bleeding times have normal aggregation studies. We must assume that the abnormal aggregation studies are in vitro reflections of an abnormal stem cell origin that have no necessary in vivo hemostatic consequences. Aggregation abnormalities are not seen in patients with reactive thrombocytosis; therefore, these studies can be used in differential diagnosis with thrombocytosis secondary to myeloproliferative disease. Aggregation abnormalities should not be interpreted as a contraindication for surgery or an indication for platelet transfusion. However, platelet transfusion may be necessary to support a patient with a platelet function defect that is reflected in a prolonged bleeding time and a clinical hemorrhagic tendency.

Thrombocytosis

Some patients with thrombocytosis secondary to myeloproliferative disease have a thrombotic tendency that is characterized by occlusions in the cerebral and coronary arterial circulations. Occlusive disease of the extremities takes the characteristic form of erythromelalgia,[103] in which there is localized painful burning, redness, and warm congestion in the hands and feet that often progresses to acrocyanosis or necrosis in the toes and fingers. These symptoms often respond dramatically to nonsteroidal anti-inflammatory agents.

Surprisingly, a hemorrhagic tendency may be present either simultaneously or independently; when hemorrhagic complications result from thrombocytosis per se, the platelet count usually is in excess of 1 million cells/mm^3. Three lines of evidence support the idea that bleeding is caused by thrombocytosis per se and not coincident platelet dysfunction. First, these patients commonly have a normal bleeding time when they are having pathologic hemorrhage,[102] and the bleeding time is an extremely sensitive test for platelet dysfunction. Second, the bleeding tendency decreases if the platelet count is lowered by myelosuppressive therapy or thrombocytapheresis, and it is difficult to imagine how lowering the number of dysfunctional platelets would decrease a bleeding tendency. And third, platelets from such patients once were used successfully in platelet transfusion therapy. However, pathologic hemorrhage has not been reported in patients with reactive thrombocytosis. Thus, thrombocytosis alone is not sufficient to induce a hemorrhagic state. It must be admitted that we currently do not know why these patients with extreme thrombocytosis and myeloproliferative disease bleed.

Most clinicians feel that the platelet count of the patient with thrombocytosis who has demonstrated a thrombotic or hemorrhagic tendency should be lowered; this can be accomplished immediately by plateletpheresis and over time by myelosuppressive therapy. Commonly used agents are hydroxyurea and interferon-α. The management of the patient with marked elevation of the platelet count who has not demonstrated a hemorrhagic or thrombotic tendency, however, is more controversial, because these agents have not been used long enough for their long-term complications to be known. Many of these patients may remain asymptomatic for many years while maintaining a high platelet count, so the decision whether to use myelosuppressive agents is not easy. The age of the patient should be taken into consideration; the young patient has a longer projected lifespan during which a complication from therapy might develop as well as less pre-existent vascular disease on which thrombotic complications may be superimposed. Thus, one will be less likely to treat the young patient. Antiplatelet agents such as aspirin may be helpful in some cases for the thrombotic complications, but they also may increase the hemorrhagic tendency.[104]

Polycythemia

Patients with an elevated hematocrit may have both thrombotic and hemorrhagic tendencies, presumably related to increased blood viscosity. This is seen most commonly in polycythemia vera. The bleeding time almost always is normal, and symptoms improve dramatically if the hematocrit is lowered by either phlebotomy or myelosuppressive therapy. It is wise to maintain the hematocrit below 50% at all times. Surgical complications of thrombosis and hemorrhage are particularly common in this group if an operation is performed before the hematocrit has been lowered.

VASCULAR AND CONNECTIVE TISSUE DISORDERS

The clinical manifestations of vascular and connective tissue disorders may mimic those in abnormalities of platelet number or function. Certainly, determining the platelet count is indicated for any patient with purpura or ecchymoses, but knowledge of the characteristic clinical and laboratory features of these illnesses allows the clinician to proceed with the appropriate management without detailed study of platelet function.

Innocent and Benign Ecchymoses

SENILE PURPURA. Patients with this common yet benign problem complain of easy bruising, with the formation of sharply delineated, dark-blue ecchymoses, almost exclusively on the dorsal surface of the forearms either without trauma or after trivial trauma. Senile purpura usually are seen in the elderly patient whose skin has lost its elasticity; however, they also may be seen in younger patients (in their fifties) who are quite vigorous and far from senile. No laboratory study is indicated if the clinical picture is typical and nothing else suggests a hemorrhagic tendency.

UNEXPLAINED EASY BRUISING. This problem lacks a suitable name. Many individuals, generally women from 15 to 50 years old, complain of unwarranted ecchymoses, particularly on their extremities, and on examination, ecchymoses are indeed present. There are no other findings in the patient's history to suggest a hemorrhagic tendency. The vast majority of these patients also do not show any coagulation abnormality when studied in detail, and they can undergo surgery without difficulty. Therefore, if there are no other findings in the history to suggest a hemorrhagic diathesis, the evaluation of platelet function can be limited to a platelet count and bleeding time. There is no better point than this to emphasize that a carefully taken history is the most important tool in the diagnosis of the patients discussed in this chapter.

Gardner-Diamond Syndrome

The Gardner-Diamond syndrome originally was termed *the autoerythrocyte sensitization syndrome* by the physicians who described it.[105] Others have used the term *psychogenic purpura,* thereby implying a different etiology.[106] Almost invariably, the patient is a woman whose hemorrhagic symptomatology begins in the second, third, or fourth decade of life, and the manifestations begin rather abruptly, often at a time of emotional stress or after surgery or trauma. The diagnosis must be made by clinical observation, because all laboratory findings are normal. Ecchymoses commonly are preceded by subjective prodromata of local burning, tingling, or pain, and prominent painful erythema precedes or accompanies the development of the ecchymosis. These manifestations are inconspicuous or totally lacking in the spontaneous ecchymosis that forms in patients with a hemorrhagic tendency, and petechiae are not seen. The lesions may occur in any area of the body, but they are most common on the lower extremities and range from 1 to 15 cm in diameter. There is no spontaneous internal bleeding. Typically, the patient has undergone one or more surgical procedures in an attempt to relieve the myriad of systemic complaints that are characteristic; excessive bleeding with surgery is not observed.

As suggested by the variety of names ascribed to this syndrome, the etiology is uncertain. Gardner and Diamond originally observed that the intracutaneous injection of the patient's own blood would produce the characteristic lesion, and they hypothesized that the patients had become sensitized to their own erythrocytes and the lesions resulted from a response to minute extravasations of blood occurring from the trauma of everyday life. Ratnoff has now studied 71 patients and found that more than 40%, who were otherwise typical, had negative skin tests.[106] Ratnoff further discovered that most patients shared a pattern of severe emotional disturbance characterized by hysterical and masochistic character traits, and he proposed that the syndrome be renamed *psychogenic purpura.*

Complete studies of plasma coagulation and platelet function should be carried out once both to reassure the physician and to convince the patient there is no hemorrhagic diathesis. Drug therapy has not been helpful, but psychotherapy has been in some patients, particularly if begun at an early age.

Vasculitis of Small Blood Vessels

When an inflammatory reaction involves arterioles, capillaries, or venules, a purpuric eruption can develop that may be difficult to distinguish from that which occurs in severe thrombocytopenia. Such small-vessel involvement has been referred to as *allergic, hypersensitivity, necrotizing,* or *leukocytoclastic vasculitis.*

Characteristically, as in thrombocytopenia, the purpura is more severe in the lower extremities; however, it often is raised and accompanied by erythema, edema, pain, itching, burning, and ulceration (all features that are not seen with thrombocytopenia). Because disorders of platelet function are not accompanied by such florid formation of petechiae, their presence with a normal platelet count usually indicates vasculitis. There is no hemorrhagic risk if surgery should be required.

In most instances, such vasculitis probably results from circulating immune complexes that fix complement to the wall of the small vessel.[107] Thus, immunoglobulin and complement components can be demonstrated by immunofluorescence. Presumably, activated complement components initiate the inflammatory reaction, and any internal organ, as well as the skin, can be involved. Such a process may be seen either as part of a drug reaction or serum sickness; as secondary to connective tissue or lymphoproliferative disease; with certain infectious diseases such as infective endocarditis, meningococcemia, gonococcemia, and Rocky Mountain spotted fever; and in three other relatively well-defined diseases: cryoglobulinemia purpura,[108] hyperglobulinemic purpura of Waldenström,[109] and anaphylactoid (Schönlein-Henoch) purpura.[110]

Noninflammatory Blood Vessel Abnormalities

One heterogeneous group of disorders has pathologic bleeding and purpura that results from noninflammatory abnormalities of blood vessels as a common denominator. These disorders include amyloidosis, scurvy, hereditary hemorrhagic telangiectasia, and other heritable disorders of connective tissue.

AMYLOIDOSIS. Petechiae and purpura are common in patients with amyloidosis.[111] However, in contrast to thrombocytopenic purpura and the purpura in vasculitis syndromes, the purpura in amyloidosis is more common in the upper part of the body (most commonly the face, neck, and periorbital region). It often is brought on by activities that involve the Valsalva maneuver, such as vomiting and coughing, and hemorrhage in the mucous membranes of the mouth and from the gastrointestinal tract also may be seen. Skin biopsies have indicated there is infiltration of vessel walls with amyloid, and it is assumed that this leads to weakening that results in hemorrhage when the intravascular pressure is increased.

SCURVY. A hemorrhagic tendency is seen with severe deficiency of ascorbic acid, and scurvy is still seen, particularly in single men whose diet contains inadequate fresh fruits and vegetables.[112] In addition to the classic, minute perifollicular hemorrhage seen in dependent portions of the body, intradermal, intramuscular, and subperiosteal hemorrhage occurs as well. Ascorbic acid is necessary for the formation and maintenance of connective tissue, and hemorrhage apparently results from the inadequate connective tissue support of the vasculature.

HEREDITARY HEMORRHAGIC TELANGIECTASIA (OSLER-WEBER-RENDU DISEASE).

Hereditary hemorrhagic telangiectasia is an autosomal dominant condition characterized by the development of localized dilatations of capillaries and venules of the skin and mucous membranes.[113] The lesions are 1 to 3 mm in diameter and blanch with pressure. It is typical for lesions to accumulate gradually over decades, and patients may be free of symptoms or suffer only recurrent epistaxis until early adult life, when bleeding becomes more frequent and severe. The nose remains the most common site, but oral, gastrointestinal, genitourinary, pulmonary, and cerebral bleeding are seen as well. Approximately 10% to 20% of these patients have pulmonary arteriovenous fistulas, which may produce cyanosis, polycythemia, and clubbing; in fact, 50% to 70% of such fistulas are seen in patients with this illness.

On physical examination, the lesions are most prominent on the skin of the face and on the mucous membranes of the mouth and nose. The liver and spleen may be enlarged as a result of vascular malformations, and findings from laboratory studies of hemostasis are all normal. The bleeding is due entirely to the anatomic lesions.

Treatment is palliative. Bleeding commonly is profuse enough to require transfusion of red blood cells, and a patient may have continuing gastrointestinal blood loss at a rate approaching 1 L/day. The need for transfusion can be reduced by the intravenous infusion of iron dextran if oral iron replacement is insufficient.

OTHER HERITABLE DISORDERS OF CONNECTIVE TISSUE.

These diseases result from inherited defects of the body's supporting structures, leading to malfunction of the skin, bones, joints, and blood vessels.[114] In three of the diseases, these defects lead to hemorrhagic manifestations that suggest a coagulation or platelet disorder. First, the Ehlers-Danlos syndrome, which has an autosomal dominant mode of inheritance, is characterized by hyperplastic, fragile skin and hyperextensible joints. The second, osteogenesis imperfecta, also has an autosomal dominant inheritance and is characterized by liability to bone fracture, blue sclerae, and otosclerosis leading to deafness. In both of these syndromes, easy bruising and hematoma formation in the skin are common, and patients with the Ehlers-Danlos syndrome also bleed from the gums and gastrointestinal tract as well as post partum.

The third disease, pseudoxanthoma elasticum, is much rarer and has an autosomal recessive inheritance. Hemorrhage, most commonly gastrointestinal, often is the most important problem that these patients present clinically; subarachnoid, genitourinary, and nasal bleeding is observed but is less common. Repeated bleeding episodes may remain unexplained until the other manifestations of the disease are recognized, and thickened, grooved skin (most typically in the face and neck) is the most easily detected manifestation. Angioid streaks in the ocular fundus as well as premature peripheral and coronary arterial insufficiency are the other major manifestations.

REFERENCES

1. Gaydos LA, Freireich EJ, Mantel N. The quantitative relation between platelet count and hemorrhage in patients with acute leukemia. N Eng J Med 1962;266:905.
2. Thompson CG, Jakubowski JA. The pathophysiology and clinical relevance of platelet heterogeneity. Blood 1988;72:1.
3. Aster RH, Jandl JH. Platelet sequestration in man. I. Methods. J Clin Invest 1964;43:843.
4. Vicari A, Banfi G, Bonini PA. EDTA-dependent pseudothrombocytopaenia: a 12-month epidemiological study. Scand J Clin Lab Invest 1988;48:537.
5. Hoffman R. Regulation of megakaryocytopoiesis. Blood 1989; 74:1196.
6. Rodeghiero F, Avvisati G, Castaman G, Barbui T, Mandelli F. Early deaths and anti-hemorrhagic treatments in acute promyelocytic leukemia. A GIMEMA retrospective study in 268 consecutive patients. Blood 1990;75:2112.
7. May SJ, Smith SA, Jacobs A, Williams A, Baily-Wood R. The myelodysplastic syndrome: analysis of laboratory characteristics in relation to the FAB classification. Br J Haematol 1985; 59:311.
8. Coffier B, Adeleine P, Viala JJ, et al. Dysmyelopoietic syndromes. Cancer 1983;52:83.
9. Efira A, Cauchie P, Rauis M, de Maertelaere E. Platelet survival in myelodysplastic syndromes. Acta Haematol 1986;76:124.
10. De Planque MM, Van Krieken JHJM, Kluin-Nelemans HC, et al. Bone marrow histopathology of patients with severe aplastic anaemia before treatment and at follow-up. Br J Haematol 1989;72:439.
11. Hall JG, Levin J, Kuhn UP, Ottenheimer EJ, Van Berkun KAP, McKusick VA. Thrombocytopenia with absent radius (TAR). Medicine 1969;48:411.
12. Hanson SR, Slichter SJ. Platelet kinetics in patients with bone marrow hypoplasia: evidence for a fixed platelet requirement. Blood 1985;66:1105.
13. Stoll DB, Blum S, Pasquale D, Murphy S. Thrombocytopenia with decreased megakaryocytes. Ann Intern Med 1981;94:170.
14. Manoharan A, Williams NT, Sparrow R. Acquired amegakaryocytic thrombocytopenia: report of a case and review of literature. Q J Med 1989;70:243.
15. Camitta BM, Thomas ED, Nathan DG, et al. A prospective study of androgens and bone marrow transplantation for treatment of severe aplastic anemia. Blood 1979;53:504.
16. Speck G, Gratwohl A, Nissen C, et al. Treatment of severe aplastic anemia. Exp Hematol 1986;14:126.

17. Doney K, Storb R, Buckner CD, et al. Treatment of aplastic anemia with antithymocyte globulin, high-dose corticosteroids, and androgens. Exp Hematol 1987;15:239.

18. Bishop JF, McGrath K, Wolf MM, et al. Clinical factors influencing the efficacy of pooled platelet transfusions. Blood 1988;71:383.

19. Consensus Conference. Platelet transfusion therapy. JAMA 1987;257:1777.

20. Meryman HT. Transfusion-induced alloimmunization and immunosuppression and the effects of leukocyte depletion. Transfusion Med Reviews 1989;3:180.

21. Bolan CD, Alving BM. Pharmacologic agents in the management of bleeding disorders. Transfusion 1990;30:541.

22. Wadenvik H, Denfors I, Kutti J. Splenic blood flow and intrasplenic platelet kinetics in relation to spleen volume. Br J Haematol 1987;67:181.

23. El-Khishen MA, Henderson JM, Millikan WJ, et al. Splenectomy is contraindicated for thrombocytopenia secondary to portal hypertension. Surg Gynecol Obstet 1985;160:233.

24. Holme S, Simmonds M, Ballek R, et al. Comparative measurements of platelet size by Coulter counter, microscopy of blood smears and light-transmission studies. J Lab Clin Med 1981;97:610.

25. Menitove JE, Pereira J, Hoffman R, et al. Cyclic thrombocytopenia of apparent autoimmune etiology. Blood 1989;73:1561.

26. George JN. Platelet immunoglobulin G: its significance for the evaluation of thrombocytopenia and for understanding the origin of α-granule proteins. Blood 1990;76:859.

27. Kiefel V, Santoso S, Weisheit M, et al. Monoclonal antibody-specific immunobilization of platelet antigens (MAIPA): a new tool for the identification of platelet-reactive antibodies. Blood 1987;70:1722.

28. McMillian R. Antigen-specific assays in immune thrombocytopenia. Transfusion Med Reviews 4:136, 1990.

29. Tani P, Berchtold P, McMillian R. Autoantibodies in chronic ITP. Blut 1989;59:44.

30. Ballem PJ, Segal GM, Stratton JR, et al. Mechanism of thrombocytopenia in chronic autoimmune thrombocytopenic purpura. J Clin Invest 1987;80:33.

31. Tong M, Seth P, Penington DG. Proplatelets and stress platelets. Blood 1987;69:522.

32. McMillian R. Chronic idiopathic thrombocytopenic purpura. N Engl J Med 1981;304:1135.

33. Stuart MJ, Kelton JG, Allen JB. Abnormal platelet function and arachidonate metabolism in chronic idiopathic thrombocytopenic purpura. Blood 1981;58:326.

34. Samuels P, Bussel JB, Braitman LE, et al. Estimation of the risk of thrombocytopenia in the offspring of pregnant women with presumed immune thrombocytopenic purpura. N Engl J Med 1990;323:229.

35. Scioscia AL, Grannum PAT, Copel JA. The use of percutaneous umbilical blood sampling in immune thrombocytopenic purpura. Am J Obstet Gynecol 1988;159:1066.

36. Burrow RF, Kelton JG. Incidentally detected thrombocytopenia in healthy mothers and their infants. N Engl J Med 1988;319:142.

37. Stoll D, Cines DB, Aster RH, Murphy S. Platelet kinetics in patients with idiopathic thrombocytopenic purpura and moderate thrombocytopenia. Blood 1985;65:584.

38. Gernsheimer T, Stratton J, Ballen PJ, et al. Mechanisms of response to treatment in autoimmune thrombocytopenic purpura. N Engl J Med 1989;320:974.

39. Pizzuto J, Ambirz R. Therapeutic experience on 934 adults with idiopathic thrombocytopenic purpura: multicentric trial of the Cooperative Latin American Group on Hemostasis and Thrombosis. Blood 1984;64:1179.

40. Bussel JB, Pham LC. Intravenous treatment with gamma-globulin in adults with immune thrombocytopenic purpura: review of the literature. Vox Sang 1987;52:206.

41. Bussel JB, Pham LC, Aledort L. Maintenance treatment of adults with chronic refractory immune thrombocytopenic purpura using repeated intravenous infusions of gammaglobulin. Blood 1988;72:121.

42. Quiquandon I, Fenaux P, Caulier MT, et al. Reevaluation of the role of azathioprine in the treatment of adult chronic idiopathic thrombocytopenic purpura: a report on 53 cases. Br J Haematol 1990;74:223.

43. Ahn YS, Rocha R, Mylvaganam R, et al. Long-term danazol therapy in autoimmune thrombocytopenia: unmaintained remission and age-dependent response in women. Ann Intern Med 1989;111:723.

44. Fenaux P, Quiquandon I, Caulier MT, et al. Slow infusions of vinblastine in the treatment of adult idiopathic thrombocytopenic purpura: a report on 43 cases. Blut 1990;60:238.

45. Proctor SJ, Jackson G, Carey P, et al. Improvement of platelet counts in steroid-unresponsive idiopathic immune thrombocytopenic purpura after short-course therapy with recombinant α2b interferon. Blood 1989;74:1894.

46. Carr JM, Kruskall MS, Kaye JA, et al. Efficacy of platelet transfusions in immune thrombocytopenia. Am J Med 1986;80:1051.

47. Scadden DT, Zon LI, Groopman JE. Pathophysiology and management of HIV-associated hematologic disorders. Blood 1989;74:1455.

48. Holzman RS, Walsh CM, Karpatkin S. Risk for the acquired immunodeficiency syndrome among thrombocytopenic and nonthrombocytopenic homosexual men seropositive for the human immunodeficiency virus. Ann Intern Med 1987;106:383.

49. Ballem PJ, Belzberg A, Devine D, et al. Pathophysiology of thrombocytopenia associated with HIV infection in homosexual men. Blut 1989;59:111.

50. Walsh CM, Nardi MA, Karpatkin S. On the mechanism of thrombocytopenic purpura in sexually active homosexual men. N Engl J Med 1984;311:635.

51. Stricker RB, Abrams DI, Corash L, et al. Target platelet antigen in homosexual men with immune thrombocytopenia. N Engl J Med 1985;313:1375.

52. Bettaieb A, Oksenhendler E, Fromont P, et al. Immunochemical analysis of platelet autoantibodies in HIV-related thrombocytopenic purpura: a study of 68 patients. Br J Haematol 1989;73:241.

53. Oksenhendler E, Bierling P, Farcet JP, et al. Response to therapy in 37 patients with HIV-related thrombocytopenic purpura. Br J Haematol 1987;66:491.

54. Ragni MV, Bontempo FA, Myers DJ, et al. Hemorrhagic sequelae of immune thrombocytopenic purpura in human immunodeficiency virus–infected hemophiliacs. Blood 1990;75:1267.

55. Jouhikainen T, Kekomaki R, Leirisalo-Repo M, et al. Platelet autoantibodies detected by immunoblotting in systemic lupus erythematosus: association with the lupus anticoagulant, and with history of thrombosis and thrombocytopenia. Eur J Haematol 1990;44:234.

56. Hall S, McCormic JL, Greipp PR, et al. Splenectomy does not cure the thrombocytopenia of systemic lupus erythematosus. Ann Intern Med 1985;102:325.

57. Xiros N, Binder T, Anger B, et al. Idiopathic thrombocytopenic purpura and autoimmune hemolytic anemia in Hodgkin's disease. Eur J Haematol 1988;40:437.

58. Lawrence HJ, Greenberg BR. Autoimmune thrombocytopenia in sarcoidosis. Am J Med 1985;79:761.

59. Carey RW, McGinnis A, Jacobson BM, et al. Idiopathic thrombocytopenic purpura complicating chronic lymphocytic leukemia. Arch Intern Med 1976;136:62.

60. Schwartz KA, Slichter SJ, Harker LA. Immune-mediated platelet destruction and thrombocytopenia in patients with solid tumors. Br J Haematol 1982;51:17.

61. Winiarski J. Antibodies to platelet membrane glycoprotein antigens in three cases of infectious mononucleosis–induced thrombocytopenic purpura. Eur J Haematol 1989;43:29.

62. Conley ME, Park CL, Douglas SD. Childhood common variable immunodeficiency with autoimmune disease. J Pediatrics 1986;108:915.

63. First LR, Smith BR, Lipton J, et al. Isolated thrombocytopenia after allogeneic bone marrow transplantation: existence of transient and chronic thrombocytopenic syndromes. Blood 1985;65:368.

64. Anasetti C, Rybka W, Sullivan KM, et al. Graft-v-host disease is associated with autoimmune-like thrombocytopenia. Blood 1989;73:1054.

65. Hackett T, Kelton JG, Powers P. Drug-induced platelet destruction. Semin Thromb Hemost 1982;8:116.

66. Smith ME, Reid DM, Jones CE, et al. Binding of quinine- and quinidine-dependent drug antibodies to platelets is mediated by the fab domain of the immunoglobulin G and is not Fc dependent. J Clin Invest 1987;79:912.

67. Christie DJ, Mullen PC, Aster RH. Quinine and quinidine platelet antibodies can react with GPIIb/IIIa. Br J Haematol 1987;67:213.

68. Sheridan D, Carter C, Kelton JG. A diagnostic test for heparin-induced thrombocytopenia. Blood 1986;67:27.

69. King DJ, Kelton JG. Heparin-associated thrombocytopenia. Ann Intern Med 1984;100:535.

70. Coblyn JS, Weinblatt M, Holdsworth D, et al. Gold-induced thrombocytopenia. Ann Intern Med 1981;95:178.

71. Mueller-Eckhardt C. Annotation. Post-transfusion purpura. Br J Haematol 1986;64:419.

72. Simon TL, Collins J, Kunicki TJ, et al. Posttransfusion purpura associated with alloantibody specific for the platelet antigen, Pen[a]. Am J Hematol 1988;29:38.

73. Mueller-Eckhardt C, Kiefel V. High-dose IgG for post-transfusion purpura—revisited. Blut 1988;57:163.

74. Brecher ME, Moore SB, Letendre L. Posttransfusion purpura: the therapeutic value of P1[A1]-negative platelets. Transfusion 1990;30:433.

75. Bussel JB, Richard MD, Berkowitz L, et al. Antenatal treatment of neonatal alloimmune thrombocytopenia. N Engl J Med 1988;319:1374.

76. Mueller-Eckhardt C, Grubert A, Kiefel V, et al. 348 Cases of suspected neonatal alloimmune thrombocytopenia. Lancet, 1989;1:363.

77. Kaplan C, Daffos F, Forestier F, et al. Management of alloimmune thrombocytopenia: antenatal diagnosis and in utero transfusion of maternal platelets. Blood 1988;72:340.

78. Neame PB, Kelton JG, Walker IR, et al. Thrombocytopenia in septicemia: the role of disseminated intravascular coagulation. Blood 1980;56:88.

79. Lichtin AE, Schreiber AD, Hurwitz S, et al. Efficacy of intensive plasmapheresis in thrombotic thrombocytopenic purpura. Arch Intern Med 1987;147:2122.

80. Liu ET, Linker CA, Shuman MA. Management of treatment failures in thrombotic thrombocytopenic purpura. Am J Hematol 1986;23:347.

81. Lesesne JB, Rothschild N, Erickson B, et al. Cancer-associated hemolytic-uremic syndrome: analysis of 85 cases from a national registry. J Clin Oncol 1989;7:781.

82. Reed RL, Ciavarella D, Heimbach DM, et al. Prophylactic platelet administration during massive transfusion. Ann Surg 1986;203:40.

83. Gibson B, Hunter D, Neame PB, Kelton JG. Thrombocytopenia in preeclampsia and eclampsia. Semin Thromb Hemost 1982;8:234.

84. Thiagarajah S, Bourgeois FJ, Harber GM, et al. Thrombocytopenia in preeclampsia: associated abnormalities and management principles. Am J Obstet Gynecol 1984;150:1.

85. Murphy S. Hereditary thrombocytopenia. Clin Haematol 1972;1:359.

86. Corash L, Shafer B, Blaese MR. Platelet-associated immunoglobulin, platelet size, and the effect of splenectomy in the Wiskott-Aldrich syndrome. Blood 1985;65:1439.

87. Greinacher A, Mueller-Eckhardt C: Hereditary types of thrombocytopenia with giant platelets and inclusion bodies in the leukocytes. Blut 1990;60:53.

88. Najean Y, Lecompte T. Genetic thrombocytopenia with autosomal dominant transmission: a review of 54 cases. Br J Haematol 1990;74:203.

89. George JN, Shattil SJ. The clinical importance of acquired abnormalities of platelet function. N Engl J Med 1991; 324:27.

90. Kunicki TJ. Platelet membrane glycoproteins and their function: an overview. Blut 1989;59:30.

91. Channing Rougers RP, Levin J. A critical reappraisal of the bleeding time. Semin Thromb Hemost 1990;16:1.

92. George JN, Reimann TA, Moake JL. Bernard-Soulier disease: a study of four patients and their parents. Br J Haematol 1981;48:459.

93. Weiss HJ, Tschopp TB, Baumgartner HR, et al. Decreased adhesion of giant (Bernard-Soulier) platelets to subendothelium. Am J Med 1974;57:920.

94. Kaneshiro MM, Mielke CH, Kasper CK, et al. Bleeding time after aspirin in disorders of intrinsic clotting. N Engl J Med 1969;281:1039.

95. Remaley AT, Kennedy JM, Laposata M. Evaluation of the clinical utility of platelet aggregation studies. Am J Hematol 1989;31:188.

96. Nieuwenhuis HK, Akkerman JN, Sixma JJ. Patients with a prolonged bleeding time and normal aggregation tests may have storage pool deficiency: studies on one hundred six patients. Blood 1987;70:620.

97. Israels SJ, McNicol A, Robertson C, Gerrard JM. Platelet storage pool deficiency: diagnosis in patients with prolonged bleeding times and normal platelet aggregation. Br J Haematol 1990;75:118.

98. George JN, Caen JP, Nurden AT. Glanzmann's thrombasthenia: the spectrum of clinical disease. Blood 1990;75:1383.

99. Brown CH, Bradshaw W, Natelson EA, et al. Defective platelet function following the administration of penicillin compounds. Blood 1976;47:949.

100. Perkins HA, MacKenzie MR, Fudenberg HH. Hemostatic defects in dysproteinemias. Blood 1970;35:695.

101. Woodman RC, Harker LA: Bleeding complications associated with cardiopulmonary bypass. Blood 1990;76:1680.

102. Murphy S, Davis JL, Walsh PN, et al. Template bleeding time and clinical hemorrhage in myeloproliferative disease. Arch Intern Med 1978;138:1251.

103. Michiels JJ, Abels J, Steketee J, et al. Erythromelalgia caused by platelet-mediated arteriolar inflammation and thrombosis in thrombocythemia. Ann Intern Med 1985;102:466.

104. Schafer AI. Bleeding and thrombosis in the myeloproliferative disorers. Blood 1984;64:1.

105. Gardner FH, Diamond LK. Autoerythrocyte sensitization: a form of purpura producing painful bruising following autosensitization to red blood cells in certain women. Blood 1955; 10:675.

106. Ratnoff OD. Psychogenic purpura (autoerythrocyte sensitization): an unsolved dilemma. Am J Med 1989;87:3N.

107. Fauci AS, Haynes BF, Katz P. The spectrum of vasculitis. Ann Intern Med 1978;89:660.
108. Gorevic PD, Kassab JH, Levo Y, et al. Mixed cryoglobulinemia: clinical aspects and long-term follow-up of 40 patients. Am J Med 1980;69:287.
109. Capra JD, Winchester RJ, Kunkle GH. Hypergammaglobulinemic purpura. Medicine 1971;50:125.
110. Cream JJ, Gumpel JM, Peachey RDG. Schonlein-Henoch purpura in the adult: a study of 77 adults with anaphylactoid or Schonlein-Henoch purpura. Q J Med 1970;39:461.
111. Kyle RA, Bayrd ED. Amyloidosis: review of 236 cases. Medicine 1975;54:271.
112. Wallerstein RO, Wallerstein RO Jr. Scurvy. Semin Hematol 1976;13:211.
113. Perry WH. Clinical spectrum of hereditary hemorrhagic telangiectasia (Osler-Weber-Rendu Disease). Am J Med 1987;82:989.
114. Nydegger UE, Miescher PA. Bleeding due to vascular disorders. Semin Hematol 1980;17:178.

18

Coagulation Factors

Craig M. Kessler, M.D., and William R. Bell, M.D.

Effective hemostasis is accomplished through an integrated sequence of both vascular and intravascular functions. When the continuity of the vessel wall is broken, small arteries and veins normally undergo localized vasoconstriction that impedes blood flow and facilitates the accumulation of platelets for the subsequent formation of the platelet hemostatic plug. The process of vasoconstriction appears to be a manifestation of neural reflexes involving the smooth muscles of both arterioles and venules, and it is potentiated by epinephrine and serotonin, biogenic amines, and prostaglandin derivatives that are released at the site of injury by aggregated platelets.[1] Blood loss within fascial planes and closed tissue spaces also may be minimized by the extrinsic pressure exerted on the vessel following the extravascular accumulation of blood.

Disruption of the endothelial surface of blood vessels exposes collagen fibers and connective tissue, and these provide surfaces that promote platelet adherence, aggregation, and subsequent release reaction. Substances liberated from the platelets further stimulate platelet aggregation (e.g., adenosine diphosphate and thromboxane A_2), maintain vasoconstriction (e.g., serotonin and prostaglandin derivatives), and participate in blood coagulation (e.g., platelet factors III and IV). In addition, the release reaction modifies platelet membranes in a manner that renders phospholipid available for coagulation, and the thrombin elaborated by the coagulation mechanism is a potent agent in the induction of the platelet release reaction.

Stabilization and transition of the platelet plug both require the participation of the blood coagulation system, which leads to the eventual formation of fibrin.

Because most knowledge concerning blood coagulation has been gained under artificial in vitro laboratory conditions and then extrapolated to clinical settings, many gaps exist in our comprehension of the blood clotting mechanism. Usually, this complex system is conceptualized either as a waterfall or a cascade to emphasize the sequential interactions of clot-promoting substances,[2,3] and these schema accommodate amplification and negative feedback mechanisms, provide the coagulation process with critical sites of control, and allow for interactions of end products and by-products with other systems (e.g., activation of the kallikrein/kinin system by fragments of coagulation factor XII). Each of the proteins and other substances involved in blood coagulation (Table 18.1) has been assigned a Roman numeral (by the International Committee on Nomenclature of Blood Clotting Factors) and can be represented diagrammatically as in Figure 18.1. Factor VI was deleted when it was discovered to be identical to activated factor V (Va).

The coagulation process can be activated and proceed either via the intrinsic or extrinsic systems (Fig. 18.1). Both sequential pathways advance independently through their initial interactions, but they eventually follow a common course. The activity of both is important in vivo, and the concept of separate systems provides a practical means for evaluating laboratory and clinical coagulation abnormalities.

The extrinsic coagulation pathway is initiated when tissue extracts with lipid–protein properties are released from the membranes of endothelial/subcutaneous cells following injury or insult. These substances, collectively designated *tissue thromboplastin* or *tissue factor*,

TABLE 18.1. Factors Involved in Blood Coagulation

	I	II	III	IV	V	VII
Common synonym	Fibrinogen	Prothrombin	Thrombo-plastin	Calcium	Proaccelerin, plasma ac-globulin	Serum prothrombin conversion accelerator, proconvertin
Molecular weight, d	340,000	70,000		40	330,000	48,000 to 100,000
Site of biosynthesis	Liver	Liver	All body tissues		Liver	Liver
Biologic half-life, h	95 to 120	72			12 to 36	4 to 6
Activity						
Plasma	Present	Present		Present	Present	Present
Serum	Absent	Absent		Present	Absent	Present
Activity level required for normal hemostasis, *% normal*	20	20			10 to 20	10
Volume of distribution*	2.5	1.5 to 2.5			2.0	2.0 to 4.0
Inheritance of deficiency state	Autosomal recessive	Autosomal recessive	Not reported		Autosomal recessive	Autosomal recessive
Incidence of inherited deficiency, *prevalence per million*	0.5	0.5			0.5	0.5
Biochemistry	Glycoprotein	Serine protease, glycoprotein, α-globulin Vitamin K dependent	Lipoprotein	Divalent cation	Glycoprotein (labile)	Glycoprotein α- Or β-globulin, serine protease Vitamin K dependent
Replacement therapy	Cryoprecipitate stored plasma, lyophilized fibrinogen	Fresh or fresh-frozen plasma, prothrombin-complex concentrate			Fresh or fresh-frozen plasma	Fresh, fresh-frozen, or stored plasma, prothrombin-complex concentrate
Gene located on chromosome	4q26–q28	11p11q12				13q34

Note: Factors II, VII, IX, and X depend on vitamin K for postribosomal modification following synthesis of the inactive precursor proenzyme factor.

*The number indicated multiplied by the plasma volume is the total volume in which the factor is located.

VIII	IX	X	XI	XII	XIII	vWF
Antihemophilic globulin, antihemophilic factor	Plasma thromboplastin component, Christmas factor	Stuart-Prower factor	Plasma thrombo-plastin antecedent	Hageman factor	Fibrin stabilizing factor	
2,000,000 (procoagulant subunit-200,000)	55,000 to 70,000	55,000 to 100,000	160,000 to 200,000	80,000 to 100,000	350,000	30,000,000
? Endothelium ? Reticulo-endothelial cells	Liver	Liver	± Liver	?	± Liver, megakaryo-cytes	Vascular endothelial megakaryo-cytes
6 to 10 (initial) 15 to 18 (secondary)	6 to 10 (initial) 25 to 30 (secondary)	40 to 50	50 to 80	50 to 60	95 to 120	18 to 24
Present Absent	Present Present	Present Present	Present Present	Present Present	Present Decreased trace quantities	Present Absent
30 to 40	30 to 40	10 to 20	10 to 20	< 10	1 to 2	30 to 40
1.0 to 1.5	2.0 to 3.0	1.0	1.0		1.0 to 2.0	1.0 to 1.5
Hemophilia A sex-linked recessive Von Willebrand disease—autosomal dominant	Sex-linked recessive	Autosomal recessive	Autosomal recessive (dominant)	Autosomal recessive	Autosomal recessive	Autosomal dominant
60.0 to 80.0	15.0 to 20.0	< 0.5	< 1.0	< 1.0	< 0.5	80.0 to 100.0
65 to 100						
Glycoprotein, α- or β-globulin	α- Or β-globulin, serine protease Vitamin K dependent	Vitamin K dependent Glycoprotein, α-globulin, serine protease	β- Or γ-globulin, serine protease	Sialoglyco-protein, β- or γ-globulin, serine protease	γ₂-Globulin	Glycoprotein, α-β globulin
Factor VIII concentrate, purified factor VII, cryo-precipitate, fresh or fresh-frozen plasma	Fresh or fresh-frozen plasma, prothrombin complex concentrate	Fresh or fresh-frozen plasma, prothrombin complex concentrate	Fresh, fresh-frozen, or stored plasma	Fresh, fresh-frozen, or stored plasma	Fresh, fresh-frozen, or stored plasma	Cryprecipitate, fresh-frozen plasma
Xq28	Xq26–27	13q34				12pter-12

by the hepatocyte. The modified factor is then available for activation by other specific activated factors in the cascade. vWF = von Willebrand

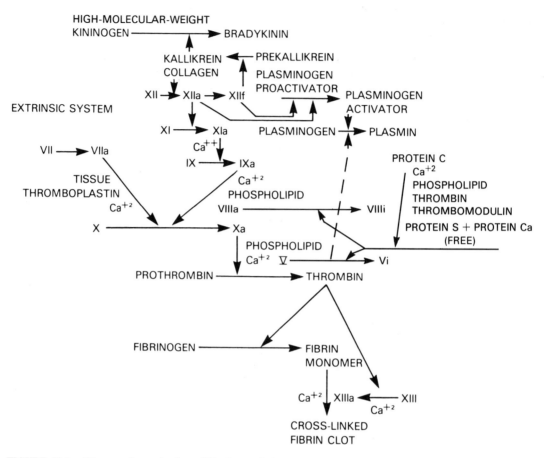

FIGURE 18.1. The cascade mechanism of blood coagulation.

are ubiquitously present in the adventitia of blood vessels and many other cells, and they complex with circulating factor VIIa. The factor VIIa/tissue factor complex in the presence of calcium ions subsequently initiates coagulation by activating either factor X or IX within the extrinsic pathway (Fig. 18.1), and this activation of factor X by the factor VIIa/tissue factor complex is regulated by a specific plasma inhibitor, termed the *extrinsic pathway inhibitor* or *the lipoprotein-associated coagulation inhibitor,* which complexes with factor Xa and inhibits the expression of factor VIIa/tissue factor complex–mediated coagulation when blood comes in contact with cell surfaces that contain tissue factor (e.g., endothelial cells and platelets). In vitro evidence suggests that factor X can be activated less rapidly through the interaction of kallikrein with factor VII.[4] However, the physiologic significance of this reaction has not been determined; the physiochemical properties of factor VII are presented in Table 18.1.

The intrinsic coagulation pathway involves more protein–protein interactions and thus proceeds considerably slower than the extrinsic system (Fig. 18.1). Intrinsic clotting was demonstrated originally in vitro by allowing plasma to clot in a glass test tube;[5] it now is appreciated that the plasma component affected by the high negative charge of glass is factor XII (Hageman factor), a sialoglycoprotein with a molecular weight of 80,000 to 100,000 d. Apparently, activation is accomplished without a change in the molecular structure; however, conformational modifications are induced by in vitro activators of factor XII (*e.g.,* collagen, endotoxin, platelet and endothelial membranes) and by ellagic acid, trypsin, or heparin. Whether prekallikrein (Fletcher factor) and high-molecular-weight kininogen (Williams, Fitzgerald, Flaujeac, Warren, and Reid factors) are necessary to activate factor XII in vivo or for expression of the coagulant properties of factor XIIa remains unclear. However, plasmin enzymatically

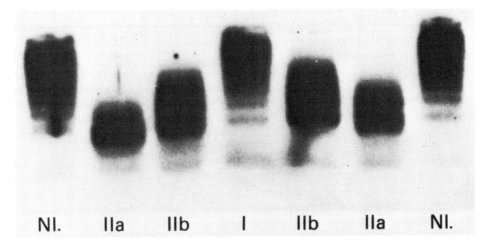

FIGURE 18.2. The multimeric structure of factor VIII (von Willebrand factor [fVIII/vWF]) in patients' plasma. These proteins were separated by electrophoresis and examined by autoradiography after incubation with ^{125}I-labelled rabbit and anti-VIIIR:Ag. The point of application is at the top and the anode at the bottom. Normal (*Nl*) plasma contains a series of fVIII/vWF multimers ranging in weight between 0.85×10^6 and 20×10^6 d. The absence of both larger multimers from type IIB(*II$_b$*)vWd as well as the large and intermediate forms from type IIA(*II$_a$*)vWd are evident.

cleaves factor XIIa to produce factor XII fragments (XIIf), which complete the feedback loop for the regulation of factor XII activation in the kinin system (Fig. 18.1).

Two substrates are susceptible to the actions of factor XIIa: plasminogen proactivator; and factor XI (plasma thromboplastin antecedent) (Fig. 18.1), a serine protease glycoprotein with a molecular weight of 160,000 to 200,000 d. Presumably, factor XI is synthesized in the liver, and its activation by factor XIIa is catalyzed by high-molecular-weight kininogen. Evidence indicates that factor XI also can be activated by other, less well-defined mechanisms that are questionably significant. Factor XIa converts factor IX (Christmas factor, plasma thromboplastin component) to its activated form (IXa) in the presence of calcium ions (Fig. 18.1). Factor IX has a molecular weight of 55,000 to 70,000 d, and its hepatic synthesis is vitamin K–dependent. Factor IX activation can be accomplished in vitro through interactions with activated Stuart-Prower Factor (Xa), kallikrein, and the reaction product of tissue thromboplastin and factor VII.[6-8] Hypothetically, these alternative means of activating factor IX may assume physiologic importance in patients who manifest only mild hemorrhagic symptoms despite deficiencies of factor XI, factor IX, Fletcher factor, or high-molecular-weight kininogen.

Factor VIII (antihemophilic globulin) is the next coagulation protein in the intrinsic pathway (Fig. 18.1);

its deficiency (VIII:C) is associated with classic hemophilia A. The intact factor VIII molecule is a glycoprotein composed of a low-molecular-weight subunit (230,000 d) that possesses procoagulant activity (VIII:C). It circulates normally in the plasma and is complexed with a very high-molecular-weight protein (up to 30 million d) (Fig. 18.2) designated *the von Willebrand factor antigen* (VIII:Ag or vWF) because of its immunoprecipitation by heterologous antiserum raised in rabbits immunized with purified von Willebrand factor protein (the deficient protein in von Willebrand disease). Von Willebrand factor protein does not participate in humoral coagulation per se, but it does mediate both the platelet interactions with the components of the subendothelial matrix, initiating platelet adhesion at the site of vessel injury, and the subsequent platelet–platelet interactions leading to the formation of the hemostatic platelet plug. Von Willebrand factor protein activity is expressed in vitro as a ristocetin cofactor, because this activity promotes platelet agglutination that can be quantitated following addition of the antibiotic ristocetin to fresh or formalinized normal platelets. Typical von Willebrand disease is characterized by bleeding and simultaneous reductions in the plasma levels of both von Willebrand factor antigen and activity, which are present at normal concentrations in classic hemophilia A. The procoagulant factor VIII:C activity is reduced in both hemophilia A and von Willebrand disease, but usually to a much greater degree in hemophilia A (Table

TABLE 18.2.   The Laboratory Expression of Hemophilia A and von Willebrand Disease

| | Hemophilia A | Von Willebrand Disease | | |
		Type I	Type IIA	Type IIB
VIII:C	Decreased	Decreased	Normal or decreased	Normal or decreased
VIIIR:Ag	Normal	Decreased or absent	Normal or decreased	Normal or decreased
VIII:RCoF	Normal	Greatly decreased	Usually decreased	Usually decreased
Ritocetin-induced PRP aggregation	Normal	Abnormally decreased	Abnormally decreased	Hyperresponsive
Bleeding time	Normal	Increased	Increased	Increased
Two-dimensional immunoelectrophoresis of VIIIR:Ag	Normal	Normal (if detectable)	Anodal shift	Anodal shift
Analysis of FVIII/vWF structure	Normal	Normal (if detectable)	Loss of high and intermediate-molecular-weight multimeric forms	Loss of highest-molecular-weight multimeric forms
Therapy	Cryoprecipitate or FVIII concentrate	FFP or cryoprecipitate	FFP or cryoprecipitate	FFP or cryoprecipitate

Note: FFP = fresh-frozen plasma; PRP = platelet-rich plasma.

18.2). It is hypothesized that circulating factor VIII is stabilized by its complex formation with von Willebrand factor protein in a manner allowing for its complete functional expression and survival.

The site of factor VIII protein synthesis is believed to be primarily in the liver. Transplants of normal livers into several patients with severe hemophilia A have resulted in significant elevations of circulating factor VIII procoagulant activity as well as the subsequent ability to achieve adequate hemostasis without therapeutic or prophylactic factor VIII replacement.[9] Von Willebrand factor protein primarily is synthesized/processed in the Golgi complex and stored in the Weibel-Palade body component of the endothelial cell. It is produced as a noncovalently linked single molecule, proteolytically modified with the release of a cleaved polypeptide (designated *von Willebrand factor II*), and is assembled then into multimers via a process mediated by the presence of von Willebrand factor II.[10]

Factor VIII procoagulant protein functions as an essential coenzyme in the intrinsic clotting pathway by complexing with factor IXa, phospholipid, and calcium ions to mediate the activation of factor X (Fig. 18.1). Factor Xa and thrombin, which eventually are elaborated in trace amounts, enhance factor VIII activity in plasma, and when larger amounts of thrombin are produced, factor VIII is inactivated.[11] Factor VIIIa also is inactivated by the direct proteolytic cleavage of activated protein C (a vitamin K–dependent anticoagulant protein synthesized in the liver and activated by thrombin) complexed with free protein S (another vitamin K–dependent protein synthesized in the liver, en-

dothelial cells, and the megakaryocytes). Plasmin inactivates factor VIII and von Willebrand factor proteins readily in plasma as well, and factor VIII has sequence homology with factor V and ceruloplasmin, a noncoagulation protein.

Factor X activation can be accomplished by the products derived from either the intrinsic or extrinsic pathway (Fig. 18.1); as such, it represents the beginning of the common pathway of coagulation. In vitro assays are based on the direct conversion of factor X to Xa by proteases such as trypsin or Russell viper venom. Factor X (Stuart-Prower factor) is a glycoprotein with a molecular weight of 59,000 d and is composed of two polypeptide chains, one heavy and one light. Activation is achieved in vivo on the surfaces of both platelets and endothelial cells by proteolytic cleavage of the heavy chain either with factors IXa and VIIIa or the factor VIIa/tissue factor complex; the resulting factor Xa is a serum protease inhibited by antithrombin III–heparin complexes that are produced during anticoagulation. This interaction forms the rationale for using low doses of heparin to provide effective prophylaxis against thrombotic events. One microgram of the inhibitor–heparin complex can neutralize 32 units of factor Xa and thus indirectly prevent the formation of 1600 units of thrombin that otherwise would be available for subsequent clot formation.[12]

Laboratory evidence suggests that factor Xa may potentiate the activities of both factor VII and IX.[6,13] More important, factor Xa can bind to a phospholipid membrane surface, where it can cleave peptides from the prothrombin molecule (factor II) in the presence of calcium ions to generate thrombin. Factor V (proaccelerin) is necessary in this reaction as well, and it is the next clotting protein involved in the common pathway.

Efforts both to purify and to characterize factor V have been hampered by its inherent instability and lability. With a molecular weight of approximately 300,000 d, this glycoprotein participates in prothrombin activation as a catalyst of factor Xa activity, possibly by increasing the affinities of both factor Xa and prothrombin for the phospholipid template where thrombin eventually is generated.[14]

Prothrombin (factor II) is a single-chain glycoprotein with a molecular weight of 70,000 d. When activated, the prothrombin molecule undergoes proteolytic cleavage at two sites, yielding a two-chain molecule that is linked by a disulfide bond; this new product is thrombin. Although factor Xa alone can convert prothrombin to thrombin, the participation of phospholipid and calcium ions in the presence of factor V increases 100-fold both the rate and the efficiency of thrombin formation.[15] This requirement for phospholipid may be instrumental in concentrating subsequent thrombin generation at sites where phospholipid from injured endothelial cells and adherent platelets will be available.

Thrombin, the two-chain derivative of the prothrombin molecule, has a molecular weight of approximately 37,000 d, and its proteolytic properties induce the conversion of fibrinogen to fibrin to produce the initial visible manifestation of coagulation: the soluble fibrin clot. In addition, thrombin influences the activities of factors V, VIII, XIII, and plasmin. When complexed with its specific endothelial receptor thrombomodulin, thrombin activates protein C, which in the presence of its cofactor (free protein S) inactivates factors Va and VIIIa and thus impedes further thrombin generation. Thrombin complexed to thrombomodulin loses its ability to cleave the fibrinopeptides A and B from fibrinogen to produce fibrin, and thrombin also affects platelet function by inducing viscous metamorphosis as well as the release reaction with subsequent aggregation.

Fibrinogen (factor I) is the primary target of the proteolytic activity of thrombin. Its molecular weight is 340,000 d, and its concentration in plasma is 300 mg/dl, which is greater than any other protein involved in the coagulation pathway. Fibrinogen is a dimeric glycoprotein consisting of three pairs of nonidentical chains (A/α, B/β, and γ) that are held together by disulfide bonds; the letters *A* and *B* represent the peptides located on the central amino terminal ends of the α and β chains, respectively. These peptides are cleaved specifically by thrombin at arginine–glycine bonds to produce the gelatinous clot of soluble fibrin monomers (Figs. 18.1 and 18.3) and are designated *fibrinopeptides A and B*.

The final phase of the coagulation cascade is the stabilization and cross-linking of soluble fibrin monomers and polymers, and this is accomplished by factor XIII, fibrin stabilizing factor (Figs. 18.1 and 18.3), which is synthesized primarily in the liver and megakaryocyte. Factor XIII circulates as a proenzyme that is composed of two pairs of different polypeptide chains, designated *a* and *b*. Intact factor XIII possesses a molecular weight of approximately 300,000 d and is converted to its active transglutaminase form in the presence of both calcium ions and thrombin. Factor XIIIa catalyzes an irreversible amide-exchange reaction between the γ-glutamine and ε-lysine side chains of adjacent fibrin monomers, which results in cross-linking between γ and γ-chains, γ and α-chains, and α and α-chains of fibrin. This strengthens the clot structure and renders it insoluble in 5M urea or monochloracetic acid.

Both fibrinogen and fibrin serve as physiologic targets of plasmin, the fibrin(ogen)olytic enzyme that is derived from plasminogen (Fig. 18.2). Complete degradation of fibrinogen and fibrin proceeds through three stages. Stage 1 plasmic digests contain fragment X, formed by cleaving a small portion of the carboxyterminal end of the A/α-chain. Fibrinopeptide B is removed from fibrinogen during this stage of digestion, but this reaction does not pertain to fibrin that previously has lost both fibrinopeptides through interaction with thrombin. Fibrinogen fragment X is the only fibrinogen degradation product that retains its coagulability on addition of thrombin. Stage 2 involves the asymmetric cleavage of fragment X to form one mole each of fragment D and fragment Y, and during stage 3, fragment Y is digested further to yield another mole of fragment D and one of fragment E. The plasmic degradation products of crossed-linked fibrin (i.e., after factor XIIIa cross-links γ-chains of adjacent fibrin monomers) can be distinguished from those of fibrinogen by the presence of the D-dimer, which is derived from the cross-linked γ–γ-chains of fibrin. Both the D and E plasmic degradation fragments of noncross-linked fibrin essentially appear to be identical to those derived from fibrinogen; however, plasmic degradation of noncross-linked fibrin yields a B/β 15–42 fragment from the B/β-chain in contrast to a B/β 1–42 fragment cleaved from fibrinogen. This difference reflects the action of thrombin on the intact fibrinogen molecule that results in the release of a B/β 1–14 fragment from the β-chain.

The physiologic functions of the degradation products remain speculative, but in vitro evidence indicates that products of fibrinogen proteolysis interfere with fibrin monomer polymerization as well as the release of fibrinopeptides from fibrinogen by thrombin.[16,17] In addition, both fibrin and fibrinogen degradation products inhibit

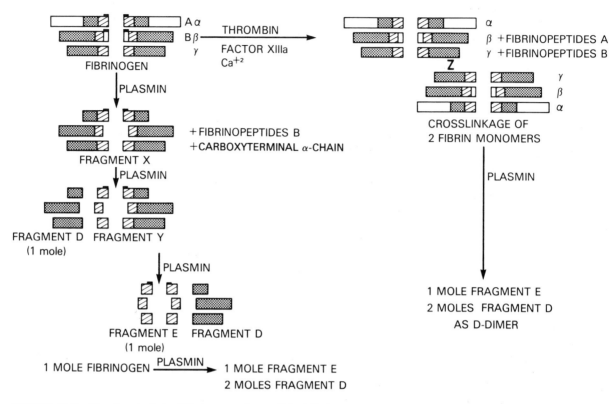

FIGURE 18.3.   The plasminolysis of fibrinogen and cross-linked fibrin.

platelet adhesiveness and aggregation.[18] Data also suggest that fibrinogen synthesis is stimulated significantly by stage 3 digestion products of fibrinogen plasminolysis.[19]

By counterbalancing the effects of blood coagulation, the mechanism of fibrinolysis homeostatically maintains the lumen patency of blood vessels in the event of thrombus formation. Lysis of the fibrin clot depends on the hydrolytic properties of plasmin, a nonspecific proteolytic enzyme generated from activation of the proenzyme plasminogen; naturally occurring activators of this enzyme reaction are present in the plasma and vascular endothelium. They also can be prepared for therapeutic purposes by recombinant DNA techniques (tissue-type plasminogen activator and single-chain urokinase), ex vivo embryonic renal parenchymal cell cultures (two-chain urokinase), and purification from in vitro bacterial sources (streptokinase). Factor XIIa and prekallikrein (Fletcher factor) are involved as well in plasminogen activation in vitro, but their physiologic importance in vivo remains unclear. The plasminogen activators are adsorbed onto the fibrin clot with varying degrees of specificity, and they penetrate into its mesh in a manner that allows the generated plasmin to remain inaccessible to rapidly neutralizing inhibitors. The most efficient and specific inhibitor of plasmin is α_2-antiplasmin, which is pivotal in the regulation of both physiologic and pharmacologically induced fibrinolysis. In addition, fibrinolysis may be modulated by the actions of plasminogen activator inhibitors 1 (from endothelial cells and platelets) and 2 (from human placenta and macrophages); plasminogen activator inhibitor is the most efficient inhibitor of tissue plasminogen activator. The integrin thrombospondin and histidine-rich glycoprotein play an uncertain role in the regulation of fibrinolysis in vivo, and in addition to fibrinogen and fibrin, plasmin hydrolyzes a number of other plasma proteins, including clotting factors V, VIII:C and von Willebrand factor protein, factor XII, and the first component of complement.

Coagulation factors II, VII, IX, X, and XI as well as factor XIIa fragments, thrombin, and plasmin are classified as serine proteases, because each possesses a serine residue at its enzymatically active site. The physiologic activities of these serine proteases are modulated by endogenous circulating proteinase inhibitors that probably form irreversible covalent complexes with the proteases and secondarily prevent participation of the active serine sites in enzymatic reactions. The natural protease inhibitors include C1-esterase inhibitor, α_1-antitrypsin, α_1-antichymotrypsin, inter-α-trypsin inhibitor, α_2-antiplasmin, α_2-macroglobulin, and antithrombin III; the last three are considered the most important. The influence of heparin on antithrombin III function is discussed elsewhere.

Factors II, VII, IX, and X as well as proteins C, S, and Z are vitamin K–dependent proteins that are synthesized in the liver along with fibrinogen, factor V, factor VIII, and probably factors XI and XIII. Vitamin K–dependent clotting factors are nonfunctional in the presence of vitamin K antagonists, such as the coumarin anticoagulants, and these agents block the vitamin K–dependent formation of γ-carboxylated glutamic acid residues on the amino terminal ends of the molecule. This residue normally binds calcium ions which in turn link the clotting factors to a phospholipid template for activation. Vitamin K deficiency is difficult to achieve by dietary restriction alone; however, in combination with malabsorption and/or antibiotic destruction of the intestinal flora that normally synthesize vitamin K_2, decreased intake assumes an important role.

LABORATORY EVALUATION OF COAGULATION

Laboratory assessment of coagulation should complement a complete history and physical examination. Special attention should be focused on the family history.

The majority of coagulation tests performed in vitro depend on either the visual or mechanical detection of a fibrin clot; this end point requires an adequate amount of normally functioning fibrinogen. An insensitive but useful bedside screening test for assessing clotting function is the whole-blood clotting time, usually performed according to Lee and White.[20] An abnormally prolonged clotting time reflects either a severe deficiency of the coagulation factors involved in the intrinsic and common pathways or the presence of heparin or acquired endogenous circulating anticoagulants. Marked thrombocytopenia and deficiencies of factors VII and XIII usually do not affect the test.

The nonactivated partial thromboplastin time (PTT) monitors the activity of factors in the intrinsic and common pathways, and abnormal results usually indicate a reduction of clotting factor function to below 15% to 20% of normal. In addition, the partial thromboplastin time (nonactivated) is prolonged by heparin or pathologically induced circulating inhibitors directed toward components of the intrinsic or common systems. The test is insensitive to platelet function and deficiencies in factors VII and XIII. The activated partial

thromboplastin time (APTT) is a modification of the partial thromboplastin time (nonactivated) in which artificial reagents, such as kaolin or ellagic acid, are employed to activate rapidly the intrinsic system.

The prothrombin time measures coagulation factor activity in the extrinsic and common pathways. It reflects the activity of the vitamin K–dependent factors VII, X, and II, but not factor IX as the intrinsic pathway is bypassed in this instance. (The B^m or B^+ variant of factor IX deficiency is associated with a prolonged prothrombin time.[21]) The prothrombin time may be prolonged slightly by the anticoagulant action of heparin, and it is affected significantly by the coumarin anticoagulants.

The thrombin time measures the rate required to form a fibrin clot from fibrinogen after exogenous thrombin is added to plasma. The test is prolonged by fibrinogen levels depressed below 20–30 mg/dl, dysfibrinogenemias, and substances that exhibit antithrombin activity. (These substances include heparin, fibrinogen–fibrin degradation products, and circulating anticoagulants.) The activity of other clotting factors do not affect the thrombin time.

Specific in vitro assays have been developed for each of the coagulation factors. Many of these techniques are based on the ability of the test plasma to correct the clotting abnormality of the substrate plasma, which is selectively deficient in the factor being evaluated. The substrate plasma often is obtained from patients with documented congenital deficiencies, and specific immunologic assays of the coagulation factors have been added to the diagnostic armamentarium as well.

The thromboplastin generation test involves a complex procedure to confirm the existence of a coagulation defect; however, the abnormality may not be localized specifically. This test has no advantage over the others described and seldom is used.

Division of the coagulation process into the intrinsic, extrinsic, and common pathways is artificial, but it does provide a useful approach to the definitive diagnosis of coagulation disorders. A prolonged activated partial thromboplastin time associated with a normal prothrombin time localizes the coagulation defect to the intrinsic pathway and factors VIII, IX, XI, XII, which together comprise more than 95% of all hereditary coagulopathies. Multiple deficiencies of intrinsic system factors may prolong the activated partial thromboplastin time to a significantly greater degree than any single factor deficiency. Deficiencies of prekallikrein (Fletcher factor), high-molecular-weight kininogen (Fitzgerald, Williams, Flaujeac, Warren, and Reid factors), as well as Passovoy factor also prolong the activated partial thromboplastin time, and these newly described coagulation factors participate at various points in the intrinsic pathway. Bleeding disorders that are characterized by prolongation of both the activated partial thromboplastin time and prothrombin time indicate deficiencies in the common pathway (factors I, II, V, or X); these abnormalities are identified individually by specific factor assays. Isolated factor VII deficiency is reflected in a normal partial thromboplastin time (nonactivated) and activated partial thromboplastin time but a prolonged prothrombin time. When the prothrombin time, activated partial thromboplastin time, thrombin time, and fibrinogen concentrations are normal in a patient with a history of bleeding, factor XIII deficiency must be considered, but the activity of this factor is not detected by other screening tests and requires its own specific assay. Variants of von Willebrand disease and mild factor XI deficiency rarely are associated with normal activated partial thromboplastin time and may fall into this laboratory category as well; however, specific factor procoagulant and antigen assays can confirm their presence.

Plasma samples associated with abnormalities in the screening tests of coagulation function may contain circulating anticoagulants. Abnormalities caused by clotting factor deficiencies characteristically are corrected by the addition of normal plasma to the test plasma; however, when plasma containing circulating inhibitors is added to normal plasma, abnormal coagulation studies persist. Often, these changes become more obvious following the incubation of normal plasma with that containing the inhibitors at 37°C for 1 hour or when progressively diluting the inhibitor plasma.

COAGULATION DISORDERS

Factor I

Hereditary afibrinogenemia (deficiency of fibrinogen) is an extremely rare, autosomal recessive disorder that is associated with a high degree of consanguinity. Its clinical features usually are manifested at birth, with persistent hemorrhage from the umbilical cord and/or circumcision site; thereafter, affected individuals may experience easy bruising, epistaxis, gingival bleeding, and excessive abnormal hemorrhage following trauma or surgery. Defective healing of wounds, abnormal scar formation, and increased frequency of spontaneous first-trimester abortions also have been reported, but hemarthroses and menstrual difficulty are rare.

Laboratory findings include a decreased rate of sedimentation and a prolonged bleeding time. Because the routine screening coagulation tests (prothrombin time, activated partial thromboplastin time, and thrombin time) depend on the presence of fibrinogen to form the fibrin clot, these tests are all strikingly abnormal in this disorder. Although fibrinogen cannot be detected in this disorder with assays that measure clottable protein, no trace amounts may be identified in affected plasmas that are subjected to immunoelectrophoresis. This suggests that the basic defect in this disorder is one of impaired or inadequate hepatic synthesis or failure to release fibrinogen from the hepatocyte. Platelet dysfunction has been observed and is attributed to the absence of fibrinogen to interact with platelet membrane glycoproteins, and anecdotal reports indicate that the intravenous administration of desmopressin may correct the abnormally prolonged bleeding time and the platelet aggregation defects observed in association with afibrinogenemia.

Occasionally, individuals are hypofibrinogenemic, with fibrinogen levels always less than 100 mg/dl. This usually is adequate to produce normal coagulation measurements and few clinical symptoms, and these patients may represent heterozygotes of afibrinogenemia parents or may have dysfibrinogenemia or hypodysfibrinogenemia.

Treatment of afibrinogenemia may be indicated prophylactically before and during surgical procedures and therapeutically to terminate episodes of persistent hemorrhage. This can be achieved by infusions of fresh-frozen plasma or cryoprecipitate that is enriched with fibrinogen; the use of fibrinogen concentrates has been associated with an unacceptable risk of hepatitis. Fibrinogen infused into afibrinogenemic individuals has a normal circulating half-life.

Recent epidemiologic observations have suggested that elevated plasma fibrinogen concentrations may predispose individuals to coronary artery disease, perhaps in conjunction with increased factor VII levels. Further observations are necessary to confirm this association as well as to establish a firm cause-and-effect relationship.

Hereditary dysfibrinogenemias usually are inherited in an autosomal dominant manner. Approximately 120 abnormal fibrinogens have been described. However, the molecular lesions in most of these qualitatively defective fibrinogens have not been identified, so it is possible some redundancy in their designations may exist. Specific structural abnormalities have been demonstrated in a minority of the dysfibrinogenemias. Usually, the localization of the molecular defect has explained the biochemical abnormality of the dysfibrinogenemia, so that defects in the amino terminal portion of the A/α-chain may lead to aberrant thrombin cleavage (fibrinogen Detroit) and that γ-chain mutations may produce defective fibrin polymerization and cross-linking (fibrinogens Baltimore I and Paris I). The majority of dysfibrinogenemias produce asymptomatic clinical courses and are discovered fortuitously; others have been associated with abnormal bleeding (fibrinogens Bethesda I, Giessen I, Detroit, etc.), increased thrombotic complications (fibrinogens Baltimore I, Nancy, etc.), defective wound healing and dehiscence (fibrinogens Paris I, Cleveland I, etc.), and recurrent spontaneous abortions (fibrinogens Bethesda III, Metz, Marburg, etc.).

Acquired dysfibrinogenemias have been reported in association with severe liver disease. In particular, they have been associated with hepatomas, hepatitis, and metastatic carcinomas.

Many of the dysfibrinogenemias can be detected in the laboratory, because their defective fibrinopeptide release by thrombin, their abnormal fibrin monomer polymerization, and their ineffectively cross-linked fibrin polymers often produce abnormally prolonged prothrombin times, activated partial thromboplastin times, and thrombin times. In addition, plasma fibrinogen concentrations determined chronometrically (time-dependent thrombin generation of fibrin) may be decreased, while levels of fibrinogen/fibrin degradation products may be increased. Fibrinogen concentrations determined as either thrombin-clottable or immunologically recognizable protein usually are much greater than the chronometrically determined levels. Purified procoagulant enzymes derived from snake venoms (e.g., reptilase and ancrod) can be substituted for thrombin in the thrombin time assay and provide information concerning fibrinopeptide release from abnormal fibrinogens. Dysfibrinogens also may be analyzed for their carbohydrate content (particularly sialic acid) and their structure on polyacrylamide gel electrophoresis, but these techniques provide variable results and do not help to identify specifically the molecular defect.

Experience with replacement therapy in patients with dysfibrinogenemia is limited by dysfibrinogenemia's rare occurrence and the relative lack of associated symptomatology. If therapy is required, fresh-frozen plasma and cryoprecipitate are the preferred sources of fibrinogen, and rarely, replacement therapy may be complicated by thrombotic episodes.

Factor II

Inherited in an autosomal recessive fashion, hypoprothrombinemia (deficiency of prothrombin) is the rarest of the hereditary coagulation disorders. Clinical bleeding is mild. Congenital dysprothrombinemias also have been reported, and several have been characterized by reduced (15% to 50% of normal) biologic prothrombin activity but normal immunologic activity.

Acquired hypoprothrombinemia may accompany defective vitamin K absorption or utilization. This is observed in liver disease, malabsorption of the fat-soluble vitamins, and administration of the oral anticoagulants of coumarin derivatives.

Prolonged prothrombin time, activated partial thromboplastin time, and variable clotting times are noted in laboratory specimens that are deficient in factor II. Bleeding times usually are normal, and a two-stage prothrombin assay is necessary to confirm hypoprothrombinemia.

When replacement therapy is needed in hypoprothrombinemia, fresh-frozen plasma or purified prothrombin-complex concentrates can be used; the latter is associated with a high incidence of hepatitis and may be thrombogenic, particularly when administered to patients with pre-existing hepatic dysfunction.

Factor III and Factor IV

No reported congenital or acquired coagulopathies have been produced by deficiencies of factors III (thromboplastin) or IV (calcium). Thromboplastin is ubiquitous to most body tissues, and calcium ions are required only in trace amounts for coagulation. Before levels of this decreased cation could fall low enough to affect coagulation, other calcium-dependent body functions (myocardium) would fail, and death would ensue.

Factor V

Hereditary proaccelerin deficiency is a rare, autosomal recessive coagulopathy that occasionally is associated with other congenital defects. Homozygous individuals possess factor V levels that are 9% to 10% of normal, and they demonstrate variable degrees of bleeding tendencies that may correlate with the level of factor V in the individual's platelets. Several instances of fatal hemorrhage resulting from tooth extractions as well as menses have been reported. Hemarthroses almost never occur, and because Factor V is involved in the common pathway of clotting, its deficiency produces an abnormal activated partial thromboplastin time and prothrombin time. Unexplainably, the bleeding time is prolonged in some affected individuals.

Heterozygous individuals generally have adequate levels of factor V to remain asymptomatic. Combined deficiencies of factors V and VIII have been identified more frequently than would be expected by chance alone, and deficiencies of factor V may be acquired during disseminated intravascular coagulation.

Replacement therapy in factor V deficiency (excluding disseminated intravascular coagulation) requires fresh-frozen plasma; the characteristic lability and short plasma half-life (12 to 36 hours) of factor V lead to a rapid loss of proaccelerin activity in stored plasma. Transfusions of normal platelets, which have factor V absorbed to their membranes, also have been used as replacement therapy.

Factor VII

Factor VII (serum prothrombin conversion accelerator, proconvertin) deficiency is an uncommon autosomal recessive coagulopathy that is associated with abnormal bleeding and thrombotic tendencies. Homozygous individuals usually have less than 10% of normal factor VII activity and experience mild to severe symptoms, including hemarthroses; heterozygous individuals demonstrate decreased factor VII levels but are asymptomatic. Deep venous thrombosis and pulmonary emboli have been reported in several affected individuals, and in addition, there is a high frequency of factor VII deficiency in patients with Dubin-Johnson syndrome.[22] Acquired factor VII deficiency is seen in newborn babies, during anticoagulation therapy with vitamin K antagonists, in hepatic disease, and with vitamin K depletion.

Factor VII deficiency affects only the extrinsic clotting system and is reflected by a prolonged prothrombin time with normal activated partial thromboplastin time and thrombin time. Immunologic detection of factor VII antigen has been described in several patients with absent biologic activity, and replacement therapy can be accomplished by the infusion of stored plasma. Factor VII also is contained in the first generation prothrombin-complex concentrates but may be absent from new formulations.

Factor VIII

Factor VIII (antihemophilic factor, antihemophilic globulin) deficiency (classic hemophilia or hemophilia A) is inherited as a sex-linked recessive disorder and is probably the second most-common severe congenital coagulopathy. Hemorrhagic complications may become obvious shortly after birth with circumcision and then increase in both severity and frequency with age and activity. The severity of bleeding symptoms appears to be related to the degree of factor VIII:C deficiency; severely affected individuals (factor VIII:C procoagulant activity lower than 1% of normal) experience repeated and often spontaneous hemorrhagic episodes, most commonly hemarthroses. Repeated involvement of the joints ultimately produces crippling deformities and arthritides that may require surgical intervention for synovectomy or joint replacement. The knees are involved most frequently, followed by the elbows, ankles, and less commonly, the wrists, shoulders, and hips. Other hemorrhagic manifestations of severe hemophilia A include bleeding into the subcutaneous and intramuscular compartments, hematuria, epistaxis, intracranial bleeding, gingival bleeding, hematemesis, and melena; these may occur either spontaneously or following minimal trauma.

Soft tissue hemorrhage into closed spaces may compromise the sensory or motor function of nerves, dissect along fascial planes to compress vital structures (i.e., trachea, intestines), or form blood-filled loculations (pseudotumors) that may increase gradually in size and subsequently destroy the adjacent soft tissue and bone. Retroperitoneal hemorrhage may mimic acute appendicitis or other causes of an acute abdomen, and hematuria is not uncommon, is usually microscopic and asymptomatic, and resolves spontaneously without treatment. Occasionally, gastrointestinal bleeding occurs but this should not be attributed to the coagulopathy until the presence of pathologic lesions has been discounted. Intracranial hemorrhage is associated with high mortality and requires both prompt diagnosis and aggressive treatment.

Hemophiliacs with slightly less-severe deficiencies of factor VIII:C activity (1% to 5% of normal) or mild deficiencies (6% to 60% of normal) rarely experience spontaneous hemorrhagic episodes, but these individuals may become symptomatic following trauma or surgery. The degree of factor VIII activity deficiency remains constant throughout the life of the affected individual.

The presence of hemophilia A is determined by a prolonged activated partial thromboplastin time unless the factor VIII level is more than 20% to 30% of normal. Whole blood clotting times are usually abnormal; however, prothrombin time, bleeding times, and thrombin time are normal. Specific assay for factor VIII procoagulant activity indicates a significant reduction in level, and the factor VIII–related antigen (as detected immunologically with heterologous antibody) is normal. Detection of female carriers related to patients with hemophilia is based on obtaining factor VIII activity measurements that are of intermediate to normal values and match values observed in the proband. A ratio of procoagulant activity to factor VIII antigen level less than 0.75 suggests the carrier state in family members of a patient with congenital deficiency. The detection of restriction fragment length polymorphisms has increased the sensitivity of carrier-state determinations in both obligate and nonobligate carriers, particularly when the restriction fragment length polymorphism pattern matches that observed in a male relative who is affected. Although hemophilia A can occur in female children of a female carrier and affected male, in females with Turner syndrome, or in females with a high degree of lyonization and X mosaicism, this is an exceedingly unusual event. The diagnosis of hemophilia A in a female requires the exclusion of von Willebrand disease, a coagulopathy transmitted most frequently in an autosomal dominant manner.

The adequacy and promptness of replacement therapy in hemophilia A determine the subsequent morbidity and mortality of this disorder. For the majority of superficial soft tissues and hemarthroses, factor VIII levels should be raised to between 25% to 30% of normal; this can be accomplished with cryoprecipitate or factor VIII concentrates. Alternatively, the infusion of desmopressin at a dose of 0.3 μg/kg in individuals with moderate or mild hemophilia A usually will raise and sustain the factor VIII activity at adequate levels, thus obviating blood-derived products. When factor VIII activity levels between 30% and 50% are required, as in major soft tissue or visceral bleeds and in minor surgical procedures, cryoprecipitate or factor VIII concentrates should be used unless desmopressin has been shown previously to achieve adequate factor VIII levels in individuals who are either moderately or mildly affected. For major surgery as well as documented or clinically suspected central nervous system hemorrhage, factor VIII activities of 80% to 100% are considered adequate; however, because of the great risks of intracerebral bleeding, replacement to concentrations of at least 100% should be attempted, which is achieved most promptly and efficiently with factor VIII concentrates. One unit of factor VIII replacement per kilogram should raise the plasma factor VIII activity level by 2% (0.02 unit/ml plasma); repeat dosing should be calculated on an 8 to 12 hour circulating half-life for factor VIII.

Individuals with hemophilia are obligate recipients of blood products containing their deficient clotting factor to maintain both the quality and length of their lives; as such, they have been exposed to numerous pathogenic blood-borne viruses. Virtually all individuals with severe hemophilia have evidence of serum antibodies against hepatitis surface antigen and non-A, non-B hepatitis, and 60% to 90% have antibodies against the human immunodeficiency virus as well. In addition, approximately 7%–25% of all those with hemophilia in the United States have had the diagnosis of acquired immunodeficiency syndrome (AIDS) confirmed. Fortunately, all of the factor VIII concentrate preparations currently available employ viral attenuation or elimination techniques that render the products virtually hepatitis- and human immunodeficiency virus (HIV)-free. No individual with hemophilia born after 1986 should experience these problems.

Circulating inhibitors to factor VIII may develop in approximately 10% of those with hemophilia who are exposed over long periods to factor VIII replacement. The effects of inhibitors present in low titers (less than 5 Bethesda units) usually can be overcome by infusions of factor VIII concentrate in large doses. For the high responders, with greater than 10 Bethesda units of inhibitor, porcine factor VIII and the nonactivated or activated prothrombin complex concentrates should be used; in desperate situations, extracorporeal circulation of the patient's plasma over columns employing sepharose coated with staphlococcal protein A has been attempted, with variable success, to remove the IgG antibody functioning as the inhibitor. Interestingly, HIV-seropositive individuals occasionally may lose their inhibitors spontaneously over time.

Von Willebrand Disease

Von Willebrand disease usually is inherited as an autosomal dominant disorder with variable penetrance. It probably is the most common of the congenital coagulopathies, with a prevalence estimated to be as high as 0.4% to 1.0% of the general population. A particularly severe form of this disease may be transmitted as an autosomal recessive abnormality; however, the prevalence in this case is considerably rarer. Typically, von Willebrand disease is characterized by epistaxis as well as mucosal and gastrointestinal hemorrhage, which occasionally may be exacerbated by the concomitant presence of angiodysplasia and hereditary hemorrhagic telangiectasia (Osler-Weber-Rendu syndrome), and spontaneous hemarthroses are rare except in the most severe forms. The diagnosis classically is established in males and females who exhibit prolonged bleeding times, abnormal ristocetin cofactor assays, defective ristocetin-induced platelet agglutination, reduced concentrations of von Willebrand factor protein antigen ($_v$Wf:Ag), and mild to moderate deficiencies in factor VIII coagulant activity (VIII:c) that also prolongs the activated partial thromboplastin time. Results of the screening assays to establish the diagnosis of von Willebrand disease may be normal at times in the same patient, and the assays should be repeated on multiple occasions before excluding the diagnosis in individuals whose clinical symptomatology is otherwise consistent.

Numerous subtypes or variants of von Willebrand disease have been described, based on the examination of the multimeric composition of the von Willebrand antigen by agarose gel electrophoresis of patient plasma samples. Whereas classic von Willebrand disease involves the diminished biosynthesis of the von Willebrand factor protein by endothelial cells and megakaryocytes, the variants of this disease result from the abnormal biosynthesis or processing of the von Willebrand factor protein so that the highest-molecular-weight multimer subunits are either absent or reduced. The most common of these variants is designated *type IIA,* in which both the largest and intermediate multimers of von Willebrand factor protein are missing, and *type IIB,* in which the largest multimers are absent. Furthermore, these variants may be suspected when discordance exists between the normal or slightly decreased levels of von Willebrand antigen and the more markedly decreased levels of von Willebrand factor activity. Type IIB von Willebrand disease variant is characterized by hyperresponsiveness to low concentrations of ristocetin in the ristocetin-induced platelet agglutination assay. An additional variant of von Willebrand disease, the so-called *pseudo* or *platelet type* von Willebrand disease, has a multimeric composition indistinguishable from type IIB, but its pathophysiology is due to the increased binding affinity of these multimers to the patient's platelets (the GP1b receptor site is abnormal in platelets) rather than to the synthesis of an intrinsically abnormal von Willebrand factor protein.

The goal of treatment is to normalize the bleeding time, factor VIII coagulant activity, and von Willebrand factor activity (ristocetin cofactor assay). The degree of abnormality in these assays, however, may not correlate with the clinical severity, thus indicating that both the amount and intactness of von Willebrand factor protein either contained in and released from the platelets may influence the character of the disease. Cryoprecipitate has been the mainstay of replacement therapy in von Willebrand disease, because it contains high concentrations of von Willebrand factor protein with the normal complement of molecular weight multimers. The amount to be infused is determined empirically, and infusions of either normal or hemophilic plasma or cryoprecipitate produce significantly higher and longer-lasting levels of factor VIII coagulant activity than would be predicted from the amount of factor VIII activity administered. Unfortunately, use of cryoprecipitate is complicated by the potential transmission of blood-borne viruses; thus, in some patients, use of specific viral attenuated factor VIII concentrates that contain high levels of ristocetin cofactor activity and/or multimerically intact von Willebrand factor protein should be considered. Desmopressin can be used intravenously at a dose of 0.3 µg/kg in patients with both moderately and mildly severe von Willebrand disease with few side effects, and repeat administration is based on the circulating survival times of the corrected laboratory parameters as well as the clinical response to treatment. Patients should be pretested with this agent before major surgery to determine the adequacy of response; some may develop tachyphylaxis with re-peated use. Desmopressin response in patients with type IIA disease varies, and the use of desmopressin in type IIB disease is contraindicated as it may induce spontaneous intravascular platelet aggregation with subsequent significant thrombocytopenia. Acute angina and thromboembolic phenomena rarely have been reported with its use. Because desmopressin stimulates the release of tissue plasminogen activator from the endothelial cell, the concomitant use of antifibrinolytic agents (e.g., ϵ-aminocaproic acid or tranexamic acid) is recommended for dental extractions or surgical procedures on mucous membranes.

Acquired von Willebrand disease[23] has been attributed most commonly to underlying autoimmune or lymphoproliferative diseases, and it may be associated with either circulating inhibitors or the increased adsorption of the von Willebrand factor protein to the surface of malignant lymphocytes. Some patients with myeloproliferative disorders also may have laboratory and clinical evidence of acquired von Willebrand disease that results from the excessive proteolytic degradation of otherwise normal von Willebrand factor protein.

A sixth type of this disease process designated von Willebrand Normandy has recently been described. In this type of the disease the von Willebrand protein does not properly bind VIII:c resulting in reduced levels of Factor VIII:c.

Factor IX

Congenital deficiency of factor IX (plasma thromboplastin component, Christmas factor) is termed *Christmas disease* or *hemophilia B*. It is both clinically and genetically similar to hemophilia A but occurs less frequently. Homozygous females are rare, but symptoms may occur in females with X-chromosome abnormalities such as Turner syndrome (XO). Combined deficiencies of factor VIII and IX have been described as well. Hemophilia B appears to be a heterogenous group of disorders, with the most common type characterized by depressed levels of factor IX coagulant activity and normal factor IX antigen as detected by specific heterologous antibodies; factor IX deficiency with absence of the factor IX antigen is associated with milder symptoms. Numerous genetic variants of hemophilia B have been described, and one, designated *hemophila B^m*, accounts for up to 15% of all hemophilia B cases and consists of an abnormal factor IX acting as a competitive inhibitor of factor VII.[21] Plasma from patients with hemophilia B^m manifests a prolonged activated partial thromboplastin time and prothrombin time (using bovine brain as a source of thromboplastin) despite normal levels of all coagulation factors except factor IX.

Factor IX levels in homozygous hemophilia B usually are not as depressed as levels in hemophilia A, and activity lower than 1% of normal is uncommon. Carriers for hemophilia B are detected by their intermediate depressions of factor IX activity, but much more accurate results have been obtained by using DNA probes and restriction fragment length polymorphism analysis on specimens from patients known to be affected and from both obligate and suspected carriers as well as on chorionic villous sampling specimens of the fetus. Laboratory diagnosis for hemophilia B is characterized by a prolonged activated partial thromboplastin time but normal prothrombin time and thrombin time. Bleeding times usually also are normal. Specific factor IX assays reveal the deficiency.

Treatment of hemophilia B is approached similarly to that for hemophilia A. Replacement is achieved both promptly and efficiently with fresh-frozen plasma or nonactivated or activated prothrombin complex concentrates, which contain all of the vitamin K–dependent clotting factors (including factor IX). One unit/kg of factor IX should raise the circulating plasma activity of factor IX by 1%/ml plasma; the repeated dosing is based on the circulating survival time of factor IX of 18 to 24 hours. Unfortunately, the currently available factor IX–replacement products appear to have varying potentials to transmit both hepatitis B and non-A, non-B hepatitis. All products have been heat-treated, so the risk of transmitting HIV virtually has been eliminated. Furthermore, the prothrombin complex concentrates may be thrombogenic when administered frequently, and future availability of highly purified and more effectively viral-attenuated factor IX products will prevent both of these toxicities. Factor IX is not present in cryoprecipitate and cannot be induced in vivo by infusions of desmopressin. Circulating inhibitors also may appear but are rare.

Acquired factor IX deficiency occasionally occurs with hepatic disease, administration of coumarin anticoagulants, and nephrotic syndrome with proteinuria of greater than 10 g/day. Combined factor IX and X deficiencies have been reported in amyloidosis, and factor IX inhibitors have been observed in association with autoimmune diseases.[24]

Factor X

Congenital factor X (Stuart-Prower factor) deficiency is a rare, autosomal recessive disorder and clinically resembles factor VII deficiency. Several variants have been described, based on either the presence or absence of factor X antigen as detected by a specific heterolo-gous antibody. Acquired factor X deficiency occurs with vitamin K deficiency, hepatic disease, coumarin ingestion, and amyloidosis.[24,25] Laboratory tests yield prolonged prothrombin time and activated partial thromboplastin time as well as normal thrombin time and bleeding time, and specific factor X assay using Russell viper venom confirms the deficiency.

Factor XI

Factor XI (plasma thromboplastin antecedent) deficiency is a rare hereditary coagulopathy that reportedly is transmitted both as an autosomal dominant and autosomal recessive trait. The disease occurs predominantly in Jews, and the severity is variable and often remains asymptomatic until major trauma or surgery is encountered. Spontaneous hemorrhage and hemarthroses are rare; however, when bleeding does occur, its severity is unrelated to levels of factor XI.

Laboratory workup reveals prolonged activated partial thromboplastin time and whole blood clotting time. The prothrombin time is normal, and the bleeding time is rarely prolonged. The specific assay for factor XI and the activated partial thromboplastin time should be performed on fresh plasma collected in silicone-treated glassware, because factor XI is activated slightly by glass and by freezing. Replacement therapy can be accomplished with plasma infusions.

Factor XII

Factor XII (Hageman factor) deficiency usually is inherited as an autosomal recessive trait. It rarely is associated with hemorrhagic complications, but mild bleeding and easy bruising have been described in a few cases of severe deficiency. Affected individuals appear to have an increased tendency toward thromboembolic complications. The original proband (Mr. Hageman) expired following deep leg-vein thrombosis and massive pulmonary emboli; this may represent the incomplete or diminished intrinsic activation of plasminogen to plasmin by factor XII. Other investigators have suggested that factor XII inhibits platelet aggregation and that its deficiency promotes thrombogenesis through this mechanism.[26]

As with deficiencies of factors VIII, IX, and XI, Hageman factor deficiency is associated with a prolonged activated partial thromboplastin time and normal prothrombin time and thrombin time. Whole blood clotting times performed in glass also are prolonged, and although it was prolonged in the original proband, the bleeding time usually is normal. Specific assays for factor XII coagulation activity, using established factor-deficient plasma, indicate levels significantly below normal. No factor XII antigen has been demonstrated in patients affected.

Theoretically, replacement therapy is unnecessary, because clinical bleeding is rare. Nevertheless, some hematologists recommend prophylactic infusions of plasma for patients with factor XII deficiency before surgery or following trauma.

Factor XIII

Congenital factor XIII (fibrin stabilizing factor) deficiency is inherited as an autosomal recessive trait and, in most cases, becomes clinically apparent at birth with persistent umbilical bleeding. Easy bruising and hematoma formation are prominent in patients with this deficiency, but spontaneous hemorrhage, mucous membrane bleeding, and hemarthroses are rare. Wound healing is defective, and dehiscence is common. In addition, multiple spontaneous abortions have been observed in affected females.

This diagnosis should be suspected when clinical bleeding occurs in conjunction with normal screening tests of coagulations (e.g., prothrombin time, activated partial thromboplastin time, thrombin time, bleeding time, whole blood clotting time, clot retraction, and specific assays for clotting factors). In each test, the final fibrin clot appears friable and is soluble in 5M urea or 1% monochloroacetic acid. Only 1% factor XIII activity is necessary to cross-link normally fibrin clots and to render fibrin insoluble. Replacement therapy is achieved with the administration of minimal quantities of plasma; the half-life of transfused factor XIII ranges from 95 to 125 hours.

Fletcher Factor; Fitzgerald, Flaujeac, Williams, Warren, Reid Factor; Passovoy Factor

Deficiencies of Fletcher factor (prekallikrein); Fitzgerald, Flaujeac, Williams, Warren, and Reid factor (high-molecular-weight kininogen); and Passovoy factor also have been recognized. These appear to be involved in the contact phase of the intrinsic pathway of coagulation, and with the exception of Passovoy factor deficiency, all are asymptomatic. The hemorrhagic severity of Passovoy deficiency appears comparable to that seen in factor XI deficiency. Replacement therapy is accomplished with administration of fresh-frozen plasma. These deficiencies are characterized by a prolonged activated partial thromboplastin time and normal prothrombin time and thrombin time; in Fletcher factor deficiency, the activated partial thromboplastin time gradually shortens with incubation at 37° C. Specific assays for prekallikrein and high-molecular-weight kininogen confirm the deficiencies, but the abnormality present in the Passovoy defect has not been identified.

Protein C

Protein C is a vitamin K–dependent anticoagulant protein, synthesized in the liver, that modulates both coagulation and fibrinolysis. After activation by the thrombin–thrombomodulin complex on the surface of endothelial cells and platelets, protein Ca can either inactivate factors VIIIa and Va by direct proteolysis (thereby impeding further generation of thrombin) or enhance the fibrinolytic process in vivo by inactivating the primary inhibitor of plasminogen activator activity;[27,28] therefore, the inherited or acquired deficiency of protein C may be expected to result in a hypercoagulable state. The congenital heterozygous form of protein C deficiency has been detected in approximately 0.3% of the general population, but thromboembolic phenomena are recognized much less frequently. Recurrent deep venous thromboses and/or pulmonary emboli in young adults, who often have a family history of hypercoagulability and unexplained sudden death, characterizes protein C deficiency. Arterial thrombosis and cerebrovascular accidents are uncommon but may occur. The homozygous form of the disease is often fatal in utero or may result in the development of purpura fulminans in the neonate.

The use of oral coumarin anticoagulants in heterozygous deficiency states may produce areas of skin necrosis that are characterized pathologically by infarction of the venules. Coumarin-induced skin necrosis typically occurs during the first week of therapy, and it usually involves fatty tissues such as the buttocks and breasts. The penis also may be affected occasionally. This syndrome may represent the iatrogenic exacerbation of an already decreased and marginally compensated level of protein C by a drug that interferes with the production both of this and other functional vitamin K–dependent proteins. Protein C deficiency can be acquired in association with disseminated intravascular coagulation, malignancies, and severe liver disease.

Protein C antigen levels in plasma can be determined by the Laurell electroimmunoassay or enzyme-linked immunosorbent assay (ELISA) techniques. Functional protein C activity is determined in a modified activated partial thromboplastin time assay that is prolonged in proportion to the concentration of intrinsic protein C converted to activated form with specific snake venoms. Concomitant administration of heparin or coumarin may interfere with protein C determinations in plasma. Also, discordance between the immunologic levels and the functional activity levels of protein C may indicate the presence of a functionally deficient dysproteinemia (type II deficiency).[29]

Replacement therapy is accomplished by transfusions of fresh-frozen plasma or prothrombin complex concentrates, which are contaminated by all of the vitamin K–dependent proteins except factor VII. Long-term anticoagulation with heparin or coumarin is indicated for those individuals who have manifested hypercoagulable complications of protein C deficiency.

Protein S

Protein S is another vitamin K–dependent anticoagulant protein synthesized in the liver.[30,31] By complexing with activated protein C, it functions as a cofactor mediating full expression of the fibrinolytic and anticoagulant activities of protein C. Both congenital and acquired deficiencies of protein S may predispose individuals to thromboembolic complications similar to protein C deficiency, and pregnancy, oral estrogen-contraceptive administration, nephrotic syndromes, severe hepatic disease, and the presence of anticardiolipin antibodies and/or lupus-like anticoagulants are associated with acquired protein S deficiency.

Protein S antigen levels in plasma can be determined in either their free, functionally active circulating form (40%) or their nonfunctional inactive form (60%) complexed to the C4b binding protein by using Laurell electroimmunoassays, ELISA assays, or two-dimensional electrophoresis both before and after precipitating the protein S–C4b binding protein complex with polyethylene glycol. Functional assays are difficult to perform. However, new techniques are now available in kit form.

Replacement therapy of protein S is similar to protein C. The long-term treatment of the thromboembolic complications is similar to that of protein C as well.

Antithrombin III

Antithrombin III is a naturally occurring, circulating inhibitor of serine proteases, which includes factors Xa, IXa, XIa, thrombin, and plasmin. Hereditary deficiencies of this protein occur in an autosomal dominant manner, and they result in a predisposition to venous thromboembolic events in young individuals.[32] Arterial thrombotic complications are extremely rare, and acquired deficiencies are observed most commonly in association with hepatic disease, the nephrotic syndrome, and disseminated intravascular coagulation.

Plasma levels of antigenic antithrombin III are determined easily by Laurell electroimmunoassays, ELISA techniques, or radial immunodiffusion assays. Functional assays are based on modified plasma clotting tests or chromogenic substrate techniques. Replacement of antithrombin III can be accomplished by infusions of fresh-frozen plasma and, more recently, by infusions of purified antithrombin III concentrates.

Deficiencies of the other coagulation modulators, (e.g., α_2-macroglobulin, α_1-antitrypsin, heparin cofactor II, etc.) have not been associated with clinically important abnormalities in coagulation. However, α_2-antiplasmin deficiency has produced profuse bleeding complications in individuals with the congenital form and in those with the acquired disorder associated with acute promyelocytic leukemia.

CIRCULATING ANTICOAGULANTS

Acquired inhibitors of blood coagulation develop in two clinical situations.[33] First, they are encountered in individuals with congenital factor deficiencies (e.g., factors VIII and IX) who develop antibodies to the deficient factor following repeated exposure to sources of replacement therapy. The second situation involves the spontaneous development of inhibitors in individuals without pre-existing coagulation abnormalities; these inhibitors either specifically inactivate a previously activated clotting factor or interfere with the interaction of coagulation factors and/or platelets.

Acquired inhibitors of coagulation factors usually are IgG immunoglobulins (IgG4), although inhibitors of the IgM and IgA variety have been associated, but very rarely, with abnormal paraproteinemias. Thus, these antibodies may arise in immunologic disorders such as multiple myeloma, macroglobulinemias, ulcerative colitis, and autoimmune diseases. Rarely, a curious unexplained inhibitor of factor VIII develops postpartum; in addition, circulating anticoagulants have been related to the use of antibiotics and phenytoin (Dilantin, Parke-Davis, Morris Plains, NJ). Factor VIII inhibitors have been described with penicillin administration, and aminoglycosides have been implicated in the spontaneous development of factor V inhibitors. Antibodies against factor XIII have occurred in association with use of isoniazid, but in most instances, inhibitors induced by drugs eventually disappear when administration of the medication is stopped.

The most commonly encountered acquired circulating inhibitor of coagulation is the lupus anticoagulant, which is an abnormal immunoglobulin directed against the phospholipid components of platelet membranes and the prothrombin activator complex (at the site of factor

Xa, factor V, and calcium conversion of prothrombin to thrombin in the common pathway). This inhibitor, therefore, has the potential to affect both coagulation and platelet function. Despite its designation, the lupus anticoagulant occurs in only 5% to 10% of patients affected with systemic lupus erythematosus; it also has been observed in other collagen vascular disorders, autoimmune processes, malignancies, and AIDS. Bleeding complications are associated uncommonly with the typical lupus anticoagulant unless concurrent hypoprothrombinemia or qualitative or quantitative platelet abnormalities exist. The hypoprothrombinemia is due to the rapid clearance of circulating prothrombin-inhibitor complexes from the plasma rather than to a synthetic defect or direct inhibition of prothrombin activity. Thrombocytopenia and interference with platelet function manifested by abnormal aggregation studies probably reflect the direct effects of the inhibitor interaction with platelet membrane-associated phospholipids. Paradoxically, the lupus anticoagulant may produce hypercoagulability with both venous and arterial thromboembolic events, and in women of childbearing age, it may result in recurrent spontaneous miscarriages.

Other circulating anticoagulants have been described less frequently in association with systemic lupus erythematosus and appear to be directed specifically against clotting factors such as factors VIII, XI, and XII; these coagulation inhibitors are much more likely to produce clinically significant hemorrhagic complications than the typical lupus anticoagulant. In addition, acquired von Willebrand disease has been observed as well.

Abnormalities found by laboratory tests performed in the presence of a circulating anticoagulant depend on the site of the inhibitor's action; characteristically, an abnormal test does not normalize when normal plasma is mixed with the sample that contains the inhibitor. Incubation of the mixture at 37° C for 1 hour may exaggerate the abnormality, but the inhibitory effects of the typical lupus anticoagulant are not time-dependent. In contrast, correction does occur when mixing experiments are performed in true clotting factor deficiencies. The functional expression of the typical lupus anticoagulant can be detected specifically in the tissue thromboplastin inhibition assay and the Russell viper venom time, and prolongations of the activated activated partial thromboplastin time commonly are noted. Abnormal prothrombin times also may reflect hypoprothrombinemia. The activated partial thromboplastin time may normalize after adsorbing the inhibitor onto platelet membranes, and the immunologic expression of the typical lupus anticoagulant is reflected in the anticardiolipin antibody assay. High serum titers of anticardiolipin antibodies may be present in the absence of abnormal coagulation assays and vice versa. The clinical manifestations may occur with abnormalities in one or both types of assays as well.

Treatment of the typical lupus anticoagulant is not indicated unless bleeding or hypercoagulability occur. Corticosteroids may be used to suppress production of the abnormal immunoglobulin, and cytoxic agents also may be necessary. Transfusions of fresh-frozen plasma and platelets may be ineffective. In addition, daily doses of aspirin also have been shown to reduce the frequency of fetal wastage in pregnant women with evidence of lupus anticoagulant and/or anticardiolipin antibodies in some studies.

DISSEMINATED INTRAVASCULAR COAGULATION

Disseminated intravascular coagulation (DIC) is a complex pathologic bleeding syndrome,[34] and only the basic concepts and principles are discussed here. DIC is associated with the intravascular formation of fibrin thrombi and is accompanied by reduction in clotting factors, platelets, and fibrinogen; this process results in the simultaneous activation of the fibrinolytic system. A variety of etiologies precipitate this disorder, including endotoxemias, septicemias, hypotension, disseminated carcinomas and leukemias, obstetric complications, and immune complex diseases. The initiating mechanisms probably involve activation of factor XII, release of thromboplastic substances, or promotion of the platelet release reaction, and spontaneous activation of the fibrinolytic system defends against intravascular deposition of fibrin and also generates degradation products of both fibrinogen and fibrin.

The hemorrhagic complications of DIC can be attributed to depletion of fibrinogen, platelets, and other clotting factors as well as to the anticoagulant effects of the degradation products. Laboratory tests usually reveal a prolonged activated partial thromboplastin time, prothrombin time, and thrombin time, and the platelet count and factors I, V, and VIII are depressed. However, the titer of fibrinogen–fibrin degradation products is elevated. Many of these proteins unfortunately are acute-phase reactants and their levels initially elevated; therefore, a striking reduction may yield values within the normal range. Other helpful diagnostic indicators of DIC include the presence of fragmented erythrocytes on the peripheral blood smear and the rapid lysis of a whole blood clot. This rapid lysis may primarily be due to a decreased fibrinogen concentration. ELISA assays are available to detect elevated plasma levels of fibrinopeptide A and the prothrombin fragment 1.2 peptide, both of which are indirect indicators of increased thrombin activity, and in addition, assays that detect the generation of B/β 15–42 peptides from noncross-linked fibrin can be utilized to monitor plasmin effects in vivo.

Disseminated intravascular coagulation is an acquired secondary manifestation of other disease states; therefore, its treatment should be aimed specifically at the underlying cause. The use of heparin is a debatable issue, because no prospective, randomized, controlled studies have been performed and would be difficult to accomplish as well because of the typical clinical complexity and life-threatening nature of the illness. The use of heparin both to reduce consumption of clotting factors and to impede thrombin generation probably should be reserved as a temporizing measure while awaiting the effects of therapy for the underlying disease to become evident; the effectiveness of heparin therapy in this situation can be assessed by observing for normalization of the previously depressed fibrinogen and platelet levels. Recently, some investigators have advocated the empiric use of antithrombin III concentrates in the treatment of DIC, because plasma levels of antithrombin III typically are depressed in this disorder. However, again, no controlled studies have confirmed the usefulness of this in decreasing either the mortality or duration of DIC. Infusions of fresh-frozen plasma or cryoprecipitate may be beneficial during DIC to replace volume, and both fibrinogen and platelet transfusions may be needed to maintain adequate hemostasis. Concomitant treatment of the underlying disease state (with or without heparin) should accompany replacement of these components. The administration of ε-aminocaproic acid or tranexamic acid as fibrinolytic inhibitors should be approached with caution, because both may exacerbate the pre-existing hypercoagulability. These agents may be particularly helpful to prevent the bleeding complications associated with acute promyelocytic leukemia as an acquired deficiency of α_2-antiplasmin may exist, resulting in a hyperplasminemic state.

Disseminated intravascular coagulation can be precipitated by many underlying disease states. Some of these include malignant neoplasms, infections, obstetric complications, crush injuries, prolonged hypotension, snake bites, and endothelematous or cavernous hemangiomas (Kasabach-Merritt syndrome). Chronic DIC may complicate occult or obvious malignancies and is characterized by recurrent and migratory thromboembolic phenomena, including deep venous thrombosis and arterial emboli due to nonbacterial thrombotic endocarditis (Trousseau syndrome). Coumarin failure may be encountered in the prevention of thrombotic episodes associated with the Trousseau syndrome, and the administration of heparin may be a necessary adjunctive therapy on a long-term basis until chemotherapy has controlled the elaboration of thromboplastin-like substances by the underlying malignancy.

REFERENCES

1. Vene JR, Anggard EE, Botting RM. Regulatory functions of the vascular endothelium. N Engl J Med 1990;323:27–36.
2. Davie EW, Ratnoff OD. Waterfall sequence for intrinsic blood clotting. Science 1964;145:1310.
3. MacFarlane RG. An enzyme cascade in the blood clotting mechanism, and its function as a biochemical amplifier. Nature 1964;202:498.
4. Gjonnaess H. Cold-promoted activation of factor VIII: IV. Relation to the coagulation system. Thromb Diath Haemorrh 1972;28:194.
5. Conley CL, Hartmann RC, Morse WI II. The clotting behavior of human "platelet-free" plasma: evidence for the existence of a "plasma thromboplastin." J Clin Invest 1949;28:340.
6. Kalousek F, Koningsberg W, Nemerson Y. Activation of factor IX by activated factor X: a link between the extrinsic and intrinsic coagulation system. FEBS Lett 1975;50:382.
7. Ratnoff OD. Blood clotting mechanisms: an overview. In: Ogston D, Bennett R, eds. Pathology. New York: John Wiley & Sons, 1977:13.
8. Osterud B, Rapaport SI. Activation of factor IX by the reaction product of tissue factor and factor VII: additional pathway for initiating blood coagulation. Proc Natl Acad Sci U S A 1977;74:5260.
9. White GC, Shoemaker CB. Factor VIII gene and hemophilia A. Blood 1989;73:1–12.
10. Ewenstein BM, Inbal A, Pober JS, Handin RI. Molecular studies of von Willebrand disease. Blood 1990;75:1466–72.
11. Legaz ME, Weinstein MJ, Helderbrant CM, Davie EW. Isolation, subunit structure, and proteolytic modification of bovine factor VIII. Ann N Y Acad Sci 1975;240:43.
12. Rosenberg RD. Actions and interactions of thrombin and heparin. N Engl J Med 1975;292:146.
13. Radcliffe RD, Nemerson Y. Activation and control of factor VII by activated factor X and thrombin. J Biol Chem 1975;250:388.
14. Gidding JC, Blood AL. Factor V activation by thrombin and its role in prothrombin conversion. Br J Haematol 1975;29:349.
15. Suttie JW, Jackson CM. Prothrombin structure, activation and biosynthesis. Physiol Rev 1977;57:1.
16. Lattallo ZS, Fletcher AP, Alkjaersig N, Sherry S. Inhibition of fibrin polymerization by fibrinogen proteolysis products. Am J Physiol 1962;202:681.
17. Latolla ZS, Budzynski AZ, Lipinski B, Kowalski E. Inhibition of thrombin and of fibrin polymerization, two activities derived from plasmin digested fibrinogen. Nature 1964;203:1184.
18. Kowalski E, Kopec M, Wegrzynowicz Z. Influence of fibrinogen degradation products (FDP) on platelet aggregation, adhesiveness, and viscous metamorphosis. Thromb Diath Haemorrh 1964;10:406.
19. Kessler CM, Bell WR. Effect of homologous thrombin and fibrinogen degradation products on fibrinogen synthesis in rabbits. J Lab Clin Med 1979;93:768.
20. Lee RI, White PD. A clinical study of the coagulation time of blood. Am J Med Sci 1913;145:495.
21. Hougie C, Twomey JJ. Hemophilia B^m: a new type of factor IX deficiency. Lancet 1967;i:698.
22. Seligsohn U, Shani M, Ramot B, Adam A, Sheba CH. Dubin-Johnson syndrome in Israel: II. Association with factor VII deficiency. Q J Med 1970;39:569.
23. Rosborough TK, Swaim WR. Acquired von Willebrand's disease platelet-release defect and angiodysplasia. Am J Med 1978;65:96.
24. McPherson RA, Onstad JW, Ugoretz RJ, Wolf PL. Coagulopathy in amyloidosis: combined deficiency of factors IX and X. Am J Hematol 1977;3:225.

25. Pechet L, Kastrul JJ. Amyloidosis associated with factor X (Stuart) deficiency: case report. Ann Intern Med 1964;61:315.

26. Aznar J, Fernandez Pavon A. Letter: thromboembolic accidents in patients with congenital deficiency of factor XII. Thromb Diath Haemorrh 1974;31:525.

27. Marlar RA, Griffin JH. Deficiency of protein C inhibitor in combined factor V/VIII deficiency disease. J Clin Invest 1980;66:1186.

28. Stenflo J. A new vitamin K–dependent protein. J Biol Chem 1976;251:355.

29. Esmon CT. The role of protein C and thrombomodulin in regulation of blood coagulation. J Biol Chem 1989;264:4743–6.

30. Engesser L, Broekmans AW, Briet E, Brymmer EJP, Bertina RM. Hereditary protein S deficiency: clinical manifestations. Ann Intern Med 1987;106:677.

31. Walker FJ. Protein S and the regulation of activated protein C. Semin Thromb Hemost 1984;10:131.

32. Rosenberg RD, ed. Role of antithrombin III in coagulation disorders: state-of-the-art review. Am J Med 1989;87(3B):3B1S–3B67S.

33. Shapiro SS, Hulten M. Acquired inhibitors to the blood coagulation factors. Semin Thromb Hemost 1975;1:366.

34. Bell WR. Disseminated intravascular coagulation. Johns Hopkins Med J 1980;146:289.

19

Antithrombotic Therapy

Craig M. Kessler, M.D., and William R. Bell, M.D.

Homeostatic regulation of the coagulation mechanism depends on dynamic interactions between the sequential activation of circulating proenzymes (which comprise the clotting cascade) and the induction of fibrinolytic enzymes that are necessary to prevent a hypercoagulable state. The contributions of both platelets and endogenous circulating plasma inhibitors (e.g., antithrombin III, α_2-macroglobulins, antiplasmin, α_1-antitrypsin), C_1-inactivator, and inter-α-antitrypsin are important to both systems, and antithrombotic therapy is based on interference of the intricate physiologic balance at key sites in the coagulation cascade scheme.

There are four recognized classes of antithrombotic agents. The most commonly employed antithrombotic agents are the anticoagulants, which include heparin and the coumarin–indanedione compounds; these agents have been available and used extensively for the past 35 years. More recently, agents that alter platelet function in vitro (platelet antiaggregating drugs) have been given considerable attention and, to some extent, have been evaluated in clinical trials. As a result of both improved biochemic purification techniques and widespread, properly designed clinical trials, renewed interest has been generated in the third class, thrombolytic agents, and the fourth class, defibrinogenating agents, which remove fibrinogen from the circulating blood. Antithrombotic regimens that employ drugs from any of these categories must be individualized both to the clinical circumstances and to the patient's response. The therapeutic effectiveness of each agent must be assessed regularly, with any appropriate alterations made in the dosage schedule, and one should be aware that hereditary or acquired deficiencies of either coagulation or platelet function will increase the sensitivity of patients to the antithrombotic properties of these agents.

ANTICOAGULANTS

Anticoagulants reduce the coagulability of blood by producing defects in the coagulation cascade. Both heparin and the coumarin–indanedione compounds are discussed.

Heparin

Heparin, a highly anionic mucopolysaccharide, was discovered fortuitously in 1916 during the search for natural procoagulant substrates; it since has become the most commonly employed parenterally administered anticoagulant in clinical medicine. Heparin is produced in the mast cells of most animals, and it is particularly abundant in the liver, lungs, and intestines. Commercial preparations usually are extracted from porcine and bovine alimentary tract and bovine lung. Heparin is effective as both an in vivo and in vitro anticoagulant, and it may be detected as a circulating anticoagulant in the laboratory. It has been documented to interfere with blood clotting at multiple critical steps in the coagulation cascade (as listed in Table 19.1), and heparin's therapeutic effects are attributed to its ability to complex with and thereby both potentiate and accelerate the activity of antithrombin III, the primary natural inhibitor of coagulation factor activation.[1,2] In the presence of this circulating α_2-globulin, much smaller quantities of heparin are required to inhibit the initiation of clotting than

TABLE 19.1. Heparin

Generic Name	Heparin sodium
Chemistry	Heterogeneous, densely anionic mucopolysaccharide containing sulfaminic linkages
Molecular Weight	Between 6000 and 20,000 d
Commercial Names	Heparin sodium
	Liquaemin sodium
	Lipo-Hepin
	Panheprin
Antocoagulant Activity	Inhibits proteolytic action of thrombin on fibrinogen; interferes with platelet release reaction and viscous metamorphosis induced by thrombin; inhibits activation of coagulation factors XI, X, IX, and VIII; potentiates anticoagulated effects of thrombin–antithrombin III complex
Administration and Usual Adult Dose	
Intravenous (continuous infusion)	300 to 600 U/kg every 24 hours immediately following loading dose of 10,000 U
Intermittent bolus	75 to 150 U/kg every 4 to 6 hours beginning 4 to 6 hours after loading dose of 10,000 U
Subcutaneous	8000 to 10,000 U every 8 hours to 12,000 to 20,000 U every 12 hours
Low-dose therapy	5000 U every 8 hours or 5000 to 10,000 U every 12 hours (beginning 2 hours before abdominal surgery)

would be to inhibit fibrin formation after the elaboration of thrombin from prothrombin; this forms the rationale for low-dose heparin therapy in the prophylaxis of venous thromboembolism.[3] Also, because of its strong negative charge, heparin can neutralize directly the proteins involved in the clotting cascade, but it does not depress or alter the biosynthesis of any coagulation factor.

Other pharmacologic considerations include heparin's anticomplement activity, antilipemic action secondary to the release of lipoprotein lipase, and ability to release histaminase. In addition, heparin does not cross the placenta, and it is not secreted into breast milk.

Method of Administration

Because it is not absorbed sufficiently after oral administration, heparin must be given parenterally to achieve sufficient blood levels; the intramuscular route is not recommended because of variable absorption as well as the possibility of localized hematoma formation. Subcutaneous injection of heparin, usually into the abdominal-wall fat pad, also may be complicated by erratic absorption, local hemorrhage, and discomfort from long-term administration. Nevertheless, subcutaneous injection commonly is employed in the low-dose heparin regimen and for long-term anticoagulation in outpatients. Therapeutic levels are achieved 2 to 4 hours after subcutaneous instillation, but the anticoagulant effect is achieved almost immediately after intravenous injection. Intermittent bolus therapy provides excellent transient effects, but this must be repeated at 4- to 6-hour intervals to maintain adequate levels as the half-life of heparin in the circulation is approximately 90 minutes. The continuous intravenous infusion of heparin produces a sustained therapeutic blood level of medication (and with less heparin required) and may provide more effective and safer anticoagulation (less bleeding) than intermittent doses.[4] Investigators also have employed the intrapulmonary administration of an aerosolized heparin with therapeutic prolongation of the clotting time, but this technique remains experimental.[5]

DOSAGE AND MONITORING OF THERAPY. The objective of heparin therapy is to achieve the maximum inhibition of coagulation with the minimum risk of hemorrhage. Unfortunately, variability in patient response and the relative insensitivity of the clotting assays available in measuring heparin's therapeutic effect on coagulation make this task difficult. The whole blood clotting time (the Lee-White clotting time, employing plain, clean glass tubes) appears to provide the most accurate predictive information regarding adequacy of the antithrombotic effects of routine heparin therapy, but this is cumbersome, both time- and labor-intensive, and has been replaced in most centers by the activated partial thromboplastin time (APTT). For the treatment of acute thromboembolic events, sufficient heparin should be administered to prolong the APTT from 1.5 to 2.5 times the normal control value, measured immediately before the institution of heparin. This approach is empiric, because a sufficient number of studies have not utilized the APTT to define the degree of prolongation that provides the optimal antithrombotic (as opposed to anticoagulant) effects of heparin; nevertheless, when followed, these guidelines have proven to be effective. When the whole blood clotting time is used to monitor anticoagulation, the heparin dose should be adjusted to maintain the clotting time at more than 20 minutes but less than 45 minutes. In monitoring therapy, it must be remembered that both the reproducibility and the accuracy of the APTT or Lee-White clotting time depend on the quality of venepuncture as well as the manner by which the blood sample was handled before assay.[6,7] Therapeutic levels of heparin rarely prolong the prothrombin time but usually do prolong the thrombin time, and the prolonged thrombin times and APTTs produced by heparin therapy can be corrected in vitro following addition of protamine sulfate or toluidine blue. Furthermore, the reptilase time assay, which employs a snake venom instead of thrombin to form a fibrin clot, is not inhibited by heparin but may be prolonged by circulating fibrinogen/fibrin split products, dysfibrinogens, and both abnormal qualitative and quantitative immunoglobulins.

The technique selected to monitor therapy (by constant infusion) should be repeated initially every 6 hours until a satisfactory therapeutic dose of heparin is achieved. Thereafter, the monitoring technique should be repeated at 12-hour intervals for 3 days, and at this point, if the clotting times are reproducible in the therapeutic range with a stable dose and no evidence of bleeding exists, then monitoring can be repeated at 24-hour intervals for the duration of therapy. If the intermittent intravenous bolus method of administration is used, the monitoring assay should be performed immediately before doses of heparin are given. For the intermittent subcutaneous approach, the APTT should be repeated 6 hours after each 12-hour heparin dose.

Monitoring should be performed with the indicated frequency until adequate therapeutic levels of heparin are achieved and maintained for the initial 3 to 4 days of therapy; then, it should be performed once daily for the duration of therapy. Monitoring techniques are intended both to ensure adequate antithrombotic anticoagulant efficacy as well as minimize hemorrhagic complications.

For the continuous infusion method of administration, an intravenous loading dose of 5000 to 10000 units of heparin (in 10 to 20 ml of diluent) is given slowly; this is followed immediately by the infusion of heparin delivered at a constant rate (150 to 300 units/kg in 250 to 500 ml of 5% dextrose administered over 12 hours). Intravenous intermittent heparin therapy is carried out most conveniently using an indwelling "heparin lock"; a loading dose similar to that used in the continuous method is administered and then followed by 75 to 150 units/kg in 10 to 20 ml of 5% dextrose every 4 to 6 hours. The subcutaneous route of administration requires 10,000 to 25,000 units of heparin every 6 to 12 hours, depending on the results of the monitoring assays, and the most commonly used subcutaneous regimen recommends the administration of 10,000 to 15,000 units of heparin every 12 hours, adjusted to maintain the APTT at 1.5 to 2.0 times normal 6 hours after the preceding dose. This technique has been shown to effectively prophylax against recurrent deep venous thrombosis and pulmonary emboli without producing significant hemorrhagic complications.

The schedule for low-dose heparin therapy is 5000 units subcutaneously every 8 hours (or 5000 to 10,000 units every 12 hours). If surgery is involved, then the regimen should be initiated 2 hours before the procedure and be continued for 8 to 10 days postoperatively (until the patient is ambulatory). Investigations indicate that this technique of administration provides effective prophylaxis for the development of deep venous thrombosis and subsequent fatal pulmonary emboli following general surgery.[8,9] Its use in total hip replacement, open prostatectomies, biliary tract surgery, and myocardial infarction therapy, however, is much less impressive and may produce significant bleeding. Monitoring tests are not helpful, because the low doses usually do not influence the coagulation assays. However, hematocrit values should be followed, and the patient should be observed for possible urinary and gastrointestinal bleeding.

Although age and gender (elderly females being the most sensitive) are important considerations, drug interactions are the most prevalent of factors that affect heparin dosage.[10] The use of aspirin or other antiplatelet medications (e.g., indomethacin and dipyridamole) may precipitate hemorrhage despite a presumably safe heparin dose, and digitalis, tetracyclines, nicotine, and antihistamines may inhibit heparin activity. In addition, resistance to heparin may be associated with febrile states, right-sided heart failure, carcinoma, myocardial infarction, and acute thrombosis.

COMPLICATIONS. The most common complication of heparin therapy is spontaneous hemorrhage, the frequency of which is proportional to the dose and may range as high as 20% to 30%;[11] therefore, any contemplated invasive diagnostic or therapeutic procedure should be deferred until the effect of the heparin has dissipated. Other reactions include transient alopecia, dysesthesia pedis, and development of osteoporosis with spontaneous fractures in some patients on high doses over prolonged periods. Both local and systemic hypersensitivity reactions may include fever, urticaria, bronchospasm, rhinorrhea, and conjunctivitis, and the development of significant thrombocytopenia (occasionally associated with disseminated intravascular coagulopathy and major venous and/or arterial thromboembolic phenomena) has been observed within the first 5 to 7 days of heparin anticoagulation therapy.[12]

Heparin-associated thrombocytopenia (HAT) varies in severity, may be heparin lot–related, and may result from the spontaneous aggregation of platelets in vivo (possibly via an immune mechanism). Nevertheless, HAT may occur in patients who never received heparin previously and may not necessarily recur on future reexposure. HAT most commonly is associated with the use of heparin from bovine-derived sources, but 3% to 5% of cases have been observed after the administration of porcine mucosal heparin. HAT resolves over 3 to 7 days after discontinuation of heparin, and it may necessitate either substituting porcine sources of heparin in the interim, beginning coumarin anticoagulation, or employing prostacycline analogues. Recently, the infusion of the defibrinating agent, ancrod, has been used successfully in the treatment of HAT. The diagnosis of HAT often is confirmed by in vitro platelet aggregation assays, where the addition of exogenous heparin to the patient's platelet-rich plasma or to normal platelet-rich plasma to which the patient's platelet-poor plasma has been added will spontaneously induce platelet aggregation.

Protamine sulfate is the recommended antidote when serious hemorrhage necessitates the prompt reversal of heparin's effect. By forming stable complexes, 1.0 mg of protamine sulfate can neutralize 100 units (approximately 1.0 mg) of heparin circulating in the body. However, because protamine sulfate has potential anticoagulant properties if excess amounts are administered, the calculated dose should be equivalent to one half of the previous heparin dose (in milligrams) and should be administered intravenously at a rate not exceeding 5 mg/min. No more than 50 mg should be given per single injection, and additional doses of protamine sulfate should not be given unless the clotting tests used to monitor heparin's effect indicate residual hyperheparinemia. Other heparin antagonists include lysozyme, hexadimethrine bromide (Polybrene, Abbott Laboratories, North Chicago, IL), toluidine blue, fuchsin, and clupeine, but these are not used clinically. Transfusions of whole blood, plasma, or platelets also are not effective antagonists of the anticoagulant properties of heparin.

Recent studies have been performed with low-molecular-weight heparins (fractionated from standard heparin preparations, peptides fractionated from heparin, and synthetic peptides of heparin fragments), and these preparations predominantly contain the low-molecular-weight fractions that interact efficiently with antithrombin III and eliminate the high-molecular-weight fractions that interact with platelets. The incidence of HAT should be minimized significantly with these preparations, and the safety margin for parenteral anticoagulation should be enhanced greatly. Thus far, clinical studies have confirmed the safety and efficacy of low-molecular-weight heparins, but randomized, controlled studies have not yet established their superiority over conventional heparin. The anticoagulant effects of low-molecular-weight heparin administered in therapeutic doses are undetectable by the APTT, and antifactor Xa activity determinations correlate best with the antithrombotic potential and safety margin of these products.

Coumarin–Indanedione Oral Anticoagulants

This class of anticoagulants inhibits blood clotting through their actions on vitamin K, a fat-soluble substance necessary for the normal biosynthesis of prothrombin (factor II), factor VII, factor IX, and factor X. Vitamin K functions as the crucial mediator of intrahepatic carboxylation of glutamine acid residues in the inert precursors of these coagulant proteins, and this process provides binding sites for calcium ions, which in turn promote binding of the inert coagulant proteins to phospholipid surfaces for subsequent activation.[13,14] Therefore, these vitamin K antagonists derive their anticoagulation properties from altering the structure of the inactive precursor coagulant proteins (which results in loss of biologic function) rather than by depressing their hepatic synthesis. The inactive precursor coagulant proteins, designated *protein induced by vitamin K antagonist,* may be detected during coumarin–indanedione therapy and are similar antigenically to their activated forms. The oral anticoagulants manifest their pharmacologic effects in vivo only, and, unlike heparin, they possess no in vitro anticoagulant activity. Miscellaneous effects of the coumarin–indanedione drugs include increased urinary excretion of uric acid, slight impairment of thyroid activity, and dilation of the coronary arteries with enhanced blood flow to the myocardium.

METHOD OF ADMINISTRATION. Although many coumarin–indanedione preparations are available for clinical oral anticoagulation, warfarin (Coumadin, Du Pont Pharmaceuticals, Wilmington, DE) is the most commonly used in the United States, and it is the only one that also can be used intravenously. The indanedione derivatives are more popular elsewhere, and in clinical studies, they appear to be associated with increased frequency of side-effects.[15,16] Bishydroxycoumarin (Dicumarol, Abbott Laboratories, North Chicago, IL) may be the least toxic of all the coumarin congeners; however, its delayed and erratic absorption as well as prolonged duration of action are undesirable.[15] In contrast, warfarin is absorbed rapidly and almost completely from the alimentary tract and has an acceptable half-life.

Following their absorption from the gastrointestinal tract, the coumarin–indanedione derivatives are bound almost entirely to albumin.[17] They then accumulate predominantly in the liver, where they can exert their pharmacologic effects and be metabolized for excretion into the bile, and the drug metabolites are reabsorbed from the intestine and finally eliminated in the urine. A therapeutic response to oral anticoagulant administration does not become evident until the coagulant activity of pre-existing vitamin K–dependent factors decreases. This requires several days, and it is dependent on the biologic half-lives of the individual circulating factors. The half-life is shortest for factor VII and is sequentially longer for factors IX, X, and II. The biologic function of the other vitamin K–dependent proteins, proteins C and S, also are affected by coumarin-type drugs.

DOSAGE AND MONITORING OF THERAPY. The anticoagulant effect of the coumarin–indanedione derivatives is measured most reliably by the one-stage prothrombin time.[15,16,18] This monitors the extrinsic pathway of the coagulation cascade and is influenced by alterations in factors II, V, VII, and X. Factor IX is not measured directly by the test, but its activity parallels that of the others during drug therapy. It also should be noted that the one-stage prothrombin test crudely reflects the plasma fibrinogen concentration, which must be adequate to produce a clot end point for the assay.

The philosophy for what constitutes effective and adequate anticoagulation with minimal hemorrhagic complications is changing after recent clinical studies indicated that therapeutic and prophylactic coumarin regimens employing lower dose intensity have been successful in minimizing bleeding complications as well as preventing thrombotic or embolic episodes, with prothrombin times maintained at 1.2 to 1.5 times control levels. The traditional approach of maintaining the therapeutic prothrombin time between 1.5 to 2.5 times the control level was effective in preventing thrombosis, but it also was associated with up to a 27% frequency of major bleeding problems. In addition, the current rabbit-brain thromboplastin reagents used to determine the prothrombin time in most U.S. laboratories appears to be less sensitive to coumarin's effects than the original

reagents that were used to establish the traditional treatment criteria, and when coumarin derivatives are used in conjunction with heparin administration, special considerations for monitoring must be employed. Baseline APTTs (or Lee-White clotting times) should be obtained before institution of the anticoagulants; because the prothrombin time usually is not unaffected (or just minimally prolonged) with therapeutic levels of heparin, this remains an excellent assay to monitor and adjust the adequacy of coumarin doses during concomitant heparin administration. In contrast, the APTT is influenced by both heparin and coumarin drugs and should be maintained within the therapeutic range by adjusting the heparin dose. After 5 to 7 days of overlap therapy with heparin and coumarin when the prothrombin time is in the therapeutic range, the heparin can be discontinued, but the overlap period is recommended to avoid the development of coumarin-induced skin necrosis, which in some patients may be due to the early depletion of protein C associated with the initiation of oral anticoagulation. Oral anticoagulants also may prolong the whole blood clotting and recalcification time slightly, but the bleeding time is unaffected.

Two approaches are available to initiate therapy with coumarin–indanedione preparations. The first advocates the administration of a large loading dose (e.g., warfarin, 25 to 60 mg) followed 36 hours later by a daily maintenance dose (e.g., 2 to 15 mg) based on prothrombin time results. After the loading dose, there is a rapid depression of factor VII activity, and this is reflected in the prolonged prothrombin time and occurs before any changes can be detected in the levels of the other vitamin K–dependent factors. Whether effective antithrombotic activity can be produced by an isolated decrease in factor VII is speculative, particularly because concomitant severe decreases in proteins C and S also occur and could induce hypercoagulability. In a few patients, the loading dose method also may be associated with an increased likelihood of hemorrhagic complications.

The alternative approach to initiation involves much smaller doses (e.g., warfarin, 10 to 15 mg daily) that are still adequate to depress factor VII activity but with less danger of hemorrhage. The subsequent daily doses, usually ranging from 2 to 5 mg, are determined by results of the prothrombin time. No significant difference in the long-term antithrombotic effectiveness of these two methods has been documented, but recent clinical studies indicate that oral anticoagulant administration initiated either simultaneously or within 24 to 48 hours after beginning full-dose heparinization and with a 5- to 7-day overlap produces safe and effective treatment, allows earlier patient discharge from the hospital, prevents the development of coumarin-induced skin necrosis, and provides adequate anticoagulation coverage if HAT develops. With any approach, however, the dosage must be monitored using daily prothrombin times until a maintenance dose of anticoagulant is established; subsequently, monitoring should be performed at 1 week and then at 2- to 3-week intervals.

Many factors can influence the therapeutic effectiveness of oral anticoagulants. The most common involves interactions with other drugs (Table 19.2),[19,20] which may affect the absorption, excretion, or metabolism of vitamin K or coumarin and may alter the albumin binding of coumarin derivatives. Several second-generation cephalosporin derivatives, such as moxalactam and cefamandole, contain a N-methylthiotetrazole side ring that interferes with the vitamin K–dependent γ-carboxylation of coagulation factors and prolongs the prothrombin time. Levels of proteins C and S may be depressed during the administration of these antibiotics as well.

In addition, systemic conditions associated with steatorrhea, biliary obstruction, compromised hepatic and cardiac function, and hypoalbuminemia may influence anticoagulant action. Warfarin hypersensitivity occasionally is encountered in older patients, and a rare, inherited autosomal dominant resistance to the effects of coumarin–indanedione drugs has been described in two kindreds.[21,22] Also, the antithrombotic effects of oral anticoagulants can be influenced significantly by the concomitant use of heparin or antiplatelet medications such as aspirin.

The existence of a "rebound phenomenon" following the cessation of oral anticoagulant therapy is controversial. Its advocates claim that thromboembolic events are more likely to occur unless there is a gradual reduction in the dosage over 48 to 72 hours. However, its opponents know the long half-lives of the coumarin–indanedione agents (ranging from 40 to 75 hours) obviate further tapering of dosage.

As with heparin, hemorrhage is the most commonly encountered complication of oral anticoagulation using coumarin–indanedione agents, with an estimated 0.2% chance per year of a fatal hemorrhagic episode. Occasionally, occult gastrointestinal carcinomas have been unmasked during therapy,[23] but other toxic effects are rare and include alopecia, dermatitis, urticaria, erythema, the syndrome of coumarin-induced skin necrosis (a condition that involves localized microvasculature thrombosis occurring after 7 to 10 days of therapy which may be caused by the early depression of protein C levels by coumarin), and the "purple toes" syndrome that occurs after long-term therapy. The indanedione derivates in particular are associated with leukopenia, agranulocytosis, pyrexia, hepatitis, nephropathy, and innocuous red-orange discoloration of urine. The oral anticoagulants are secreted into breast milk; therefore, breast-feeding is not recommended even though the prothrombin times usually are unaltered in nursing infants of mothers taking anticoagulants. In addition, oral anticoagulants can cross the placenta, and their administration during the latter part of pregnancy is known to cause fetal or placental hemorrhage. Their use early in gestation has been associated with multiple congenital anomalies as well.[24–31]

Surreptitious self-administration of oral anticoagulants occasionally is seen in psychiatrically disturbed people; usually, these patients are women in paramedical occupations. Warfarin-containing insecticides are the anticoagulants most frequently ingested accidentally by children.

ANTIDOTES. Vitamin K_1 is the specific antidote for the anticoagulant effects of the coumarin–indanedione derivatives. Vitamin K_1 preparations can be administered either orally, intramuscularly, or intravenously at a rate not to exceed 5 mg/min, and therapeutic results occur within 4 to 6 hours after intravenous administration. Prothrombin times return to baseline levels within 12 to 24 hours after large doses of vitamin K_1 (50 to 100 mg) are given to reverse completely life-threatening hemorrhage induced by coumarin excess; in cases of less urgent hemorrhage, where the patient is to remain on anticoagulant therapy after the reversal of the hemorrhage, lower doses of vitamin K_1 (5 to 10 mg) are sufficient. Transfusions of fresh-frozen plasma can counteract the effects of oral anticoagulation in patients with severe hepatic disease, in whom vitamin K is ineffective, or in individuals whose bleeding is of such magnitude that immediate correction of the prothrombin time is mandatory. Although plasma concentrates of factors II, VII, IX, and X (Proplex, Hyland Division, Baxter Healthcare Corporation, Glendale, CA; Konyne, Miles-Cutter, West Haven, CT) are effective antagonists of the coumarin–indanedione drugs, they also are associated with a high risk of hepatitis, may be thrombogenic, and should be used only in extreme situations.

ANTIPLATELET DRUGS

Drugs that interfere with platelet function have generated considerable interest because of both their theoretic usefulness as antithrombotic agents and their clinical advantages of oral administration and minimal toxicity.[32] For example, aspirin (acetylsalicylic acid) is a potent in vitro inhibitor of platelet aggregation by collagen, epinephrine, and adenosine diphosphate; in vivo, it prolongs the bleeding time but does not affect platelet

TABLE 19.2. Common Interactions of Drugs With Coumarin–Indanedione Anticoagulants

Type of Drug	Generic Name (Trade Name)	Mechanism	Effect on Coumarin–Indanedione Activity
Anabolic steroid	Methandrostenolone (Dianabol) Norethandrolone (Nilevar) Oxymetholone (Anadrol-50) Nandrolone (Deca-Durabolin)	? Impaired synthesis of vitamin K–dependent clotting factors by increasing affinity of receptor site for anticoagulant	Potentiating

Sedative	Barbiturates
	  Amobarbital (Amytal)
	  Secobarbital (Seconal)
	  Phenobarbital
		Induction of hepatic microsomal enzymes that catabolize coumarin–indanedione derivatives	Inibitory

Hypnotic, anticonvulsant	Glutethimide (Doriden) Ethchlorvynol (Placidyl)		Potentiating
	Phenytoin (Dilantin)	Delay of hepatic catabolism of oral anticoagulants	
Antilipemic	Clofibrate (Atromid-S)	Displacement of anticoagulant from albumin binding sites	Potentiating
	D-Thyroxine (Choloxin)	Possibly, increase in affinity of anticoagulants for their hepatic binding sites	Potentiating
	Cholestyramine (Questran)	Interference with absorption of vitamin K and warfarin from the gut	Potentiating
Antipyretic and anti-inflammatory	Salicylates	Inhibition of vitamin K–dependent factors (in large doses)	Potentiating
	Phenylbutazone (Butazolidin) Oxyphenbutazone (Tandearil)	Displacement of anticoagulant from albumin binding sites	
	Acetaminophen	Unknown	Very minor potentiation (preferable to salicylates as antipyretic or analgesic during anticoagulant therapy)
Antifungal	Griscofulvin (Fulvicin, Grifulvin, Grisactin)	Interference with absorption of oral anticoagulant; induction of hepatic microsomal enzymes for metabolism or oral anticoagulants	Inhibitory
Antibiotic	Nalidixic acid (NegGram) Sulfonamides, long-acting	Displacement of oral anticoagulant from albumin binding sites	Potentiating
	Chloramphenicol (Chloromycetin) Chlortetracycline Neomycin	Probably, reduction of bacterial source of vitamin K synthesis	Potentiating (only when intake of vitamin K is extremely reduced)
	Rifampin (Rifampicin, Rimactane)	Enhancement of warfarin secretion by stimulation of bile flow	Inhibitory
Diuretic	Hydrochlorothiazide (Esidrix, HydroDIURIL [does not apply to chlorothiazides])	? Decrease of binding of anticoagulant to albumin	Potentiating
	Diazoxide (Hyperstat) Ethacrynic acid (Edecrin)		Inhibitory
	Organic mercurials (Mercuhydrin, Thiomerin)	? Reduction of hepatic congestion in edematous individuals, resulting in enhancement of clotting factor synthesis ? Reduction of plasma volume and concentration of existing circulating clotting factors	
Antiarrhythmic	Quinidine, quinine derivatives	Unknown	Potentiating
Immune inhibitor	Cyclosporine	Unknown	Inactivated by coumarin compounds

Note: The benzodiazepine muscle relaxants, chloridiazepoxide (Librium) and diazepam (Valium), have not been shown to affect the anticoagulant effects of coumarin–indanedione derivatives; this also is true for the closely related hypnotic agent flurazepam (Dalmane). In addition, ethanol ingestion (in moderate quantities) in the absence of liver disease most likely does not alter oral anticoagulant effects.

survival. Aspirin interferes with prostaglandin synthesis in the platelet, presumably by acetylation of the cyclooxygenase that is necessary to synthesize mediators of the platelet release reaction,[33] and this produces a permanent defect in the platelets exposed to aspirin and can be achieved by the ingestion of very small doses. Salicylic acid, propoxyphene, and acetaminophen possess no antiplatelet activity.

Ingestion of dipyridamole does not alter either the bleeding time or in vitro platelet aggregation; however, platelet adhesiveness may be decreased in some patients. Dipyridamole is a potent phosphodiesterase inhibitor, and it suppresses the platelet release reaction by increasing platelet cyclic adenosine monophosphate. Normalization of decreased platelet survival in vivo also has been reported with its use.

Sulfinpyrazone, a competitive inhibitor of platelet prostaglandin synthesis, also normalizes decreased platelet survival and interferes with the platelet release reaction.[34] The bleeding time is unaffected following its administration, and several investigators believe that sulfinpyrazone exerts a protective effect on the vessel endothelium rather than acting directly on the platelets.

Dextran consists of low-molecular-weight glucose polymers that may retard platelet adhesiveness when administered intravenously. In vitro tests of both platelet aggregation and release reaction are inhibited by its use, and large concentrations may induce an anticoagulant effect with abnormal bleeding.

Ticlopidine is a potent antiplatelet aggregatory agent that specifically inhibits thromboxane A_2 generation in the platelet without affecting prostacyclin synthesis by the endothelial cell. Recent clinical trials suggest that this agent may be superior to aspirin in reducing the incidence of both recurrent stroke and stroke associated with pre-existing transient ischemic attacks.

Other antiplatelet agents, such as clofibrate, phenylbutazone, indomethacin, and mefenamic acid, also are available, but they have not been employed widely in clinical studies of antithrombotic therapy. The commonly used compounds originally were investigated for their potential usefulness in the treatment and prophylaxis of arterial thrombosis, and despite the large platelet component associated with the formation of arterial thrombi, the ability of antiplatelet drugs to• prevent or treat these thrombi has not been confirmed in the majority of trials.[35–37]

The efficacy of antiplatelet medications in the treatment of venous thrombosis also is disappointing. Sulfinpyrazone (but not aspirin or dipyridamole) has been shown in some reports to reduce both the incidence of transient ischemic attacks and the mortality from cerebrovascular accidents.[38,39] Retrospective epidemiologic studies have indicated significantly reduced mor-

bidity and mortality from coronary artery disease in aspirin users, but controlled prospective investigations have not yielded similar encouraging results with dipyridamole or aspirin either administered individually or in combination. Trials are underway to determine whether adequate prophylaxis can be provided by larger doses of these antiplatelet drugs.

Also, the clinical significance of decreased platelet survival has not been established; if reduced platelet lifespan predisposes to thrombus formation, then dipyridamole or sulfinpyrazone therapy should provide adequate prophylaxis in conditions associated with decreased platelet survival (i.e., severe rheumatic heart disease and the presence of prosthetic heart valves). However, if reduced platelet survival reflects platelet consumption by an existing thrombus, then antiplatelet therapy theoretically would be less effective. There also is firm evidence that thromboembolic complications in patients with prosthetic heart valves are reduced more by dipyridamole given in conjunction with warfarin than by anticoagulation alone.

Clinical investigations have been conducted to examine the effectiveness of antiplatelet agents in prophylaxis of deep venous thrombosis and pulmonary embolism as well, but the results have been disappointing. Dextran and the other antiplatelet drugs do not appear to affect significantly the incidence of postoperative thrombotic episodes, and none of the antiplatelet drugs approaches the effectiveness of either oral or parenteral anticoagulants. The data, however, are difficult to interpret because of the marked variations in the experimental models.

Therapy with antiplatelet medications requires less supervision and monitoring; however, bleeding complications may develop in patients with hemophilia, von Willebrand disease, or thrombocytopenia. These complications also may occur in those patients concurrently using anticoagulants.

THROMBOLYTIC AGENTS

Once a thrombus has formed in the circulation, anticoagulant therapy may prevent further extension of the clot but has little effect on its lysis. Both physiologic and pharmacologic thrombolysis depend on the activation of the proenzyme plasminogen to form plasmin, a nonspecific proteolytic enzyme that is directed against fibrinogen, fibrin, and various other clotting factors (factor V, factor VIII, and von Willebrand factor) as well as components of the complement system cascade. Plasmin is inhibited rapidly and specifically by α_2-antiplasmin, which along with other, less important circulating inhibitors of plasmin regulates the degree of thrombolysis in vivo.[40] Currently, there are four commercially available therapeutic agents that are used to induce thrombolytic states in vivo; their pharmacologic mechanisms, fibrin specificities, and pharmacokinetics all differ and determine their individual dosing schedules, degree of fibrinogenolysis, and probably their rapidity of lysis as well. Several experimental agents also are being studied.

Streptokinase indirectly activates plasminogen by forming a complex with circulating free plasminogen; this activator complex is the most efficient of the known plasminogen activators. However, the overall pharmacologic mechanism is relatively inefficient, because streptokinase itself has little or no fibrin specificity. Also, inadequate amounts of residual plasminogen may be available to maintain a thrombolytic state after being consumed by the clot and after complexing with streptokinase to form the plasminogen activator. The lack of fibrin specificity increases the likelihood that a systemic lytic state will be produced following streptokinase administration (i.e., significant hypofibrinogenemia and generation of fibrinogen/fibrin degradation products), and it also may contribute to the greater success reported with its use compared with the other thrombolytic agents.[41]

Streptokinase is a metabolite derived from filtrates of group C β-hemolytic streptococcus cultures; as such, this agent is antigenic and may stimulate the formation of antistreptococcal antibodies. The presence of such antibodies in plasma, acquired either from previous untreated streptococcal infections or prior exposure to streptokinase within the past 4 to 6 months, subsequently may blunt or block the generation of a thrombolytic state by streptokinase. The bacterial source of streptokinase also contributes to the high frequency of hypersensitivity reactions (up to 12%) associated with its use; consisting of urticaria, high fevers, hypotension, and rare anaphylaxis, these side effects can be minimized or even eliminated by pretreatment with acetaminophen, diphenhydramine, and hydrocortisone. For the thrombolysis of deep vein thrombosis and pulmonary embolism, streptokinase usually is administered as an intravenous bolus dose of 250,000 IU followed by a maintenance dose of 100,000 IU/hour for 24 to 72 hours in the case of deep venous thrombosis and for 12 to 24 hours in cases with pulmonary emboli. For coronary artery reperfusion, 1.5 million IU is administered over 1 hour, and loading doses of 25,000 to 250,000 IU have been followed by intra-arterial infusions of 5000 to 15,000 IU/hour for up to 48 hours in the lysis of arterial thrombi.

In an attempt to enhance the fibrin specificity of streptokinase, an anisoylated plasminogen-streptokinase activator complex (APSAC, Eminase, Smith Kline Beecham, Philadelphia, PA) has been manufactured.[42] Theoretically, the chemical acylation of the catalytic center of a purified plasminogen-streptokinase activator complex should allow the complex to bind to fibrin before any plasminogen is converted to plasmin, because the activity of the activator complex is dependent on hydrolysis of the acyl group. Thus, localized fibrinolysis should be achieved, and the plasmin generated within the clot should be protected somewhat from its specific circulating inhibitor, α_2-antiplasmin. In practice, however, the fibrin specificity of this agent has been less than expected. APSAC produces marked systemic lytic activity, and as with streptokinase, APSAC also appears to be antigenic. APSAC has been evaluated primarily for the treatment of acute myocardial infarction, with its predominant advantage being the generation of a thrombolytic state rapidly after bolus intravenous infusion. Clinical data suggest that APSAC administered within 4 hours after the onset of cardiac symptoms produces superior coronary angiographic improvement compared with continuous intravenous infusions of streptokinase; however, there were no differences between these two agents in the levels of hypofibrinogenemia produced or the frequency of hemorrhagic complications. Large, randomized clinical studies also are being conducted to compare both the efficacy and safety of APSAC versus recombinant tissue plasminogen activator (tPA) in coronary lysis.

Urokinase is produced normally in the human genitourinary tract and can be extracted either from urine or, more efficiently, from the large-scale cultures of transformed human renal cells; recently, urokinase has been synthesized through recombinant DNA technology. Urokinase directly cleaves plasminogen to form plasmin, and perhaps because of its ability to be adsorbed slightly to fibrin, it does not produce the same degree of systemic hypofibrinogenemia, hypoplasminogenemia, or hemorrhagic complications as streptokinase. Urokinase is not antigenic and rarely produces allergic reactions, fevers, and so on, and it can be readministered at any time without neutralization by circulating antibodies. For the treatment of pulmonary embolus and deep venous thrombosis, urokinase is administered as a bolus dose of 2,000 IU/pound over 15 to 20 minutes, followed by continuous intravenous infusion of 2,000 IU/pound/hour for 12 to 24 hours. For deep venous thrombosis, the infusions were maintained for up to 3 days. Clinical studies revealed no differences in lytic success between urokinase and streptokinase; however, urokinase is approximately 10-fold more expensive. Studies employing innovative bolus dosing of urokinase for the treatment of pulmonary embolus also are being conducted in an attempt to increase both lytic efficacy and clinical safety. Bolus administration of urokinase has been used successfully in the treatment of acute myocardial infarction, but controlled studies have examined urokinase in this context only with continuous infusion regimens. Results indicate that urokinase and recombinant tPA have similar efficacy and safety profiles (urokinase given as a bolus dose of 1.5 million IU followed by 1.5 million IU over 90 minutes).

Single-chain urokinase plasminogen activator (SCUPA) recently has been genetically engineered as the single-chain precursor of conventional urokinase.[43] This agent has a much higher fibrin specificity, but the duration of its lytic effect appears much shorter than with urokinase. Small preliminary studies in patients with acute myocardial infarction indicate that SCUPA can be administered safely and lysis achieved without producing significant hypofibrinogenemia or elevated fibrinogen/fibrin degradation products.

Tissue plasminogen activator is an endogenous plasminogen activator that is synthesized, stored, and released from vascular endothelial cells.[44] Recently, it has been produced through recombinant DNA technology and is available generally for clinical thrombolytic therapy having received Food and Drug Administration approval for the treatment for acute myocardial infarction and pulmonary embolus. Recombinant tPA directly cleaves plasminogen to form plasmin, a reaction that occurs particularly efficiently and rapidly in the presence of fibrin. This localized generation of plasmin on the clot surface may account for the relative degree of fibrin specificity for recombinant tPA; however, in practice, plasminogen consumption results in decreases in fibrinogen concentration, with substantial generation of fibrinogen degradation products. Reductions of α_2-antiplasmin levels are observed as well. Recombinant tPA has received most of its attention because of its rapid reperfusion of coronary artery occlusion. Despite the fact that recombinant tPA (0.75 mg/kg administered intravenously over 90 minutes) produced very rapid clot lysis and reperfusion, significantly less systemic fibrolytic effects, but more hemorrhagic complications than streptokinase, there still have been no mortality advantages observed thus far between these two agents in this situation. Recombinant tPA clearly lyses pulmonary emboli more rapidly and safely than conventional doses of urokinase, but again, no survival advantage or decreased frequency of recurrent emboli have been observed with recombinant tPA. Preliminary studies using recombinant tPA for deep venous thrombosis have yielded encouraging results, but these are no better than for other, less expensive thrombolytic agents.[45,46]

Heparinization should be instituted following termination of thrombolytic therapy and is initiated for deep venous thrombosis and pulmonary embolus when the thrombin time returns to approximately 2 times the normal baseline level. This maneuver helps to prevent rethrombosis as well as propagation of the original thrombus, and by initiating heparin at a dose of 1000 units/hour without a bolus and, subsequently, adjusting the infusion rate to achieve a therapeutic APTT of 1.5 to 2.0 times control values, bleeding complications can be minimized. Oral anticoagulation also can be started within 24 hours with at least a 5-day overlap before discontinuing heparin.

The adequacy of thrombolytic therapy is monitored routinely by fibrinogen determinations and thrombin times, which should be maintained between 2 to 5 times the normal level to avoid hemorrhagic complications. Minimal manipulation of the patient with avoidance of unnecessary invasive procedures and careful patient selection are the keys to a safe and effective thrombolytic therapy. Patients with active internal bleeding or within 2 months of recent stroke should be rejected absolutely for potential thrombolytic therapy, and those within 10 days of major surgery, obstetric delivery, or invasive diagnostic procedures (e.g., renal or hepatic biopsy) or patients with recent major gastrointestinal bleeding, recent hemorrhagic strokes (within 12 months), primary or metastatic tumors in vital organs, underlying coagulopathies, and uncontrolled hypertension are at extremely high risk for developing major complications with thrombolytic therapy and should be excluded unless the therapy is life-saving. Pregnancy is a minor relative contraindication for lytic therapy because of the high risk to both fetus and mother, and urinary pregnancy tests should be performed before therapy in any woman of childbearing potential. The presence of fresh left ventricular thrombi is another relative contraindication, as may be age of greater than 75 years. At all times, the benefit–risk ratio should be in the patient's favor before initiating thrombolytic therapy.

Bleeding is the most commonly encountered complication with thrombolytic therapy, and minor bleeding occurs in up to 40% of patients. With careful patient selection and care, this incidence can be reduced greatly. Severe, life-threatening bleeding problems occur in less than 5% of patients, and intracerebral bleeds have an overall incidence of less than 1.0% with both streptokinase and urokinase and may be 1% to 2% or higher with the new thrombolytic agents. If severe bleeding does occur, then the thrombolytic effects can be reversed rapidly by infusions of fresh-frozen plasma or cryoprecipitate; these products replenish fibrinogen, plasminogen, and α_2-antiplasmin. In addition, antifibrinolytic agents such as ϵ-aminocaproic acid (Amicar, Lederle Laboratories, Wayne, NJ) can be given in a 3- to

5-g bolus intravenously over 30 to 45 minutes, followed by 1.0 g intravenously every 4 to 6 hours to prevent further plasmin formation. Tranexamic acid (Cyklokapron, Kabi Pharmacia, Piscataway, NJ) can be administered as well.

DEFIBRINOGENATING AGENTS

Purified clotting enzymes have been extracted from several crude snake venoms, and these offer a unique approach to antithrombotic therapy. The most thoroughly studied venom fractions are ancrod, from the Malayan pit viper (*Agkistrodon rhodostoma*), and defibrase, from *Bothrops atrox moojeni*. When administered slowly and in small quantities, these agents rapidly deplete circulating fibrinogen without altering the levels of other coagulation factors, activating factor XIII, or affecting platelet function and number. Soluble nonpolymerized fibrin microclots are produced and rapidly cleared by the reticuloendothelial system.

Detailed discussion of these defibrinogenating (thrombin-like) venom extracts is beyond the scope of this chapter. However, the results of several clinical investigations have been encouraging, and these agents perhaps will become available in the future.[47-50] Ancrod is not licensed for use in this country, but it is available commercially in continental Europe, the United Kingdom, Ireland, and Canada.

REFERENCES

1. Rosenberg RD. Actions and interactions of antithrombin and heparin. N Engl J Med 1985;292:146.
2. Rosenberg RD. Heparin action. Circulation 1974;49:603.
3. Wessler S, Yin ET. Theory and practice of mini-dose heparin in surgical patients. Circulation 1973;47:671.
4. Salzman EW, Deykin D, Shapiro RM, Rosenberg R. Management of heparin therapy. N Engl J Med 1975;292:1046.
5. Jacques IB. Intrapulmonary heparin: a new procedure for anticoagulant therapy. Lancet 1976;ii:1157.
6. Makaray AZ, Waterbury L. The activated partial thromboplastin time as a monitor of heparin therapy: a warning. Johns Hopkins Med J 1977;140:311.
7. Shapiro GA, Huntzinger SW, Wilson JE. Variation among commercial activated partial thromboplastin time reagents in response to heparin. Am J Clin Pathol 1977;67:477.
8. Clagett GP, Salzman EW. Prevention of thromboembolism in surgical patients. N Engl J Med 1974;290:93.
9. International multicentre trial: prevention of fatal postoperative pulmonary embolism by low doses of heparin: an international multicentre trial. Lancet 1975;ii:45.
10. Colburn WA. Pharmacologic implications of heparin interactions with other drugs. Drug Metab Rev 1976;5:281.
11. Porter J, Jick H. Drug-related deaths among medical inpatients. JAMA 1977;237:879.
12. Bell WR, Tomasulo PA, Alving BM, Duffy TP. Thrombocytopenia occurring during the administration of heparin. Ann Intern Med 1976;85:155.
13. Stenflo J, Ganrot P. Vitamin K and the biosynthesis of prothrombin: I. Identification and purification of a dicoumarol-induced abnormal prothrombin from bovine plasma. J Biol Chem 1972;247:8160.
14. Stenflo J. Vitamin K and the biosynthesis of prothrombin: IV. Isolation of peptides containing prosthetic groups from normal prothrombin and the corresponding peptides from dicoumarol-induced prothrombin. J Biol Chem 1974;249:5527.
15. Sherry S, ed. Symposium: thrombosis and anticoagulation. Am J Med 1962;33:619.
16. Douglas AS. Anticoagulant Therapy. Philadelphia; F.A. Davis, 1962.
17. Wilding G, Blumberg BS, Vessell ES. Reduced warfarin binding of albumin variants. Science 1977;195:911.
18. Editorial: laboratory control of oral anticoagulants. Lancet 1975;i:317.
19. Koch-Weser J, Sellers EM. Drug interactions with coumarin anticoagulants. N Engl J Med 1971;285:487,547.
20. Sandler AL. Interactions of oral coumarin anticoagulants. In: Hartshort EA, ed. Handbook of Drug Interactions. Hamilton IL: Drug Intelligence Publications, 1973:82.
21. O'Reilly RA, Aggeler PM, Hoag MS, Leong LS, Kropatkin ML. Hereditary transmission of exceptional resistance to coumarin anticoagulant drugs: the first reported kindred. N Engl J Med 1964;271:809.
22. O'Reilly RA. The second reported kindred with hereditary resistance to oral anticoagulant drugs. N Engl J Med 1970;282:1448.
23. Coon WW, Willis PW III. Hemorrhagic complications of anticoagulant therapy. Arch Intern Med 1974;133:386.
24. Fillmore SJ, McDevitt E. Effects of coumarin compounds on the fetus. Ann Intern Med 1970;73:731.
25. Hirsh J, Cade JF, Gallus AS. Fetal effects of coumadin administered during pregnancy. Blood 1970;36:623.
26. Hirsh J, Cade JF, Gallus AS. Anticoagulants in pregnancy: a review of indications and complications. Am Heart J 1972;83:301.
27. Casanegra P, Aviles G, Maturana G, Dubernet J. Cardiovascular management of pregnant women with a heart valve prosthesis. Am J Cardiol 1975;36:802.
28. Pettifor JM, Benson R. Congenital malformations associated with the administration of oral anticoagulants during pregnancy. J Pediatr 1975;86:459.
29. Warkany J. A warfarin embryopathy? Am J Dis Child 1975;129:287.
30. Husted S, Andreasen F. Problems encountered in long-term treatment with anticoagulants. Acta Med Scand 1976;200:379.
31. Pauli RM, Madden JD, Kranzler KJ, Culpepper W, Port R. Warfarin therapy initiated during pregnancy and phenotypic chondrodysplasia punctata. J Pediatr 1976;88:506.
32. Stein B, Fuster V, Israel DH, et al. Platelet inhibitor agents in cardiovascular disease: an update. J Am Coll Cardiol 1989;14:813.
33. Roth GJ, Majerus PW. The mechanism of the effect of aspirin on human platelets. J Clin Invest 1977;56:624.
34. Au M, McDonald JWD. Effects of sulfinpyrazone on platelet prostaglandin synthesis and platelet release of serotonin. J Lab Clin Med 1977;89:868.
35. Mustard JF, Packham MA. Platelets, thrombosis and drugs. Drugs 1975;9:19.
36. Genton E, Gent M, Hirsh J, Harker LA. Platelet-inhibiting drugs in the prevention of clinical thrombotic disease. N Engl J Med 1975;293:1174,1236,1296.
37. Verstraete M. Are agents affecting platelet functions clinically useful? Am J Med 1976;61:897.
38. Evans G, Gent M. Effect of platelet suppressive drugs on arterial

and venous thromboembolism. In: Hirsch J, Cade JF, Gallus AS, Schonbaum E, eds. Platelets, Drugs, and Thrombosis. Basel: Karger, 1975:258.

39. Blakely JA, Gent M. Platelets, drugs, and longevity in a geriatric population. In: Hirsch J, Cade JF, Gallus AS, Schonbaum E, eds. Platelets, Drugs, and Thrombosis. Basel: Karger, 1975:284.

40. Marder VJ, Sherry S. Thrombolytic therapy: current status. N Engl J Med 1988;318:1512–20,1585–95.

41. Gruppo Italiano per L. Studio Della Soparavvenenza. GISSI-3: a factorial randomized trial of alteplase versus streptokinase and heparin versus no heparin among 12,490 patients with acute myocardial infarction. Lancet 1990;336:65–71.

42. Crabbe SJ, Grimm AM, Hopkins LE. Acylated plasminogen-streptokinase activator complex: a new approach to thrombolytic therapy. Pharmacotherapy 1990;10:115–26.

43. Primi Study Group. Randomized double-blind trial of recombinant prourokinase against streptokinase in acute myocardial infarction. Lancet 1989;i:863–8.

44. Sobel BE. Coronary thrombolyses and the new biology. J Am Coll Cardiol 1989;14:850–60.

45. Rentrop P, Blanke H, Karsel KR, Kaiser H, Kostering H, Leitz K. Selective intracoronary thrombolysis in acute myocardial infarction and unstable angina pectoris. Circulation 1981;63:307.

46. Ganz W, Buchbinder N, Marcus H, et al. Intracoronary thrombolysis in evolving myocardial infarction. Am Heart J 1981; 101:4.

47. Bell WR, Pitney WR, Goodwin JF. Therapeutic defibrination in the treatment of thrombotic disease. Lancet 1968;i:490.

48. Olsen EGJ, Pitney WR. The effect of Arvin on experimental pulmonary embolism. Br J Haematol 1969;17:425.

49. Sharp AA, Warren BA, Paxton AM, Allington MJ. Anticoagulant therapy with a purified fraction of Malayan pit viper venom. Lancet 1968;i:493.

50. Cole CW, Bormanes J. Ancrod: a practical alternative to heparin. J Vasc Surg 1988;8:59.

20

Blood Banking and Transfusion Principles

Paul M. Ness, M.D., and Thomas S. Kickler, M.D.

IMMUNOHEMATOLOGY

Blood groups are determined by the presence of antigenic substances on the surface of the red cell. These substances either are an integral part of the red cell membrane itself, such as Rh antigens, or are outward molecular extensions from the membrane, such as ABO antigens. That these antigenic determinants are present on the red cells of some people and absent from those of others is a result of genetic heterogeneity. Antibodies to red cells occur in human subjects or animals who lack these antigens even when there has been no known exposure to these particular antigens, and such "naturally occurring" antibodies are thought to result from exposure to substances with similar antigenic determinants either in the environment or in foods.[1]

The blood groups of human red cells remain constant throughout life, except for uncommon circumstances when they are modified by disease, and their inheritance follows mendelian genetic laws. The function of blood group antigens on the red cell generally is unknown; however, we are becoming increasingly aware of the associations between disease states and antigenic patterns on red cells. For example, there is a known association between a susceptibility to malaria and the Duffy blood group, and there are unusual Kell antigen groups in some patients with chronic granulomatous disease.[2,3] In some cases, the absence of a blood group produces abnormalities of red cell function, such as the compensated hemolytic state found in patients who lack any Rh antigens (i.e., Rh null disease).[4]

Although the functions of blood group antigens remain speculative, their importance in clinical medicine cannot be questioned. The application of blood group serology is essential for the safety of blood transfusions as well as tissue transplantations. Blood groups are important markers in both genetic and anthropologic studies, and in addition, blood group identification is useful in paternity testing and forensic medicine.

Our knowledge of the biochemistry of blood groups is expanding rapidly for some groups but is still rudimentary for others. In some instances, antigenic determinants similar to blood group antigens are found on substances present in body fluids, such as milk and plasma, and in cyst fluid; these substances can be purified to obtain adequate amounts of blood group antigen for biochemic analysis and have facilitated an understanding of the ABO, Lewis, and P blood groups. Antigens that are found only on the red cell membrane have proven difficult to purify in quantities sufficient for study, but some, such as Rh, recently have been subjected to biochemic analysis and now are better understood.

Serologic Identification of Blood Group Antigens

The interaction of red cell blood groups and antibodies directed against these antigens usually is detected by agglutination methods in the blood bank. Agglutination of red cells can be considered to have two distinct phases: the first (sensitization) where antibody makes physical contact with antigen, and the second (agglutination) where antibody-coated cells interact with each other. Some antibodies, particularly those of the IgM class, can cause agglutination of red cells directly; their pentameric structure is sufficient to bridge the distance between cells and has led to their description as *complete antibodies*. Most antibodies of the IgG class fail to agglutinate red cells unless the red cell surface charge is manipulated or bridging is enhanced by other means; these antibodies are described as *incomplete*, denoting an antibody that reacts with but fails to produce visible agglutination of erythrocytes. Agglutination by incomplete or coating antibodies can be facilitated by various means such as proteolytic enzymes, addition of albumin, or treatment with antiglobulin reagents.[5,6]

Temperature is important in blood group serology. Some antibodies are considered "warm" and react best at 37°C; these usually are the most important in transfusion and the most likely to cause adverse transfusion reactions. Other antibodies react best in the cold in vitro but still may be reactive at temperatures approaching that of the body; these "cold" antibodies that react above 30°C are considered to have a high thermal amplitude and may cause in vivo clinical problems.[7]

Blood group antibody attachment can be affected by pH as well.[8] For example, some antibodies reactive against the M antigen are enhanced at pH 5.5, whereas others are best detected at neutral pH. In addition, red cell sensitization by antibody is time-dependent, and although prolonged incubation can increase the amount of antibody coating, clinical practice often demands a quick answer. Thus, laboratory procedures are designed to produce adequate sensitization in minimal time.

The ionic strength of the reaction medium affects the rate of antibody sensitization on the red cell;[9] red cells possess a large electronegative charge that prevents spontaneous aggregation and facilitates gas exchange. The suspension of red cells in electrolyte media such as saline causes cations to form around the cell in a positively charged ionic cloud, and the resulting positive charge or zeta potential can deter binding of positively charged immunoglobulin molecules as well as hamper sensitization. The use of low ionic-strength solution has made an important practical impact on blood banking by reducing the time required for antibody detection and crossmatching incubations; it has been determined experimentally that low ionic-strength solution enhances the rate of antibody uptake but does not accelerate the second stage (agglutination).[10]

The ratio of antibody to antigen also can affect the rate of antibody attachment in red cell sensitization. Although sensitization typically is enhanced by increasing the amount of antibody, a paradoxic result can occur, with reduced sensitization by increased antibody. This prozone phenomenon must be considered in serologic investigations.[11]

Treatment of red cells with proteolytic enzymes has been shown experimentally to enhance antibody binding and red cell agglutination;[12] their mechanism of action is to remove negatively charged molecules of sialic acid and protein. Enzyme treatment also permits movement of the red cell antigens in the membrane to form antigen clusters that also enhance agglutination.[13] Enzymes enhance the reactivity of antibodies to some blood groups, such as Rh and Kidd, but prevent detection of other blood group antibodies such as MNSs and Duffy; therefore, their use must be selective and supplementary to other techniques.

Albumin also is thought to enhance agglutination reactions, but its mechanism of action is not known clearly.[14] Albumin may raise the dielectric constant of the medium and lower the zeta potential to permit agglutination, and other studies suggest that the decreased ionic strength of albumin solutions actually may enhance agglutination.

The most commonly used means of demonstrating the presence of IgG antibodies that do not agglutinate red cells directly is the antiglobulin test.[15] Antisera are prepared by injecting animals with human IgG and then harvesting the immune serum. The addition of antiglobulin serum to red cells coated with IgG will cause agglutination. If the cells are coated in vivo, the presence of IgG is determined by a direct antiglobulin (Coombs) test; when the red cells are tested in vitro with human serum, the presence of incomplete antibodies in the serum can be detected by agglutination after the addition of antiglobulin serum using the indirect antiglobulin test. Some blood group antibodies can activate the complement cascade,[16] and complement activation can lead to lysis of the red cells or result in complement sensitization without lysis. Antiglobulin serum, therefore, usually is designed to be "broad spectrum" or "polyspecific," with reactivity against human IgG as well as human complement components such as C3. The so-called monospecific reagents will react with IgG or complement components (C3 or C3d) alone.[17]

ABO System

The ABO system was the first blood group recognized, and it remains pre-eminent in blood transfusion practice. In 1900, Landsteiner tested red cells and sera from his laboratory workers and noted that the sera from some workers agglutinated the cells of others but not their own.[18] He then divided individuals into three groups (A, B, and O) based on these experiments, and in 1902, Von Decastello and Sturli found the fourth group, AB. The ABO classification is based on the detection of two antigens (A and B) on the red cells and two antibodies (anti-A and anti-B) in the serum.

A reciprocal relationship exists whereby the presence of an antigen on the red cell prohibits the presence of an antibody against that antigen in the serum, and this reciprocal relationship is the basis of routine serologic practice in the blood bank. Two antisera, anti-A and anti-B, are used to test the patient's red cells, a practice known as *front-typing* or *forward grouping*. The patient's serum also is tested with cells of known ABO group, termed *back-typing* or *reverse grouping,* and these results are compared and, typically, are confirmatory. Discrepant results, however, can be an important clue to serologic difficulties and require further investigation in all cases.

Routine ABO typing identifies four common phenotypes (Table 20.1). Red cells that react with anti-A can be characterized further by their reactions with anti-A_1, which distinguishes patients with A_1 from A_2. A_1 cells also can be identified by their reactions with plant seed lectins such as *Dolichus biflorus*. Patients with type A_2 or A_2B can form antibodies against A_1 red cells, which can cause hemolysis in rare patients, so the distinction between types A_1 and A_2 can be significant clinically. Also, rare patients with type A subgroups (such as A_3, A_m, or A_x) have even fewer antigen sites and generally are recognized because of ABO typing discrepancies.[19]

That patients routinely have anti-A, anti-B, or both in their serum if they lack the corresponding blood groups on their red cells also explains the clinical importance of recognizing the ABO blood group system. The high density of ABO antigen sites on the red cell are ready targets for the IgM anti-A or anti-B isoagglutinins, and their interaction usually causes significant destruction of red cells. ABO-incompatible blood, administered inadvertently as a result of clerical errors, remains the most common cause of fatal transfusion reactions.[20]

It therefore is highly desirable to transfuse patients only with ABO-identical blood. Patients with the uncommon AB type have been considered as universal recipients in the past because they lack anti-A and anti-B; likewise, group O red cells (universal donor) are considered safe for administration to all patients. Blood supplies generally are adequate to avoid using universal donor blood except in cases of major trauma when transfusion is mandated before blood grouping can be

completed. Group O blood is administered as red cells on these occasions to avoid the potential problem of anti-A and anti-B in the donor plasma. ABO-incompatible plasma products should be avoided if large volumes are to be administered to small-blood-volume recipients.

The expression of ABO antigens both on the red cell and in body fluids results from the interactions of several genetic loci and the subsequent interaction with precursor substances of their gene products.[18,21] ABO specificity on the red cell arises from glycosphingolipid molecules that are inserted into the red cell membrane, but expression of ABO antigens requires the presence of another gene, *H*. ABO antigens are expressed on glycoproteins that occur in body fluid secretions if the secretor gene *Se* is present. The Lewis gene, *Le*, also acts on the oligosaccharide chain that determines *A, B,* and *H* gene activity; these genes are closely related, act on the same precursor substances, but are not linked. *ABO* genes have been localized to chromosome 9 in humans. The *Le, Se,* and *H* gene loci are on chromosome 19.

ABO specificity is determined by the conjugation of sugar molecules to an oligosaccharide chain, and the specific ABO gene product is an enzyme transferase that couples monosaccharides in a characteristic sequence to confer blood group specificity. ABO expression requires the preliminary action of a transferase, resulting from the presence of the *H* gene, which conjugates a fucose molecule to the precursor chain. Patients who lack H substance are considered to be genotype *hh* and cannot add the fucose to produce H substance. The presence of this fucose molecule is required for the action of specific ABO transferase; therefore, individuals who lack H cannot produce ABO antigens. The *hh* genotype results in the rare Bombay phenotype, and these patients lack H substance and ABO antigens on the red cells and produce antibodies against H, A, and B, permitting transfusion only with blood from donors with the Bombay phenotype.[22]

H substance is a precursor molecule for the action of ABO gene products. If the *A* gene is present, a transferase is produced and attaches *N*-acetylgalactosamine to the H substance, thus producing A antigen; in the presence of the *B* gene, a different transferase enzyme

TABLE 20.1. ABO Grouping

Cells Tested With		Serum Tested With		Interpretation	Frequency in U.S. Population (%)	
Anti-A	Anti-B	A Cells	B Cells	ABO Group	White	Black
0	0	+	+	O	45	49
+	0	0	+	A	40	27
0	+	+	0	B	11	20
+	+	0	0	AB	4	4

adds galactose to produce B substance. The third possible gene, *O*, is an amorph and produces no transferase, so the H substance remains unmodified. The *A*, *B*, and *O* genes are codominant; one cannot determine whether a patient who types as group A is homozygous *AA* or heterozygous *AO* without family studies or the measurement of transferase activity.

A third gene, *Se* (secretor), determines whether ABO specificity will be found only on red cells or additionally in body fluid secretions. The presence of the *Se* gene in approximately 85% of the general population permits the attachment of the oligosaccharides determining the ABH to the peptide chains; these glycoprotein molecules are water soluble and result in ABH specificity in body fluids. Patients who lack the *Se* gene (genotype, *sese*) do not have soluble ABO antigens, but their red cells do have normal ABO expression resulting from glycolipid antigen sites.

The Lewis gene product is a transferase that also acts on the oligosaccharide chain determining ABO specificity. The presence of the *Le* gene facilitates incorporation of a fucose residue to *N*-acetylgalactosamine, and the Lewis antigens that appear on the red cell surface as well as in secretions depend on the presence or absence of both *Lele* genes and *Sese* genes. In patients who are nonsecretors (*sese*) but who inherit the *Le* gene, the red cells have the Le^a antigen. If the patient inherits the *Se* gene, the molecule produced has fucose on the terminal galactose as well as the adjacent *N*-acetylgalactosamine, creating the molecule Le^b on the red cell. Lewis antigens on the red cells result from the passive adsorption of these substances from soluble glycoproteins in the plasma.[23] Also, red cells from patients who lack the *Le* gene and whose red cells are Le(a−b−) can be converted to Le(a+) by incubation with plasma from a Le(a+) donor.

The Rh System

The awareness of the blood group system termed *Rh* began in 1939, when Levine and Stetson published a case where the mother of a stillborn baby had a transfusion reaction after receiving the husband's ABO-compatible blood.[24] The mother's serum was found to react with the husband's red cells, and with approximately 80% of other ABO-compatible donors. These findings suggested that the mother's immune system had recognized and made antibody to a foreign antigen on the father's red cells and that the baby had inherited the father's antigen. In 1940, Landsteiner and Wiener found additional evidence when they discovered that sera raised in rabbits and guinea pigs who had been injected with rhesus monkey red cells would agglutinate rhesus cells as well as 80% of the red cells from Caucasian blood donors;[25] they designated the donors whose cells reacted with their sera as *Rh positive*. Wiener and Peters later demonstrated the presence of anti-Rh antibody in the sera of a patient who had transfusion reactions with ABO-compatible blood,[26] and these findings led to the association of Rh incompatibility and erythroblastosis fetalis and were the discoveries forecasting the importance of the Rh blood group in routine transfusion.

Although the Rh system now has been shown to contain at least 30 different specificities, the original specificity identified, Rh$_o$(D), remains the most important. Unlike the ABO system, antibodies to the D antigen only arise after stimulation from incompatible pregnancies or transfusions. The antigen can be detected on red cells in routine practice, but the extra assurance that is possible for ABO through back-typing the serum is not possible for RH. It also has been found that small aliquots of less than 1 ml of D-positive red cells can immunize Rh negative recipients, and 50% of the 75% of Rh negative patients receiving Rh positive blood will produce anti-D antibody.[27] For these reasons, donor blood and patient's red cells are typed routinely for the D antigen; it also is routine that Rh negative recipients receive Rh negative blood products. The donor classification of Rh positive or negative is determined solely by the presence or absence of the D antigen on the red cells.

The genetics and biochemistry of the Rh system are areas of active research. Rh antigens are found only on red cells and are not secreted in body fluids, so material for biochemical investigations is difficult to obtain. That patients with no detectable Rh antigens (Rh null) have red cell membrane abnormalities suggests that Rh antigens are an integral part of the membrane. The D antigen is associated with a transmembrane polypeptide that is absent in Rh null cells, and the presence of the D antigen has been found to be an autosomal dominant trait. In addition, the *Rh* gene has been localized to chromosome 1 by other studies.[28]

Further attempts to characterize sera from patients with transfusion reactions revealed other antigens that are associated with the principal Rh antigen, Rh$_o$(D). In addition, it was soon recognized that four other specificities could be determined and played a clinical role in transfusion; these antigens are called rh′(C), rh″(E), hr′(c), and hr″(e). These antigens also are the result of the *Rh* gene or system of genes on chromosome 1, and they behave as mendelian codominants (e.g., a patient can be homozygous *CC*, heterozygous *Cc*, or homozygous *cc*). The gene that produces the D antigen is autosomal dominant as well, but a corresponding d antigen has not been found. Patients who are homozygous for D have never made an antibody (anti-d), leading to the current theory that the *d* gene is an amorph similar to the *O* gene in the ABO system.

The five principal Rh antigens appear to be inherited either through the action of a single gene locus with multiple alleles or by several closely linked genes. That certain antigens commonly are expressed together, such as c and e in the absence of D, suggested to Wiener that one gene with many alleles was inherited. Wiener's theory proposes that the gene product is a single molecular entity, termed an *agglutinogen,* that is characterized by multiple antigenic sites, and the Rh-Hr terminology is derived from this theory.[29] Fisher and Race postulated that the Rh system is composed of three closely linked genes that code individually for D or d, C or c, and E or e,[30] and the resulting terminology uses CDE notation. Still a third terminology, proposed by Rosenfield et al.,[31] uses numeric nomenclature and is not based on any particular gene structure theory. Because the debate among proponents of the Fisher and Race or the Wiener system has not been resolved by experimental evidence, most immunohematologists use a combination of the two notations systems (Table 20.2).

In clinical practice, only five reagent antisera are used (anti-D, -C, -E, -c, and -e). For most transfusion-related work, evaluation with anti-D alone is sufficient; the other four antisera are used for antibody investigations, family studies, and paternity testing. One can characterize red cells for Rh phenotype by these five antisera, and a Rh genotype then can be predicted based on genotype studies from families of known racial backgrounds (Table 20.2). That d is amorphic as well as the resulting inability to distinguish a patient who is homozygous for D from a patient who is heterozygous, complicates the prediction of Rh genotype from serologic testing.

The distinction between Rh positive and negative cells usually is simple, but it is complicated by the fact that some Rh positive cells react only weakly with anti-D antisera. Rh typing is performed with antisera that agglutinates most Rh positive red cells directly, but occasional Rh positive cells can be shown to possess Rh₀(D) antigen only with the addition of antiglobulin serum. This weakened expression of the Rh₀(D) antigen is termed *Du.* In practice, donor blood with the Du phenotype is less immunogenic than Rh positive blood that is identified by standard agglutination practices.[32] The transfusion of patients with the Du phenotype is controversial; the safest approach is the use of Rh negative blood.

The Rh blood system plays an important role in transfusion. Because the Rh₀(D) antigen is highly immunogenic and the 85% of donors who possess the antigen can immunize readily the 15% of patients who lack the antigen, Rh positive blood products should be administered only to Rh positive recipients. Even though the antigen is limited to red cells and is not known to be present in the plasma, white cells, or platelets, many of these blood products are contaminated with red cells. Therefore, Rh positive platelets or granulocytes should be avoided in Rh negative recipients; frozen plasma products do not contain enough red cells to be a clinical problem. The other common cause of Rh immunization, Rh incompatible pregnancy, can be modified by the ability of passive immunity, arising from the injection of anti-D antibody to prevent the immunization of Rh negative mothers from the small amounts of blood passed from their Rh positive babies at delivery.[33] The routine administration of anti-D to Rh negative mothers postpartum reduces the risk of immunization from approximately 15% of mothers at risk to approximately 1%,[34] and this reduction in sensitization has lowered both the incidence of hemolytic disease in newborn babies due to anti-Rh₀(D) and fetal morbidity and mortality.

Other Blood Groups

In addition to those of the ABO and Rh systems, there are at least 500 other blood group antigens that can be detected on the surface of red blood cells, and they can be divided in two groups: antigens whose absence commonly is accompanied by naturally occurring antibodies, and antigens where alloantibodies are found only with previous immunization. The former commonly are not associated with transfusion problems, because the antibodies generally do not cause immune red cell destruction. The latter group can cause hemolysis and clinical problems, but these antigens are less immunogenic than Rh₀(D). When these antibodies are present, incompatible blood is avoided, but no routine attempt is made to administer donor blood that matches the patient's phenotype unless prior immunization has occurred. Occasionally, these blood groups and their

TABLE 20.2. Rh Gene Frequencies

Wiener	Fisher-Race	U.S. Frequency (%)	
		White	Black
R¹	CDe	42	17
r	cde	37	26
R²	cDE	14	11
R⁰	cDe	4	44
r′	Cde	2	2
r″	cdE	1	1
Rᶻ	CDE	1	1
rʸ	CdE	1	1

antibodies accompany hematologic disease in noteworthy patterns (Table 20.3).

The Lewis blood group system has been described previously in conjunction with ABO. Both anti-Le[a] and anti-Le[b] can occur naturally and rarely are of clinical concern. Because these antibodies usually are IgM and cannot cross the placenta, and also because Lewis antigens are developed poorly on the cord red cells, Lewis antibodies do not cause hemolytic disease of the newborn. The antibodies usually do not react at 37°C, so compatible blood can be found by crossmatching at 37°C. Lewis antibodies also are detected commonly during pregnancy, when red cells tend to lose Lewis antigen strength. In general, the presence of Lewis antibodies is a nuisance that can impede red cell transfusions; Lewis incompatibility, however, has been shown to be related to renal allograft survival and may play a future role in transplant donor selection.[35]

The P system has been characterized biochemically largely due to its presence in hydatid cyst fluids.[36] It rarely is related to transfusion problems unless the patient is of the rare p phenotype. Patients with the unusual hemolytic syndrome of paroxysmal cold hemoglobinuria have an autoantibody characterized by the Donath-Landsteiner test that usually has P specificity.[37]

The MNSs system is a complicated blood group whose biochemistry is unfolding under current investigation.[38] Certain antibodies to its antigens (anti-M, anti-N) usually occur naturally and are unlikely to produce transfusion difficulties; anti-S, -s, and -U (an uncommon antibody occurring in blacks whose red cells are negative for the S and s antigens) usually are immune antibodies and can cause both hemolytic disease of the newborn and transfusion reactions.

The Ii system differs from other blood groups in several ways. The i antigen is abundant on fetal and newborn red cells, but I antigen strength increases gradually and becomes predominant before 2 years of age.[39] There is considerable variability, however, with rare adults (1 in 10,000) remaining predominantly i throughout life. In patients with bone marrow stress, there may be increased reactivity of i on the red cells with normal I reactivity,[40] and many healthy blood donors have cold-reacting autoantibodies with anti-I activity in their sera that are without clinical significance. In patients with cold agglutinin disease, autoantibodies to I antigen increase in titer and thermal amplitude and may cause in vivo hemolysis; many of these pathologic cold antibodies are monoclonal and occur in association with lymphoproliferative diseases. Also, the cold agglutinin syndrome associated with viral syndromes can have polyclonal anti-I (mycoplasma infections) or anti-i (infectious mononucleosis).[41]

The Kell, Kidd, and Duffy systems are polymorphic blood groups that frequently are implicated in transfusion reactions or hemolytic disease of the newborn after the Rh system has been cleared of suspicion. Antibodies to these antigens usually are IgG, and these antibodies can cause severe reactions even though their presence may be difficult to detect. Antibodies to Kidd antigens are notorious for weak or evanescent reactions, but they can be enhanced by enzymes or detected using homozygous cells. Duffy antibodies can cause serious reactions, and their in vitro reactivity is weakened when the red cell targets are treated with proteolytic enzymes (an important differential point in serology). Also of additional interest is that cells which are negative for the common Duffy antigens (Fy[a] and Fy[b]) are resistant to invasion by malaria parasites.[2] The Kell system has an unusual association with hematologic disease, and a weakened expression of Kell antigens on the red cells (the McLeod phenotype) has been found in some young males with chronic granulomatous disease, an X-linked disorder affecting granulocytes. Patients with the McLeod phenotype may have abnormalities of their red cells and blood film with many acanthocytes; the common link is the lack of a precursor antigen Kx, which is required for normal granulocyte function and Kell antigen expression. Patients can have chronic granulomatous disease without red cell antigen abnormalities, in concert with

TABLE 20.3. Other Blood Groups

Blood Group	Common Antigens	Clinical Significance	Other Associations
Lewis	Le[a], Le[b]	Rare	Transplantation antigen
P	P$_1$, P$_2$, p	Rare	PCH specificity
MNSsU	M, N, S, s, U	M, N-rare	
		S, s, U-common	
Ii	I, i	Rare (unless autoantibody)	Cold hemolytic anemia
			Marrow stress
Kell	K, k	Common	CGD
Kidd	Jk[a], Jk[b]	Common	
Duffy	Fy[a], Fy[b]	Common	Malaria

the McLeod phenotype, or may have abnormal red cells without granulocyte dysfunction.[3]

PRINCIPLES OF TRANSFUSION THERAPY

To use blood products appropriately, one must know what products are available as well as their respective therapeutic advantages. Every transfusion carries a risk of isoimmunization, incompatibility, and hepatitis transmission; as with any therapy administered to a patient, the potential benefit should be weighed against the potential risk before prescribing the blood components. When a transfusion is considered essential, there is much that the blood bank can do to ensure its safety. However, the requesting physician also can help to minimize the risk by following two basic transfusion principles. First, patients should receive only specific blood components to correct the deficiency without supplying unnecessary cells or plasma proteins that may lead to complications. Second, it is unnecessary to correct a deficiency to normal levels; rather, physiologic levels only should be restored, allowing the patient's own homeostatic mechanisms to make any additional correction following short-term treatment. This approach minimizes the number of transfusions received and thereby reduces the exposure risk.

Modern medical and surgical practice generally has been guided by the practice of transfusing patients when the hemoglobin falls below 10 g/dl, but this guideline probably is too liberal for the majority of patients. Clinical observations of patients with chronic anemic conditions, such as those associated with renal failure or sickle cell anemia, suggest that hemoglobin values of 7 to 8 g/dl do not always lead to clinical impairment. Reports detailing several series of patients who refused blood transfusions also suggest that many major operations are tolerated without adverse effect.[42]

The decision to transfuse a specific patient requires the consideration of the duration of the anemia, the blood volume loss, and any conditions that might impair oxygen delivery to the tissues. Those patients with impaired pulmonary function, peripheral vascular disease, poor cardiac output, or cardiac ischemia may need to be transfused at a higher hemoglobin concentration than if these conditions were absent. Also, for uncompromised patients, delaying transfusion until hemoglobin values of 7 g/dl are reached may be appropriate.[42]

Red Blood Cell Products

A variety of red cell products currently are available for transfusion; Table 20.4 lists these products along

TABLE 20.4.   Indications for Products Containing Red Cells

Red Blood Cells Product	Clinical Use
Whole blood	Simultaneous correction of anemia and blood volume
	Exchange transfusion
Red cell concentrates	Correction of anemia
Leukocyte-poor red cells	Prevention of febrile transfusion reactions
	Reduction in HLA alloimmunization
Washed red cells	Severe allergic transfusion reactions
Frozen-deglycerolized red cells	Same as leukocyte-poor or washed red cells
	Long-term storage for autologous transfusion
	Storage of rare phenotypes

with their clinical use. Each has particular characteristics that determine its effectiveness in a given clinical situation.

WHOLE BLOOD. Massive hemorrhage is best treated with whole blood, because both red cells and plasma are replaced simultaneously. Prompt correction of the intravascular volume depletion is important to prevent the sequelae of prolonged hypotension (i.e., acidosis, disseminated intravascular coagulation, renal failure). Other red cell products also may be used instead of whole blood when in combination with volume expanders (i.e., crystalloid, plasma, or plasma derivatives such as albumin or plasma protein fraction).

One theoretic concern that has developed about transfusion of stored whole blood is the ability to maintain adequate hemostasis. After 24 hours, blood stored at 4°C lacks viable platelets, and replacement of lost blood with platelet-free blood could result in dilution of the recipient's platelet count. In the massively transfused patient, this dilutional thrombocytopenia has not been found to be significant clinically until 15 or 20 units have been given;[43] if thrombocytopenia does develop, platelet concentrates can be administered to raise the platelet count above 50,000 cells/mm^3.

The other hemostatic change that occurs on storage is a gradual decrease in the levels of coagulation factors V and VIII. By day 21 of storage, factor V levels range from 20% to 60% of normal; factor VIII levels range from 20% to 50%.[44] The clinical significance of these deficiencies is minimal if one recalls that the level of factor V required for surgical hemostasis is approximately 15% of normal and that of factor VIII 30% to 40%.[45] The other coagulation factors are stable in stored blood; hence, in the uncompromised recipient, whole blood will maintain clotting factors at adequate levels for hemostasis.

These considerations do not preclude the necessity of monitoring the coagulation profiles of patients receiving massive transfusions. When hemostatic insufficiency does develop, therapy is assessed best by monitoring the platelet count, prothrombin time, partial thromboplastin time, and fibrinogen, and when the urgency of the situation is such that empiric transfusion therapy is necessary, platelet concentrates (6 to 8 units) should be given after the transfusion of 15 units of whole blood. Routine administration of fresh-frozen plasma also has been advocated, but no evidence is available to support this recommendation.

RED CELL CONCENTRATES. Packed red cells are obtained from a unit of whole blood by removing the plasma, and they are preserved for 35 days when collected into citrate-phosphate-dextrose-adenine (CPD-A). The resultant unit of red cells has a volume of approximately 300 ml and a hematocrit between 65% and 80%. Red cells are the component of choice when the restoration of oxygen-carrying capacity alone is required; if the patient has chronic anemia, congestive heart failure, or is elderly, then transfusing with red cells minimizes the volume expansion and maximally improves the oxygen delivery. A second advantage is that nonhemolytic transfusion reactions occur less frequently after the transfusion of packed cells than with whole blood.[46] Some red cell concentrates are collected into an extended preservative solution that allows storage for up to 42 days, and these red cells have virtually all of the plasma removed and a volume of 350 ml because of the additive solution.

FROZEN RED CELLS. Red cells can be frozen effectively with a cryoprotective agent such as glycerol and stored for several years,[47] but the indications for this product are limited. Freezing red cells can provide an inventory of phenotyped red cells for transfusion to patients with complex antibody problems or for those patients who require rare blood types; freezing also provides a mechanism for storing autologous units that may be used in future surgery or with patients who are unlikely to have compatible blood available. The freezing and subsequent deglycerolization procedure removes IgA protein and leukocyte antigens, so frozen cells are useful in reducing immunologic reactions. However, other potential advantages, such as the prevention either of hepatitis transmission or of graft-versus-host disease in immunodeficient recipients, have not materialized.[48,49]

LEUKOCYTE-POOR BLOOD. Patients receiving multiple transfusions as well as multiparous women may develop antibodies to leukocytes. When transfused with incompatible leukocytes contained in red cell units, febrile reactions may occur, and to prevent these reactions, leukocyte-poor red cells prepared by differential centrifugation, filtration, or cell washing are recommended. Most reactions are prevented by removing at least 70% of the leukocytes.[50] If severe febrile transfusion reactions still occur, then frozen red cells are used.

WASHED RED CELLS. Washing red cells with isotonic saline solution removes almost all plasma and nonred-cell constituents. This product is indicated for patients with severe allergic reactions to plasma constituents; in particular, those patients with IgA deficiency should receive washed cells.

Blood Derivatives

Human serum albumin is the most commonly used plasma volume expander. This is produced by fractionating plasma and collecting Cohn Fraction V. The most widely available product is a 25% solution, and in the manufacturing process, heating inactivates any viruses, so there is no risk of hepatitis. The primary indication for its administration is volume expansion; however, much debate exists whether crystalloid solutions alone are not equally effective in correcting hypovolemia. Other possible indications are cardiac bypass pump priming, fluid replacement for burn patients, adult respiratory distress syndrome, and acute nephrosis.[51,52]

If during the fractionation of plasma both Cohn Fraction V (albumin) and Cohn Fraction IV are not separated further, then the product is termed *plasma protein fraction*. This product can be used for the same indications as albumin. Plasma protein factor has been implicated in causing severe hypotension when rapidly infused, but this hypotensive effect is mediated by prekallikrein activator, which acts on kininogen to produce bradykinin.[53]

Clinical Considerations When Transfusing Stored Blood

The preservation of blood in the liquid state is achieved by storage at from 1°C to 6°C and by the addition of anticoagulant preservatives that allow the red cells to maintain adenosine triphosphate. Until recently, however, the only available preservative solutions were acid citrate dextrose and citrate-phosphate-dextrose (CPD), but CPD-A now has been introduced as the standard anticoagulant preservative, extending the available storage time to 35 days.[54] These storage conditions lead to several biochemical and functional changes in the erythrocytes that potentially may affect the recipient; hence, it is important to know the altered characteristics of stored blood so these potential adverse effects of transfusion can be monitored.

HEMOGLOBIN FUNCTION. The initial pH of blood collected in CPD-A is 7.55, falling to 6.71 by day 35 as a result of the accumulation of hydrogen ions generated from the metabolism of glucose to lactate.[55] As the pH decreases, the 2,3-diphosphoglycerate (2,3-DPG) levels also fall because of the decreased enzymatic activity of hexokinase, phosphofructokinase, and DPG-mutase. The 2,3-DPG plays an important role in oxygen delivery to the tissues because of its stabilizing effect on the deoxyhemoglobin conformation of hemoglobin, thus facilitating the oxygen delivery.

When blood is stored in CPD-A, adequate 2,3-DPG levels are maintained for 12 to 14 days but then decline gradually to less than 5% of the initial value. This stored blood, now depleted of 2,3-DPG, has an increased oxygen affinity and is less efficient at oxygen delivery. However, the clinical importance of transfused erythrocytes with low 2,3-DPG levels is unclear.

In the recipient, transfused red cells regenerate 2,3-DPG levels up to at least 50% of normal within several hours.[56] After 24 hours, the oxygen–hemoglobin affinity is corrected to near normal.[57] In the patient who is able to increase cardiac output, adequate oxygen delivery is maintained despite these biochemic changes that affect hemoglobin function, and studies of resuscitation in seriously injured male soldiers showed adequate oxygen delivery to tissue after three blood-volume exchanges of 2,3-DPG–depleted erythrocytes.[58] However, Dennis et al.[59] have suggested that patients with compromised homeostatic mechanisms may be affected adversely by the transfusion of red cells with increased oxygen affinity. Further work is needed to clarify these theoretical concerns, but at present, it appears that transfusion with stored blood is adequate to meet the oxygen-delivery requirements for the vast majority of patients undergoing transfusion.

ACID LOAD. Stored blood demonstrates the biochemical changes of both metabolic acidosis (plasma HCO_3—8—12 mEq) and respiratory acidosis (P_{CO_2}—104—130 torr). The respiratory element is eliminated readily by the lungs, resulting in no elevation of Pa_{CO_2} in patients receiving transfusions; however, the metabolic component, or acid load, has been of concern. When blood was stored in acid citrate dextrose, the hydrogen ion load was sufficiently great that administration of sodium bicarbonate was advocated if several units were transfused rapidly. This practice is no longer necessary because of the lower acid load of CPD blood; if a patient is massively transfused and concern exists about the ability to buffer the acid load of stored blood, then close monitoring of the acid–base status is recommended rather than blind administration of sodium bicarbonate.

POTASSIUM. The plasma potassium concentration in packed cells stored in CPD-A for 35 days is approximately 78 mEq/L, compared with 5 mEq/L in freshly collected blood.[55] This accumulation of potassium occurs from intracellular leakage due to the storage inhibition of ion transport. In addition to the potassium load from intracellular leakage, a second contribution is made by the early destruction of nonviable erythrocytes. This value at 35 days may appear dangerously high, but it should be recalled that the total plasma volume in red cell concentrates is less than 70 ml. Therefore, the total load of potassium per unit of red cells is only 5.5 mEq. Also, whole blood at expiration date has a slightly higher load, 8.2 mEq, than packed cells. Because of these factors, patients who cannot tolerate an excess potassium load should be transfused with blood that is less than 5 days old.

CITRATE TOXICITY. Citrate-phosphate-dextrose with adenine contains trisodium citrate (0.368 g/100 ml of blood) and citric acid (0.046 g/100 ml of blood). Citrate, being an active binder of calcium, potentially may decrease the blood recipient's ionized calcium, and this depletion may cause problems after rapid infusions of blood to patients with either hepatic dysfunction or neonatal immaturity. Therefore, citrate toxicity has been of great concern to physicians performing massive transfusions or exchange transfusion. However, Howland et al.[60] were unable to document citrate toxicity in massively transfused patients; they believe the value of calcium replacement in adult transfusion practices is doubtful. The occurrence of citrate toxicity in neonates is well documented, particularly in exchange transfusions, but this problem can be minimized by performing exchanges at slow rates.

Besides citrate's effect on calcium, its administration will affect the acid–base balance. Because citrate is metabolized to bicarbonate, 1 unit of whole blood will generate 22.8 mEq of this base; this contribution has a positive effect in counterbalancing the administration of blood with a low pH. Also, the occurrence of a resulting mild metabolic alkalosis will mitigate the tendency of transfusion-induced hyperkalemia.

MICROAGGREGATES. In stored blood, aggregates of both leukocytes and platelets up to 200 μg form.[61] In patients who have received a massive transfusion of blood, hypoxia commonly develops and is directly proportional in severity to the volume of blood transfused; one possible cause is the pulmonary deposition of debris from stored transfused blood. In a series of patients with severe trauma who were given stored blood administered through microaggregate filters to eliminate the aggregates, it was shown that pulmonary insufficiency could be reduced,[62] and studies in animals have led to questions concerning the relationship of pulmonary insufficiency and the microaggregates found in stored blood.[63] Opinions vary concerning the necessity of administering blood through special filters when transfusing a large volume, but one reasonable suggestion is that the filters should be used when more than 5 units of blood are given.[64]

ADVERSE EFFECTS OF TRANSFUSION

Transfusion Reactions

ACUTE HEMOLYTIC TRANSFUSION REACTIONS. The signs and symptoms of an acute hemolytic transfusion reaction are triggered by the interaction of an antibody, generally of the IgM class, with transfused red cells, leading to the activation of complement and intravascular hemolysis. This type of hemolytic reaction occurs most frequently when ABO-incompatible blood is mistakenly transfused; the most serious sequelae of hemolytic transfusion reactions are acute renal failure and disseminated intravascular coagulopathy (DIC), which is most likely initiated by the intravascular hemolysis of the incompatible red cells and the antigen–antibody complex activation of the coagulation process. However, despite intensive study of the pathogenesis of the acute renal failure, some uncertainty remains. There is general agreement it is postischemic in origin and etiologically unrelated to hemoglobin toxicity. The decreased renal blood flow, particularly to the cortical area, may be related to the release of vasoconstrictor substances that lead to decreased microcirculation and increased stasis, but it is far from clear whether DIC plays a major role in inducing the renal failure from acute hemolytic reactions.[65]

The initial signs and symptoms of a hemolytic transfusion reaction vary; the most frequent are fever and chills. Vague symptoms of either backache or flushing also may be the only initial manifestation. In unconscious patients, the only signs may be hypotension and bleeding at surgical or venipuncture sites, and if sufficient incompatible red cells are transfused, then hypotension and oliguria progressing to anuria may ensue.[66]

When a hemolytic reaction is suspected, the transfusion should be stopped and samples of both the transfused blood and the patient's posttransfusion blood sent to the blood bank for investigation. In general, two simple tests are sufficient to confirm or exclude acute hemolysis: visual inspection of the patient's serum for hemoglobin, and a direct Coombs test (whose results should be available in approximately 30 minutes). However, initial treatment should not be delayed pending these results.

Aggressive treatment of hypotension as well as maintenance of adequate renal blood flow are the goals of therapy for hemolytic transfusion reactions. To promote urine output, 0.9% saline should be administered with intravenous furosemide, which improves the cortical blood flow. Mannitol, an osmotic diuretic, previously was used frequently, but some debate exists concerning its usefulness. If anuria develops, then the patient should be managed for acute renal failure (i.e., fluid restriction, observation of electrolytes, and dialysis may be required).

The management of hemorrhagic complications of a hemolytic reaction should be individualized. It has been recommended that heparin be used for the treatment of DIC;[67] however, one should note that most patients with severe reactions will improve without any heparin therapy. If severe coagulation deficiencies develop, with clinical bleeding, then appropriate blood component therapy should be given.

DELAYED TRANSFUSION REACTIONS. This type of hemolytic reaction usually is mild and occurs several days after the transfusion. The hemolysis results from an anamnestic response to the transfused red cell antigens in a previously immunized recipient. The alloantibody, usually an IgG, formed after the primary response may decrease to undetectable levels, but as the rechallenged recipient produces increasing amounts of antibody, the transfused red cells are coated, which leads to shortened survival from extravascular destruction. The most frequent presenting symptoms are fever, unexplained fall in hemoglobin level, and jaundice. Renal failure is unusual. Also, the direct Coombs test is positive until the transfused blood is destroyed, and serum alloantibody usually becomes detectable. Blood that lacks the antigens against which the alloantibodies have formed is required for future transfusions.

NONHEMOLYTIC FEBRILE TRANSFUSION REACTIONS. Recipients who have been multiply transfused or had multiple pregnancies are likely to experience febrile transfusion reactions. These occur because patients become sensitized to granulocyte, lymphocyte, or platelet antigens.[50] The development of fever and/or chills during transfusion is an indication to stop the procedure, because an acute hemolytic transfusion may present first as fever. A second possible, but rare, cause of fever developing during transfusion is bacterial contamination of the blood product; therefore, it is best that these conditions be ruled out before proceeding with the transfusion. After the initial febrile reactions, not all patients will experience similar reactions, but if a patient has had two or more reactions, then leukocyte-poor red cells should be administered.

URTICARIA. The etiology of urticarial reactions is unclear. If hives are not accompanied by any other symptom or sign, then the transfusion may be resumed without laboratory testing. If hives develop, however, it is suggested that the transfusion be slowed or stopped and antihistamines administered; once the patient has improved, the transfusion may resume. Pretreatment with antihistamines usually is adequate to prevent future occurrences.

ANAPHYLACTIC TRANSFUSION REACTIONS. Anaphylactic reactions to blood products are rare. They occur most commonly in patients with IgA deficiency who have antibodies to IgA. Approximately 1 in 700 people are IgA deficient, and when the absence of IgA is documented in an individual who has experienced an anaphylactic transfusion reaction, measurement of anti-IgA can further confirm the hypersensitivity.[68] To prevent further reactions in these sensitized patients, only blood products free of IgA should be transfused. Washed or frozen-deglycerolized red cells may be used for red cell replacement; if plasma is required, it must be obtained from IgA-deficient donors. Small amounts of IgA are present in albumin preparations and significantly larger amounts in plasma protein fractions, so these blood derivatives should be avoided in IgA-deficient, sensitized patients.

Infectious Agents Transmitted by Transfusion

VIRAL HEPATITIS. Viral hepatitis is one of the most serious posttransfusion complications, and despite both the elimination of commercial blood donors and the screening of donor blood for hepatitis B surface antigen, posttransfusion hepatitis still develops in as many as 10% of all transfusion recipients. Type B hepatitis accounts for only 10% of cases, with the remainder attributed to non-A, non-B hepatitis.[69] Although transmitted in a similar fashion to hepatitis B, non-A, non-B hepatitis is subclinical and anicteric in most cases; furthermore, non-A, non-B hepatitis following transfusion has a propensity toward chronicity.[70] The Transfusion Transmission Virus Study[71] demonstrated that the posttransfusion incidence of non-A, non-B hepatitis may be reduced by screening donors for elevation of alanine aminotransferase activity and antibody to hepa-

titis B core antigen, and this study suggests that indirect methods of screening could be useful to reduce posttransfusion hepatitis. Because a specific test for non-A, non-B hepatitis was not available, alanine aminotransferase and anti–hepatitis B core screening of blood donors were introduced in 1986. In 1988, a virus called hepatitis C virus was discovered,[72] and a review of previous posttransfusion cases of hepatitis demonstrated that the majority of cases of non-A, non-B hepatitis were caused by this agent.[73] A specific test for anti–hepatitis C virus was instituted in 1990 for blood donor screening.

CYTOMEGALOVIRUS. After the transfusion of blood, recipients may develop a mild febrile illness, splenomegaly, and reactive lymphocytes in the blood. This illness was described originally in cardiac surgery patients who had received large amounts of fresh blood; hence, it was called postperfusion syndrome. It subsequently was observed that transfused blood could transmit cytomegalovirus (CMV) leading to this syndrome.[74] Although CMV infection was attributed initially to fresh blood transfusions, it also occurs after the transfusion of stored blood. Patients who are immune-suppressed, such as those receiving solid organ or bone marrow transplants, are at greatest risk of CMV infection; CMV infection also is a problem for low-birth-weight neonates whose mothers lack antibody to CMV.[75] To prevent CMV transmission to patients at high risk for posttransfusion infection, blood components from donors who are negative for CMV antibodies should be transfused.

MALARIA. Malaria parasites can survive in stored blood and be transmitted to the recipient. Regulations eliminating prospective donors who have either had malaria in the last 3 years or traveled in endemic areas have made this adverse effect of transfusion rare. Nonetheless, the diagnosis of malaria should be considered in patients with paroxysmal fever following transfusion.

ACQUIRED IMMUNODEFICIENCY SYNDROME. In 1982, a case of acquired immunodeficiency syndrome (AIDS) in a neonate who received blood from a donor who later developed AIDS first raised the question of AIDS transmission by transfusion.[76] Transmission by blood transfusion is now well documented, with approximately 2% of reported AIDS cases associated with blood transfusion. AIDS also has occurred in many hemophiliacs who have been treated with factor VIII concentrates.[77] These events occurred before a test for the antibody to human immunodeficiency virus (HIV) became available in 1985; presently, the risk of AIDS as a result of transfusion has been reduced to between 1 in 50,000 and 1 in 150,000 units.[78] This has been accomplished by a four-part program including voluntary blood donations, a careful medical history to eliminate high-risk donors, a sensitive test for anti-HIV, and a confidential self-exclusion procedure. Heat-treated factor concentrates as well as solvent/detergent-treated and monoclonal factor VIII concentrates have eliminated AIDS as a risk for hemophiliacs; however, because the incubation period for AIDS may be very long, a thorough transfusion history should be obtained from any patient developing AIDS.

HUMAN T-CELL LYMPHOTROPIC VIRUS TYPE I. This is a retrovirus associated with cases of adult T-cell leukemia/lymphoma and a neuropathy termed *tropical spastic paraparesis*.[79,80] Because asymptomatic blood donors can transmit this virus, resulting in seroconversion and possible illness in transfusion recipients, screening for human T-cell lymphotropic virus type I in blood donors was initiated in 1989. Several cases of neuropathy have been reported in recipients of blood transfused before the availability of testing.

OTHER INFECTIONS. Syphilis transmission has been reduced by using both stored blood and serologic testing of donors. Other diseases transmitted by blood products include Chagas' disease, toxoplasmosis, filariasis, and leishmaniasis.[81]

Other Delayed Complications of Blood Transfusion

TRANSFUSION HEMOSIDEROSIS. Each unit of blood contains approximately 250 mg of iron. Therefore, in those patients receiving long-term transfusion for congenital anemias or aplastic anemia, the iron load can become deleteriously high, and the accumulation of iron in the heart, liver, and endocrine organs eventually leads to dysfunction. Iron chelation may reduce deposited iron, and a new approach is the use of neocytes in conjunction with chelation therapy to help decrease the rate of iron accumulation.[82]

GRAFT-VERSUS-HOST DISEASE. Immunocompetent donor lymphocytes may survive the storage of red cell products and are found in the greatest numbers in white cell or platelet products.[83,84] These lymphoid cells may engraft in immunosuppressed recipients, leading to graft-versus-host disease, but irradiating blood products for recipients considered susceptible to graft-versus-host reactions eliminates the hazard. If transfusions from related blood donors are given to normal recipients with similar HLA types as the donor, transfused lymphocytes also may engraft, leading to graft-versus-host disease; for this reason, when transfusions from close

relatives are used, irradiation of the transfusion product is recommended as well.[85]

REDUCING THE RISK OF TRANSFUSION

With the growing awareness of the risks of transfusion, especially the virally transmitted diseases, a variety of approaches to reduce the number of transfusion exposures have become popular. Autologous blood transfusions effectively eliminate the risks of transfusion, and the most widely used form of autologous transfusion requires presurgery blood donation. Autologous blood donation generally is well tolerated and usually can lead to the collection of as many as 4 to 6 units of blood. Intraoperatively shed blood from sterile sites also can be a source of autologous blood, and a third approach to autologous transfusion is hemodilution. Just before surgery, units of blood can be collected and the reduced blood volume replaced with crystalloid. When bleeding occurs, the autologous blood may be transfused.

With the availability of recombinant erythropoietin, patients with hypoproliferative anemias caused by the deficiency of endogenous erythropoietin may have their anemia treated by the administration of recombinant erythropoietin. This approach has been especially effective in patients with the anemia of end stage renal failure, and it appears that other forms of anemia associated with malignancy or chronic disease also may benefit from erythropoietin administration.[86]

REFERENCES

1. Springer GF, Horton RE, Forbes M. Origin of anti-human blood group B agglutinins in white leghorn chicks. J Exp Med 1959;110:221.
2. Miller LH, Mason SJ, Dvorak JA, McGinniss MH, Rothmann IK. Erythrocyte receptors for *Plasmodium knowlesi* malaria: the Duffy blood group determinants. Science 1977;189:561.
3. Marsh WL, Oyen R, Nichols ME, Allen FH. Chronic granulomatous disease and the Kell blood groups. Br J Haematol 1975;29:247.
4. Sturgeon P. Hematological observations on the anemia associated with blood type Rh null. Blood 1970;36:310.
5. Voak D, Cawley JC, Emmines JP, Barker CR. The role of enzymes and albumin in haemagglutination reactions: a serological ultra-structural study with ferritin-labeled anti-D. Vox Sang 1974;27:156.
6. Hughes-Jones NC, Polley MJ, Telford R, Gardner B, Kleinschmidt G. Optimal conditions for detecting blood group antibodies by the antiglobulin test. Vox Sang 1964;9:385.
7. Giblett ER. Blood group alloantibodies: an assessment of some laboratory practices. Transfusion 1977;17:299.
8. Beattie KM, Zuelzer WW. The frequency and properties of pH-dependent anti-M. Transfusion 1965;5:322.
9. Low B, Messeter L. Antiglobulin test in low ionic strength salt solution for rapid antibody screening and crossmatching. Vox Sang 1974;26:53.

10. Leikola J, Perkins HA. Red cell antibodies and low ionic strength: a study with enzyme-linked antiglobulin test. Transfusion 1980;20:244.

11. Renton PM, Hancock JA. Rh antibodies and the prozone phenomenon. J Clin Pathol 1958;11:49.

12. Pollack W, Hager HJ, Reckel R, Toren DA, Singher HO. A study of the forces involved in the second stage of hemagglutination. Transfusion 1965;5:158.

13. Victoria EJ, Muchmore EA, Sudora EJ, Masouredis SP. The role of antigen mobility in the anti-Rho(D)-induced agglutination. J Clin Invest 1975;56:292.

14. Morton JA, Pickles MM. The proteolytic enzyme test in the detection of incomplete antibodies. J Clin Pathol 1951;4:189.

15. Coombs RRA, Mourant AE, Race RR. A new test for the detection of weak and "incomplete" Rh agglutinins. Br J Exp Pathol 1945;26:225.

16. Gillialand BC, Leddy JP, Vaughn JH. The detection of cell-bound antibody on complement-coated human red cells. J Clin Invest 1970;49:898.

17. Petz LD, Garratty G. Antiglobulin sera—past, present, and future. Transfusion 1978;18:257.

18. Widmann FK, ed. Technical Manual of the American Association of Blood Banks, 8th Ed. Washington, DC: American Association of Blood Banks, 1981:105–23.

19. Issitt PD, Issitt CH. Applied Blood Group Serology, 2nd Ed. Oxnard, CA: Spectra Biologicals, 1975.

20. Myhre BA. Fatalities from blood transfusion. JAMA 1980;244:1333.

21. Watkins WM. Blood group substances: their nature and genetics. In: Surgenor D, Mac N, eds. The Red Blood Cell, Vol. 1, 2nd Ed. New York: Academic Press, 1974:293–360.

22. Bhatia HM, Sathe MS. Incidence of Bombay (Oh) phenotype and weaker variants of A and B antigens in Bombay (India). Vox Sang 1974;27:524.

23. Marcus DM, Cass LE. Glycosphingolipids with Lewis blood group activity: uptake by human erythrocytes. Science 1969;164:553.

24. Levine P, Stetson RE. An unusual case of intragroup agglutination. JAMA 1939;113:126.

25. Landsteiner K, Wiener AS. An agglutinable factor in human blood recognized by immune sera for Rhesus blood. Proc Soc Exp Biol N Y 1940;43:223.

26. Wiener AS, Peters HR. Hemolytic reactions following transfusions of blood of the homologous group, with three cases in which the same agglutinogen was responsible. Ann Intern Med 1940;13:2306.

27. Pollack W, Ascari WQ, Kochesky RJ, O'Connor RR, Ho TY, Tripodi D. Studies on Rh Prophylaxis. I. Relationship between dose of anti-Rh and size of antigenic structures. Transfusion 1971;11:333.

28. Ruddle F, Ricciati FA, McMorris FA. Somatic cell genetic assignment of peptidase C and the Rh linkage group to chromosome no. 1. Science 1972;176:1429.

29. Wiener AS. Genetic theory of the Rh blood types. Proc Soc Exp Biol N Y 1943;54:316.

30. Race RR. The Rh genotypes and Fisher's theory. Blood 1978;3(suppl 2):27.

31. Rosenfield RE, Allen FH Jr, Swisher SN, Kochwa S. A review of Rh serology and presentation of a new terminology. Transfusion 1962;2:287.

32. Schmidt PJ, Morrison EG, Shohl J. The antigenicity of the Rho(D^u) blood factor. Blood 1962;20:196.

33. Pollack W, Ascari WQ, Crispan JF, O'Connor RR, Ho TY. Studies in Rh prophylaxis. II. Rh immune prophylaxis after tranfusion with Rh positive blood. Transfusion 1970;11:340.

34. Bowman JM. Suppression of Rh isoimmunization, a review. Obstet Gynecol 1978;52:384.

35. Oriol R, Opelz G, Chan C, Terasaki PL. The Lewis system and kidney transplantation. Transplantation 1980;29:397.

36. Naiki M, Fong J, Ledeen R, Marcus DM. Structure of the human erythrocyte blood group P_1 glycosphingolipid. Biochemistry 1975;14:4831.

37. Levine P, Celano MJ, Falkowski F. The specificity of the antibody in paroxysmal cold hemoglobinuria. Transfusion 1963;3:278.

38. Springer GF, Desai PR. Human blood group MN and precursor specificities: structural and biological aspects. Carbohydr Res 1975;40:183.

39. Marsh WL. Anti-i: a cold antibody defining the iI relationship in human red cells. Br J Haematol 1961;7:200.

40. Hillman RS, Giblett ER. Red cell membrane alteration associated with "marrow stress." J Clin Invest 1965;44:1730.

41. Rosenfield RE, Schmidt PJ, Calvo RC, McGuinniss MH. Anti-i: a frequent cold agglutinin in infectious mononucleosis. Vox Sang 1965;10:631.

42. Perioperative Red Cell Transfusion. National Institutes of Health Consensus Development Conference Statement. Vol. 7, No. 4, June 27–29, 1988:1–17.

43. Krevans JR, Jackson DP. Hemorrhagic disorder following massive whole blood transfusions. JAMA 1955;159:171.

44. Rapaport GI, Ames SB, Mikkelsen S. The levels of anti-hemophilic globulin and proaccelerin in fresh and bank blood. Am J Clin Pathol 1959;31:297.

45. Rizza CR. Management of patients with coagulation factor deficiencies. In: Biggs R, ed. Human Blood Coagulation, Hemostasis and Thrombosis. Oxford: Blackwell, 1976:392.

46. Milner LV, Butcher K. Transfusion reactions reported after transfusions of red blood cells and of whole blood. Transfusion 1978;18:493.

47. Meryman HT. The cryopreservation of blood cells for clinical use. Prog Hematol 1979;11:193.

48. Alter HJ, Tabor E, Meryman H, et al. Transmission of hepatitis-B virus by transfusion of frozen-deglycerolized red blood cells. N Engl J Med 1978;298:637.

49. Kurtz SR, Van Deinse WH, Valeri CR. The immunocompetence of residual leukocytes at various stages of red cell cryopreservation with 40% w/v glycerol in an ionic medium at −80°C. Transfusion 1978;18:441.

50. Perkins HA, Payne R, Ferguson J, Wood M. Non-hemolytic febrile transfusion reactions. Quantitative effects of blood components with emphasis on isoantigenic incompatibility of leukocytes. Vox Sang 1966;11:578.

51. Tullis JL. Albumin 1. Background and use. JAMA 1977;237:335.

52. Tullis JL. Albumin 2. Guidelines for clinical use. JAMA 1977;237:460.

53. Alving B, Hojima Y, Pisano JJ, et al. Hypotension associated with prekallikrein activator in plasma protein fraction. N Engl J Med 1978;299:66.

54. Zuck TF, Bensinger TA, Peck CC, et al. The in vivo survival of red blood cells stored in modified CPD with adenine: report of a multi-institutional cooperative effort. Transfusion 1977;17:374.

55. Moore GL, Peck CC, Sohmer PR, Zuck TF. Some properties of blood stored in anticoagulant CPDA-1 solutions. A brief summary. Transfusion 1981;21:135.

56. Valeri CR, Hirsch NM. Restoration in vivo of erythrocyte adenosine triphosphate, 2,3-diphosphoglycerate, potassium ion and sodium ion concentrations following the transfusion of acid-citrate dextrose stored human red blood cells. J Lab Clin Med 1969;73:722.

57. Valtis DJ, Kennedy AD. Defective gas-transport function of stored red blood cells. Lancet 1954;i:119.

58. Collins JA. Problems associated with the massive transfusion of stored blood. Surgery 1974;75:274.

59. Dennis RC, Vito L, Weisel RD, et al. Improved myocardial performance following high 2,3-diphosphoglycerate red cell transfusion. Surgery 1975;77:741.

60. Howland WS, Bellville JW, Zucker MB, et al. Massive blood transfusion. V. Failure to demonstrate citrate intoxication. Surg Gynecol Obstet 1957;105:529.

61. Swank RL. Alterations of blood on storage: measurement of adhesiveness of aging platelets and leukocytes and their removal by filtration. N Engl J Med 1961;265:728.

62. Reul GJ, Beall AC, Greenfield SD. Protection of the pulmonary vasculature by fine screen blood filtration. Chest 1974;66:4.

63. Tobey RE. Kopriva CJ, Homer LD, et al. Pulmonary gas exchange following hemorrhagic shock and massive transfusion in the baboon. Ann Surg 1974;179:316.

64. Solis RT, Walker BD. International forum: does a relationship exist between massive blood transfusion and the adult respiratory distress syndrome? Vox Sang 1977;32:319.

65. Goldfinger D. Acute hemolytic transfusion reactions—a fresh look at pathogenesis and considerations regarding therapy. Transfusion 1977;17:85.

66. Pineda AA, Brzica SM, Taswell H. Hemolytic transfusion reaction. Mayo Clin Proc 1978;53:378.

67. Rock RC, Bove JR, Nemerson Y. Heparin treatment of intravascular coagulation accompanying hemolytic transfusion reactions. Transfusion 1969;9:57.

68. Vyas GN, Perkins HA, Fudenberg HH. Anaphylactoid transfusion reaction associated with anti-IgA. Lancet 1968;ii:312.

69. Aach RD, Lander JJ, Sherman LA, et al. Transfusion-transmitted viruses: interim analysis of hepatitis among transfused and nontransfused patients. In: Vyas GN, Cohen SN, Schmid R, eds. Viral Hepatitis. Philadelphia: Franklin Institute Press, 1978:383–96.

70. Aach RD, Kahn RA. Post-transfusion hepatitis: current perspectives. Ann Intern Med 1980;92:539.

71. Aach RD, et al. The transfusion-transmitted viruses study: serum alanine aminotransferase of donors in relation to the risk of non-A, non-B hepatitis in recipients. N Engl J Med 1981;304:989.

72. Choo QL, Kuo G, Weiner AJ, Overby LR, Bradley DW, Houghton M. Isolation of a cDNA clone derived from a blood-borne non-A, non-B hepatitis genome. Science 1989;244:359–62.

73. Alter HJ, Purcell RH, Shih JW, et al. Detection of antibody to hepatitis C virus in prospectively followed transfusion recipients with acute and chronic non-A, non-B hepatitis. N Engl J Med 1989;321:1494–500.

74. Foster KM. Post-transfusion mononucleosis. Aust Ann Med 1966;15:305.

75. Yeager AS, Grumet FC, Hafleigh EB, Arvin AM, Bradley JS, Prober CG. Prevention of transfusion-acquired cytomegalovirus infections in newborn infants. J Pediatr 1982;98:281–7.

76. Possible transfusion-associated acquired immune deficiency syndrome (AIDS)—California. MMWR 1982;31:652–5.

77. Eyster ME, Goedert JJ, Sarngadharau MG, Weiss SH, Gallo RC, Blattner WA. Development and early natural history of HTLV-III antibodies in persons with hemophilia. JAMA 1985;253:2219–23.

78. Cohen ND, Munoz A, Ness PM, et al. Transmission of human T-cell leukemia virus type I (HTLV-I) by transfusion among patients undergoing cardiac surgery. N Engl J Med 1989;320:1172–6.

79. Poiesz BJ, Ruscetti FW, Reitz MS, et al. Isolation of a new type C retrovirus (HTLV) in primary uncultured cells of a patient with Sezary T-cell leukemia. Nature 1981;294:268–71.

80. Gessain A, Barin F, Vernant JC, et al. Antibodies to human T-lymphotropic virus type-I in patients with tropical spastic paraparesis. Lancet 1985;ii:407–10.

81. Wolfe MS. Parasites other than malaria, transmissible by blood transfusion. In: Greenwalt TS, Jamieson GA, eds. Transmissible Disease and Blood Transfusion. New York: Grune & Stratton, 1975:267.

82. Propper RD, Button LN, Nathan DG. New approach to the transfusion management of thalassemia. Blood 1980;55:1.

83. Dinsmore RE, Straus DJ, Pollack MS, et al. Fatal graft-versus-host disease following blood transfusion in Hodgkin's disease documented by HLA typing. Blood 1980;55:831.

84. Cohen D, Weinstein H, Misham M, Yankee R. Non-fatal graft-versus-host disease occurring after transfusion with leukocytes and platelets obtained from normal donors. Blood 1979;53:1059.

85. Vogelsang G. Transfusion associated graft versus host disease in nonimmunocompromised hosts. Transfusion 1990;30:101.

86. Eschbach JW, Egrie JC, Downing MR, et al. Correction of the anemia of end stage renal disease with recombinant human erythropoietin. Results of a combined phase I and II clinical trial. New Engl J Med 1987;316:73.

21

The Management of Bone Marrow Suppression

Hayden G. Braine, M.D.

Bone marrow toxicity is the most common adverse effect of cancer chemotherapy; in fact, it was the myelotoxicity that suggested application of the drugs currently employed in the treatment of acute leukemia, lymphoma, and multiple myeloma. In general, antineoplastic agents do not exert a selective toxicity on any specific myeloid cell line (Table 21.1).[1] Anemia, thrombocytopenia, and leukopenia are encountered with most cytotoxic drugs. Impairment of erythropoiesis generally is manageable. Because of the long lifespan of the erythrocyte, intermittent pulses of chemotherapy do not result in the rapid onset of profound anemia; furthermore, red cell transfusion offers palliative therapy and recombinant human erythropoietin the possibility of either preventing or correcting anemia without transfusion. Thrombocytopenia and neutropenia, however, have been more difficult to manage. Before an understanding of the pathophysiology of marrow failure was reached, death from leukopenia or thrombocytopenia was common, but with current practice, long periods of profound thrombocytopenia or neutropenia now can be managed successfully.

PRINCIPLES OF THE HEMATOLOGIC TOXICITY OF CANCER CHEMOTHERAPY

All current anticancer drugs have a very narrow therapeutic ratio, and they are used at doses that are toxic to normal tissues. Most antineoplastic agents either exert or express their toxicity on cells that are actively in the cell cycle. Because of their rapid turnover and short cycle, the mucous membrane cells of the gastrointestinal tract as well as the cells of the hematopoietic system are the two most common tissues that limit the dose escalation of antineoplastic agents. To minimize the toxicity to normal tissue while maximizing the anticancer activity, three major therapeutic strategies have been employed.

Combination chemotherapy is the first. By employing combinations of drugs with different dose-limiting toxicities, one is able to achieve additive anticancer effects with an acceptable clinical toxicity. Furthermore, each drug, working through a different biochemical mechanism, inhibits the emergence of drug resistance.

High-dose therapy is the second strategy. To allow the maximum anticancer activity and to prevent the development of drug resistance, each drug is used at its maximum tolerated dosage. This usually means using the drugs at dosages where there is some mucocutaneous or hematologic toxicity.

In the third strategy, treatment regimens usually are given in a pulsed or cyclical manner (cyclical pulse therapy). This maximizes the anticancer effect related to the peak drug levels, and it allows a recruitment of cells into cycle. With many agents, treatment in a cyclical manner minimizes the immunosuppressive effects of the drug while maintaining a good antitumor response.

The MOPP regimen (nitrogen *m*ustard, *O*ncovin [vincristine], *p*rednisone, and *p*rocarbazine) used in the treatment of advanced-stage Hodgkin disease is a good example of how these principles are applied.[2] Nitrogen mustard is a strong emetic with dose-related myelotox-

TABLE 21.1. The Hematologic Toxicity of Commonly Used Antineoplastic Agents

Agent	Degree of Toxicity at Commonly Used Dosages		
	Minimal	Moderate	Marked
Alkaloids			
Vincristine	G,P		
Vinblastine	G,P		
VP-16	P	G	
Antibiotics			
Actinomycin			G,P
Doxorubicin			G,P
Mitomycin-C			G,P
Bleomycin	G,P		
Antimetabolites			
Methotrexate		G,P	
5-Fluorouracil	G,P		
Cytosine arabinoside		G,P	
Alkylating Agents			
Cyclophosphamide		P	G
Melphalan		G,P	
Busulfan*			G,P
Carmustine*			G,P
Lomustine*			G,P
Cisplatin		G,P	
Miscellaneous			
Dacarbazine		G,P	
Procarbazine		G,P	
L-Asparaginase	G,P		
Prednisone	G,P		

Source: DeVita et al. 1982[1]
*May cause irreversible toxicity.
Note: G = toxicity to granulopoiesis; P = toxicity to thrombopoiesis.

icity, and procarbazine has mild myelotoxicity and neurotoxicity. Vincristine and prednisone have no myelotoxicity. Their dose-limiting toxicities relate to neurotoxicity (vincristine) and altered glucose metabolism, salt balance, and immunosuppression (prednisone). Each drug is given at its maximum tolerated dosage (Table 21.2).

Nitrogen mustard and vincristine are given intravenously on days 1 and 8. The prednisone and procarbazine then are given daily for 14 days. Following this 2-week cycle, the patient is observed with weekly blood counts, and the degree of both neutropenia and thrombocytopenia are evaluated. The dosages of the subsequent cycles are selected based on the myelotoxicity experienced with the first cycle (Table 21.3).These cycles are repeated until either a complete remission is achieved or resistance to therapy is documented. Depending on the stage of the disease, MOPP also can be integrated with gamma radiation to lymph node areas.

Combination therapies based on similar principles have been effective in many other cancers, including both acute and chronic leukemias, testicular carcinoma, non-Hodgkin lymphoma, breast cancer, and many cancers of children.

Despite close observation, inadvertent excess toxicity is encountered; it is not unusual to encounter some degree of leukopenia and thrombocytopenia with the MOPP regimen. In such situations, both prompt diagnosis and appropriate management are required to minimize morbidity and mortality.

Alternatively, the dose schedules of antineoplastic therapy deliberately may be increased to myelotoxic levels. This strategy may be required when normal marrow elements have been replaced by tumor, as in the case of newly diagnosed acute leukemia,[3] and in such a situation with diminished myeloid reserves, nonmyelotoxic therapy is not possible. Myeloablative therapy also has been employed to increase the antitumor effect; brief periods of severe pancytopenia are induced deliberately to maximize the anticancer effect in such situations. This is the strategy employed in bone marrow transplantation for malignancy.[4,5] Myeloablative chemo/radiotherapy is followed by bone marrow infusion, and in the 2 to 3 weeks before a functioning marrow proliferates and differentiates, clinical care must be directed at the management of marrow failure.

TIMING OF THE CLINICAL SIGNS OF HEMATOLOGIC TOXICITY SECONDARY TO CANCER CHEMOTHERAPY

The effect of cytotoxic therapy is not seen immediately in the peripheral blood. In general, cytotoxic agents affect only those cells that are actively in the cell cycle; committed, terminally differentiated cells are relatively protected from the cytotoxic effect. The circulating platelet has a lifespan of approximately 9 days; thus, even if all thrombopoiesis is ablated by therapy, clinically significant thrombocytopenia will not develop for 5 to 7 days.[6-8] However, the circulating neutrophil has a peripheral blood transit time of only 12 hours. Following a pulse of cytotoxic therapy, the nadir of neutropenia does not develop until 7 to 10 days after treatment; this is because a large reservoir of postmitotic metamyelocytes and bands that are refractory to cytotoxic therapy exists in the marrow. This cellular compartment, beginning at the metamyelocyte, can support neutrophil production for approximately 6 days, and at that time, severe neutropenia will develop because of the cytotoxic effect of therapy on the myeloblast, promyelocyte, and myelocyte. When chemotherapy is discontinued, regeneration of the neutrophil compartment from committed

TABLE 21.2. The MOPP Regimen†

Agent	Day													
	1	2	3	4	5	6	7	8	9	10	11	12	13	14
Nitrogen mustard (6 mg/m^2 IV)	X							X						
Oncovin (1.4 mg/m^2 IV)	X							X						
Procarbazine (100 mg/m^2 PO)	X	X	X	X	X	X	X	X	X	X	X	X	X	X
Prednisone* (40 mg/m^2 PO)		X	X	X	X	X	X	X	X	X	X	X	X	X

Source: Reproduced, with permission, from DeVita et al. 1970[2]
*Given on cycles 1 and 4 only.
†Each 2-week course repeated monthly for 6 months.
Note: IV = intravenously; PO = orally.

TABLE 21.3. Dose Adjustments for MOPP

Peripheral Blood Counts on Day 28		Percentage of Dose Given on Last Cycle		
Leukocyte Count/mm^3	Platelet Count/mm^3	Nitrogen Mustard	Procarbazine	Oncovin
> 4000	> 100,000	100	100	100
3000 to 4000	> 100,000	50	50	100
2000 to 3000	50,000 to 100,000	25	25	100
1000 to 2000	> 50,000	25	25	50
< 1000	< 5000	0	0	0

Note: Predisone is not adjusted for myelotoxicity.

progenitors can begin, and recovery will occur in the peripheral blood after 10 to 14 days (Fig. 21.1).[9,10] Using this model, one sees that both the duration and the degree of myelotoxicity are dose dependent, whereas the day of nadir of the cell deficits is relatively independent of the dose. For example, a dose of cyclophosphamide of 30 mg/kg will produce a moderate degree of leukopenia (1500 leukocytes/mm^3), with a nadir on day 10; with a dose of 120 mg/kg, severe neutropenia develops, but the nadir occurs on the same day.[11]

Most cytotoxic agents appear to have minimal effect on the totipotential hematopoietic stem cell; however, there are notable exceptions. The nitrosoureas (carmustine and lomustine), busulfan, and gamma irradiation affect the hematopoietic stem cell,[1] and this toxicity is manifested by pancytopenia 4 to 6 weeks after therapy and can be irreversible. Therefore, these agents must be used more conservatively than other drugs having reversible hematologic toxicity.

The clinical management of thrombocytopenia and neutropenia following cytotoxic therapy is based on these kinetics. Depending on the drugs used, the dose, and the schedule, varying degrees of pancytopenia can be anticipated. If a patient develops leukopenia following a single intravenous administration of a drug such as cyclophosphamide and recovery can be anticipated within 14 days, then support can be expected to be of short duration; however, when 7- to 10-day infusions of cytosine arabinoside are used in the management of acute myelocytic leukemia, periods of pancytopenia lasting 21 to 28 days can be expected and support must be modified for this longer duration.

MANAGEMENT OF THROMBOCYTOPENIA SECONDARY TO MARROW FAILURE

Thrombocytopenia and Clinical Hemorrhage

The role of the circulating platelet in hemostasis has been well described. Physiologically, humans appear to have a large reserve of platelets. Platelet counts of 100,000 cells/mm^3 or lower are associated with a proportional decrease in template bleeding times. This was first described by Harker and Slichter,[12] who noted a bleeding time of approximately 5 minutes at 100,000 platelets/mm^3 and a proportional decrease such that, at 10,000 platelets/mm^3, the bleeding time was prolonged to approximately 30 minutes. However, there was no

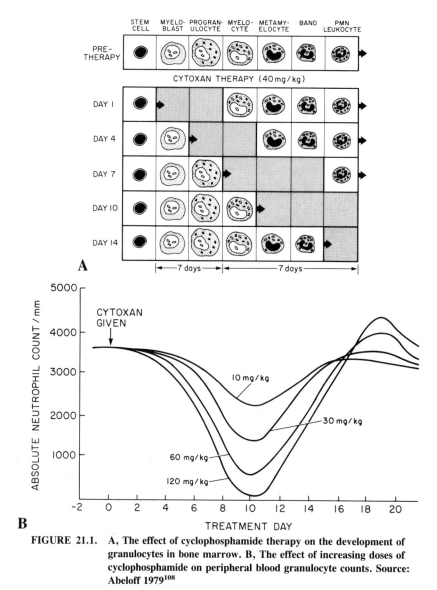

FIGURE 21.1. **A,** The effect of cyclophosphamide therapy on the development of granulocytes in bone marrow. **B,** The effect of increasing doses of cyclophosphamide on peripheral blood granulocyte counts. Source: Abeloff 1979[108]

proportionate shortening of the bleeding time for platelet counts above 100,000 cells/mm^3. In addition, for counts below 10,000 cells/mm^3, the bleeding time was quite variable, ranging from 30 minutes to over 1 hour.

Measurement of spontaneous gastrointestinal blood loss during thrombocytopenia indicates that clinically important hemorrhage may not develop consistently until severe thrombocytopenia is present. Slichter and Harker[13] measured spontaneous gastrointestinal blood loss using chromium 51–labelled red cells in a population of 20 patients with thrombocytopenia. At platelet counts above 10,000 cells/mm^3, blood loss averaged less than 5 ml/day; when counts were between 5000 and

10,000 cells/mm^3, blood loss increased to 9 ml/day. However, when platelet counts were below 5000 cells/mm^3, blood loss increased to greater than 50 ml/day.

Clinical observations of significant hemorrhage generally have confirmed these physiologic findings. Before the advent of effective platelet transfusion, hemorrhage accounted for over 50% of the deaths of patients with acute leukemia.[14] In many cases, hemorrhage was abrupt and rapidly fatal; this was true particularly for intracranial hemorrhages, the most serious hemorrhage site in the patient with thrombocytopenia. Since the advent of effective platelet transfusion, however, mortality from hemorrhage during the treatment of acute leukemia has been reduced to less than 5%.[14] Because of the clear efficacy of platelet transfusion, there have been only two prospective, randomized, controlled evaluations concerning this. In one study, patients with thrombocytopenia were transfused with "high doses" versus "low doses" of platelets; serious bleeding occurred in 1.3% and 3.7% of patients, respectively. Both groups, however, were superior to the 11.8% incidence in historical controls.[15] Another trial compared platelet-rich plasma to platelet-free fresh plasma in patients with thrombocytopenia and acute leukemia, but this study was terminated because of increased morbidity and mortality in the plasma-therapy group.[16]

To determine when prophylactic platelet transfusions should be performed, many have attempted to define a platelet threshold for clinical hemorrhage. Gaydos et al.[17] reviewed the transfusion experience in the treatment of acute leukemia at the National Institutes of Health in the early 1960s.[17] Patients with platelet counts below 100,000 cells/mm^3 were noted to have an increase in minor hemorrhage, but serious, life-threatening complications were not noticeably greater than those of patients without thrombocytopenia until the platelet count was below 20,000 cells/mm^3. Patients with counts below 5000 cells/mm^3 manifested some bleeding abnormality during 30% of the days at risk, and 10% of the days with levels below 5000 platelets/mm^3 were associated with serious, potentially life-threatening bleeding. However, despite this general trend toward more serious bleeding at the lower platelet counts, the authors were unable to identify a clear platelet-count threshold for clinical hemorrhage.

Indications for Platelet Transfusion

It is clear that in patients with thrombocytopenia secondary to marrow failure, platelet counts below 5000/mm^3 should be avoided. Traditionally, oncologists have elected to initiate prophylactic platelet transfusions in patients with counts below 20,000 platelets/mm^3; it should be appreciated that when this approach was established in the 1970s, there was no easily available, consistent supply of platelet concentrates for transfusion. Platelets frequently had to be ordered 24 hours in advance, and consequently, establishing a platelet count above 20,000 cells/mm^3 created a safety buffer. Today, when platelets are readily available, a lower threshold for prophylactic transfusion seems to be acceptable.

Two studies have attempted to address in a controlled manner this question of the role of prophylactic platelet transfusion.[18,19] Patients in these studies were assigned to either prophylactic platelet transfusion for counts below 20,000/mm^3 or emergent transfusion for significant hemorrhage. In both studies, patients assigned to prophylactic transfusions received more platelet transfusions without any reduction in morbidity or mortality secondary to hemorrhage; however, these studies were small and may not have had the power to detect small differences between groups. Furthermore, the treatment regimens employed were not as intensive as current regimens, and the study patients may not have had as high a risk of hemorrhage as do current patients. For these reasons, most oncologists continue prophylaxis for platelet counts below 20,000/mm^3 in patients with thrombocytopenia secondary to bone marrow failure.

Indications for platelet transfusion are not limited to severe thrombocytopenia. Platelet transfusion for patients with platelet counts over 20,000/mm^3 can be indicated when there is an acquired or hereditary[20] cause of platelet dysfunction (Table 21.4). In these situations, abnormal platelet function can predispose patients to hemorrhage despite normal platelet numbers; in such patients, evaluation of the template bleeding time may be helpful. If a prolonged bleeding time can be documented despite a normal platelet count, then platelet transfusion may be indicated for hemorrhage.

Determination of the bleeding time also may be helpful in identifying some patients with severely low platelet counts who also have normal bleeding times. This has been observed in patients with immune thrombocytopenia purpura who may have a normal bleeding time even with platelet counts below 10,000/mm^3;[12] these patients apparently have a marked increase in platelet production, with a proportional increase in larger, younger platelets. These platelets seem able to achieve hemostasis better than the senescent platelets observed in patients with thrombocytopenia and platelet-production deficits.

Thrombocytopenia alone is not an indication for platelet transfusion. When evaluating a patient for platelet transfusion, one must consider the etiology of the thrombocytopenia; if there is not a clear antecedent cause for the thrombocytopenia, such as chemotherapy, a bone marrow biopsy and aspirate is indicated. Plentiful megakaryocytes suggest increased consumption as the cause of the thrombocytopenia, and in such circum-

TABLE 21.4.   Acquired Functional Platelet Disorders that May Indicate Platelet Transfusion

Aspirin
Nonsteroidal anti-inflammatory agents
High-dose penicillin and semisynthetic penicillin therapy
Disseminated intravascular coagulation
Uremia
Myeloproliferative disorders

stances, platelet transfusion should be reserved for those patients with clinical evidence of hemorrhage. However, if thrombocytopenia is caused by decreased platelet production, then the circulating platelet count is a good predictor of hemorrhage. In this circumstance, one must estimate the anticipated degree of thrombocytopenia. If platelet counts below 5000/mm^3 are anticipated, then prophylactic platelet transfusion is reasonable. The selection of the platelet-count threshold for transfusion will depend on each patient's clinical status; for example, afebrile patients with stable thrombocytopenia may be prophylaxed at 10,000 platelets/mm^3. Patients with fever, impairment of platelet function secondary to uremia, or petechiae may need prophylaxis at a higher count.

PLATELET CONCENTRATES AND TRANSFUSION

Methods of Collection

Platelet concentrates for transfusion can be produced by fractionation of single units from whole blood or by plateletpheresis of a single donor using one of several commercially available blood cell separators; platelets prepared from single units of whole blood are the most commonly used concentrate in the United States today. Following donation, each unit of blood is processed by differential centrifugation to obtain a platelet concentrate. First, platelet-rich plasma is prepared by centrifugation, and then is centrifuged at a higher speed that pellets the platelets and leaves nearly cell-free plasma. The pelleted platelets subsequently are resuspended in 50 ml of donor plasma.[21,22] Federal standards require that 75% of the platelet concentrates prepared in this manner have more than 5.5×10^{10} platelets,[23] but in practice, most units prepared in this manner have 6 to 7×10^{10} platelets. (Still, it has become common practice to refer to 5.5×10^{10} platelets as a *unit* of platelets.) To prepare a single transfusion for an adult using these concentrates requires that 6 to 10 units of platelets from 6 to 10 individual units of blood be pooled together; thus, this concentrate for transfusion is referred to as *pooled platelets* or *multiple-donor platelets*. This is in contrast to "single donor" platelet concentrates, which are prepared from one donor by automated plateletpheresis.

Platelet concentrates prepared by plateletpheresis have been available since the mid-1960s. Initially, manual techniques were used, and these involved removing serial units of whole blood, separating out platelets by centrifugation, and then returning plasma and red cells to the donor. Manual plateletpheresis was tedious and labor intensive. The introduction of semiautomated blood cell separators in the early 1970s made

plateletpheresis easier to perform.[24,25] These systems usually required bilateral venipuncture to obtain a blood flow of 40 to 60 ml/min into the cell separator. Before centrifugation, donor blood was mixed with a solution of acid citrate dextrose, which functioned as a calcium-binding anticoagulant, and the blood was then separated by centrifugation and fractions of red cells, plasma, and platelets obtained. The red cells and plasma were returned to the donor via the second venipuncture and the citrate anticoagulant neutralized by the donor's endogenous calcium.

Early cell separators had several limitations, however. Tubing sets were disposable, but they required multiple connections with the risk of contamination during assembly. Thus, these collection systems were termed *open systems*, and storage was limited to 24 hours or less. This contrasts with the integrally connected blood-bag systems used for whole blood collection that allowed fractionation without connections and thus were termed *closed systems*. Platelets prepared in closed systems could be stored for 3 to 8 days depending on the type of plastic bags used. Secondly, initial apheresis equipment required a relatively large extracorporeal volume of blood in the separator, and this increased the risk of hypovolemia. Finally, the early systems also collected large numbers of lymphocytes, and this placed the repetitive donor at a theoretic risk of some degree of leukocyte depletion and exposed the recipient to the hazards of leukocyte-rich products. Second- and third-generation cell separators largely have eliminated these adverse considerations.[25–28] Extracorporeal blood volume now is low (in the range of 100 to 200 ml), disposable-tubing sets and centrifugation chambers are integrally connected to allow collection in a closed system, and leukocyte contamination per platelet concentrate can be reduced to below 1×10^8 leukocytes.

Over the years, there has been considerable discussion regarding the relative merits of single-donor apheresis products versus pooled platelet concentrates. The single-donor product has the advantage of fewer blood-donor exposures per platelet transfusion (Table 21.5), and this has the theoretic benefit of reducing the hazard of transfusion-transmitted diseases such as the acquired immunodeficiency syndrome, hepatitis, and cytomegalovirus (CMV) infections. Today, however, these risks are small; furthermore, they cannot be avoided completely, even with the use of single-donor platelets. Single-donor platelets also have the benefit of being associated with fewer febrile transfusion reactions, but the main advantage of single-donor platelets is that they allow the collection of clinically useful numbers of platelets from specially selected donors. The production of HLA-matched platelets for the alloimmune patient, or

TABLE 21.5. The Relative Advantages of Pooled Platelet Concentrates Versus Single-Donor Platelet Concentrates

Pooled Platelet Concentrates Prepared from Single Units of Whole Blood	Single-Donor Platelet Concentrates Prepared by Plateletpheresis
Least cost to produce	Fewer donor exposures per patient
	Less hazard of infectious disease
	Fewer transfusion reactions
Generally available	
Makes maximal use of available blood components	May be prepared from specially selected donors
Effective in patients with oligospecific anti-HLA antibodies	HLA-matched platelets
	CMV-seronegative platelets

TABLE 21.6. Factors Affecting the Viability of Platelets During Storage

Factor	Effect
Plastics used to make containers	Many surfaces induce platelet adhesion. Specific plastics must be used.
pH	CO_2 production during storage acidifies concentrates. pH ≤ 6.0 irreversibly damages platelets. Microporous collection bags allow more gas exchange.
Temperature	20°C to 24°C optimal. Cold injures platelets.
Platelets and leukocytes in concentrate	Higher concentrations of cells may acidify products faster.
Method of agitation	Flatbed horizontal agitation generally preferred to reduce platelet aggregation.
Time to centrifugation (multiple-donor only)	To preserve best function, separate platelets from whole blood within 6 hours of collection

CMV-negative platelets from CMV-seronegative platelet donors, can be achieved easily only by plateletpheresis, and in these special circumstances, there is no substitute for the single-donor platelet. However, for the nonalloimmunized, general patient population, it is unclear if the added expense and logistic difficulties of running a plateletpheresis program outweighs the lower costs and general availability of platelets that can be made as a by-product of whole blood processing. Furthermore, single-donor platelets may result in absolute transfusion failure in patients with oligospecific HLA antibodies; thus, a single-donor platelet concentrate from a donor with the HLA-A2 antigen may be destroyed completely by a recipient with a monospecific anti-A2 antibody. If 6 to 8 units of pooled platelets were given to such a patient, it would be anticipated that 60% to 70% of the units would not have A2 and would survive normally. Thus, in certain specific circumstances, apheresis platelets paradoxically may result in more transfusion failure.

Storage of Platelet Concentrates

One of the major challenges in clinical platelet transfusion has been developing techniques to allow the long-term storage of platelets. The platelet is exquisitely sensitive to a number of factors that can result in aggregation and irreversible loss of functional platelets (Table 21.6).[21,22,29–32] Platelets will adhere to many surfaces; thus, it was not until the introduction of the polyvinyl chloride blood bag that the separation of platelets from whole blood became feasible. Furthermore, it was noted that cold storage of platelets resulted in membrane changes which altered their function.[29] One of the most important factors in platelet storage was the prevention of acidification of the concentrates. Platelets and leukocytes collected in these concentrates are active metabolically, and glycolysis produces carbon dioxide. Over time, this results in acidification of the concentrates.[32] Concentrates with pHs below 6.0 at the end of storage have been found to be ineffective, so to maintain a pH above 6.0, platelet storage initially was limited to 3 days after collection. However, the production of newer plastics, with a molecular structure that allows carbon dioxide diffusion through the bag, allows maintenance of a normal pH for periods of 5 to 7 days.[33] Finally, it also was noted that platelets must be agitated gently to prevent adhesions to either the surface of the container or other platelets; at this time, most platelet concentrates usually are agitated during storage with a gentle, horizontal movement on a flatbed rotator.

The clinician should be aware of these variables to evaluate better the outcome of transfusion failure. In general, platelet storage for shorter periods of time will result in more viable platelets. Those stored up to 5 days will lose 20% to 30% of the viable platelets, and selected units may have an even greater loss. Thus, a significant cause of clinical transfusion failure may be the use of improperly manufactured or stored platelets. Close communication between the clinic and the blood bank is required to ensure that transfusion failures are not from use of nonviable platelets. Federal regulations require that blood collection centers count four platelet concentrates per month for platelet content,[23] so it is not general practice to count the content of all platelet concentrates. Documentation of the platelet content may be desirable on a more frequent basis when patients become refractory to platelet transfusion.

Indications for Platelet Transfusion

As discussed previously, thrombocytopenia secondary to marrow failure results in varying degrees of risk for hemorrhage depending on the circulating platelet count. To minimize this risk, either a prophylactic or an emergent platelet transfusion strategy can be undertaken. The emergent strategy, widely used in Europe and supported by several published studies,[18,19] reserves platelet transfusion until the first clinical evidence of hemorrhage, such as petechiae, epistaxis, bleeding from venipuncture sites, or hematuria; the prophylactic strategy sets a threshold value, usually 10,000 to 20,000 platelets/mm^3, and initiates transfusion at such levels. Higher levels (generally above 50,000/mm^3) are employed when invasive procedures such as surgery, thoracentesis, or lumbar puncture are undertaken.

Selection of the Dose of Platelet Concentrates for Transfusion

Historically, the dose of platelets chosen for transfusion has been somewhat arbitrary. In general, the strategy of platelet transfusion has been to raise the patient's count to above 50,000/mm^3, which should result in a substantial improvement in the patient's bleeding time. To achieve this level of platelets when beginning with a pretransfusion count of 10,000/mm^3 usually requires 4 to 6 units/m^2. Another rule of thumb has been to administer 1 unit/10 kg of recipient weight. Additional units should be used if higher posttransfusion counts are required.

Evaluation of Platelet Transfusion

Platelet transfusions should be monitored by obtaining 10-to-60-minute and 18-to-24-hour posttransfusion platelet counts.[34,35] One-hour posttransfusion platelet counts are used to determine platelet recovery, and the 18-to-24-hour counts are used to evaluate platelet survival. Both platelet recovery and survival should be determined with each patient's first platelet transfusion, then at regular intervals; to do this, a corrected posttransfusion platelet increment should be determined. The corrected count increment (CCI)[36] can be determined by the following formula:

$$CCI = \frac{\dfrac{(\text{Posttransfusion Count} - \text{Pretransfusion Count})}{(\text{Patient Body Surface Area in m}^2)}}{\text{Platelets} \times 10^{11}}$$

A normal 1-hour posttransfusion CCI is between 7500 and 15,000. Clinically, this means that 1 unit of platelets (1.0×10^{11}) will raise a 1-m^2 patient's platelet count by 7500 to 15,000 platelets/mm^3. This recovery takes into account that approximately 30% of platelets are sequestered in the spleen at any time; patients without spleens should be expected to achieve counts approximately 30% higher.[37] Also, splenomegaly will reduce the 1-hour CCI but not the 18-to-24-hour survival.

Platelet CCI recoveries at 18 to 24 hours after transfusion usually are between 3700 and 5000. This is less than would be expected with a normal 7-to-9-day platelet survival, because platelet survival in patients with thrombocytopenia generally is shortened. In the range of 10,000 to 50,000 platelets/mm^3, platelet survivals can be expected to be less than 4 days.[37]

Patients are classified as refractory to platelet transfusion if they fail to achieve a CCI greater than 7500 within one hour after transfusion using a platelet product that has been stored less than 48 hours, is ABO compatible with the recipient, and has had its platelet content determined by count at the time of issue. Multiple clinical conditions result in the platelet refractory state, and factors affecting the 1-hour posttransfusion CCI include splenomegaly, disseminated intravascular coagulation, autoimmune thrombocytopenia, and alloimmunization to both HLA and non-HLA platelet antigens (Table 21.7).[34] The clinical factors affecting the 18-to-24-hour posttransfusion platelet survival are more numerous. In the usual clinical situation, many also may be present simultaneously, and several studies have attempted to determine the most important clinical variables affecting posttransfusion platelet survival. The patient's primary disease has been shown to affect survival, and patients undergoing therapy for acute leukemia and bone marrow transplantation commonly develop the platelet refractory state. Additionally, intensive cytotoxic therapy has been shown to be associated with platelet refractoriness. Several studies have indicated that fever, infection, and bleeding independently affect platelet survival as well.[38-40]

Fortunately, fewer factors affect the 1-hour recovery than the 18-to-24-hour survival of platelets.[34,35] This can be helpful clinically, as splenomegaly can be evaluated by physical and laboratory examination and disseminated intravascular coagulation evaluated by determination of fibrinogen and the presence of fibrin split products. Thus, failure to achieve a 1-hour CCI of 7500 or higher without the presence of splenomegaly or disseminated intravascular coagulation strongly indicates an alloimmune or autoimmune cause for transfusion failure.[34]

It is critically important to establish if the platelet refractory state is secondary to alloimmunization as this can be addressed with HLA-matched platelet transfusions.[40,41] The determination of circulating lymphocytotoxic antibody has proven to be most useful in determining the need for HLA-matched platelets.[42] Patients' sera are tested against panels of lymphocytes from 20 to 40 different donors, and cytotoxicity is determined by complement lysis and trypan blue viability. Strongly cytotoxic antibodies nearly always are directed against HLA class I (HLA-A and HLA-B) specificities; as this is the antibody group most commonly involved in the

alloimmune destruction of platelets, lymphocytotoxic antibody testing has proven to be of considerable value. In our experience, lymphocytotoxic antibody testing has over an 85% positive-predictive value, with less than a 7.5% false-negative rate. However, as no test is 100% predictive, even patients refractory to platelet transfusion who manifest a negative lymphocytotoxic antibody test should be given at least one test transfusion with an HLA-matched product to assure this is not the cause of the platelet refractory state.

PLATELET TRANSFUSION FAILURE SECONDARY TO ALLOIMMUNIZATION

Platelet Antigen Systems

Three major antigen systems are involved in alloimmune platelet destruction. These are the ABO, HLA, and the platelet-specific antigen systems that are designated *human platelet antigens* (HPA).

It only recently has been appreciated that the ABO system can have a major impact on the outcome of platelet transfusion; it was felt initially that ABO incompatibility accounted for less than a 20% loss of platelets when ABO-incompatible transfusions were given.[43] More recently, however, it has become apparent that with A incompatibility (platelet donor type A/recipient type anti-A), posttransfusion platelet recovery can be less than 10% of that expected.[44] Whenever possible, platelet transfusions should be ABO compatible with the recipient. (The Rh antigen system has no known effect on platelet transfusion.)

Platelet-specific antigen systems now are recognized to be the major antigen system involved in posttransfusion purpura. HPA systems include HPA-1 (P1^1, Zw), HPA-2 (Ko), HPA-3 (BAK), HPA-4 (Yuk,Pen), and HPA-5 (Bv,Zav). Theoretically, HPA systems could be a major factor in posttransfusion alloimmunization, but clinically, this appears not to be the case. It is the general feeling that HPA systems account for less than 5% of posttransfusion alloimmunization;[44] this probably relates to the low frequency of homozygous individuals who are HPA-negative and could be sensitized to HPA-positive transfusion. For example, the phenotypic frequency in Caucasians of HPA-1a is estimated at 98%, HPA-2a at 97.6%, and HPA-3a at 90.8%.[45]

Presently, studies indicate that most posttransfusion alloantibodies are directed at antigens of the HLA-A and -B loci.[41] HLA-A and -B antigens are expressed variably on platelets,[46] and the major mechanism of platelet destruction by alloantibodies is antibody-mediated clearance through the reticuloendothelial system. Transfused platelets bind antigen-specific circulating anti-HLA antibodies, which are then recognized by Fc

TABLE 21.7.   Clinical Variables Decreasing Posttransfusion Platelet Recovery and Survival

1-Hour Recovery	24-Hour Recovery
Splenomegaly	Splenomegaly
Severe DIC	DIC
Severe autoimmune thrombocytopenia	Autoimmune thrombocytopenia
Alloimmunization	Alloimmunization
	Chemotherapy
	Fever
	Patient diagnosis
	Infection
	Bleeding

Note: DIC = disseminated intravascular coagulation

TABLE 21.8. Factors Affecting Alloimmunization to Class I Antigens on Platelets

Factor	Comment
Number of transfusions or pregnancies	Exposure to more antigens
Leukocyte content of blood transfusions	Platelets lack class II antigens required for alloimmunization

Treatment factors
  1° disease
  Chemotherapy
	Immunosuppression blunts alloimmune response

Patient factors
  ? Immune response
  Genes
	20% to 60% of patients will not become alloimmunized despite multiple transfusions

receptors on phagocytic reticuloendothelial cells in the spleen and liver, and depending on the recipient antibody titer and the antigen density on the platelet, removal can occur within 1 hour of transfusion or more slowly over several days. Early alloimmune responses first tend to affect platelet 18-to-24-hour survival and the 1-hour posttransfusion platelet recovery second. IgG, IgA, and IgM antiplatelet antibodies have been documented, but IgG antibodies appear to be involved the most consistently in posttransfusion alloimmunization.[47] In addition to HLA antigen-specific antibodies, platelets may adsorb immune complexes to their surface, and these complexes then may be recognized by the reticuloendothelial system and lead to platelet destruction.[48]

Posttransfusion alloimmunization to HLA antigens is a complex interaction between several factors, including antigen presentation and recipient immune responsiveness (Table 21.8). The number of antigenic exposures seems to have varying effects on alloimmunization. Two studies have shown that single-donor platelets are less alloimmunogenic than multiple-donor platelets,[49,50] and this may relate to fewer antigenic exposures per treatment course that occurs when single donor platelets are used. However, when patients with leukemia receive more than 10 to 20 transfusions, a dose-response relationship between transfusion and alloimmunization does not seem to exist. In our experience, only 29% of patients undergoing induction therapy for acute myelocytic leukemia became alloimmunized as evidenced by the development of lymphocytotoxic antibody, and 24 of these 26 patients who became alloimmunized did so within the first 6 weeks of transfusion. Further transfusion produced little additional alloimmunization; Dutcher et al.[51] have made similar observations. This suggests that not all patients can be alloimmunized, but in one study, over 80% of patients with aplastic anemia developed posttransfusion alloimmunization. Intensively treated patients with cancer had half that incidence.[52,53] Thus, the development of posttrans-

fusion alloimmunization is a complex interrelationship between antigen exposure, innate patient immune responsiveness, and any concurrent immunosuppression.

Paradoxically, platelets themselves are not antigenic with respect to HLA-A and -B (class I) antigens. To respond to class I HLA antigens, the recipient's immune system must be presented with cells that express both class I and class II (HLA-D,Dr) antigens.[54] Platelets, lacking class II antigens, are not highly immunogenic, so it appears that leukocytes expressing both class I and II antigens that are in the platelet concentrates are the sensitizing cells. This has led to strategies to prevent alloimmunization by leukocyte depletion of platelet products[55] or modification of leukocytes in platelet concentrates by ultraviolet (UV) light.[56]

Prevention of Posttransfusion Alloimmunization

One unit of whole blood contains approximately 1×10^9 leukocytes. Depending on the method of manufacture, platelet concentrates may contain from 1×10^7 to 1×10^8 leukocytes.[21,22] Studies in animals, and some in humans, have indicated that as few as 1×10^6 leukocytes can stimulate an immune response;[57] it is felt currently that to be clinically effective in preventing posttransfusion alloimmunization, leukocyte depletion must result in fewer than 5×10^6 cells/transfusion. There have been six randomized trials of leukocyte depletion to prevent posttransfusion alloimmunization,[49,58–62] but none has eliminated posttransfusion alloimmunization completely. Four of the six documented less alloimmunization by in vitro measurement of anti-HLA (lymphocytotoxic) antibody; however, only three documented an improved clinical response to transfusion. A major cause of these mixed results undoubtedly relates to the difficulty of depleting the blood products of leukocytes. Both centrifugation and early filtration techniques could reduce leukocyte contamination by only 2 logs (99%), but the recent development of platelet and red cell filters capable of 3–4 log reductions of white cells may prove to be more effective in preventing alloimmunization.[63]

One alternate approach for preventing alloimmunization has been UV irradiation of platelet products before transfusion. In the dog model of bone marrow transplant as well as early human transfusion trials, the exposure of platelet concentrates to UV radiation rendered the transfusion non-immunogenic.[54] This apparently relates to molecular changes within dendritic leukocytes in the blood product when exposed to UV light.[56] These leukocytes are, for a period of at least 24 hours, rendered hypoantigenic. Platelets so radiated seem to have near-normal function, and this raises the possibility of preventing alloimmunization by UV irradiation of platelet products. At this time, however, this technique has not been tested in large clinical trials. In addition, this technique would not be applicable to treatment of red cell concentrates that do not allow penetration of UV light. Although these technologies offer the hope of reducing posttransfusion alloimmunization, there always will remain some patients who, either through transfusion or pregnancy, become alloimmunized to platelets, and these patients will require the use of HLA-matched platelets.

MANAGEMENT OF POSTTRANSFUSION ALLOIMMUNIZATION

HLA Matching

In 1969, Yankee et al.[41] reported the correction of posttransfusion alloimmunization using unrelated platelet donors selected by what we currently recognize as the HLA-A and -B locus antigens of the major histocompatibility complex. The feasibility of widespread application of this knowledge was limited by the heterogeneity of the HLA-A and -B locus antigens; over 20 HLA-A locus and over 30 HLA-B locus antigens are recognized. Phenotypes representing 2 HLA-A locus and 2 HLA-B locus antigens are highly pleomorphic, and it was estimated that to identify a clinically useful number of donors for the majority of alloimmunized patients, a donor pool ranging from 5000 to over 50,000 would be required.[64]

Fortunately, there is a high degree of homology among certain HLA antigens, and this homology defines several cross-reacting HLA antigen groups. Duquesnoy et al.[65] were the first to document that this degree of cross-reactivity can be helpful clinically. Patients who were refractory to multiple-donor platelet concentrates were transfused with platelets that were selected for varying degrees of HLA match (Table 21.9). HLA-matching platelets from unrelated donors must be se-

TABLE 21.9. Degrees of HLA Matching for Platelet Transfusion*

Degree of Match	Example of Donor HLA Type
A	A1, A2, B8, B12
B1U	A1, B8, B12
B2U	A1, B8
B1X	A1, A28, B8, B12
B2X	A11, A28, B8, B12
B2UX	A11, B8, B12
C	One-antigen mismatch
D	Two-antigen mismatch

*Recipients A1, A2, B8, B12.

lected by their HLA phenotype, and when four different HLA specificities are demonstrated in one donor, it is fairly certain that the complete phenotype has been defined. However, when only two or three antigens can be defined, the antigen(s) lacking may be due to homozygosity or to the presence of an undetected, potentially mismatched antigen. Thus, a B2U transfusion from a donor who was phenotypically homozygous at the HLA-A and -B loci (for example, A1, B8) may be as good as an A match or as bad as a two-antigen match for a recipient with an HLA type such as A1, A2, B8, B12.

The degree of the match also can be characterized by the number of antigens that are included because of their apparent homology with recipient antigens. In the example previously given, HLA-A11 is close antigenically to A1, and HLA-A28 is similar antigenically to A2. A unit mismatch for these two antigens would be termed *B2X*. Duquesnoy et al. were able to document that in clinically refractory patients, there was a wide variation in response, regardless of the degree of HLA match between the donor and the recipient; however, the mean platelet recovery for A matches was similar to fairly distant B2U and B2X matches. These observations greatly expanded the ability to provide effective HLA-matched transfusion support, and using these degrees of cross-reactivity, donor pools as small as 1000 would contain sufficient individuals to support the majority of patients with HLA-mediated transfusion alloimmunization.

Platelet Crossmatching

Despite the use of matched HLA products, transfusion failures are still a major problem. In some studies, over 30% of A-matched platelet transfusions fail; this is felt to be related to platelet-specific antigens. Furthermore, many one- or two-antigen mismatched transfusions give normal posttransfusion increments.[66] For these reasons, many attempts have been made to develop an in vitro platelet crossmatching system that would identify compatible donors on a serologic basis. Multiple platelet crossmatching systems have been proposed, but no single system has gained wide application. This probably relates to problems with the sensitivity and specificity of the tests themselves and that the platelet refractory state is rather heterogenous with respect to etiology. Few patients present with a refractoriness to platelet transfusions based purely on alloimmunization, and with this clinical variability, it is difficult to document the superiority of one crossmatching system over another. In clinically stable patients who respond to HLA-matched platelets, platelet crossmatching can be highly predictive of transfusion outcome.[67] However, in the usual unstable clinical situation, with multiple reasons for platelet transfusion failure, platelet crossmatching has not proven to be highly useful.

Other Techniques

Many strategies have been employed to manage patients with severe alloimmunization. Massive transfusion, splenectomy, and treatment with high-dose steroids have proven ineffective;[64,68] likewise, plasmapheresis to remove circulating antibodies has not been effective.[69,70] Treatment with high dose of intravenous γ-globulin sufficient to saturate Fc receptors of the reticuloendothelial system recently has proven effective in the management of autoimmune thrombocytopenia purpura. However, application of high-dose intravenous γ-globulin to the management of posttransfusion alloimmunization has proven less effective. In one study, modest increases in 1-hour posttransfusion platelet recovery could be achieved, but 18-to-24-hour survival was not affected.[71]

Cryopreservation of autologous platelets also have been employed to manage alloimmunization. While effective, this technique is difficult, and freeze/thaw platelet loss can approach 50%. Furthermore, one must have the opportunity to collect large numbers of autologous platelets before their need.[72]

A Management Algorithm

The optimal management of a patient requiring platelet transfusion is complex, and there is no single best manner to assure a successful platelet transfusion outcome. Most centers involved in intensive transfusion, however, use an algorithm similar to that shown in Figure 21.2. Patients undergoing transfusion with either single- or multiple-donor platelets should be monitored with frequent 1-hour posttransfusion platelet increments, and patients manifesting a transfusion failure as

indicated by a CCI below 7500 should be transfused with fresh (less than 48 hours old) ABO-compatible platelets; if this corrects the posttransfusion CCI, then simply maintaining ABO compatibility and platelet freshness should be adequate. However, patients who obtain a CCI below 7500 with fresh ABO-compatible platelets must be considered for HLA-matched platelet transfusion support. If lymphocytotoxic antibody can be identified, it is most likely that alloimmune refractoriness is present, and such patients should receive either HLA-matched or crossmatched compatible platelets. Patients showing no lymphocytotoxic antibody, however, also may benefit from HLA-matched platelets. Thus, a platelet transfusion with an HLA-A, -B1U, or -B2U platelet is indicated. If a normal CCI can be obtained with an HLA-A, -B1U, or -B2U concentrate, then the patient should continue receiving HLA-matched platelets. Patients who fail an HLA challenge may have some degree of HLA-related refractoriness, but other problems may preclude response to HLA-matched platelets. In such patients, attempts should be made to improve their clinical status (lower fever, institute appropriate antibiotic therapy, etc.). If bleeding develops, some have suggested transfusion with frequent small doses of platelets to a maximum of 24 units in a 24-hour period for an average adult; if autoimmune thrombocytopenia is suspected, a trial with intravenous γ-globulin or prednisone may be indicated. Transfusion failure secondary to splenomegaly may be corrected by splenectomy, but in the presence of refractory thrombocytopenia because of bone marrow failure, this is frequently contraindicated due to the inability to maintain hemostasis. Some also have attempted to improve hemostasis in patients with refractory platelet transfusion and bleeding thrombocytopenia by use of the fibrinolytic inhibitor ε-aminocaproic acid.[73] However, a recent trial of tranexamic acid, another fibrinolytic inhibitor was shown not to prevent hemorrhage.[74]

MANAGEMENT OF ANEMIA SECONDARY TO MARROW FAILURE

Following myeloablative therapy, the proliferative compartment of red cell production also is damaged; however, the consequences of decreased red cell production are not as acute as those of the decreased production of platelets or leukocytes. Because of the long half-life of a circulating erythrocyte, anemia is slower to develop, but with appropriately timed sequences of therapy, total red cell loss may be moderate. Furthermore, the consequences of anemia are more subtle. Whereas thrombocytopenia can result in acute morbidity and mortality, the consequences of anemia are longer term.

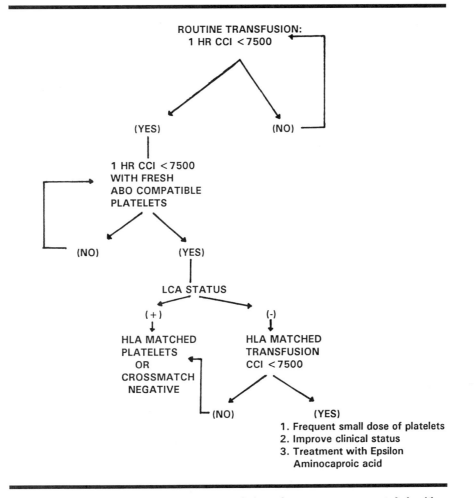

FIGURE 21.2. **The management of platelet transfusion refractory state: a suggested algorithm.**
Note: **CCI = corrected count increment; LCA = lymphocytotoxic antibody.**

A specific patient's ability to tolerate anemia is quite variable. In general, patients with hematocrits below hemoglobin levels less than 6 g/dl are symptomatic,[75] and such degrees of anemia ultimately result in tissue hypoxia and death. Lesser degrees of anemia, however, can be well tolerated. Acute drops in hemoglobin can result in symptomatic hypoxia, but more gradual reductions in hemoglobin can be compensated for by various mechanisms. Previously, a hematocrit below 30 (hemoglobin of 10 g/dl) was considered a minimal value for the induction of general anesthesia; more recently, however, it has been recognized that this is a rather arbitrary cutoff. An individual patient's response to anemia depends on multiple factors, and patients with good pulmonary and cardiac function but without an increased tissue requirement for oxygen can tolerate significant degrees of anemia. This is true particularly when patients are at bed rest in the hospital. However, patients with either acute or chronic pulmonary insufficiency as well as impaired cardiac vascular or increased tissue requirements for oxygen may require higher levels of circulating hemoglobin.

A recent consensus of transfusion specialists has recommended transfusion criteria to be individualized to the specific patient.[76] In situations of acute blood loss, transfusion should be adjusted to the estimated loss. In situations of bone marrow failure, however, the decision to transfuse erythrocytes is more difficult. In healthy adults younger than 50 years of age and with normal pulmonary and cardiac reserve, maintenance of the hematocrit above 25% may be well tolerated; older patients without specific medical problems may require hematocrits in the 30% range. Patients with impaired pulmonary function or cardiac reserve, or those who require increased oxygen perfusion of tissues such as patients with ischemic vascular disease, may require maintenance of a hematocrit above 35%. Further details regarding the principle of red cell support as well as the use of the hormone erythropoietin are provided elsewhere in this book.

MANAGEMENT OF GRANULOCYTOPENIA SECONDARY TO MARROW FAILURE

Characteristics of Infection

In the 1960s, during the early trials of cytotoxic therapy for acute leukemia, it became apparent that granulocytopenia was associated with acute morbidity and mortality.[77] It also soon was appreciated that the development of leukopenia below 1000 white cells/mm^3 was associated both with fever and a high incidence of gram-negative sepsis, and in one study, over 20% of the episodes of fever during neutropenia were associated with gram-negative bacteremia.[78] Without adequate antibiotic therapy, this condition was frequently fatal.

Evaluation of the patient with neutropenia is complicated by subtle changes in the physical signs of infection during periods of inadequate white cell production. The development of exudates and fluctuance is dependent on granulocyte function, but fever has been a consistent characteristic of infection in these patients. Redness, swelling, and pain also persist during neutropenia. Without the presence of an exudate, infections in the patient with neutropenia may be confused with viral infections, and this has been particularly hazardous as infections in these patients characteristically are caused by bacterial agents, especially gram-negative rods.[79] Infection with *Pseudomonas aerugenosa* in the patient with neutropenia has been particularly feared, because vascular collapse is associated with this infection.[80] However, infections with other gram-negative rods, such as *Escherichia coli*, *Klebsiella* species, and *Proteus* species, are serious as well.[81] With both the development of broad-spectrum antibiotic coverage of fever and the use of indwelling catheters for long-term intravenous therapy, infection with gram-positive organisms, particularly *Staphylococcus epidermidis*, recently has become more prominent.[82]

The clinical sites of infection observed in the neutropenic host are different than those observed in the noncompromised host as well. Neutropenic infections are common in moist intertriginous areas that normally are colonized with bacteria and traumatized during daily activity; such infection sites include axillary, inguinal,

or periungual sites in the skin. In the gastrointestinal tract, gingivitis, esophagitis, and perirectal infections are common, and because of the lack of granulocytes to establish local control, pneumonia in the neutropenic patient can be multilobar with minimal signs of consolidation. The difficulty of diagnosis as well as the overwhelming consequences of undertreatment have led to a reliance on empiric therapy in the patient with severe neutropenia.[79]

Granulocyte Transfusion

In view of the morbidity and mortality, transfusion replacement therapy with granulocyte concentrates would seem to be a logical therapeutic approach; in fact, it was for the purpose of granulocyte collection that clinical blood cell separators first were developed. However, the isolation of granulocytes from normal blood donors has proven to be most difficult. The density of the normal circulating granulocyte is such that separation from red cells is difficult, and to separate the red cells from granulocytes by using centrifugation methodologies, hydroxyethyl starch or a dextran agent must be added. The hydroxyethyl starch structures the red cell mass in rouleau in the cell separator so that granulocytes are excluded and forced into the buffy layer containing the platelets and lymphocytes.[83] In a 2- or 3-hour donation employing hydroxyethyl starch, granulocyte concentrates containing from 1 to 2 × 10^{10} neutrophils can be achieved, and with the addition of pretreating donors with corticosteroids to induce leukocytosis, granulocyte yields can be doubled.

Over the last decade, over 100,000 leukapheresis procedures have been performed without serious toxicity to donors. However, granulocyte donation has more potential morbidity for donors than plateletpheresis. Donation periods are longer than for leukapheresis, frequently 2 to 3 hours, and in addition, hydroxyethyl starch must be used. This long, branched glucose polymer is metabolized slowly by the body,[83] and residual hydroxyethyl starch can be detected in the donor for several years after the donation. Also, donation of granulocyte several times a week over several weeks has resulted in severe pruritus secondary to elevated hydroxyethyl starch levels. The use of steroids for leukapheresis is problematic as well, as premedication with steroids can result in acute steroid side effects, including gastric hyperacidity, insomnia, and hyperactivity. For these reasons, both leukapheresis and leukotransfusion should be undertaken only in the indicated circumstances.[84]

One of the major deterrents to effective granulocyte transfusion has been the difficulty of collecting adequate numbers to substitute for clinical needs. A normal bone marrow produces approximately 10^{11} granulocytes/day,[9,10] and this can be increased several-fold during infection. However, even when employing hydroxyethyl starch and with mobilization of the donors' granulocyte marginating pooled with steroids, only doses of from 2 to 4×10^{10} granulocytes can be collected; transfusion of these low numbers is insufficient to replace the normal circulating granulocyte numbers. Hence, granulocyte transfusion usually is not associated with an increase in posttransfusion circulating neutrophils unless one obtains an immediate posttransfusion neutrophil count.

The second major problem in leukotransfusion is the definition of granulocyte serocompatibility. It is clear that the HLA-A and -B locus antigens are important determinants for granulocyte transfusion; in vitro studies indicate that granulocytes reacted with specific anti-HLA-A or -B locus antibodies fail to have normal diapedesis and chemotaxis.[85] Further transfusion of HLA-incompatible granulocytes has been noted to result in the failure of transfused granulocytes to target the sites of infection. Thus, alloimmunization to HLA antigens generally is considered a contraindication to granulocyte transfusion. It also is clear that there are several granulocyte-specific antigen systems. The serology of these antigens is understood poorly, and no effective crossmatch test is available. Hence, idiosyncratic toxicity or therapeutic failure on an immunologic basis is not uncommon with granulocyte transfusions.

Initial studies of granulocyte transfusions were conducted in patients undergoing chemotherapy for acute leukemia in the 1970s. At that time, effective gram-negative therapy for infection during neutropenia was not available,[86,87] and gram-negative sepsis was associated with a 50% mortality. In this situation, patients with severe neutropenia (fewer than 500 circulating granulocytes/mm^3) and positive blood cultures for gram-negative bacteria were noted to have a 50% reduction in mortality if 5 to 10 days of granulocyte transfusions could be administered. To improve on this marginal response, prophylactic granulocyte transfusion was attempted; however, in one prospective, randomized study during therapy for acute myelocytic leukemia, no therapeutic advantage of prophylactic transfusion could be demonstrated. In fact, patients receiving granulocyte transfusion had an increased incidence of pulmonary infiltrates.[88] Based on this data, we currently recommend granulocyte transfusion only for those patients who are severely neutropenic (fewer than 100 neutrophils/mm^3), have anticipated aplasia of greater than 7 days, manifest no lymphocytotoxic antibody, and have a gram-negative bacteremia or Candidemia that is resistant to antibiotic management.

The morbidity of granulocyte transfusions is considerable,[88] and febrile transfusion reactions are common. These can be severe, with fevers of 40°C or more, and premedication with either steroids or antipyretics frequently is required. Furthermore, pulmonary infiltrates are not uncommon following granulocyte transfusion. In some patients, these may represent therapeutic infiltration of infected pulmonary tissue by granulocytes; in others, they may indicate an acute leukoagglutinin pulmonary edema or a nonspecific adult respiratory distress syndrome secondary to potent biomediators released by nonviable granulocytes. One series reported synergistic toxicity between amphotericin B and granulocyte transfusions,[89] but this has not been substantiated by subsequent studies.[90] Both amphotericin B and granulocyte transfusions can result in febrile reactions and pulmonary infiltrates and therefore should be used with caution; however, there is no contraindication to their concurrent use in the same patient.

ANTIBIOTIC MANAGEMENT OF INFECTION IN NEUTROPENIA

Empiric Treatment of Fever

Historically, the initial attempts to manage infection in the patient with neutropenia by use of antibiotics were unsuccessful. Treatment with combinations of cephalosporins, kanamycin, and colistin not only were highly nephrotoxic, they only were marginally effective in treating gram-negative sepsis. With the introduction of empiric combination therapy using gentamicin and carbenicillin in the 1970s, the outcome became much more predictable,[91] and in the last decade, multiple studies have investigated various combination antibiotic therapies for the treatment of patients with febrile neutropenia.[81] No single antibiotic regimen has gained universal acceptance. Most specialists today would recommend a combination of an aminoglycoside (gentamicin or amikacin) with a β-lactam (ceftazidime) antibiotic.[92] Most investigators also prefer combination over monotherapy because of the broader spectrum of antibiotic coverage, the theoretic advantage of enhanced bacterial cytotoxicity, and a decreased emergence of resistant organisms. However, several centers recently explored the possibility of monotherapy with ceftazidime.[93] Single-agent antibiotic therapy has the advantage of being easier to administer and is both less costly and less toxic; however, the most important determinant of selecting an appropriate empiric antibiotic therapy should be an individual institution's epidemiologic patterns. Hospitals having continuing problems with resistant *Pseudomonas aeruginosa* infections would, perhaps, best continue to use combination antibiotic therapy; other hospitals with a high incidence of penicillin-resistant *Staphylococcus epidermidis* infections may add vancomycin to their empiric regimens. Still others may find monotherapy with ceftazidime effective. Thus, no single antibiotic regimen can be recommended universally for empiric use in patients with febrile neutropenia; however, there is no question that empiric antibiotic therapy of fever in patients with neutropenia is essential.

The duration of antibiotic therapy also has been subject to controversy. In general, until the granulocyte deficiency is repaired by marrow recovery, the potential for either recurrence or progression of infection is high when the antibiotic therapy is stopped. Consequently, many investigators have recommended continuing antibiotic therapy for 10 to 14 days in the patient with granulocytopenia regardless of the fever's course.[94]

Patients who defervesce following initial combination therapy and then develop recurrent fever, or those who manifest progressive fever during neutropenia, constitute a serious problem. In this population, resistant gram-negative or fungal infection is extremely common; consequently, secondary empiric therapy with more effective gram-negative antibiotic coverage or the introduction of antifungal therapy with amphotericin B usually is recommended. On the resolution of neutropenia, continuation of antibiotic therapy is not required unless a major soft tissue infection has developed. In this case, antibiotic therapy should be continued using standard principles of infectious disease therapy.

Antibiotic Prophylaxis

In view of the morbidity and mortality of established infection in the patient with neutropenia, prophylactic antibiotic therapy has seemed logical. In the majority of these patients, infections are caused by endogenous organisms, and in the hospitalized patient, these may be either normal commensal organisms or nosocomial organisms acquired after admission. In either case, the patient usually is colonized by the pathogen before the manifestation of the first infection.[95] This has led several investigators to attempt reducing the host bacterial load during neutropenia. Attempts to selectively decontaminate the gastrointestinal tract with oral nonabsorbable antibiotics, such as colistin, kanamycin, or gentamicin, were only partially effective,[96] and in addition, these regimens were tolerated poorly, with significant nausea, vomiting, and diarrhea. Furthermore, overgrowth with other resistant organisms was common.

The concept of protective isolation was developed further to include total life island systems.[97,98] With both intensive gastrointestinal and dermal decontamina-tion in conjunction with sterile diets and sterile filtered air, these units are able to decrease the number of febrile days in selected diseases, but they are unable to cause any difference in the overall survival. As the use of a total life island concept is expensive and fraught with significant psychologic difficulties, it is not used widely.

Recently, the concept of selective gastrointestinal decontamination has been introduced, and with the use of norfloxacin or ciprofloxacin, gram-negative coverage has been achieved while sparing anaerobic organisms.[99] Retention of anaerobic flora apparently inhibits colonization with resistant, nosocomially acquired organisms. In selected patient populations, these agents have been shown to delay the onset of first fever and result in a higher incidence of response to empiric antibiotic therapy for first fever; however, studies have not indicated improved survival using these agents. Nonetheless, because of their low cost and easy administration, they generally are considered an important addition to therapy.

Viral infections in the patient with isolated neutropenia have not been as overwhelmingly fatal as bacterial infections; however, infections with viruses, particularly those of the herpes simplex group, are a major cause of morbidity following cancer chemotherapy. Reactivation of latent infection can result in severe disruption of the mucosal barrier with subsequent invasion of bacterial pathogens. Fortunately, low-dose prophylactic therapy with acyclovir has proven to be almost uniformly effective in preventing the reactivation of herpes simplex infection.[100]

Prophylaxis of fungal infections in the patient with neutropenia has been more problematic.[101] Trials with myconazol and fluconazol have resulted in variable results, and at this time, routine antifungal prophylaxis generally is not recommended. However, depending on the individual institution's patient population and nosocomial data, prophylactic therapy in specific populations may be appropriate.

OTHER ADJUNCTIVE THERAPIES IN THE MANAGEMENT OF APLASIA

Hematopoietic Growth Factors

The major determinant of survival in the aplastic patient is the successful recovery of normal marrow function. In this regard, the development of therapeutic quantities of hematopoietic growth factors for use in the patient with aplasia has led to the possibility of shortening the duration of this condition. Currently, four hematopoietic growth factors are being evaluated in clinical trials;[102] these include granulocyte-macrophage colony-stimulating factor, interleukin-3 (multi-colony stimulating factor), granulocyte colony-stimulating factor, and macrophage colony-stimulating factor. Preliminary studies with both granulocyte-macrophage and granulocyte colony-stimulating factors indicate that these agents can accelerate neutrophil recovery following a variety of intensive chemotherapy regimens.[103,104] Most studies also have demonstrated a decrease in febrile days as well as in the number of microbiologically documented infections. No study, however, has indicated an improved survival. Nonetheless, it appears that these factors will become an important adjuvant in the management of bone marrow failure in selected patient populations, but their widespread use may be limited by the minimal shortening of aplasia (usually 3 to 6 days), high cost, and side effects.

Bone Marrow Transplantation

As discussed previously, myelotoxicity is the major dose-limiting toxicity with current chemoradiation therapy. Total-body irradiation or intensive therapy with stem cell ablative cytotoxics can result in irreversible aplasia. Use of hematopoietic stem cell transplantation to reverse marrow ablation has been widely developed during the last two decades, and by using allogeneic or autologous stem cells, hematopoietic recovery following myeloablative therapy can be achieved. Depending on the cell dose, in vitro treatment to remove selective lymphocyte or tumor cell populations, and any cryopreservation, the rate of hematopoietic recovery can vary; however, with an adequate dose of bone marrow cells exceeding 1×10^8 nucleated cells/kg, reconstitution of granulocytes to levels above 500 cells/mm^3 usually can be achieved within 19 days after marrow transplantation. Recovery of platelets and reticulocytes is somewhat more variable. Nonetheless, stem cell transplantation using either cells collected from the bone marrow or circulating hematopoietic stem cells can result in both accelerated and sustained engraftment following intensive cytotoxic therapy.[4,5]

Graft-Versus-Host Disease in Aplastic Patient

Transfusion support with specific cell components is essential to the successful management of the patient with aplasia. However, blood components contain a variable number of T lymphocytes that are capable of engrafting in the severely immunosuppressed host, and these cells then are capable of causing graft-versus-host disease.[105] When caused by third-party lymphocytes, this disease is characterized by a pentad of gastroenteritis, hepatitis, dermatitis, immunosuppression, and pan-

cytopenia. Gastroenteritis can be severe, with life-threatening diarrhea. Hepatitis with graft-versus-host disease is nonspecific, but the dermatitis is a characteristic erythroderma initially involving the palms, soles, and earlobes in its early stage. Overall, the syndrome of graft-versus-host disease may appear to mimic a viral infection, and diagnosis is dependent on a low threshold of suspicion and tissue biopsy.

There presently is no efficacious therapy for third-party graft-versus-host disease; therefore, clinical management must be based on prevention. Posttransfusion graft-versus-host disease has been reported in a variety of situations, and three factors apparently play crucial roles in determining which patients will develop this disease (Table 21.10). First, the blood product must have a significant number of viable T lymphocytes; certain products such as fresh-frozen plasma and frozen deglycerolized red cells have essentially no lymphocytes. Other products, such as granulocyte transfusions and certain platelet transfusions, can have over 1×10^9 viable lymphocytes/transfusion. Lymphocyte doses as low as 1×10^7/kg have been reported to cause graft-versus-host disease.

In addition to receiving a substantial number of viable lymphocytes, the host usually has been immunosuppressed. Fetuses receiving intrauterine transfusions, neonates, and children with various inherited immunodeficiency syndromes particularly are susceptible to graft-versus-host disease. Patients with acquired immune defects, such as those undergoing bone marrow transplantation, chemotherapy for acute leukemia, or treatment of Hodgkin disease, also are at risk for graft-versus-host disease.

It has been appreciated as well that the degree of HLA-matching is important. Apparently normal patients undergoing transfusion support during coronary artery bypass surgery have been reported to have died of severe third-party graft-versus-host disease. Retrospec-

TABLE 21.10. Factors Predisposing to Posttransfusion Graft-Versus-Host Disease

Factor	Comment
Type of blood product	Number of viable lymphocytes varies with product, method of collection, and storage

Recipient factors
  Size
  Degree of
    immunosuppression
	Engraftment not possible without some degree of recipient cellular immune defect

HLA type of product and host	HLA-matched products have a high chance of engrafting

tively, it was noted that these patients had received directed donations from phenotypically HLA-identical family members. Thus, it appears that under the appropriate circumstances, even immune competent patients may be at risk for graft-versus-host disease.

Graft-versus-host disease can be eliminated completely by appropriate irradiation of blood products.[106] Radiation to 5000 rads has been shown to abrogate the mixed lymphocyte culture in vitro, and doses of 1500 rads have been shown to prevent graft-versus-host disease in animal transfusion models. Based on this, irradiation of blood products to 1500 rads generally is recommended for patients who are felt to be susceptible to posttransfusion graft-versus-host disease, and gamma radiation at these low doses causes negligible functional impairment to red cells, platelets, or granulocytes.

Prevention of Posttransfusion Cytomegalovirus Infection

Cytomegalovirus is a common pathogen that usually causes minimal mortality in the immune competent adult; however, in the severely immunosuppressed patient, CMV can cause severe morbidity and mortality. In the immunocompromised host, CMV can cause interstitial pneumonitis, hepatitis, and gastroenteritis, and in addition, it has been reported in the organ transplant setting to predispose patients to opportunistic infection with fungus, bacteria, and pneumocystis. In the bone marrow transplants, CMV apparently aggravates graft-versus-host disease and can result in a delay in hematologic recovery.[107]

The broad spectrum of clinical symptoms secondary to CMV infection perhaps is related to its multiple effects on the host. First, CMV can have a direct cytolytic effect on various tissues, and this perhaps is the most important mechanism in CMV hepatitis and retinitis. In addition, CMV infection has an immunosuppressive effect on the host, which perhaps is responsible for the increased incidence of opportunistic infections in patients undergoing organ transplantation. Finally, CMV also can induce increased expression of HLA antigens on host cells.

Infection with CMV can be acquired from environmental sources or blood transfusion. In blood transfusion, the virus apparently is transmitted in the genome of nucleated white cells transfused with red cells or platelets; products with low white cell contamination, such as fresh-frozen plasma or frozen deglycerolized red cells, have a negligible risk of transmitting CMV infection. In patients who have not been exposed previously to CMV, the prevention of posttransfusion CMV infection is highly desirable. Preparation of blood components from donors who have not been infected previously with CMV, as indicated by their CMV-seronegative status, has been shown essentially to eliminate posttransfusion CMV infection, and newer filtration methods that reduce leukocyte contamination in blood products to less than 1×10^6 leukocytes/transfusion also may be effective. Clinical trials currently are in progress to determine this.

Conclusion

The management of the aplastic patient has improved markedly in the last four decades. Interdisciplinary clinical management with optimal transfusion and antibiotic therapy can support patients through 4 to 6 weeks of severe bone marrow failure, and an understanding of the pathophysiology of bone marrow failure and replacement therapy has been essential to the development of a rational management of aplasia induced during chemotherapy. However, it must be remembered that this supportive therapy only can be considered temporizing. Without the ultimate recovery of the bone marrow, complications from infections that are unresponsive to antibiotic management or cell deficits refractory to replacement therapy ultimately are fatal.

REFERENCES

1. DeVita VT Jr, Hellman S, Rosenberg SA. Cancer: Principles and Practice. Philadelphia: J.B. Lippincott, 1982.
2. DeVita VT, Serpick AA, Carbone PP. Combination chemotherapy in the treatment of Hodgkin's disease. Ann Intern Med 1970;73:891–5.
3. Geller RB, Burke PJ, Karp JE, et al. A two-step timed sequential treatment of acute myelocytic leukemia. Blood 1989; 74:1499–506.
4. Forman SJ, Blume KG. Allogeneic bone marrow transplantation for acute leukemia. Hematol Oncol Clin North Am 1990;4:517–29.
5. Kessinger A, Nademance A, Forman SJ, Armitage JO. Autologous bone marrow transplantation for Hodgkin's and non-Hodgkin's lymphoma. Hematol Oncol Clin North Am 1990; 4:577–87.
6. Harker LA, Finch CA. Thombokinetics in man. J Clin Invest 1969;48:963.
7. Aster RH, Jandl JH. Platelet sequestration in man. I. Methods. J Clin Invest 1964;43:843.
8. Scheffel U, Tsan M, Mitchell TG. Human platelets labelled with In-III 8-hydroxyquinoline: kinetics, distribution, and estimates of radiation dose. J Nucl Med 1982;23:149.
9. Warner HR, Athens JW. An analysis of granulocyte kinetics in blood and bone marrow. Ann N Y Acad Sci 1964;113:523.
10. Cronkite EP, Fliedner TM. Granulopoiesis. N Engl J Med 1967;270:1347.
11. Mullins GM, Anderson PN, Santos GW. High-dose cyclophosphamide therapy in solid tumors. Cancer 1975;36:1950–8.

12. Harker LA, Slichter SJ. Bleeding time as a screening test for evaluating platelet function. N Engl J Med 1972;287:155.

13. Slichter SJ, Harker LA. Thrombocytopenia, mechanisms, and management of defects in platelet production. Clin Haematol 1978;7:523.

14. Levine AS, Graw RG, Young RC. Management of infections in patients with leukemia and lymphosarcoma: current concepts and experimental approaches. Semin Hematol 1972;9:141–79.

15. Roy AJ, Djerassi JN. Prophylactic platelet transfusion in children with acute leukemia: a dose response study. Transfusion 1973;13:283.

16. Higby DJ, Cohen E, Holland JF, Sinks L. The prophylactic treatment of thrombocytopenic leukemia patients with platelets: a double blind study. Transfusion 1974;14:1440.

17. Gaydos LA, Freireich EJ, Mantel N. The quantitative relation between platelet count and hemorrhage in patients with leukemia. N Engl J Med 1962;266:905.

18. Aderka D, Praff G, Weinberger SM. Bleeding due to thrombocytopenia in acute leukemias and reevaluation of the prophylactic platelet transfusion policy. Am J Med Sci 1986;291:147.

19. Solomon J, Bokefkamp T, Fahey JL, et al. Platelet prophylaxis in acute nonlymphocytic leukemia. Lancet 1978;i:267.

20. Rao KA. Congenital disorders of platelet function. Hematol Oncol Clin North Am 1990;4:65–86.

21. Slichter SJ, Harker LA. Preparation and storage of platelet concentrates: I. Factors influencing the harvest of viable platelets from whole blood. Br J Haematol 1976;34:393.

22. Slichter SJ, Harker LA. Preparation and storage of platelet concentrates: II. Storage variables influencing platelet viability and function. Br J Haematol 1976;34:403.

23. Code of Federal Regulations, Food and Drugs, Title 21, Parts 600–799. Washington, D.C.: U.S. Government Printing Office, 1987.

24. Tullis JL, Tinch RJ, Baudanza P, et al. Plateletpheresis in a disposable system. Transfusion 1971;11:368.

25. Puig LI, Mazzara R, Gelabert A, Costillo R. Plateletpheresis: a comparative study of six different protocols. J Clin Apheresis 1986;3:129–32.

26. Bucholtz DH, Porten JH, Menitove JE, et al. Description and use of the CS-3000 blood cell separator for single donor platelet collection. Transfusion 1983;23:190.

27. Price TH, Ford SE, Northway MM. Alternate collection protocols for plateletpheresis using the COBE spectra (abstract). J Clin Apheresis 1989;5:49.

28. Straus RG, Halpern LN, Eckermann I. Comparison of autoserge versus surge protocols for discontinuous-flow centrifugation plateletpheresis. Transfusion 1987;27:499–501.

29. Murphy S, Gardner FH. Platelet preservation. Effect of storage temperature on maintenance of platelet viability—deleterious effect of refrigerated storage. N Engl J Med 1969;280:1094–8.

30. Holme S, Murphy S. Platelet storage at 22°C for transfusion: interrelationship of platelet density and size, medium pH, and viability after in vivo infusion. J Lab Clin Med 1983;101:161.

31. Snyder EL, Pope C, Ferri PM, Smith EO, Walter SD, Ezekowitz MD. The effect of mode of agitation and type of plastic bag on storage characteristics and in vivo kinetics of platelet concentrates. Transfusion 1986;26:125.

32. Lindberg JE, Slichter SJ, Murphy S, et al. In vitro function and in vivo viability of stored platelet concentrates. Effect of a secondary plasticizer component of PVC storage bags. Transfusion 1983;23:294.

33. Simon TL, Nelson EJ, Murphy S. Extension of platelet concentrate storage to 7 days in second-generation bags. Transfusion 1987;27:6.

34. Daly PA, Schiffer CA, Aisner J, Wiernik PH. Platelet transfu-

sion therapy: one hour post-transfusion increments are valuable in predicting the need for HLA-match preparations. JAMA 1980;243:435.

35. O'Connell B, Lee EJ, Schiffer CA. The value of 10-minute post-transfusion platelet counts. Transfusion 1988;28:66–7.

36. Lee EJ, Schiffer CA. ABO compatibility can influence the results of platelet transfusion. Results of a randomized trial. Transfusion 1989;29:384–9.

37. Hanson SR, Slichter SJ. Platelet kinetics in patients with bone marrow hypoplasia: evidence for a fixed platelet requirement. Blood 1985;66:1105.

38. Parker RD, Yamamoto LA, Miller WR. Interaction effects analysis of platelet transfusion data. Transfusion 1974;14:567–73.

39. Bishop JF, McGrath K, Wolf MM, et al. Clinical factors influencing the efficacy of pooled platelet transfusions. Blood 1988;71:383–7.

40. McFarland JG, Anderson AJ, Slichter SJ. Factors influencing the transfusion response to HLA-selected apheresis donor platelets in patients refractory to random platelet concentrates. Br J Haematol 1989;73:380–6.

41. Yankee RA, Grumet FC, Rogentine GN. Platelet transfusion therapy. The selection of compatible donors for refractory patients by lymphocyte HLA typing. N Engl J Med 1969;281:1208.

42. Hogge DE, Dutcher P, Aisner J, Schiffer CA. Lymphocytotoxic antibody is a predictor of response to random donor platelet transfusion. Am J Hematol 1983;14:363–9.

43. Duquesnoy RJ, Anderson AJ, Tomasulo PA, Aster RH. ABO compatibility and platelet transfusions of alloimmunized thrombocytopenic patients. Blood 1979;54:595.

44. Slichter SJ, Teramura G. Frequency of platelet-specific alloantibodies in platelet refractory thrombocytopenic patients (abstract). Blood 1988;72(suppl 1):286A.

45. McFarland JG, Aster RH. Platelet immunology and the HLA system. In: Rossi EC, Simon TL, Moss GS, eds. Principles of Transfusion Medicine. Baltimore: Williams & Wilkins, 1991:193–204.

46. Schiffer CA, O'Connell B, Lee EJ. Platelet transfusion therapy for alloimmunized patients: selective mismatching for HLA-B12, an antigen with variable expression on platelets. Blood 1989;74:1172.

47. Miller K, Kickler TS, Braine HG. Immunoglobulin class heterogeneity of platelet allo antibodies. Vox Sang 1984;47:421.

48. Kutti J, Zaroulis CG, Safai-Kutti S, et al. Evidence that circulating immune complexes remove transfused patients from the circulation. Am J Hematol 1981;11:255.

49. Sintnicolaas K, Sizoo W, Haije WG, et al. Delayed alloimmunization by random single donor platelet transfusions. Lancet 1981;i:750.

50. Gmur J, von Felten A, Osterwalder B, et al. Delayed alloimmunization using random single donor platelet transfusions: a prospective study in thrombocytopenic patients with acute leukemia. Blood 1983;62:473.

51. Dutcher JP, Schiffer CA, Aisner J. Alloimmunization following platelet transfusion: the absence of a dose response relationship. Blood 1980;57:395.

52. Tosato G, Appelbaum FR, Deisseroth AB. HLA-matched platelet transfusion therapy of severe aplastic anemia. Blood 1978;52:846.

53. Holohan TV, Terasaki PI, Deisseroth AB. Suppression of transfusion-related alloimmunization in intensively treated cancer patients. Blood 1981;58:122.

54. Slichter SJ, Deeg HJ, Kennedy MS. Prevention of platelet alloimmunization in dogs with systemic cyclosporine and by

UV-irradiation or cyclosporine-loading of donor platelets. Blood 1987;69:414.

55. Eernisse JG, Brand A. Prevention of platelet refractoriness due to HLA antibodies by administration of leukocyte-poor blood components. Exp Hematol 1981;9:77.

56. Kripke ML. Immunologic unresponsiveness induced by ultraviolet radiation. Immunol Rev 1984;80:87.

57. Fisher M, Chapman JK, Ting A, Morris PJ. Alloimmunization to HLA antigens following transfusion with leukocyte-poor and purified platelet suspensions. Vox Sang 1985;49:331–5.

58. Schiffer CA, Dutcher JP, Aisner J, et al. A randomized trial of leukocyte-depleted platelet transfusions to modify alloimmunization in patients with leukemia. Blood 1983;62:815.

59. Sniecinski I, O'Donnell MR, Nowicki B, Hill LR. Prevention of refractoriness and HLA-alloimmunization using filtered blood products. Blood 1988;71:1402.

60. Andreu G, Dewailly J, Leberre C, et al. Prevention of HLA-immunization with leukocyte-poor packed red cells and platelet concentrated obtained by filtration. Blood 1988;72:964.

61. Saarinen UM, Kekomaki R, Siimes MA, Myllyla G. Effective prophylaxis against platelet refractoriness in multi-transfused patients by use of leukocyte free blood components. Blood 1990;75:512.

62. Brand A, Claas FHJ, Voogt PJ, et al. Alloimmunization after leukocyte-depleted multiple random donor platelet transfusions. Vox Sang 1988;54:160.

63. Meryman HT. Transfusion induced alloimmunization and immunosuppression and the effects of leukocyte depletion. Trans Med Rev 1989;3:180–93.

64. Slichter SJ. Controversies in platelet transfusion therapy. Annu Rev Med 1980;31:509–40.

65. Duquesnoy RJ, Filip DJ, Rodey GE, Rimm AA, Aster RH. Successful transfusion of platelets mismatched for HLA-A antigens to alloimmunized thrombocytopenic patients. Am J Hematol 1977;2:219.

66. Kickler TS, Ness PM. Platelet crossmatching for the alloimmunized patient. In: McCarthy LJ, Menitove JE, eds. Immunologic Aspects of Platelet Transfusion. Arlington, VA: American Association of Blood Banks, 1985:71–81.

67. Kickler TS, Braine HG, Ness PM. The predictive value of crossmatching platelet transfusion for alloimmunized patients. Transfusion 1985;25:385.

68. Hogge DE, Dutcher JP, Aisner J, Schiffer CA. The ineffectiveness of random donor platelet transfusion in splenectomized, alloimmunized recipients. Blood 1984;64:253–6.

69. Besinger WI, Buckner CD, Clift RA, Slichter SJ, Thomas ED. Plasma exchange for platelet alloimmunization. Transplantation 1986;41:602–5.

70. Nagasawa T, Kim BK, Baldini MG. Temporary suppression of circulating antiplatelet antibodies by the massive infusion of fresh, stored, or lyophilized platelets. Transfusion 1978;18:429.

71. Kickler T, Braine HG, Piantadosi S, Ness PM, Herman JH, Rothko K. A randomized placebo controlled trial of intravenous gammaglobulin in alloimmunized thrombocytopenia patients. Blood 1990;75:313–6.

72. Schiffer CA, Aisner J, Wiernik PH. Frozen autologous platelet transfusions for patients with leukemia. N Engl J Med 1978;299:7.

73. Bartholomew JR, Solgia R, Bell WR. Control of bleeding in patients with immune thrombocytopenia with aminocaproic acid. Arch Intern Med 1989;149:1959–61.

74. Fricke W, Alling D, Kimball J, Griffith P, Klein H. Lack of efficacy of tranexamic acid in thrombocytopenic bleeding. Transfusion 1991;31:345–8.

75. Elwood PC, Waters WE, Greene WSW, et al. Symptoms and circulating hemoglobin level. J Chronic Dis 1969;21:615–28.

76. Perioperative Red Cell Transfusion. National Institutes of Health Consensus Development Conference Statement, Vol. 7, No. 4, June 27–29, 1988.

77. Bodey GP, Buckley M, Sathe YS, Freireich EJ. Quantitative relationships between circulating leukocytes and infection in patients with acute leukemia. Ann Intern Med 1966;64:328.

78. Burke PJ, Braine HG, Rathbun HK, Owens AH Jr. The clinical significance and management of fever in acute myelocytic leukemia. Johns Hopkins Med J 1976;139:1–12.

79. Sickles EA, Greene WH, Wiernik PH. Clinical presentation of infection in granulocytopenic patients. Arch Intern Med 1975;135:715–9.

80. Schimpff SC, Green WH, Young VM, et al. Pseudomonas septicemia: incidence, epidemiology, prevention and therapy in patients with advanced cancer. Eur J Cancer 1973;9:449–55.

81. Klastersky J, Zimmer SH, Calandra T, et al. Empiric antimicrobial therapy for febrile granulocytopenic cancer patients: lessons from four EORTC trials. Eur J Cancer Clin Oncol 1988;24:S35–S45.

82. Wade JC, Schimpff SC, Newman KA, et al. *Staphylococcus epidermidis:* an increasing cause of infection in patients with granulocytopenia. Ann Intern Med 1987;97:503–8.

83. Mishler JM. Hydroxyethyl starch as an experimental adjunct to leukocyte separation by centrifugal means: review of safety and efficacy. Transfusion 1975;15:449.

84. Higby DJ, Mishler JM, Rhomberg W, Nicora RW, Holland JF. The effect of single or double doses of dexamethasone on granulocyte collection with the continuous flow centrifuge. Vox Sang 1975;28:243.

85. Dutcher JP, Schiffer CA, Johnston GS. The effect of histocompatibility factors on the migration of transfused ^{111}Indium-Labeled granulocytes. Blood 1981;58(suppl):181A.

86. Herzig RH, Herzig GP, Graw RG Jr, Bull MI, Ray RK. Successful granulocyte therapy for gram-negative septicemia. N Engl J Med 1977;296:701.

87. Alavi BJ, Root RK, Djerassi I, et al. A randomized clinical trial of granulocyte transfusions for infection in acute leukemia. N Engl J Med 1977;296:706.

88. Strauss RG, Connett JE, Gale RP. A controlled trial of prophylactic granulocyte transfusions during initial induction chemotherapy for acute myelogenous leukemia. N Engl J Med 1981;305:597.

89. Boxer LA, Ingraham LM, Allen J. Amphotericin B promotes leukocyte aggregation of nylon-wool-fiber-treated polymorphonuclear leukocytes. Blood 1981;58:518.

90. Dana BW, Durie BGM, White RF. Concomitant administration of granulocyte transfusions and amphotericin B in neutropenic patients: absence of significant pulmonary toxicity. Blood 1981;57:90.

91. Schimpff S, Satterlee WM, Young VM, et al. Empiric therapy with carbenicillin and gentamicin for febrile patients with cancer and granulocytopenia. N Engl J Med 1971;284:1061–5.

92. The EORTC International Antimicrobial Therapy Cooperative Group. Ceftazidime combined with a short or long course of amikacin for empirical therapy of gram-negative bacteremia in cancer patients with granulocytopenia. N Engl J Med 1987;317:1692.

93. Pizzo PA, Hathorn JW, Hiemenz JW, et al. A randomized trial comparing ceftazidime alone with combination antibiotic therapy in cancer patients with fever and neutropenia. N Engl J Med 1986;315:552.

94. Pizzo PA. After empiric therapy: what to do until the granulocyte comes back. Rev Infect Dis 1987;9:214.

95. Schimpff SC, Young VM, Greene WH, et al. Origin of infection in acute nonlymphocytic leukemia: significance of hospital acquisition of potential pathogens. Ann Intern Med 1972;77:707.

96. Schimpff SC. Infection prevention during profound granulocytopenia: new approaches to alimentary canal microbial suppression. Ann Intern Med 1980;93:358–61.

97. Levine AS, Siegel SE, Schreiber AD, et al. Protected environments and prophylactic antibiotics: a prospective controlled study of their utility in the therapy of acute leukemia. N Engl J Med 1973;288:477–83.

98. Schimpff SC, Greene WH, Young VM, et al. Infection prevention in acute nonlymphocytic leukemia: laminar air flow room reverse isolation with oral, nonabsorbable antibiotic prophylaxis. Ann Intern Med 1975;82:351–8.

99. Karp JE, Merz WG, Hendricksen C, et al. Oral norfloxacin for prevention of gram-negative bacterial infections in patients with acute leukemia and granulocytopenia: a randomized, double-blind, placebo-controlled trial. Ann Intern Med 1987; 106:1–7.

100. Saral R, Burns WH, Laskin OL, et al. Acyclovir prophylaxis of herpes simplex virus infections: a randomized double-blind controlled trial in bone marrow-transplant recipients. N Engl J Med 1981;305:63.

101. Neunier F. Prevention of mycoses in immunocompromised patients. Rev Infect Dis 1987;9:408.

102. Cannistra SA, Griffin JD. Regulation of the production and function of granulocytes and monocytes. Semin Hematol 1988;25:173–88.

103. Neidhart J, Mangalik A, Kohler W, et al. Granulocyte colony-stimulating factor stimulates recovery of granulocytes in patients receiving dose-intensive chemotherapy without bone marrow transplantation. J Clin Oncol 1989;7:1685–92.

104. Antman KS, Griffin JD, Elias A, et al. Effect of recombinant human granulocyte-macrophage colony-stimulating factor on chemotherapy-induced myelosuppression. N Engl J Med 1988;319:593–8.

105. Holland PV. Prevention of transfusion-associated graft-versus-host disease. Arch Pathol Lab Med 1989;113:285–91.

106. Pritchard SL, Rodgers PC. Rationale and recommendations for the irradiation of blood products. CRC Crit Rev Oncol Hematol 1987;7:115–24.

107. Braine HG. Cytomegalovirus infection in clinical transplantation: the role of transfusion support using donors seronegative for cytomegalovirus. In: Kurtz SR, Baldwin ML, Sirchia G, eds. Controversies in Transfusion Medicine Immune Complications and Cytomegalovirus Transmission. Arlington, VA: American Association of Blood Banks, 1990.

108. Abeloff MD. ed. Complication of cancer. Baltimore: Johns Hopkins University Press, 1979:151–2.

22

Bone Marrow Transplantation

R. Bradley Slease, M.D.

Studies performed in animals over 25 years ago confirmed the existence of pluripotent bone marrow cells that are capable of reconstituting all hematopoietic cell lines.[1,2] Although not recognizable morphologically, these selfrenewing stem cells can be obtained in sufficient numbers from normal human donors to reestablish normal hematopoiesis in compatible recipients with irreversibly damaged marrow. Bone marrow transplantation (BMT) has become an increasingly common approach for the treatment of hematopoietic failure and various malignancies, and it has emerged as the treatment of choice for such diverse conditions as severe aplastic anemia and relapsed acute leukemia[3] and is the only known curative therapy for chronic myelogenous leukemia.[4]

GENERAL PRINCIPLES

Histocompatibility and Donor Selection

Donor selection for allogeneic marrow transplants (grafts between genetically nonidentical individuals) requires a careful evaluation of the prospective donor–recipient histocompatibility. In all mammalian species studied, a complex genetic region has been identified that encodes the recognition and effector responses to foreign tissue antigens.[5] The major histocompatibility complex in humans is a genetic region located on the short arm of chromosome 6,[6] and these genes code for the HLA antigens, which are polymorphic cell surface glycoproteins found on most nucleated cells.

The HLA antigens are divided in two major classes. Class I antigens, which are encoded by genes at the

HLA-A, HLA-B, and HLA-C loci, are glycoproteins of approximately 45 kd that are defined serologically;[7] multiple alleles have been identified for each of these loci, making this one of the most polymorphic genetic regions yet characterized. The major histocompatibility complex class II molecules, which also are highly polymorphic cell surface glycoproteins, are encoded by at least five gene loci within the HLA-D region, the most well-characterized of which are the DR, DQ, and DP loci. These antigens are less ubiquitous than the class I molecules, being expressed primarily on B and activated T lymphocytes, monocyte–macrophages, endothelial cells, and some early hematopoietic progenitors. Compatibility at the HLA-D region is determined by mixed lymphocyte culture reactivity, and HLA-DR and -DQ antigens are identified by serologic techniques.

The functions of both class I and class II MHC glycoproteins have not been defined completely, but HLA heterogeneity confers individuality and provides for the restriction of immune responsiveness. HLA antigens play important roles in the pathogenesis of graft rejection as well as in the unique problem of allogeneic BMT, graft-versus-host disease (GVHD), as distinguished from other organ transplants. The clinical manifestations of GVHD are discussed later.

The success of allogeneic marrow engraftment as well as both the incidence and severity of GVHD are related closely to the degree of donor–recipient HLA disparity.[8] Traditionally, marrow grafts are performed between genotypically HLA-identical siblings;[3] however, with a probability of 0.25 for any two siblings to be HLA-identical, only approximately 30% of potential recipients will have a compatible sibling donor. Recent data indicate that marrow from a family member with identity at five of six measured HLA antigens (HLA-A, -B, and -DR) may be used with little detrimental impact on survival, thus increasing by perhaps 10% the number of patients who might receive family-donor transplants.[9] Still, the majority of recipients will not have a suitable donor, and in this situation, the patient's own marrow may be used (autologous BMT) provided there is a neoplasm not involving the marrow at the time of procurement. Alternatively, an unrelated donor may be identified whose HLA type is matched closely to the recipient. Registries of HLA-typed potential marrow donors have been established worldwide, and several hundred allografts have been performed using phenotypically HLA-matched or partially matched unrelated donors. The success of these transplants is related both to the degree of HLA disparity as well as the recipient's underlying disease status.[10]

Technique of Marrow Procurement and Grafting

A volume of 700 to 1200 cm^3 of bone marrow is obtained by multiple needle aspirations of the iliac crests and then filtered through stainless-steel screens to produce a single cell suspension.[11] For allogeneic transplants, the marrow is infused intravenously into the recipient without further processing if the ABO blood groups are compatible; in cases of major ABO donor–recipient incompatibility, donor erythrocytes are depleted before marrow infusion either using a cell separator or by simple centrifugation.[12]

Some centers employ methods to deplete T lymphocytes from the donor marrow pre-BMT to prevent or reduce the severity of GVHD. These techniques, which include monoclonal antibody incubation,[13] lectin binding,[14] and elutriation,[15] are effective but generally have not improved overall patient survival because of an increased incidence of both graft failure and recurrent malignancy.[16–19]

For autologous transplantation, marrow is obtained when it morphologically is free of tumor, and some centers employ methods to "purge" or cleanse the marrow of occult tumor contamination. These techniques include incubation with cytotoxic agents,[20] fluorescent lipophilic dyes,[21] and monoclonal antibodies with differential specificities for tumor cells.[22,23] To maintain marrow viability for up to several years, autologous marrow cells are concentrated, mixed with the cryoprotectant agent dimethylsulfoxide, cryopreserved by controlled-rate freezing at temperature reductions of 1°C/min to −80°C, then stored in liquid nitrogen (−196°C).[24] Cryopreserved marrow is administered by intravenous infusion after rapid thawing at 37°C.

The morbidity that is associated with bone marrow harvesting has been minimal. At the University of Oklahoma, the procedure has been performed routinely as outpatient surgery on more than 350 donors without significant complications, and a review of more than 3000 marrow harvests worldwide, with a complication rate of 0.27% and no fatalities, confirms these findings.[25]

Alternative Sources of Hematopoietic Stem Cells

It now is well established that hematopoietic stem cells circulate in the peripheral blood,[26] and these cells have been utilized successfully for autologous transplantation in a number of patients whose marrow had been damaged by previous therapy or contaminated by tumor.[27,28] Although procurement of sufficient peripheral blood stem cells is cumbersome (usually involving 8 to 12 leukaphereses), the technique does allow high-dose therapy to be utilized for some patients who are not candidates for marrow harvesting.

Preliminary evidence indicates that marrow cells that are maintained in long-term culture can restore hematopoiesis in human recipients.[29] Because it appears that malignant cells do not survive in these cultures, this approach has been used as a method of decontaminating autologous marrow in patients with acute nonlymphocytic leukemia (ANLL)[29] and chronic myelogenous leukemia.[30]

Recipient Preparation

Pretransplant conditioning regimens vary considerably with the type of the transplant and the underlying disease. For disorders of bone marrow failure such as severe aplastic anemia, the preparative therapy only need be sufficiently immunosuppressive to allow the engraftment of allogeneic marrow; this generally is accomplished with cyclophosphamide alone at a dose of 200 mg/kg.[31] For patients with severe aplastic anemia undergoing identical twin (syngeneic) transplantation[32] or children with severe combined immunodeficiency receiving HLA-identical allogeneic marrow,[33] pretransplant immunosuppression often is unnecessary. Conversely, patients with severe aplastic anemia who are heavily presensitized to blood products[34] as well as those with other nonneoplastic hematopoietic disorders (i.e., thalassemia,[35] paroxysmal nocturnal hemoglobinuria,[36] and storage diseases[37,38]) may require additional conditioning to prevent graft failure.

Preparative therapy for the hematologic malignancies usually consists of one or more high-dose cytotoxic drugs plus total-body irradiation. By far, the most extensive experience has been with the combination of cyclophosphamide and single-dose or fractionated total-body irradiation.[39,40] Other drugs such as cytosine arabinoside and etoposide also have been used with total-body irradiation,[41,42] but extramedullary toxicity becomes prohibitive when more than two drugs are added to radiation. The combination of high-dose busulfan and cyclophosphamide without total-body irradiation (developed by Santos et al.[43] and modified by Tutschka et al.[44]) appears to be as effective as cyclophosphamide with total-body irradiation for both acute leukemias and chronic myelogenous leukemia.

Conditioning regimens for patients with hematologic malignancies or solid tumors who undergo autologous BMT vary considerably depending on the disease type and the prior therapy. Because total-body irradiation results in an unacceptably high incidence of interstitial pneumonitis in patients who have had previous mediastinal irradiation, conditioning regimens for such patients typically include drugs alone. One commonly used combination for Hodgkin disease and malignant lymphoma consists of high-dose cyclophosphamide, carmustine, and etoposide.[45,46] Other agents either used singly or in combination include melphalan,[47] thiotepa,[48] cisplatin,[49] and carboplatin.[50]

Supportive Care

Patients undergoing BMT may be cared for in regular, private hospital rooms or in more protected environments utilizing laminar airflow isolation with a filtered air supply. Although expensive, laminar airflow rooms along with selective gut decontamination may result in a reduced incidence of neutropenic infection and GVHD.[51,52] Regardless of the type of room, care should be delivered by an experienced, dedicated nursing staff.

The period of marrow aplasia usually lasts from 10 days to 4 weeks after BMT, and during this time, blood components are given to maintain adequate hemoglobin levels and platelet counts above 20,000 cells/mm^3. Prophylactic platelet transfusions have made serious bleeding a rare complication in BMT. Blood products also are irradiated to prevent the transfusion of immunocompetent T lymphocytes that might result in GVHD, and recipients who are seronegative for previous cytomegalovirus (CMV) infection only receive seronegative blood components.[53] Infusions of the recombinant hematopoietic growth factors, granulocyte-macrophage colony-stimulating factor and granulocyte colony-stimulating factor, may shorten the neutropenia after BMT, and other cytokines such as interleukin-3 show promise for promoting pluripotent stem cell growth.[54–57] Preliminary evidence suggests that these agents also may reduce BMT-related morbidity.

Virtually all patients who undergo BMT require temporary parenteral nutritional support to meet protein and caloric needs.[58] The requirements of parenteral hyperalimentation, frequent blood components, and antimicrobial drugs necessitate reliable central venous access, and multilumen silastic central venous catheters that are tunneled subcutaneously and inserted into the cephalic or subclavian veins are used.[59] Despite occasional catheter-related thrombosis or infection, these devices are indispensible in patient management.

CLINICAL RESULTS

For a number of diseases such as acute leukemia, chronic myelogenous leukemia, aplastic anemia, and thalassemia major, clinical experience with allogeneic BMT has been extensive and its role well-defined. For others, only small series or anecdotal reports are available. Similarly, many patients with malignant lymphomas and Hodgkin disease have undergone autologous BMT, but its place in the management of other hematologic malignancies and solid tumors is less clear. Table 22.1 summarizes current indications for BMT, listed by their reported success rate. Also, Figure 22.1 shows the typical survival curves of patients undergoing BMT for the commonly transplanted hematologic malignancies.

Acute Leukemias

The pioneering work of the Seattle transplant team in the early 1970s demonstrated that approximately 10% of patients with far-advanced ANLL or acute lymphocytic leukemia (ALL) could be cured with high-dose chemoradiotherapy followed by the infusion of HLA-identical sibling bone marrow.[60] Failure generally resulted from leukemic relapse (65% to 75% of failures) or GVHD. Although more recent improvements in BMT supportive care have produced somewhat better results in this group, survival remains poor, with fewer than 20% still alive after 5 years.[61]

Nevertheless, encouraged by the experience in advanced leukemia, several transplant teams began to employ allogeneic BMT for ANLL that was in first or subsequent complete remission. Such patients have had considerably better long-term disease-free survival, with approximately 50% of those transplanted during first complete remission still alive and free of leukemia 5 years after transplantation;[61–63] actuarial risk of relapse in this group is in the 20% to 25% range, with nearly all relapses occurring in the first 3 years post-BMT. Patient age is an important determinant of long-term survival, and those under 25 years of age who were transplanted in first complete remission have a 60% probability of being

TABLE 22.1. Current Indications for Bone Marrow Transplantation

Survival	Disease	Status	Allogeneic	Autologous
≥ 50% long-term survival	Acute leukemias	CR$_1$	+	+
	Chronic myelogenous leukemia	Chronic phase	+	−
	Lymphomas/Hodgkin disease	Sensitive relapse	+	+
	Severe aplastic anemia	−	+	−
	Severe combined immunodeficiency	−	+	−
	Thalassemia major	−	+	−
20% to 50% long-term survival	Acute leukemias	CR$_2$/early relapse	+	+
	Chronic myelogenous leukemia	Accelerated phase	+	−
	Myelodysplasia	−	+	−
	Neuroblastoma	Sensitive relapse	+	+
	Breast carcinoma	Sensitive relapse	−	+
	Testicular carcinoma	Sensitive relapse	−	+
< 20% long-term survival	Acute leukemias	Advanced disease	+	−
	Chronic myelogenous leukemia	Blast phase	+	−
	Lymphomas/Hodgkin disease	Resistant relapse	+	+
	Glioblastoma	Untreated	−	+
Anecdotal success (case reports or small series)	Multiple myeloma	Sensitive relapse	+	+
	Hairy-cell leukemia	−	+	−
	Acute myelosclerosis	Untreated	+	−
	Lymphomatoid granulomatosis	Sensitive relapse	+	−
	Sarcomas	Sensitive relapse	−	+
	Osteopetrosis	−	+	−
	Wiskott-Aldrich syndrome	−	+	−
	Paroxysmal nocturnal hemoglobinuria	−	+	−
	Sickle cell anemia	−	+	−
	Pure red cell aplasia	−	+	−
	Hereditary leukocyte disorders	−	+	−
	Hereditary storage diseases	−	+	−

Note: CR$_1$ = first complete remission; CR$_2$ = subsequent complete remission.

leukemia-free at 5 years versus approximately 40% for older individuals.[62] For those with ANLL in subsequent complete remission or early first relapse, allogeneic BMT is less successful. The relapse rate is approximately 50%, but 25% to 30% of these otherwise incurable patients do remain alive at 5 years.[61,62]

The major question for patients under 50 years of age who have ANLL and an HLA-identical sibling is not whether, but when, to perform allogeneic BMT. Some centers recently reported improved results using intensive postremission therapy without transplantation,[64,65] but such an approach has not been without considerable toxicity, including a number of treatment-related deaths. Trials comparing allogeneic BMT with conventional postremission therapy for patients in first complete remission have shown consistently both disease-free and overall survival advantages for transplanted patients, but these differences have not always reached statistical significance.[66–68] Other studies reported in preliminary form have documented similar results;[69,70] still others are ongoing. With continued improvements in both conventional ANLL postremission therapy as well as in both transplant preparative and supportive regimens, it is unlikely that either current or past trials will settle this controversy. Based on the available data, however, it seems reasonable to offer transplantation to all patients under 30 years of age who are in first complete remission and have an HLA-identical sibling. Because older individuals may have a higher rate of BMT-related complications, including infection, interstitial pneumonia, and GVHD,[71–73] perhaps only those between 30 and 55 years of age and with one or more high-risk factors for relapse should be transplanted during first complete remission. Others over 30 years of age might be treated conventionally and transplanted (should the leukemia recur) in early first relapse or subsequent complete remission. Further improvements in GVHD prophylaxis and BMT supportive care, how-

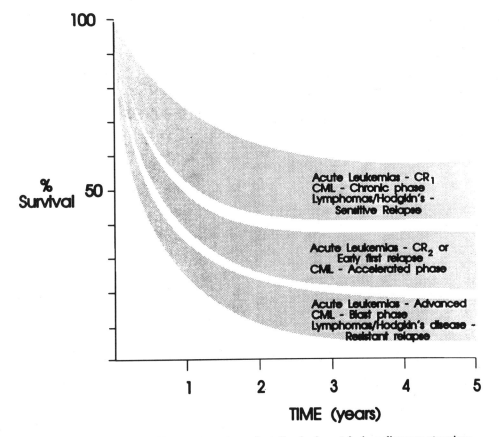

FIGURE 22.1. The results of bone marrow transplantation for hematologic malignancy at various stages of disease. *Note:* CML = chronic myelogenous leukemia; CR_1 = first complete remission; CR_2 = subsequent complete remission.

ever, may alter these recommendations, and recent studies have demonstrated excellent results of allogeneic BMT in older patients.[72–74]

The outcome of allogeneic BMT for ALL is similar, stage for stage, to that reported for ANLL,[62] but because of the curative potential of chemotherapy alone in children with standard-risk ALL, BMT usually is carried out after first relapse, most often in subsequent complete remission. Only patients with disease features indicative of a high risk for relapse (i.e., the t(9;22) chromosomal translocation, central nervous system involvement, B cell or L_3 phenotype, or age of over 18 years) are typically transplanted during first complete remission. Failure may result from infection, toxicity of the preparative regimen, or GVHD, but as in the case of ANLL, the most frequent cause is leukemic relapse.[75]

Autologous BMT also may be performed for acute leukemia using marrow harvested during complete remission and, in some centers, treated to remove contaminating leukemic cells. Preliminary results demonstrate surprisingly similar survival as compared with allogeneic transplants performed at the same disease stages.[75–78] Relapse rates are higher after autologous BMT and are not clearly reduced by purging techniques, but the morbidity and mortality from GVHD is avoided. The precise role of autologous BMT remains to be defined by ongoing prospective trials, but the two most important unanswered questions are: 1) what is the relative efficacy of autografting as compared with allogeneic BMT, particularly when the donor is unrelated or a partially mismatched family member; and 2) does any currently available purging method actually decrease the relapse rate and improve survival as compared with unmanipulated marrow? Hopefully, these answers will be forthcoming in the next decade.

Chronic Myelogenous Leukemia

Allogeneic bone marrow transplantation is the only known potentially curative therapy for chronic myelogenous leukemia. A variety of preparative regimens have been evaluated, but none are clearly superior to the cyclophosphamide and total-body irradiation combination used at Seattle[79] and other centers.[80,81] The best results have been achieved when transplants are carried out during the chronic phase of the illness, with approximately 50% of these patients achieving long-term disease-free survival.[62] Actuarial clinical relapse rates post-BMT are only 15% to 20%, but sensitive detection methods have demonstrated the persistence of typical chronic myelogenous leukemia messenger RNA transcripts in some long-term, cytogenetically normal survivors.[82] The clinical significance of this observation remains uncertain. The Seattle BMT team recently reported improved disease-free survival for patients receiving allogeneic BMT during the first year after the diagnosis of chronic-phase chronic myelogenous leukemia,[83] but these results have not yet been corroborated by other groups.

If allogeneic transplantation is performed for accelerated- or blast-phase chronic myelogenous leukemia, the results are much less favorable. Relapse rates are over 50%, and long-term survival is only 15% to 25%.[62] Therefore, patients with chronic myelogenous leukemia who are under 50 to 55 years of age and have an HLA-identical donor should strongly consider allografting early in the chronic phase.

Lymphomas and Hodgkin Disease

Although a significant percentage of patients with intermediate- or high-grade lymphomas and Hodgkin disease are cured by primary therapy, those who fail to achieve a complete remission or who relapse after the initial chemotherapy rarely are cured by standard-dose salvage regimens. However, high-dose chemotherapy or chemoradiotherapy with BMT can render many of these patients disease-free. Approximately 50% of those transplanted after responding to salvage therapy ("sensitive relapse") have achieved long-term survival,[84,85] but patients with lymphoma that is refractory to primary or salvage chemotherapy have had much poorer results, with fewer than 10% attaining durable remissions.

The vast majority of the more than 500 marrow grafts performed annually for lymphoma and Hodgkin disease are autologous, and despite concerns regarding tumor contamination of the autologous marrow, there seems to be little difference in either the overall survival or the relapse rate between autologous and allogeneic transplants.[86] Moreover, relapse rates after autologous grafts are not reduced clearly by purging techniques. Also, most relapses occur at sites of previous disease, suggesting failure of the preparative regimen rather than reinfusion of malignant cells.

Other Hematologic Malignancies

A small number of patients with hairy-cell leukemia,[73] multiple myeloma,[87] and acute myelosclerosis[88] have achieved prolonged remissions after myeloablative therapy followed by BMT. A larger experience has been reported for myelodysplasia, and it demonstrates a projected 45% 3-year disease-free survival for 59 patients undergoing allogeneic marrow grafts.[89] Considering the poor prognosis with conventional therapy, allogeneic BMT is almost certainly the treatment of choice for patients with myelodysplasia who are 55 years of age or younger and have a suitable donor.

Solid Tumors

Chemotherapy dose intensification with autologous marrow support has been tested in a variety of solid tumors. Initially, only patients with refractory neoplasia were selected, and the overall results were disappointing. Nevertheless, response rates generally were high, and a few patients with neuroblastoma or high-grade glioma became long-term survivors. Preparative regimens included either melphalan,[90] carmustine,[91] and cyclophosphamide[92] alone, or combinations of alkylating agents with or without antimetabolites[48,93–95] or total-body irradiation.[96,97]

More recently, transplant teams have used high-dose therapy with autologous stem cell support earlier in the natural history of certain neoplasms; the most encouraging results have been observed in patients whose tumors have responded to standard-dose chemotherapy and then receive high-dose treatment as "consolidation." Prolonged, unmaintained remissions have been reported in 20% to 50% of patients so treated who have advanced carcinomas of the breast[98,99] and testis,[100] neuroblastoma,[101,102] and some sarcomas.[103,104] Currently, available data supports a role for this approach in carefully selected patients, and further improvements in both preparative regimens and supportive care (including the use of cytokines to enhance hematopoietic recovery) may expand the role of dose-intensive therapy for both these and other solid tumors.

Nonmalignant Diseases

Any disorder resulting from the failure or abnormality of tissues that are derived from hematopoietic stem cells theoretically might be corrected by allogeneic BMT; indeed, such diverse conditions as paroxysmal nocturnal hemoglobinuria[105] and congenital osteopetrosis[106] have been treated successfully with transplantation. However, the most extensive clinical experience by far, has been accumulated for severe aplastic anemia.

After preparative immunosuppression (usually with high-dose cyclophosphamide alone), nearly 90% of patients with severe aplastic anemia who are receiving transplants of HLA-identical sibling marrow will achieve sustained engraftment, and 60% will become long-term survivors.[62] If transplantation is performed before the recipient has been transfused, then the success rate is over 80%; however, heavily pretransfused, "sensitized" patients have only a 45% to 50% probability of long-term survival.[107] Age also is a predictor, with those over the age of 40 years having poorer survival, primarily because of GVHD and other transplant-related toxicity. Because immunosuppressive therapy with agents such as antithymocyte globulin may induce remissions in some patients with severe aplastic anemia, this approach might be considered initially for older patients, but the problem with this choice is that extensive transfusion support is necessary to sustain patients during a trial of immunosuppressive therapy. If immunosuppression fails, then subsequent allogeneic BMT is less likely to be successful.

Marrow transplantation is the treatment of choice for children with congenital forms of severe combined immunodeficiency, and approximately 60% of these children who receive transplants with HLA-identical sibling marrow have achieved long-term survival with correction of both humoral and cellular immune defects.[108] When a histocompatible donor is unavailable, T cell–depleted haploidentical marrow from a family member may be used, but the immunologic reconstitution is slower and may be incomplete.[109]

Thalassemia major can be corrected by allogeneic BMT as well, with over 70% of patients surviving if grafted before the age of 16 years. For children transplanted before developing clinical evidence of hepatic iron overload, survival is greater than 90%.[110] Because of the long-term complications of iron excess as well as the problems associated with chelation therapy, marrow transplantation should be strongly considered at an early age for children with this disease who also have histocompatible donors. In addition, successful marrow grafts have been reported for small numbers of patients with Wiskott-Aldrich syndrome,[111] Fanconi anemia,[112] constitutional pure red cell aplasia,[113] congenital disorders of phagocytosis,[108] and certain storage diseases.[108,114]

COMPLICATIONS OF MARROW TRANSPLANTATION

Infections

Measures designed to prevent infection both during and after BMT have been partially successful. Prophylactic trimethoprim–sulfamethoxazole given during the conditioning regimen and after engraftment virtually has eliminated *Pneumocystis carinii* as a cause of fatal interstitial pneumonia.[115] Parenteral acyclovir significantly reduces the incidence of herpes simplex virus reactivation and may help prevent varicella zoster reactivation,[116] and the oral quinolones norfloxacin and ciprofloxacin reportedly decrease the frequency of gram-negative infections.[117,118] Fungal infections have proven more difficult to prevent, but the incidence of invasive aspergillosis is reduced by high-efficiency particulate air filtration systems.[119]

Despite these strategies for infection prophylaxis, most patients still become febrile during the period of marrow aplasia. Recent analyses of early post-BMT infections indicate that gram-positive bacteria now are the more common initial infecting agents than gram-negative organisms, perhaps because of the widespread use of central venous catheters and prophylactic antimicrobials;[120] fungal infections, particularly those due to *Candida* species, also remain a major cause of morbidity. Despite the aggressive intervention at first fever with broad-spectrum antibiotics and empiric systemic antifungal therapy for those who fail to defervesce, approximately 5% of patients receiving transplants die from infection early in the post-BMT period.

During the 6 months after recovery of hematopoiesis, viruses are the most frequent cause of morbidity and mortality from infection. Herpes simplex and varicella zoster reactivation may occur, but these can be managed with acyclovir.

Cytomegalovirus-associated interstitial pneumonia, also usually caused by the activation of latent virus,[121] is a major clinical problem as well, occurring in 10% to 20% of patients receiving allogeneic transplants for malignancy. This complication is unusual in patients who are seronegative for CMV antibody pre-BMT if exclusively seronegative blood products and/or high-titer intravenous immunoglobulin are given.[122,123] It also is less frequent in patients receiving autologous transplants, in allogeneic marrow recipients who do not develop GVHD, and in those receiving less-intensive preparative regimens. The new drug ganciclovir, along with high-dose immunoglobulin infusions, may reduce the high mortality rate from CMV interstitial pneumonia if begun early during the course of the illness,[124] and studies currently are underway to determine if prophylactic ganciclovir can prevent CMV activation in seropositive patients receiving transplants.

Apart from the reactivation of varicella zoster and herpes simplex viruses, late infections after BMT are likely to occur only in those patients with chronic GVHD. These infections typically are caused by gram-positive bacteria, particularly *Streptococcus pneumoniae*, but they also may be due to gram-negative or fungal organisms.[125]

Preparative Regimen-Related Toxicities

When intensive preparative regimens are used, particularly those containing total-body irradiation, busulfan, or carmustine, veno-occlusive disease of the liver may occur in 15% to 40% of patients and is fatal in 5% to 10%.[126] No specific therapy is available. This complication is especially frequent in patients with pre-existing liver disease[127] and in those receiving second transplants.[128]

Mucosal damage also is related to regimen intensity, and patients with severe mucositis may have a higher risk of infection from enteric pathogens. The incidence of radiation-related interstitial pneumonia has declined with the introduction of fractionated rather than single-dose total-body irradiation,[129] as has the frequency of cataracts.[130] Also, leukoencephalopathy sometimes has been observed in children with previous cranial irradiation, particularly if they have had intensive intrathecal chemotherapy for leptomeningeal leukemia.[131]

Hemolytic anemia may occur in the early postengraftment period, particularly in recipients of ABO-incompatible allogeneic marrow,[132] but this also may be due to minor red cell antigen mismatch.[133] Curiously, Coombs-negative hemolysis occasionally has been observed following autologous BMT.[85]

Long-term consequences of total-body irradiation include infertility,[134] retarded growth and development in children,[135] and hypothyroidism.[136] Late second malignancies thus far have been surprisingly rare.[137]

Graft Failure or Rejection

After receiving allogeneic marrow grafts, most patients become complete hematopoietic chimeras (i.e., all blood cells are of donor origin). However, the persistence of some host hematopoiesis may be detected long after the transplant, particularly in recipients of T lymphocyte–depleted marrow.[138,139]

The complete failure of engraftment or marrow rejection is rare (< 1%) when unmanipulated, HLA-identical sibling marrow is used in sufficient quantity after adequately intensive conditioning. However, when partially mismatched or T cell–depleted marrow is employed, graft failure may occur in 10% to 15% of patients.[140,141]

Mechanisms of allogeneic marrow rejection are understood incompletely. Donor T lymphocytes apparently are important for the eradication of host cells that cause rejection. In some cases, these host mediators appear to be cytolytic T lymphocytes or natural killer cells,[142] but in others, host antibodies with anti–donor cell specificities have been documented.[143] Another recent study implicated the deficient production of

hematopoietic cytokines by marrow stromal cells as a cause of graft failure.[144] Whatever the etiology, however, allograft failure carries a grim prognosis, and second transplants after initial graft failure are successful only in a small percentage of cases.

Unmanipulated autologous grafts rarely fail, but patients who are transplanted for acute leukemia often experience a very slow hematopoietic recovery. Recent evidence suggests that hematopoietic cytokines such as granulocyte-macrophage colony-stimulating factor may stimulate neutrophil production in such patients.[145] Autologous marrow purged with cytotoxic agents also may engraft more slowly,[146] and studies are underway to determine whether growth factors may be of benefit in this situation as well.

Graft-Versus-Host Disease

A unique feature of allogeneic BMT is the capacity for immunocompetent donor-derived T cells to react against host tissues. The resulting clinicopathologic syndrome of GVHD occurs in both acute and chronic forms, and each has distinct features.[3,147–152]

Acute GVHD develops within the first 100 days post-BMT. Target organs are the skin, liver, and gastrointestinal tract, and the clinical illness varies in its severity from a mild, self-limited erythematous rash to a fatal illness with extensive desquamation, severe diarrhea and/or ileus, and hepatic failure. The 40% to 50% of matched allograft recipients who develop clinically significant acute GVHD (i.e., more than a transient rash) have a much higher incidence of transplant-related mortality, primarily due to infectious complications. Figure 22.2 shows the actuarial long-term survival of 357 patients transplanted for aplastic anemia who developed little or no acute GVHD; long-term survival was 81% ± 5% in this group, but only 34% ± 7% (P < 0.0001) for 249 patients with moderate to severe acute GVHD.[62] Risk factors that are predictive for development of significant acute GVHD include donor–recipient histoincompatibility, gender mismatch (especially parous or transfused female donors), recipient age of over 30 years, and no prophylaxis against GVHD.[153]

When given during the immediate posttransplant period, both methotrexate[3] and cyclosporine[154] are effective in preventing or decreasing the severity of GVHD. When the drugs are combined, the incidence is reduced further.[155] The addition of corticosteroids to cyclosporine also may provide increased prophylactic benefit,[44,154] but whether laminar airflow isolation and gut decontamination decrease the frequency of acute GVHD remains controversial.[52,153]

As discussed previously, the depletion of T lymphocytes from allogeneic marrow before transplantation is

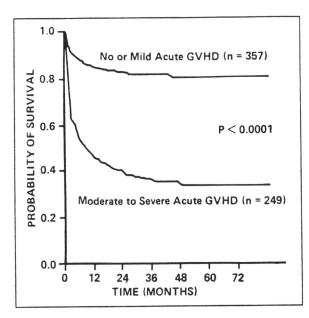

FIGURE 22.2. **The actuarial probability of survival among patients with severe aplastic anemia according to the severity of acute graft-versus-host disease (_GVHD_) in patients at risk (i.e., survival > 21 days with engraftment).** _Source:_ **Bortin et al. 1988[62]**

very effective in preventing acute GVHD.[13,19] Unfortunately, T-cell removal has not improved the overall patient survival because of an increased incidence of graft failure and relapsed neoplasia. Indeed, it appears that moderate to severe acute GVHD is associated with a significant "graft-versus-leukemia" effect (i.e., a substantial reduction in the leukemic relapse rate as compared with patients having no acute GVHD).[156,157] The increased frequency of relapse with T cell–depleted marrow grafts suggests that both the antileukemic effect as well as the acute GVHD are mediated by T lymphocytes.

Studies in animal models indicate that the graft-versus-leukemia effect may be separable from clinical GVHD,[158] and efforts to exploit this concept in human trials have been initiated. Preliminary data involving the selective depletion of donor CD8-bearing lymphocytes appear encouraging in allografts for chronic myelogenous leukemia.[159]

Therapy for established acute GVHD is limited. Corticosteroids often are beneficial in ameliorating the skin manifestations, but severe gastrointestinal or hepatic disease does not respond as well. Antithymocyte globulin, cyclosporine, and monoclonal anti–T cell antibodies occasionally are helpful in steroid-resistant

acute GVHD,[147,160] and promising preliminary results have been reported for infusions of anti-CD5 antibody–ricin A chain immunotoxin conjugate[161] and of anti-interleukin-2 receptor monoclonal antibody.[162]

Approximately 40% of allogeneic transplant survivors will develop chronic GVHD, which is a distinct clinical entity that usually begins 3 to 18 months posttransplant.[163] Patients who have had moderate to severe acute GVHD are at the highest risk for developing the chronic form, but it occasionally may occur also in patients with no history of the acute disease. The incidence of chronic GVHD increases along with patient age.

Clinically, chronic GVHD may affect the same target organs as the acute illness (skin, liver, and gut) but also typically causes keratoconjunctivitis, stomatitis, and often is associated with recurrent sinopulmonary infections.[150] Severe involvement also may lead to generalized wasting, pulmonary insufficiency from small airways obstruction, esophageal or vaginal strictures, and joint contractures from scleroderma-like skin changes.[164,165] As in autoimmune disorders, multiple autoantibodies may be found,[166] but effective immune function is depressed.[167] Untreated, extensive chronic GVHD has a high mortality (often from infection with gram-positive encapsulated organisms), but the early introduction of corticosteroids either with or without cyclosporine have improved the outlook significantly.[168] After control of the disease is achieved, therapy often can be discontinued after 9 to 24 months and, in other patients, tapered and maintained at mildly immunosuppressive doses.

THE FUTURE OF BONE MARROW TRANSPLANTATION

With improvements in both preparative treatment and supportive care, the applications for BMT have expanded considerably during the past 15 years. Although still formidable, acute transplant-related mortality has been reduced, and BMT now is a serious option for patients with chronic but ultimately fatal disorders such as thalassemia major and chronic-phase CML. Further improvements, such as reducing the risk of infection by shortening the pancytopenic period with hematopoietic growth factors, more specific approaches to the prevention and therapy of GVHD, as well as development of more effective but less toxic preparative regimens, are under active clinical investigation. When conditioning programs can eradicate reliably in vivo neoplasia, effective marrow ex vivo purging techniques will become increasingly important for autologous BMT to be more successful. To broaden the applicability of allogeneic BMT to donor–recipient pairs with more than one

HLA-antigen mismatch, specific methods of marrow T-cell depletion must be developed that do not impair engraftment or increase the risk of relapse. Given the advances of the past 25 years, it is not unreasonable to assume that many of these new approaches will be introduced within the next decade.

One of the great unfulfilled promises for BMT is use as a vehicle for gene transfer therapy. Using retroviral vectors, successful gene transfer has been accomplished in animals, including primates,[169] and it now is feasible that genetic disorders involving pluripotent hematopoietic stem cells could be corrected with gene therapy. Remaining problems include low gene-expression efficiency and providing a growth advantage for the genetically altered cells without undue risk to the recipient. When these obstacles are overcome, gene transfer may become a realistic clinical option for many genetic diseases.[170]

REFERENCES

1. Till JE, McCulloch EA. A direct measurement of radiation sensitivity of normal mouse bone marrow cells. Radiat Res 1961;14:213.

2. Becker AJ, McCulloch EA, Till JE. Cytological demonstration of the clonal nature of spleen colonies. J Cell Physiol 1967;69:65.

3. Thomas ED, Storb R, Clift RA, et al. Bone-marrow transplantation. N Engl J Med 1975;29:832,895.

4. Goldman JM. Bone marrow transplantation for chronic myeloid leukemia. Hematol Oncol 1987;5:265.

5. Snell GD, Dausset J, Nathenson S. Histocompatibility. New York: Academic Press, 1976.

6. McKusick VA, Ruddle FH. The status of the gene map of the human chromosomes. Science 1977;196:390.

7. Bach FH, van Rood JJ. The major histocompatibility complex. N Engl J Med 1976;295:806.

8. Anasetti C, Amos D, Beatty PG, et al. Effect of HLA compatibility on engraftment of bone marrow transplants in patients with leukemia or lymphoma. N Engl J Med 1989;320:197.

9. Beatty PG, Clift RA, Mickelson EM, et al. Marrow transplantation from related donors other than HLA-identical siblings. N Engl J Med 1985;313:765.

10. Ash RC, Casper JT, Chitamber CR, et al. Successful allogeneic transplantation of T-cell-depleted bone marrow from closely HLA-matched unrelated donors. N Engl J Med 1990;322:485.

11. Thomas ED, Storb R. Technique for human marrow grafting. Blood 1970;36:507.

12. Brain HG, Sensenbrenner LL, Tutschka PJ. Bone marrow transplantation with major ABO blood group incompatibility using erythrocyte depletion of marrow prior to infusion. Blood 1982;60:420.

13. Vallera DA, Ash RC, Zanjani ED, et al. Anti-T cell reagents for human bone marrow transplantation: ricin linked to three monoclonal antibodies. Science 1983;22:512.

14. Reisner Y, Kapoor N, Kirkpatrick D, et al. Transplantation for severe combined immunodeficiency with HLA-A,B,D,DR incompatible parental marrow cells fractionated by soybean agglutinin and sheep red blood cells. Blood 1983;61:34.

15. Wagner JE, Donnenberg AD, Noga SJ, et al. Lymphocyte depletion of donor bone marrow by counterflow centrifugal elutriation: results of a phase I clinical trial. Blood 1988; 72:1168.

16. Kernan NA, Flomenberg N, Dupont B, O'Reilly RJ. Graft rejection in recipients of T-cell-depleted HLA-nonidentical marrow transplants for leukemia. Transplantation 1987;43:842.

17. Martin PJ, Hansen JA, Buckner CE, et al. Effects of in vitro depletion of T cells in HLA-identical allogeneic marrow grafts. Blood 1985;66:664.

18. Mitsuyasa RT, Champlin RE, Gale RP, et al. Treatment of donor bone marrow with monoclonal anti-T-cell antibody and complement for the prevention of graft-versus-host disease. Ann Intern Med 1986;105:20.

19. Horowitz MM, Gale RP, Sondel PM, et al. Graft-versus-leukemia reactions after bone marrow transplantation. Blood 1990;75:555.

20. Kaizer H, Stuart RK, Brookmeyer R, et al. Autologous bone marrow transplantation in acute leukemia: a phase I study of in vitro treatment of marrow with 4-hydroperoxycyclophosphamide to purge tumor cells. Blood 1985;65:1504.

21. Sieber F, Rao S, Rowley SD, Sieber-Blum M. Dye-mediated photolysis of human neuroblastoma cells: implications for autologous bone marrow transplantation. Blood 1986;68:32.

22. Ritz J, Sallan SE, Bast RC Jr, et al. Autologous bone-marrow transplantation in CALLA-positive acute lymphoblastic leukaemia after in-vitro treatment with J5 monoclonal antibody and complement. Lancet 1982;ii:60.

23. Ball ED, Mills LE, Cornwell GG, et al. Autologous bone marrow transplantation for acute myeloid leukemia using monoclonal antibody-purged bone marrow. Blood 1990;75:1199.

24. Epstein RB, Slease RB. Bone marrow transplantation. In: Nyhus LM, ed. Surgery Annual. Norwalk, CT: Appleton-Century-Crofts, 1985:23.

25. Bortin MM, Buckner CD. Major complications of marrow harvesting for transplantation. Exp Hematol 1983;11:916.

26. Epstein RB, Sarpel SC. Circulating hematopoietic stem cells. In: Gale RP, Fox CF, eds. Biology of Bone Marrow Transplantation. ICN-UCLA Symposia on Molecular and Cellular Biology XVII. New York: Academic Press, 1980:405.

27. Korbling M, Martin H, Fliedner TM, et al. Autologous blood stem cell transplantation. In: Gale RP, Champlin R, eds. Progress in Bone Marrow Transplantation. New York: Alan R. Liss, 1987:877.

28. Smith DM, Kessinger A, Lobo F, et al. Peripheral blood stem cell collection and toxicity. In: Dicke KA, Spitzer G, Jagannath S, Evinger-Hodges M-J, eds. Autologous Bone Marrow Transplantation: Proceedings of the Fourth International Symposium. Houston: University of Texas M.D. Anderson Cancer Center, 1989:697.

29. Chang J, Morgenstern G, Deakin D, et al. Reconstitution of hematopoietic system with autologous marrow taken during relapse of acute meyloblastic leukaemia and grown in long-term culture. Lancet 1986;i:294.

30. Barnett MJ, Eaves CJ, Phillips GL, et al. Rapid reconstitution of Philadelphia-chromosome-negative hematopoiesis in patients with chronic myeloid leukemia transplanted with cultured autologous bone marrow to support intensive therapy. Blood 1988;72:379A.

31. Storb R, Thomas ED, Buckner CD, et al. Marrow transplantation for aplastic anemia. Semin Hematol 1984;221:27.

32. Champlin RE, Feig SA, Sparkes RS, et al. Bone marrow transplantation from identical twins in the treatment of aplastic anaemia: implication for the pathogenesis of the disease. Br J Haematol 1984;56:455.

33. Good RA, Kapoor N, Pahwa RN, et al. Current approaches to the primary immunodeficiencies. In: Fougereau M, Dausset J,

eds. Immunology 1980 (Progress in Immunology IV). New York: Academic Press, 1981:907.

34. Champlin RE, Horowitz MM, van Bekkum DW, et al. Graft failure following bone marrow transplantation for severe aplastic anemia: risk factors and treatment results. Blood 1989; 73:606.

35. Thomas ED, Buckner CD, Sanders JE, et al. Marrow transplantation for thalassemia. Lancet 1982;ii:227.

36. Antin JH, Ginsburg D, Smith BR, et al. Bone marrow transplantation for paroxysmal nocturnal hemoglobinuria: eradication of the PNH-clone and documentation of complete lymphohematopoietic engraftment. Blood 1985;66:1247.

37. Rappeport JM, Ginns EI. Bone marrow transplantation in severe Gaucher's disease. N Engl J Med 1984;311:84.

38. Krivit W, Pierpont ME, Ayaz K, et al. Bone marrow transplantation in the Maroteaux-Lamy syndrome (mucopolysaccharidosis type VI). N Engl J Med 1984;311:1606.

39. Peterson FB, Buckner CD. Allogeneic and autologous bone marrow transplantation for acute leukemia and malignant lymphoma: current status. Hematol Oncol 1987;5:233.

40. Thomas ED. Marrow transplantation for malignant diseases. J Clin Oncol 1983;1:517.

41. Coccia PF, Strandjord SE, Warkentin PI, et al. High-dose cytosine arabinoside and fractionated total-body irradiation: an improved preparative regimen for bone marrow transplantation of children with acute lymphoblastic leukemia in remission. Blood 1988;71:888.

42. Blume KG, Forman SJ, O'Donnell MR, et al. Total body irradiation and high-dose etoposide: a new preparatory regimen for bone marrow transplantation in patients with advanced hematologic malignancies. Blood 1987;69:1015.

43. Santos GW, Tutschka PJ, Brookmeyer R, et al. Marrow transplantation for acute nonlymphoblastic leukemia after treatment with busulfan and cyclophosphamide. N Engl J Med 1983; 309:1347.

44. Tutschka PJ, Copelan EA, Klein JP. Bone marrow transplantation for leukemia following a new busulfan and cyclophosphamide regimen. Blood 1987;70:1382.

45. Dicke KA, Jagannath S, Spitzer G, et al. The role of autologous bone marrow transplantation in various malignancies. Semin Hematol 1984;21:109.

46. Phillips GL, Conners JM. Bone marrow transplantation for malignant lymphoma. In: Gale RP, Champlin R, eds. Progress in Bone Marrow Transplantation. New York: Alan R. Liss, 1987:799.

47. Maraninchi D, Abecasis M, Gastaut J-A, et al. High-dose melphalan and autologous bone marrow transplant for relapsed acute leukaemia. Cancer Chemother Pharmacol 1983;10:109.

48. Williams SF, Bitran JD, Kaminer L, et al. A phase I-II study of bialkylator chemotherapy, high-dose thiotepa, and cyclophosphamide with autologous bone marrow reinfusion in patients with advanced cancer. J Clin Oncol 1987;5:260–5.

49. Eder JP, Antman K, Peters W, et al. High-dose combination alkylating agent chemotherapy with autologous bone marrow support for metastatic breast cancer. J Clin Oncol 1986; 4:1592–7.

50. Shea TC, Flaherty M, Elias A, et al. A phase I clinical and pharmacokinetic study of carboplatin and autologous bone marrow support. J Clin Oncol 1989;7:651.

51. Buckner CD. Clift RA, Sanders JE, et al. Protective environment for marrow transplant recipients: a prospective study. Ann Intern Med 1978;89:893.

52. Storb R, Prentice RL, Buckner CD, et al. Graft-versus-host disease and survival in patients with aplastic anemia treated by marrow grafts from HLA-identical siblings: beneficial effect of a protective environment. N Engl J Med 1983;308:302.

53. Bowden RA, Sayers M, Flournoy N, et al. Cytomegalovirus immune globulin and seronegative blood products to prevent primary cytomegalovirus infection after marrow transplant. N Engl J Med 1986;314:1006.

54. Brandt BJ, Peters WP, Atwater SK, et al. Effect of recombinant human granulocyte-macrophage colony-stimulating factor on hematopoietic reconstitution after high dose chemotherapy and autologous bone marrow transplantation. N Engl J Med 1988; 318:869.

55. Nemunaitis J, Singer JW, Buckner CD, et al. Use of recombinant human granulocyte-macrophage colony-stimulating factor in autologous marrow transplantation for lymphoid malignancies. Blood 1988;72:834.

56. Taylor KM, Jagannath S, Spitzer G, et al. Recombinant human granulocyte colony-stimulating factor hastens granulocyte recovery after high-dose chemotherapy and autologous bone marrow transplantation in Hodgkin's disease. J Clin Oncol 1989;7:1791.

57. Donahue RE, Seehra J, Metzger M, et al. Human IL-3 and GM-CSF act synergistically in stimulating hematopoiesis in primates. Science 1983;241:1820.

58. Weisdorf SA, Lysne J, Wind D, et al. Positive effect of prophylactic total parenteral nutrition on long-term outcome of bone marrow transplantation. Transplantation 1987;43:833.

59. Hickman RO, Buckner CD, Clift RA, et al. A modified right atrial catheter for access to the venous system in marrow transplant recipients. Surg Gynecol Obstet 1979;148:871.

60. Thomas ED, Buckner CD, Banaji M, et al. One hundred patients with acute leukemia treated by chemotherapy, total body irradiation and allogeneic marrow transplantation. Blood 1977; 49:511.

61. Clift RA, Buckner CD, Thomas ED, et al. The treatment of acute nonlymphoblastic leukemia by allogeneic marrow transplantation. Bone Marrow Transplantation 1987;2:243.

62. Bortin MM, Horowitz MM, Gale RP. Current status of bone marrow transplantation in humans: report from the International Bone Marrow Transplant Registry. Nat Immun Cell Growth Regul 1988;7:334.

63. Gratwohl A, Hermans J, Lyklema A, Zwaan FE. Bone marrow transplantation for leukaemia in Europe: report from the Leukaemia Working Party 1987. Bone Marrow Transplantation 1987;2:15.

64. Tallman MS, Appelbaum FR, Amos D. Evaluation of intensive post-remission chemotherapy for adults with acute nonlymphocytic leukemia using high-dose cytosine arabinoside with L-asparaginase and amsacrine with etoposide. J Clin Oncol 1987;5:918.

65. Gale RP, Foon KA. Therapy of acute myelogenous leukemia. Semin Hematol 1987;24:40.

66. Appelbaum FR, Fisher LD, Thomas ED, et al. Chemotherapy v. marrow transplantation for adults with acute nonlymphocytic leukemia: a five-year follow-up. Blood 1988;72:179.

67. Champlin RE, Ho WG, Gale RP, et al. Treatment of acute myelogenous leukemia: a prospective controlled trial of bone marrow transplantation versus consolidation chemotherapy. Ann Intern Med 1985;102:285.

68. Conde E, Iriondo A, Rayon C, et al. Allogeneic bone marrow transplantation versus intensification chemotherapy for acute myelogenous leukemia in first remission: a prospective controlled trial. Br J Haematol 1988;69:219.

69. Appelbaum FR, Hewlett J, Kopecky K, et al. Prospective comparative study of bone marrow transplantation (BMT) versus continued chemotherapy for adult nonlymphocytic leukemia (ANL): a Southwest Oncology Group Study. Blood 1986; 68:216A.

70. Nesbit M, Buckley J, Lampkin B, et al. Comparison of alloge-

neic bone marrow transplantation (BMT) with maintenance chemotherapy in previously untreated childhood acute non-lymphocytic leukemia (ANLL). Proc Am Soc Clin Oncol 1987;6:163.

71. Gale RP, Bortin MM, van Bekkum DW, et al. Risk factors for acute graft-versus-host disease. Br J Haematol 1987;67:397.

72. Blume KG, Forman SJ, Nademanee AP, et al. Bone marrow transplantation for hematologic malignancies in patients aged 30 years or older. J Clin Oncol 1986;4:1489.

73. Klingemann H-G, Storb R, Fefer A, et al. Marrow transplantation in patients aged 45 years and older. Blood 1986;67:770.

74. Weisdorf DJ, McGlave PH, Ramsay NKC, et al. Allogeneic bone marrow transplantation for acute leukaemia: comparative outcomes for adults and children. Br J Haematol 1988;69:351.

75. Ramsay NKC, Kersey JH. Indications for marrow transplantation in acute lymphoblastic leukemia. Blood 1990;75:815.

76. Buckner CD, Sanders JE, Hill R, et al. Allogeneic versus autologous marrow transplantation for patients with acute lymphoblastic leukemia in first or second marrow remission. In: Dicke KA, Spitzer G, Jagannath S, Evinger-Hodges M-J, eds. Autologous Bone Marrow Transplantation: Proceedings of the Fourth International Symposium. Houston: University of Texas M.D. Anderson Cancer Center Hospital and Tumor Institute, 1989:145.

77. Burnett AK, Mackinnon S, Morrison A. Autologous transplantation of unpurged bone marrow during first remission of acute myeloid leukemia. In: Dicke KA, Spitzer G, Jagannath S, eds. Autologous Bone Marrow Transplantation: Proceedings of the Third International Symposium. Houston: University of Texas M.D. Anderson Hospital and Tumor Institute, 1987:23.

78. Yeager AM, Kaizer H, Santos GW, et al. Autologous bone marrow transplantation in patients with acute nonlymphocytic leukemia, using ex vivo marrow treatment with 4-hydroperoxy-cyclophosphamide. N Engl J Med 1986;315:141.

79. Thomas ED, Clift RA, Fefer A, et al. Marrow transplantation for the treatment of chronic myelogenous leukemia. Ann Intern Med 1986;104:155.

80. Goldman JM, Apperley JF, Jones L, et al. Bone marrow transplantation for patients with chronic myeloid leukemia. N Engl J Med 1986;314:202.

81. Speck B, Bortin MM, Champlin R, et al. Allogeneic bone marrow transplantation for chronic myelogenous leukaemia. Lancet 1984;i:665.

82. Pignon JM, Henni T, Anselem S, et al. Frequent detection of minimal residual disease by use of the polymerase chain reaction in long-term survivors after bone marrow transplantation for chronic myeloid leukemia. Leukemia 1990;4:83.

83. Thomas ED, Clift RA. Indications for marrow transplantation in chronic myelogenous leukemia. Blood 1989;73:861.

84. Armitage JO. Bone marrow transplantation in the treatment of patients with lymphoma. Blood 1989;73:1749.

85. Freedman AS, Takvorian T, Anderson KC, et al. Autologous bone marrow transplantation in B-cell non-Hodgkin's lymphoma: very low treatment-related mortality in 100 patients in sensitive relapse. J Clin Oncol 1990;8:784.

86. Appelbaum FR, Sullivan KM, Buckner CD, et al. Treatment of malignant lymphoma in 100 patients with chemotherapy, total body irradiation, and marrow transplantation. J Clin Oncol 1987;5:1340.

87. Barlogie B, Alexanian R, Dicke KA, et al. High-dose chemoradiotherapy and autologous bone marrow transplantation for resistant multiple myeloma. Blood 1987;70:869.

88. Smith JW, Shulman HM, Thomas ED, et al. Bone marrow transplantation for acute myelosclerosis. Cancer 1981;48:2198.

89. Appelbaum FR, Barrall J, Storb R, et al. Bone marrow trans-

plantation for patients with myelodysplasia. Ann Intern Med 1990;112:590.

90. Graham-Pole J, Lazarus HM, Herzig RH, et al. High-dose melphalan therapy for the treatment of children with refractory neuroblastoma and Ewing sarcoma. Am J Pediatr Hematol Oncol 1984;6:17.

91. Phillips GL, Fay JW, Herzig GP, et al. Intensive 1,3-bis(2-chloroethyl)-1-nitrosourea (BCNU), NSC # 466650 and cryo-preserved autologous marrow transplantation for refractory cancer. A phase I-II study. Cancer 1983;52:1792.

92. Buckner CD, Rudolph RH, Fefer A, et al. High-dose cyclophosphamide therapy for malignant disease. Cancer 1972;29:357.

93. Slease RB, Benear JB, Selby GB, et al. High-dose combination alkylating agent therapy with autologous bone marrow rescue for refractory solid tumors. J Clin Oncol 1988;6:1314.

94. Peters WP, Eder JP, Henner WD, et al. High-dose combination alkylating agents with autologous bone marrow support: a phase I trial. J Clin Oncol 1986;4:646.

95. Slease RB, Saez RA, Selby GB, Epstein RB. High dose cyclophosphamide, etoposide, and cisplatin + BCNU with autologous bone marrow transplantation for refractory malignancies: a phase I-II study. Proc Am Soc Clin Oncol 1990;9:16.

96. Stewart P. Autologous bone marrow transplantation in metastatic breast cancer. Breast Cancer Res Treat 1982;2:85.

97. Gisselbrecht C, Lepage E, Extra J-M, et al. Inflammatory and metastatic breast cancer: cyclophosphamide and total body irradiation (TBI) with autologous bone marrow transplantation (ABMT). In: Dicke KA, Spitzer G, Jagannath S, Evinger-Hodges M-J, eds. Autologous Bone Marrow Transplantation: Proceedings of the Fourth International Symposium. Houston: University of Texas M.D. Anderson Cancer Center Hospital and Tumor Institute, 1989:363.

98. Antman K, Bearman SI, Dadvison N, et al. Dose intensive therapy in breast cancer: current status. In: Gale RP, Champlin RE, eds. New Strategies in Bone Marrow Transplantation. New York: Wiley-Liss, 1991 p. 423.

99. Frei E, Antman K, Teicher B, et al. Bone marrow autotransplantation for solid tumors—prospects. J Clin Oncol 1989;7:515.

100. Biron P, Brunat-Mentigny M, Bayle JY, et al. Centre Leon Berard experience of massive chemotherapy in non-seminomatous germ cell tumours (NSGCT): analysis of first regimens in progressive disease and VP16-IPM-CDDP (VIC) in sensitive patients. In: Dicke KA, Spitzer G, Jagannath S, Evinger-Hodges M-J, eds. Autologous Bone Marrow Transplantation: Proceedings of the Fourth International Symposium. Houston: University of Texas M.D. Anderson Cancer Center Hospital and Tumor Institute, 1989:477.

101. Philip T, Bernard JL, Zucker JM, et al. High-dose chemotherapy with bone marrow transplantation as consolidation treatment in neuroblastoma: an unselected group of stage IV over 1 year of age. J Clin Oncol 1987;5:266.

102. Hartmann O, Benhamon E, Beaujean F, et al. Repeated high-dose chemotherapy followed by purged autologous bone marrow transplantation as consolidation therapy in metastatic neuroblastoma. J Clin Oncol 1987;5:1205.

103. Hartmann O, Bouffet E, Valteau D, et al. High-dose chemo/radiotherapy and autologous bone marrow transplantation as consolidation therapy in children's metastatic Ewing's sarcoma. In: Dicke KA, Spitzer G, Jagannath S, Evinger-Hodges M-J, eds. Autologous Bone Marrow Transplantation: Proceedings of the Fourth International Symposium. Houston: University of Texas M.D. Anderson Cancer Center Hospital and Tumor Institute, 1989:609.

104. Pinkerton CR, Philip T, Hartmann O, et al. High dose chemo-radiotherapy with autologous bone marrow rescue in pediatric

soft tissue sarcomas. In: Dicke KA, Spitzer G, Jagannath S, Evinger-Hodges M-J, eds. Autologous Bone Marrow Transplantation: Proceedings of the Fourth International Symposium. Houston: University of Texas M.D. Anderson Cancer Center Hospital and Tumor Institute, 1989:617.

105. Szer J, Deeg HJ, Witherspoon RP, et al. Long-term survival after marrow transplantation for paroxysmal nocturnal hemoglobinuria with aplastic anemia. Ann Intern Med 1984;101:193.

106. Coccia PF, Krivit W, Cervenka J, et al. Successful bone-marrow transplantation for infantile malignant osteopetrosis. N Engl J Med 1980;302:701.

107. Storb R, Thomas ED, Buckner CD, et al. Marrow transplantation for aplastic anemia. Semin Hematol 1984;221:27.

108. O'Reilly RJ, Brochstein J, Dinsmore R, et al. Marrow transplantation for congenital disorders. Semin Hematol 1984;21:188.

109. Wijnaendts L, LeDeist F, Griscelli C, et al. Development of immunologic functions after bone marrow transplantation in 33 patients with severe combined immunodeficiency. Blood 1989;74:2212.

110. Lucarelli G, Galimberti M, Polchi P, et al. Bone marrow transplantation in patients with thalassemia. N Engl J Med 1990;322:417.

111. Kapoor N, Kirkpatrick D, Blaese RM, et al. Reconstitution of normal megakaryocytopoiesis and immunologic function in Wiskott-Aldrich syndrome by marrow transplantation following myeloablation and immunosuppression with busulfan and cyclophosphamide. Blood 1981;57:692.

112. Gluckman E, Berger R, Dutreix J. Bone marrow transplantation for Fanconi anemia. Semin Hematol 1984;21:20.

113. Lenarsky C, Weinberg K, Guinan E, et al. Bone marrow transplantation for constitutional pure red cell aplasia. Blood 1988;71:226.

114. Hobbs JR, Hugh-Jones K, Barett AJ, et al. Reversal of clinical features of Hurler's disease and biochemical improvement after treatment by bone marrow transplantation. Lancet 1981;ii:709.

115. Pizzo PA, Schimpff SC. Strategies for the prevention of infection in the myelosuppressed or immunosuppressed cancer patient. Cancer Treat Rep 1983;67:223.

116. Saral R, Burns WH, Laskin OL, et al. Acyclovir prophylaxis of herpes-simplex-virus infections. A randomized, double-blind, controlled trial in bone-marrow-transplant recipients. N Engl J Med 1981;305:63.

117. Karp JE, Merz WG, Hendrickson C, et al. Oral norfloxacin for prevention of gram-negative bacterial infections in patients with acute leukemia and granulocytopenia. Ann Intern Med 1987;106:1.

118. Dekker AW, Rozenberg-Arska M, Verhoef J. Infection prophylaxis in acute leukemia: a comparison of ciprofloxacin with trimethoprim-sulfamethoxazole and colistin. Ann Intern Med 1987;106:7.

119. Bodey GP, Johnston D. Microbiological evaluation of protected environments during patient occupancy. Appl Microbiol 1971;22:828.

120. Kirk JL, Greenfield RA, Slease RB, et al. Analysis of early infections complications after autologous bone marrow transplantation. Cancer 1988;62:2445.

121. Winston DJ, Huang E-S, Miller MJ, et al. Molecular epidemiology of cytomegalovirus infections associated with bone marrow transplantation. Ann Intern Med 1985;102:16.

122. Bowden RA, Sayers M, Flournoy N, et al. Cytomegalovirus immune globulin and seronegative blood products to prevent primary cytomegalovirus infection after marrow transplantation. N Engl J Med 1986;314:1006.

123. Winston DJ, Ho WG, Cheng-Hsien L, et al. Intravenous immune globulin for prevention of cytomegalovirus infection and interstitial pneumonia after bone marrow transplantation. Ann Intern Med 1987;106:12.

124. Schmidt GM, Kovacs A, Zaia JA, et al. Ganciclovir/immunoglobulin combination therapy for the treatment of human cytomegalovirus associated interstitial pneumonia in bone marrow allograft recipients. Transplantation 1988;46:905.

125. Atkinson K, Storb R, Prentice RL, et al. Analysis of late infections in 889 long-term survivors of bone marrow transplantation. Blood 1979;53:720.

126. Shulman HM, McDonald GB, Matthews D, et al. An analysis of hepatic veno-occlusive disease and centrilobular hepatic degeneration following bone marrow transplantation. Gastroenterology 1980;79:1178.

127. McDonald GB, Shulman HM, Sullivan KM, et al. Intestinal and hepatic complications of bone marrow transplantation. Gastroenterology 1986;90:460,770.

128. Sanders JE, Buckner CD, Clift RA, et al. Second marrow transplants for patients with hematologic malignancy who relapse after first transplant. Blood 1989;74:203A.

129. Meyers JD, Flournoy N, Thomas ED. Nonbacterial pneumonia after allogeneic marrow transplantation: a review of ten years' experience. Rev Infect Dis 1982;4:1119.

130. Deeg HJ, Storb R, Thomas ED. Bone marrow transplantation: a review of delayed complications. Br J Haematol 1984;57:185.

131. Thompson DB, Sanders JE, Flournoy N, et al. The risks of central nervous system relapse and leukoencephalopathy in patients receiving marrow transplants for acute leukemia. Blood 1986;67:195.

132. Suiecinski IJ, Oien L, Petz LD, Blume KG. Immunohematologic consequences of major ABO mismatched bone marrow transplantation. Transplantation 1988;45:530.

133. Hows J, Beddow K, Gordon-Smith E, et al. Donor-derived red blood cell antibodies and immune hemolysis after allogeneic bone marrow transplantation. Blood 1986;56:177.

134. Sanders JE, Buckner CD, Leonard JM, et al. Late effects on gonadal function of cyclophosphamide, total-body irradiation, and marrow transplantation. Transplantation 1983;36:2652.

135. Sanders JE, Pritchard S, Mahoney P, et al. Growth and development following marrow transplantation for leukemia. Blood 1986;68:1129.

136. Sklar CA, Kim TH, Ramsay NKC. Thyroid dysfunction among long-term survivors of bone marrow transplantation. Am J Med 1982;73:688.

137. Deeg HJ, Sanders J, Martin P, et al. Secondary malignancies after marrow transplantation. Exp Hematol 1984;12:660.

138. Bretagne S, Vidaud M, Kuentz M, et al. Mixed blood chimerism in T cell-depleted bone marrow transplant recipients: evaluation using DNA polymorphisms. Blood 1987;70:1692.

139. Roy DC, Tantravalir R, Murray C, et al. Natural history of mixed chimerism after bone marrow transplantation with CD-depleted allogeneic marrow: a stable equilibrium. Blood 1990;75:296.

140. Hansen JA, Beatty PG, Anasetti C, et al. Treatment of leukemia by marrow transplantation from donors other than HLA genotypically identical siblings. In: Gale RP, Champlin R, eds. Progress in Bone Marrow Transplantation. New York: Alan R. Liss, 1987:667.

141. Bretturini A, Gale RP. T-cell depletion in bone marrow transplantation for leukemia: current results and future directions. Bone Marrow Transplantation 1988;3:185.

142. Kernan NA, Flomberg N, Dupont B, O'Reilly R. Identification of cytotoxic T lymphocytes in patients rejecting T-cell-depleted bone marrow transplants for leukemia. Blood 1984;64:216A.

143. Barge AJ, Johnson G, Witherspoon R, Torok-Storb B. Antibody-mediated marrow failure after allogeneic bone marrow transplantation. Blood 1989;74:1477.

144. Migliaccio AR, Migliaccio G, Johnson G, et al. Comparative analysis of hematopoietic growth factors released by stromal cells from normal donors or transplanted patients. Blood 1990;75:305.

145. Nemunaitis J, Singer JW, Buckner CD, et al. Use of recombinant human granulocyte-macrophage colony-stimulating factor in autologous marrow transplantation for lymphoid malignancies. Blood 1988;72:834.

146. Rowley SD, Zuchlsdorf M, Braine HG, et al. GFU-GM content of bone marrow graft correlates with time to hematologic reconstitution following autologous bone marrow transplantation with 4-hydroperoxycyclophosphamide-purged bone marrow. Blood 1987;70:271.

147. Storb R, Thomas ED. Graft-versus-host disease in dog and man: the Seattle experience. Immunol Rev 1985;88:215.

148. Glucksberg H, Storb R, Fefer A, et al. Clinical manifestations of graft-versus-host disease in human recipients of marrow from HLA-matched sibling donors. Transplantation 1974;18:295.

149. Woodruff JM, Hansen JA, Good RA, et al. The pathology of the graft-versus-host reaction (GvHR) in adults receiving bone marrow transplants. Transplant Proc 1976;8:675.

150. Sullivan KM, Witherspoon R, Deeg HJ, et al. Chronic graft-versus-host disease in man. In: Gale RP, Champlin R, eds. Progress in Bone Marrow Transplantation. New York: Alan R. Liss, 1987:473.

151. Shulman HM, Sale GE, Lerner KG, et al. Chronic cutaneous graft-versus-host disease in man. Am J Pathol 1978;92:545.

152. Sale GE, Shulman HM, Schubert MM, et al. Oral and ophthalmic pathology of graft-versus-host disease in man: predictive value of the lip biopsy. Hum Pathol 1981;12:1022.

153. Gale RP, Bortin MM, van Bekkum DW, et al. Risk factors for acute graft-versus-host disease. Br J Haematol 1987;67:397.

154. Forman SJ, Blume KG, Krance RA, et al. A prospective randomized study of acute graft-v-host disease in 107 patients with leukemia. Methotrexate/prednisone v cyclosporine A/prednisone. Transplant Proc 1987;19:2605.

155. Storb R, Deeg HJ, Whitehead J, et al. Methotrexate and cyclosporine compared with cyclosporine alone for prophylaxis of acute graft versus host disease after marrow transplantation for leukemia. N Engl J Med 1986;314:729.

156. Weiden PL, Flournoy N, Thomas ED, et al. Antileukemic effect of graft-versus-host disease in human recipients of allogeneic marrow grafts. N Engl J Med 1979;300:1068.

157. Horowitz MM, Gale RP, Sondel PM, et al. Graft-versus-leukemia reactions after bone marrow transplantation. Blood 1990;75:555.

158. Truitt RL, LeFever AV, Shih CC-Y. Graft-versus-leukemia reactions: experimental models and clinical trials. In: Gale RP, Champlin R, eds. Progress in Bone Marrow Transplantation. New York: Alan R. Liss, 1987:219.

159. Champlin R, Lee K, Gajewski J, et al. Selective CD8 depletion of donor marrow: retention of graft-versus-leukemia effect following bone marrow transplantation (BMT) for chronic myelogenous leukemia (CML). Blood 1989;74:28A.

160. Weisdorf D, Haake R, Blazar B, et al. Treatment of moderate/severe acute graft-versus-host disease after allogeneic bone marrow transplantation: an analysis of clinical risk features and outcome. Blood 1990;75:1024.

161. Kernan NA, Byers V, Scannon PJ, et al. Treatment of steroid-resistant acute graft-versus-host disease by in vivo administration of an anti-T cell ricin A chain immunotoxin. JAMA 1988;259:3154.

162. Herve P, Wijdenes J, Bergerat JP, et al. Treatment of corticosteroid resistant acute graft-versus-host disease by in vivo administration of anti-interleukin-2 receptor monoclonal antibody (B-B10). Blood 1990;75:1017.

163. Atkinson K. Chronic graft-versus-host disease. Bone Marrow Transplantation 1990;5:69.

164. Kurzrock R, Zander A, Kanojia M, et al. Obstructive lung disease after allogeneic bone marrow transplantation. Transplantation 1984;37:156.

165. Sullivan KM, Deeg HJ, Sanders JE, et al. Late complications after marrow transplantation. Semin Hematol 1984;21:53.

166. Lister J, Messner H, Keystone E, et al. Autoantibody analysis of patients with graft-versus-host disease. J Clin Lab Immunol 1987;24:19.

167. Atkinson K, Forewell V, Storb R, et al. Analysis of late infections after human bone marrow transplantation: role of genotypic nonidentity between marrow donor and recipient and of nonspecific suppressor cells in patients with chronic graft-versus-host disease. Blood 1982;60:714.

168. Sullivan KM, Witherspoon RP, Storb R, et al. Alternating-day cyclosporine and prednisone for treatment of high-risk chronic graft-versus-host disease. Blood 1988;72:555.

169. Anderson WF, Kantoff P, Eglitis M, et al. An autologous bone marrow transplantation/gene transfer protocol in non-human primates using retroviral vectors. In: Gale RP, Champlin R, eds. Progress in Bone Marrow Transplantation. New York: Alan R. Liss, 1987:973.

170. Cline MJ. Gene therapy: current status. Am J Med 1987;83:291.

23

Nuclear Hematology

*Min-Fu Tsan, M.D., Ph.D., Donald Pasquale, M.D., and
Patricia A. McIntyre, M.D.*

The application of radioactive tracers in medicine has facilitated greatly our understanding of both the physiology and pathophysiology of diseases. This chapter describes several aspects of nuclear medicine that are useful in the diagnosis and management of patients with hematologic disorders as well as some of the recent advances in hematology made possible by the use of nuclear techniques.

ANEMIA

When dealing with patients who have anemia, the clinician must consider two factors: the rate of red cell production, and the rate of red cell removal from the circulation. When the rate of removal exceeds that of production, anemia occurs, and this may be caused by decreased red cell production, increased red cell destruction, blood loss or a combination of these factors.

The Evaluation of Red Cell Production

The rate of red cell production may be estimated by several methods. The reticulocyte count, when corrected both for the degree of anemia and the estimated lifespan of reticulocytes, is a simple and useful index of the rate of red cell production. When used in conjunction with the determination of hematocrit and reticulocyte count, examination of the bone marrow usually will provide qualitative information about the rate as well as the effectiveness of red cell production. A ferrokinetic study, however, will provide more quantitative data concerning red cell production and the site of erythropoiesis. For practical reasons, the usual measurements obtained during a ferrokinetic study conducted in a clinical laboratory consist of the half-life of the initial, rapid exponential clearance phase of the injected radioactive iron (^{59}Fe) from the plasma, the percentage of radioactive iron incorporated into the circulating red cells over the ensuing 8- to 10-day period, and external surface counting to determine semiquantitatively the initial organ localization of the infused iron as well as the subsequent clearance (or lack thereof) from these organs.

The behavior of iron transported in the subject is meaningful only if the tracer iron is bound to transferrin. Many patients referred for these studies already are iron overloaded, a consequence either of their basic disease process, previous transfusions, or iron therapy; accordingly, it is imperative that the clinician measure the patient's unsaturated iron-binding capacity before any ferrokinetic studies to ensure that if the tracer iron is given preincubated with autologous plasma, there will be sufficient unsaturated transferrin present for its binding. The conventional methods for determining unsaturated iron-binding capacity frequently do not indicate 100% saturation, because added iron binds loosely to other proteins when no transferrin binding sites are available. Therefore, unless the unsaturated iron-binding capacity is greater than 100 μg/dl, ABO-compatible plasma that tests negative for the usual panel of blood-borne pathogens (such as human immunodeficiency virus and hepatitis virus) must be obtained from a donor and used to preincubate the radioactive iron. Also, only fresh, heparinized plasma can be used, because other anticoagulants chelate the radioactive iron.

Only the early phase of plasma radioiron clearance normally is measured, so no data are obtained about the effects of labelled iron that later refluxes into the circulation from sources such as extravascular fluid compartments, nonerythroid tissue stores, and catabolized erythroid cells. Calculations of both plasma and red cell iron turnover rates from these short-term plasma clearance data are based on assumptions that the initial exponential clearance half-life is representative of the entire plasma radioiron pattern over 10 to 14 days, that there is no significant variation in the plasma iron concentration during this time, and that the rate of iron transport is constant. Such assumptions, however, frequently are not valid, so the calculation of the plasma and red cell iron turnover rates requires a much more complex and precise study of the plasma radioactive iron concentration, using multiple samples obtained over a full 10-day period. Even minor amounts of hemolysis lead to significant errors due to the extremely low concentration of radioactive iron in the later samples; therefore, this type of elaborate long-term study rarely is performed other than in research laboratories.

The normal range for the plasma radioiron clearance half-life is 60 to 140 minutes. This clearance rate can change in disease states because of alterations in the rate of erythropoiesis and in the activity of the monocyte–macrophage system (formerly termed the *reticuloendothelial system*), where iron normally is retained as storage iron. An increased clearance rate is seen in such conditions as iron deficiency anemia, anemia caused by recent blood loss, hemolytic anemia, and polycythemia vera, but generally, the clearance rate decreases markedly in patients with aplastic or hypoplastic anemia. A paradoxic increase in the rate of plasma iron clearance frequently is seen in patients with anemia caused by myelofibrosis and myeloid metaplasia, and this suggests that the measurement of plasma radioiron clearance does not differentiate between effective and ineffective erythropoiesis. This method does, however, provide a valuable quality control as it ensures that the behavior of transferrin-bound radioactive iron is being studied. When no transferrin is available for iron binding, the injected radioactive iron will be cleared from the plasma almost immediately by the monocyte–macrophage system, presumably due to colloid formation.

Determining the rate of radioactive iron incorporation into the circulating red cells estimates the effectiveness of erythropoiesis. In normal subjects, 60% to 80% of the administered dose will be incorporated into the circulating red cells after 7 to 10 days (Fig. 23.1),[1] and it is necessary to obtain more frequent samples than merely one sample at the peak time for normal incorporation. There may be immediate accelerated incorporation of radioiron into the circulating red cells in some patients with severe hemolytic anemia; however, by the seventh to tenth day, many of these labelled red cells already may have been hemolyzed. Thus, a single sample obtained at this time would indicate that the net incorporation of iron was subnormal. As Figure 23.1 shows, with the exception of iron deficiency anemia, there is a quantitative correlation between the degree of effective erythropoiesis and the percentage of red cell radioiron incorporation. In iron deficiency anemia, the actual red cell production is reduced because of substrate depletion, but when a trace amount of iron is given to these patients, there is both faster and greater incorporation into newly formed red cells.

Surface counting by a well-collimated external probe provides useful information about the initial organ localization of radioiron and the relative change in radioactivity within the organs over time; appropriate areas to count include the sacrum, precordium, liver, and spleen.[1] In normal subjects, there is a relatively rapid increase in radioactivity over the sacrum during the first few hours of the study, then a gradual decline as the radioiron is incorporated into the red cells and released into the circulation. Little radioactivity normally accumulates in the spleen and liver, and that noted over these areas in normal subjects undoubtedly represents radioiron accumulation in the adjacent areas of active marrow. Abnormal patterns of surface counting may be seen in patients with ineffective erythropoiesis or in those with significant extramedullary erythropoiesis (Fig. 23.2).[1]

The Evaluation of Red Cell Removal from the Circulation

Hemorrhage or hemolysis may reduce significantly the normal red cell lifespan of 120 days. To determine the presence of hemolysis, the clinician may measure the catabolic products of hemoglobin that are increased due to accelerated red cell destruction; alternatively, the level of circulating haptoglobin or hemopexin (the transport proteins binding hemoglobin or hemin, respectively) may be measured. The presence of abnormal red cell morphology or red cell antibodies also may provide indirect evidence of hemolysis, but the determination of red cell lifespan using radioisotopes provides a semiquantitative measurement when there is significantly reduced red cell survival.

In general, there are two types of red cell labels: those that label a cohort of cells, and those that label cells

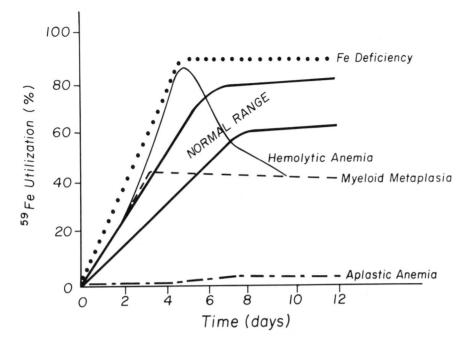

FIGURE 23.1. The utilization of radioiron by red cells in various disease states. There is a more rapid rate and total increase in iron incorporation in patients having iron deficiency anemia and hemolytic anemias; however, with the concomitant removal or destruction of the labelled cells (as shown here, a patient with autoimmune hemolytic anemia), a single sample taken at the eighth to tenth day would indicate lower-than-normal utilization of ^{59}Fe. In aplastic anemia, the incorporation of ^{59}Fe is reduced significantly. *Source:* McIntyre 1972[1] Albert Miller, illustrator.

randomly. Ideally, the cohort label would be available only to the marrow precursors of a given cell type for a specific and limited time and would not label the circulating cells; the incorporation of this label into the marrow precursors, followed by the subsequent maturation of these cells, then would result in the appearance of labelled cells of the same age in the circulation. An ideal cohort label that meets these criteria would permit determination of production rate of a given cell type, its lifespan, and its ultimate disposal within the body. None of the currently available radioisotopes for cohort labelling of red cells satisfies all these requirements; indeed, most existing cohort labels are so limited by their properties that with the exception of the iron isotopes, they are not used in routine clinical studies. Furthermore, even if such an ideal cohort label for erythrocytes was available, it is doubtful that it would be useful clinically as a full study would require more than 3 months to complete.

The radioisotopes of iron are the oldest historically and still are the most useful cohort labels for determining the initial rate of erythrocyte production. However, the body is quite conservative in handling hemoglobin iron: as soon as a labelled red cell is removed from the circulation, the heme is degraded and the label returns to the active iron pool and reappears in the new cell. This continued reutilization of ^{59}Fe makes it a less than ideal cohort label, limited to the determination of the initial rate of erythrocyte production.

Because the random method labels all cells in the sample, it is applicable only in the study of mean red cell survival. As a red cell label, ^{51}Cr has several shortcomings. Only 9% of emissions are of the gamma type and, therefore, capable of providing useful information, and ^{51}Cr elutes from normal red cells at a rate of approximately 1%/day. Also, this rate of elution varies in different disease states.[2] Because of the relatively short physical half-life of ^{99m}Tc and ^{111}In, these are unsuitable labels for red cell survival studies; thus, despite its shortcomings, ^{51}Cr-sodium chromate continues to be the main radiopharmaceutical used in the study of red cell survival. Whole blood routinely is used for ^{51}Cr

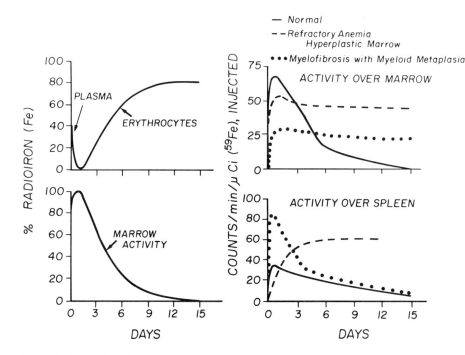

FIGURE 23.2. The relationship between blood and marrow radioactivity after intravenous injection of radioiron into a normal subject is reciprocal (*left*). As radioiron clears from the plasma, the marrow activity increases; as the marrow activity decreases, activity rises in the circulating red cell mass. Following injection of radioiron in various disease states, alterations of the normal organ localization curves occur (*right*) that may be useful diagnostically. Note the pattern of uptake but failure to release iron from the marrow in the patient with refractory anemia and hyperplastic marrow, reflecting the failure of normal erythropoiesis; in this same patient, increased deposition and retention of iron occur in the spleen as well. Decreased marrow and increased splenic uptake in the patient with myelofibrosis and myeloid metaplasia suggest effective erythropoiesis in the spleen. These curves are based on external counting over the sacrum and spleen. *Source:* McIntyre 1972[1] Albert Miller, illustrator.

labelling, but if the white blood cell count exceeds 25,000 cells/μl, then a significant portion of the ^{51}Cr will bind rapidly to these cells. In such cases, it is necessary to use a buffy coat–poor red cell suspension.[3]

Normal erythrocytes are removed from the circulation when they become senescent at a rate of approximately 1% per day. The actual mean lifespan of the normal circulating erythrocyte, therefore, is between 50 and 60 days; however, this approximately 1%/day removal of senescent red cells from the circulation, coupled with the approximately 1% elution of the ^{51}Cr label from the erythrocyte, gives the mean half-time of 25 to 35 days as measured with ^{51}Cr-labelled red cells.

Determination of the mean red cell lifespan from a label randomly applied to cells of all ages is meaningful only in a patient who is in steady state regarding the rates of both the production and destruction of red cells. If either of these rates changes, then the mean age of the circulating red cells will be changed and affect the ^{51}Cr results even though the actual longevity of each individual erythrocyte is unchanged. A constant hematocrit both before and during the period of study is one index of a steady state, and ideally, the reticulocyte count and hemoglobin concentration both should be constant for at least 2 months before the study. Inaccurate results obviously will be obtained in a patient who either is being or recently has been transfused. Because hemolysis and hemorrhage both result in an apparent shortened red cell survival, it is important to ensure there is no internal or external blood loss during the ^{51}Cr–red cell survival study. Gastrointestinal blood loss may be determined by collecting and measuring radioactivity in the patient's stool.

The study of splenic sequestration by external counting should be a routine part of the ^{51}Cr–red cell survival study. Three sites are counted: the precordium, liver, and spleen.[4] In patients with markedly enlarged spleens, it may be useful to count more than one site over the spleen, and because splenic infarction is prone to occur in enlarged spleens, counting over an infarcted area may miss the active, ongoing sequestration of red cells by the remaining spleen. In normal subjects, the spleen-to-liver ratio is about 1:1; in patients with active splenic sequestration, this ratio may vary from 2:1 to 4:1. The spleen-to-precordium ratio, however, provides a better index of the degree of splenic sequestration, because the liver in some patients also may be sequestering erythrocytes. Spleen-to-precordium ratios over 2:1 are considered abnormal. An initial and thereafter essentially constant elevation of the spleen-to-precordium ratio reflects an increased splenic blood pool, while a progressive and gradual increase indicates active and ongoing sequestration of labelled cells. Figures 23.3, 23.4, and 23.5 are examples of the patterns that may be observed with the ^{51}Cr–red cell survival and sequestration studies.[1]

Evidence that splenic sequestration may have an etiologic role in anemic disorders is of great value in selecting candidates for splenectomy. When a clear-cut example of progressive splenic sequestration is seen, it is safe to predict that the patient's hemolytic anemia will respond to splenectomy; however, it has been observed that a number of patients with no definite evidence of splenic sequestration also have an excellent response to splenectomy. This most likely is caused by inaccurate positioning of the external probe or poorly designed collimators. As a result, the evidence of splenic sequestration is not obtained properly.

Erythrokinetic Studies Using Two Isotopes

Frequently, much more complete information regarding the factors responsible for anemia may be obtained by combined studies; for example, patients with myelofibrosis and myeloid metaplasia may develop progressive anemia and increasing transfusion requirements after a prolonged, stable clinical course. One wonders whether the progressive anemia is caused by

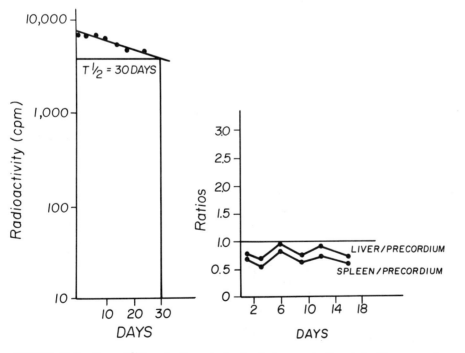

FIGURE 23.3. Normal ^{51}Cr-red cell survival and splenic sequestration study. The apparent short half-life (T½) of 30 days is due to the elution of ^{51}Cr from normal red cells at a rate of approximately 1%/day. Both the spleen/precordium and the liver/precordium ratios are below 1 throughout the course of the study. *Source:* McIntyre 1972[1] Albert Miller, illustrator.

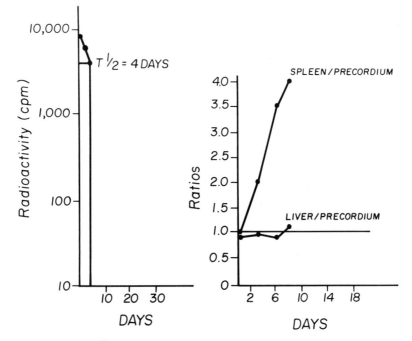

FIGURE 23.4. ^{51}Cr-red cell survival and splenic sequestration study in a patient with severe Coomb-positive autoimmune hemolytic anemia. Corticosteroid therapy was contraindicated because of severe diabetes mellitus and osteoporosis, and there is markedly shortened red cell survival with rapid, progressively increasing splenic sequestration. Splenectomy caused a prompt rise in the hematocrit to a normal level. *Note:* T½ = half-life. *Source:* McIntyre 1972[1] Albert Miller, illustrator.

depressed red cell production, increased red cell destruction by the enormous spleen, or both. Would splenectomy help this patient? In this case, combined ferrokinetic, red cell survival, and sequestration studies would be most appropriate.

Hypochromic and Microcytic Anemia

Iron deficiency continues to be the most common hematologic disorder, and in its advanced state, the patient develops microcytic and hypochromic anemia. Most often, a careful history alone will reveal the cause, but determination of the serum iron level and of the total iron-binding capacity may be useful in differentiating patients with iron deficiency anemia from those with other types of hypochromic and microcytic anemia. Iron deficiency anemia is characterized by a decreased serum iron level and an increased total iron-binding capacity; however, the total iron-binding capacity may be normal or low when the iron deficiency anemia coexists with a chronic inflammatory condition. In other types of hy-

pochromic and microcytic anemia, the serum iron level may be decreased, normal, or increased while the total iron-binding capacity is either decreased or normal. The visual estimation of stainable iron in the bone marrow commonly is used for the assessment of iron stores, but this has the disadvantage of being more invasive and less readily available than venipuncture.

Measurement of the serum ferritin level by immunoradiometric assay also may be helpful in differentiating iron deficiency anemia from other causes. In general, the serum ferritin level provides a reliable estimate of the body iron stores; markedly reduced levels are found in patients with iron deficiency and markedly elevated levels in patients with iron overload.[5] Important exceptions have been noted, however. Some patients with liver disease, inflammatory conditions, and malignant disorders (including leukemia) have disproportionately high levels of ferritin,[6,7] and variable results also are found in affected family members of patients with primary hemochromatosis.[8,9] Although a normal serum ferritin value cannot exclude iron deficiency in the

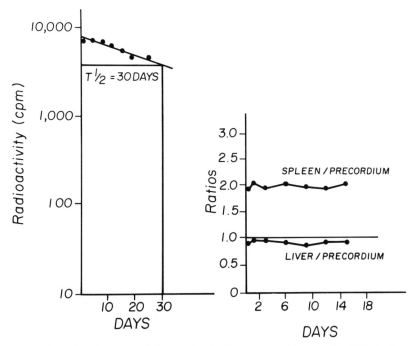

FIGURE 23.5. A patient with normal red cell survival and increased activity in the splenic pool secondary to splenomegaly. *Note:* T½ = half-life. *Source:* McIntyre 1972[1] Albert Miller, illustrator.

presence of hepatic, malignant, or inflammatory disorders, any significant decrease is indicative of decreased body iron stores.

Megaloblastic Anemia

Vitamin B_{12} deficiency as well as folate deficiency are common causes of megaloblastic anemia. Serum vitamin B_{12} levels, measured by microbiologic assays with *Euglena gracilis* or *Lactobacillus leichmannii,* are reduced markedly in vitamin B_{12} deficiency and correlate well with the clinical status of the patient; however, these microbiologic assays are tedious and time consuming. Also, special alterations in the laboratory procedure must be made if the patient is taking antibiotics or certain drugs that inhibit bacterial growth.

Radioisotope competitive protein-binding assays for the measurement of vitamin B_{12} levels are based on the principle that endogenous serum vitamin B_{12} will compete with radioactive vitamin B_{12} for binding to a limited amount of vitamin B_{12} binding protein. Because of their simplicity, these tests have replaced the conventional microbiologic assays in screening for serum vitamin B_{12} levels; however, it should be noted that when R protein is used as the vitamin B_{12} binding protein, serum vitamin B_{12} values obtained by these radioisotope dilu-

tion assays are higher than those by microbiologic assays. Also, approximately 10% of patients with vitamin B_{12} deficiency have normal serum levels,[10] due to the ability of R binding proteins to bind inactive analogues of vitamin B_{12} that normally are present in blood. When purified intrinsic factor is used as the binding protein, a good correlation between radioassay and microbiologic assay results is observed.[11] Thus, when using radioassay as a screening test for serum vitamin B_{12} levels, the clinician should use purified intrinsic factor as the binding protein.

One often-encountered problem in clinical practice is determining the significance of a low serum vitamin B_{12} level in an individual either without the typical neurologic or hematologic manifestations of vitamin B_{12} deficiency or with normal vitamin B_{12} absorption. The development of a simple radioenzymatic assay[12] for measuring serum homocysteine has improved our ability to diagnose tissue deficiency of vitamin B_{12} or folic acid, and because homocysteine is converted to methionine by an enzyme (methyltransferase) that requires both methylcobalamin and methyltetrahydrofolic acid as cofactors, a deficiency of either cofactor at the tissue level leads to increased levels of serum homocysteine.[12,13] Normal serum levels of homocysteine exclude the diagnosis of tissue deficiency of vitamin B_{12}

and folic acid, but elevated levels confirm the diagnosis of vitamin B_{12} deficiency, folate deficiency, or both.[12,13]

Several factors are important in vitamin B_{12} nutrition and absorption in humans. The same factors also apply to the absorption of tracer amounts of radioactive vitamin B_{12} used in absorption studies and include:

1. availability for human nutrition only in animal food sources,
2. cleavage of vitamin B_{12} from R binders by pancreatic proteases to allow the binding of free vitamin B_{12} to intrinsic factor produced by gastric mucosa,
3. normal ileal mucosal absorptive sites in the presence of ionic Ca^{2+} and a pH of ileal contents above 6.0, and
4. the presence of normal "transport" protein (transcobalamin II) to convey vitamin B_{12} from ileal absorptive sites to areas of active usage and storage.

Isolated, pure dietary vitamin B_{12} deficiency is very rare; therefore, the overwhelming majority of vitamin B_{12} deficiencies are caused by disorders that lead to malabsorption. The availability of radioactive vitamin B_{12} for specific testing of a patient's ability to absorb physiologic amounts of this essential nutrient consequently has been of great clinical value.

The fecal excretion test was the earliest method for measuring the absorption of radioactive vitamin B_{12}. It was often inaccurate, because it required a 7- to 10-day total stool collection. The simpler Schilling test of urinary excretion now generally is accepted as the standard method. This test requires the oral administration and retention of a vitamin B_{12} tracer dose and a transient saturation of normal binding sites in plasma, which is achieved by injecting a flushing dose of 1000 μg of nonradioactive vitamin B_{12} within 2 hours after the oral dose is administered. This results in the prompt renal excretion of a significant proportion of the absorbed tracer dose. It also is important that this tracer dose be in the range of 0.25 to 2.0 μg, similar to what might be present in a normal meal; a greater amount could be absorbed by mechanisms independent of intrinsic factor. The malabsorption of vitamin B_{12} can be documented by the appearance of less than 9% of the administered dose in the first 24-hour urine collection.

The major disadvantage of this test is its dependence on a complete 24-hour urine collection. The loss of just one urine specimen may result in falsely low results. Maximal excretion occurs between 8 and 12 hours after oral administration, and the loss of a specimen during this period may produce an abnormal test result even in a normal subject.

The 24-hour test also requires that urinary function be normal. Erroneously low values result from abnormal urinary retention, such as in men with benign prostatic hypertrophy or in patients with severe renal disease. In such patients, the amount excreted during the first 24 hours will be reduced, but significant radioactivity will continue to be excreted for the next 24 to 48 hours. The total excretion eventually will be within normal limits. For this reason, and because it often helps to determine if the first 24-hour collection was incomplete, we ask the patient to make two separate 24-hour collections after the single flushing dose, and for each 24-hour specimen, we separately measure the volume, specific gravity, and percentage of the administered dose of radioactivity. Table 23.1 shows typical results and illustrates the value of this minor modification of the Schilling test.[14]

The difficulties inherent in achieving a complete 24-hour urine collection have led some investigators to seek other methods for measuring the vitamin B_{12} absorption. In normal subjects, the liver is the primary

TABLE 23.1. Representative Results of a Schilling Test Using Two 24-Hour Urine Collections (Single Nuclide Without Intrinsic Factor)

	First Day			Second Day		
Patient	Volume, *ml*	Specific Gravity	Radioactivity, %	Volume, *ml*	Specific Gravity	Radioactivity, %
A	640	1.010	3.0	1230	1.010	0.8
B	1210	1.012	3.0	1120	1.012	0.8
C	1200	1.010	3.0	1150	1.010	4.0
D	1210	1.012	14.0	1200	1.012	0.3

Source: McIntyre 1975[14]

Note: Patient A had an incomplete first 24-hour urine collection because of the inadvertent loss of urine during cleansing enemas that had been ordered to prepare her for gastrointestinal radiographic examinations. Urinary volume on the first day was only 640 ml with a specific gravity of 1.010, which was the same as that of the second-day urine, with a volume of 1230 ml. Patient B subsequently had normal excretion when the test was repeated with the addition of a potent intrinsic factor, and the results of other studies confirmed the diagnosis of Addisonian anemia. Patient C was recognized on re-examination to have benign prostatic hypertrophy with significant bladder retention; the delayed pattern of excretion of the radioactive vitamin B_{12} was the first clinical indication of this condition. Patient D was a cooperative normal volunteer.

site of vitamin B_{12} storage, and external counting over the liver initially was thought to be an attractive alternative to the Schilling test. It was independent of both patient cooperation and the administration of a therapeutic dose of parenteral nonradioactive vitamin B_{12}.[15] However, because of problems with geometry in the external counting as well as with the abnormalities occurring in patients with liver disease, this test no longer is used widely.

Another proposed alternative was the measurement of plasma radioactivity 8 hours after administration of an oral dose of labelled vitamin B_{12}; however, false-normal results have been obtained by this test in some patients with proven pernicious anemia.[16] Thus, the Schilling test remains the test of choice for routine clinical measurements of vitamin B_{12} absorption. That choice, however, may be different if both time and special facilities permit. If a delay of 7 to 10 days is feasible, more precise quantitative measurement can be obtained by administering ^{58}Co-cyanocobalamin orally and then determining by whole-body counting the percentage of radioactivity absorbed. This method obviates fecal or urinary collections and does not depend on intact urinary function, but it does require adequate whole-body counting equipment, which is relatively insensitive to the in vivo translocations of the ^{58}Co–vitamin B_{12}. The 7- to 10-day delay before the final counting is required to ensure clearance of radioactive cobalt from the gastrointestinal tract.

An accurate measurement of vitamin B_{12} absorption also can be accomplished by the spot feces test using a double-isotope technique. This is carried out by simultaneously administering tracer amounts of radioactive vitamin B_{12} and a nonabsorbable marker such as ^{51}Cr-chromic chloride. The ratio of the two isotopes is determined both in the test dose and a single stool specimen; the change in the ratio is a function of the vitamin B_{12} absorbed. This method has been shown to correlate closely with whole-body counting,[17] and because both the whole-body counting and the spot feces test do not depend on the urinary excretion of the absorbed vitamin B_{12}, these two methods should be used to assess vitamin B_{12} absorption in anephric individuals.

The cause of vitamin B_{12} malabsorption can be determined by performing a "second stage" Schilling test, with oral administration of labelled vitamin B_{12} bound to intrinsic factor (by incubation with normal human gastric juice). Individuals with intrinsic factor deficiency (such as pernicious anemia) will absorb and excrete over 9% of the labelled vitamin B_{12}; in individuals with malabsorption due to lesions in the small bowel, less than 9% of the dose will be found in the urine. The cause also can be determined directly by using a modified Schilling test, in which vitamin B_{12} labelled with two different cobalt isotopes is administered. One form is already bound to intrinsic factor, and the other is "free." To minimize the possibility of radiolabelled vitamin B_{12} exchange, both the free and the bound vitamin B_{12} should be administered sequentially with a 2-hour separation.[18] A normal subject will excrete essentially the same amount of both isotopes, while the patient who lacks intrinsic factor will excrete greater quantities of intrinsic factor–bound vitamin B_{12}. Patients with lesions in the small bowel resulting in vitamin B_{12} malabsorption will excrete both isotopes in subnormal quantities.

In patients whose vitamin B_{12} malabsorption results from bacterial competition for host dietary vitamin B_{12}, resulting from bacterial overgrowth (small intestinal diverticula or blind loops), the malabsorption will not be corrected by intrinsic factor. Treatment with broad-spectrum antibiotics will restore the vitamin B_{12} absorption to normal in these patients, and Table 23.2 summa-

TABLE 23.2. The Use of Radioactive Vitamin B_{12} Tests for Differential Diagnosis of the Cause of Vitamin B_{12} Malabsorption

Test	Agent	Normal
First	Oral trace dose of radioactive vitamin B_{12} (*B_{12})	Normal vitamin B_{12} absorption
Second*	*B_{12} and intrinsic factor	Intrinsic factor–dependent vitamin B_{12} malabsorption‡
Third†	A) *B_{12} after a course of broad-spectrum antibiotics	Malabsorption is secondary to intestinal lesion causing bacterial overgrowth
	B) *B_{12} after withdrawal of drug	Malbsorption is induced by drug
	C) *B_{12} with addition of sodium bicarbonate and pancreatic extract	Malabsorption is secondary to pancreatic insufficiency

Source: McIntyre 1975[14]

*Performed only after the result of the preceding test was demonstrated to be abnormal.

†The type of third test (i.e., A, B, or C) is dictated by clinical information.

‡If hog intrinsic factor is used, a negative result does not completely exclude intrinsic factor–dependent malabsorption, because some subjects who were previously exposed to hog intrinsic factor (e.g., in multivitamin preparations) will be refractory to this agent but will have vitamin B_{12} malabsorption corrected by the addition of intrinsic factor from normal human gastric juice.

rizes how sequential tests aid in diagnosing the cause of vitamin B_{12} malabsorption.[14]

While normal absorption of the crystalline vitamin B_{12} given in the Schilling test excludes the malabsorption of dietary vitamin B_{12} in the vast majority of individuals, malabsorption of protein-bound vitamin B_{12} (the form found in normal diets) with normal absorption of crystalline vitamin B_{12} has been described in patients with achlorhydria (including that induced by drugs, i.e., H_2-histamine receptor blocking agents) and normal intrinsic factor production. This also has been described in individuals who have undergone gastric surgery such as vagotomy or Bilroth anastomosis.[19–22] Protein-bound vitamin B_{12} absorption can be assessed by binding labelled vitamin B_{12} to egg proteins before oral administration. Impaired absorption of an orally administered dose of labelled vitamin B_{12} also can occur in the absence of vitamin B_{12} malabsorption due to competition with unlabelled vitamin B_{12} in the gastrointestinal tract. This occurs when large daily doses of vitamin B_{12} are administered either orally or parenterally (due to biliary excretion) during the 3 days before the administration of the oral labelled dose. Likewise, vitamin B_{12} deficiency itself can cause malabsorption because of megaloblastic changes in the gastrointestinal epithelium; under this circumstance, even in the presence of added intrinsic factor, vitamin B_{12} absorption may not approach normal until several weeks after recovery. Patients with disturbed gastrointestinal functions may not be able to digest the capsule containing vitamin B_{12} and intrinsic factor, thus leading to an abnormal vitamin B_{12} absorption test. Therefore, a proper test for vitamin B_{12} absorption always should be performed with vitamin B_{12} and intrinsic factor in a liquid form.

Folate Deficiency

Unlike vitamin B_{12} deficiency, the most common cause of folate deficiency is a relative or absolute dietary deficiency. Serum folate levels are very sensitive to brief periods of dietary deprivation, and they vary directly with the recent ingestion of folate and may not correlate with tissue levels. In contrast, red cell folate levels more accurately reflect the clinical status of the patient.

As with vitamin B_{12} assays, the tedious microbiologic methods largely have been replaced by the simpler competitive protein-binding assays. Although most laboratories claim good clinical correlations, very few have performed concomitant microbiologic assays for comparison, and several studies have shown that folate values obtained by competitive protein-binding assays differ from those of microbiologic assays.[23–25] Furthermore, the only folate that currently is stable and available in high-enough specific activity is simple folic acid; the folate compound normally present in serum is 5-methyltetrahydrofolate, a reduced and substituted form of folic acid. It has been noted that patients receiving drugs which inhibit the enzyme dihydrofolate reductase may have normal serum levels as measured by these radioassays, even though they suffer from clinical folate deficiency. Thus, the optimal method for the radioassay of serum and red cell folate levels must be defined further.

ERYTHROCYTOSIS

Erythrocytosis, or increased red cell mass, usually is associated with an elevated venous hematocrit; however, elevated hematocrit does not always indicate the presence of erythrocytosis. An elevated venous hematocrit with a normal or reduced red cell mass occurs when there is decreased plasma volume. This may occur in patients who are severely dehydrated or have spurious (relative or stress) erythrocytosis. Thus, when evaluating patients with an elevated venous hematocrit of uncertain etiology, it is imperative that the clinician first determine both the red cell mass and the plasma volume.

These determinations are based on the simple radioisotope dilution technique.[26] ^{51}Cr-labelled red cells are used for measuring the red cell mass, and complete mixing of red cells after intravenous injection is essential. Ten minutes is sufficient to ensure complete mixing in normal subjects; however, in certain disease states (e.g., splenomegaly or marked erythrocytosis), mixing always is delayed. Under these circumstances, serial samples should be taken (starting at 30 minutes) until the radioactivities of the samples do not differ significantly (Table 23.3).[27] Inadequate mixing will result in an underestimation of the red cell mass. Mixing also is delayed in other patients who are clinically ill, but to a lesser extent, and a single sample at 20 to 30 minutes probably will suffice in these cases.

Iodinated albumin is the agent conventionally used for the estimation of plasma volume. However, unlike red cells, albumin does not remain solely in the intravascular space; it diffuses rapidly into the extravascular compartments. To minimize the resulting error, the clinician must take two, or preferably more, timed samples (i.e., 10, 20, and 30 minutes) from the subject, and the radioactivity in each is measured and then plotted against time on semilogarithmic paper. The best straight line is drawn through these points, using only earlier points if the later ones deviate from the initial linear slope. The zero time activity is estimated by

TABLE 23.3. The Results of the Measurement of Red Cell Volume in Patients with High Hematocrits

Patient	Hematocrit, %	Red Cell Volume, *ml/kg*					
		30 min	60 min	90 min	120 min	180 min	240 min
A	75	—	54	62	—	68	71
B	70	56	—	85	—	—	—
C	61	46	48	51	—	—	51
D	55	43	44	45	—	—	—

Source: Conley 1987[27]

Note: The red cell volume, calculated from isotope dilution in minutes after the injection of ^{51}Cr-labelled RBC, is underestimated grossly by early sampling in patients with very high hematocrits because of delayed mixing of the labelled cells.

extrapolation and is used to calculate the plasma volume. To be satisfactory, preparations of iodinated serum albumin must contain essentially no free iodine or any aggregated or otherwise denatured albumin; the presence of any of these will lead to a much more rapid tracer removal from the circulation and will result in overestimation of the plasma volume.

When the red cell or plasma volume has been measured precisely and the venous hematocrit is known, the volume of the other compartment in normal subjects can be determined if two correction factors are taken into account:

1. If the hematocrit is determined by centrifugation, then variable amounts of plasma trapping may be present. The hematocrit must be corrected for this trapped plasma to obtain the true venous hematocrit. Significant alterations in plasma trapping do occur in some diseases; however, an accurate hematocrit can be obtained using an automated blood cell counter, as hematocrit is calculated from the measured red blood cell count and mean corpuscular volume.
2. In normal subjects, there is a fixed relationship between the whole-body hematocrit and the venous hematocrit, and the average ratio of whole-body hematocrit to venous hematocrit is 0.90.

It is possible in normal subjects to estimate the total blood volume from the measurement of either red cell or plasma volume and the calculated whole-body hematocrit. This relationship is not always present, however. For instance, in patients with moderate or gross splenomegaly, the ratio of whole-body hematocrit to venous hematocrit may be increased substantially, to greater than 1.0; similarly, in patients with severe erythrocytosis, abnormalities may be present in the plasma volume as well as the red cell mass. In both these and many other clinical circumstances, the total blood volume may be estimated reliably only by measuring the red cell mass and the plasma volume simultaneously. The clinician

TABLE 23.4. Normal Blood Volume Compartment Values

	Men, *ml/kg*	Women, *ml/kg*
Total blood volume	55 to 80	50 to 75
Red cell volume*	25 to 35	20 to 30
Plasma volume†	30 to 45	30 to 45

Source: Data from Panel of Diagnostic Application of Radioisotopes in Hematology 1973[26]

*95% confidence limits

†Because of the many variables that may influence plasma volume in normal subjects, it is impossible to place confidence limits on these values.

may do this by choosing an appropriate combination of isotopes (i.e., ^{125}I-labelled human serum albumin and ^{51}Cr-labelled red cells, or ^{131}I-labelled albumin and ^{99m}Tc-labelled red cells), but a serious limitation in the interpretation of these results is that normal values for blood volume in any given subject cannot be predicted simply from such parameters as height and weight despite the many elaborate formulae or nomograms that have been proposed. In interpreting results in adults, the simplest method of calculating the values in ml/kg probably is at least as reliable as any formula or nomogram; Table 23.4 shows the normal values published by the International Committee for Standardization in Hematology.[26] Many variables, such as obesity, recent weight loss, and prolonged bed rest, make it difficult to estimate the red cell and plasma volumes directly from height and weight measurements. Because the red blood cell mass is related to the lean body mass, patients who are markedly obese or have had recent severe weight loss should have their measured values compared with those based on "ideal" or recent body weight.

BONE MARROW DISEASE

Bone marrow aspiration and biopsy are useful clinical tools for evaluating disorders of the bone marrow, but they are limited in that they sample only a small portion of the total organ. Bone marrow imaging, however, provides information on the entire blood-forming organ.

Two physiologic processes of the functional bone marrow permit scanning of that organ. First, tracer doses of transferrin-bound radioactive iron are cleared rapidly from the circulation and deposited in areas of the marrow having active erythropoiesis; these agents permit scanning of the erythroid marrow, or "erythron." Second, phagocytic cells in the marrow accumulate radiocolloids, and although a smaller percentage of injected radiocolloid accumulates in the marrow than in the liver or spleen, use of the permissible larger dose of colloids made from short-lived gamma-emitting nuclides allows scanning of the functional monocyte–macrophage system in the marrow. Table 23.5 summarizes the physical properties of these radiopharmaceuticals;[28] currently, no agents will label specifically the granulopoietic or megakaryocytic elements of the bone marrow.

Regardless of radiopharmaceutical agent used, the pattern of marrow activity distribution among normal humans is identical. In adults, the active marrow is confined to the axial skeleton and the proximal third of both humeri and femora. In young children, some degree of peripheral marrow activity, especially in the long bones of the legs, is normal. Abnormalities that can be recognized in the marrow scan pattern may include one or more of the following:

1. decrease or increase of activity in the axial or central portion of the marrow;
2. reduction or increase of activity in the proximal portions of the long bones, or extension to varying degrees of marrow activity further down the long bones (in extreme instances of marrow hyperplasia, such as in some patients with chronic and severe

hemolytic anemias, active marrow may be visualized in other osseous structures, i.e., both maxillae and mandibles);
3. focal defects, which may be single or multiple, in areas of normal marrow activity; and
4. appearance of marrow activity outside the marrow cavity (e.g., in the liver, spleen, or soft tissues—extramedullary hematopoiesis).

Figures 23.6 through 23.9 illustrate some of these marrow scan patterns.[29]

Because of the properties of iron radionuclides available, studies of the erythron by scanning techniques have been limited to only a few institutions. ^{59}Fe, widely used in ferrokinetic studies, is unsuitable for imaging the functional erythron with satisfactory spatial resolution because of its high gamma energy. However, ^{52}Fe, a short-lived nuclide, is a positron emitter, and excellent images may be obtained using a positron camera or by the administration of a substantially larger dose and use of rectilinear scanners equipped with special high-energy collimators. Several investigators have shown ^{52}Fe to be a highly satisfactory erythron imaging agent both in the presence of disease and under normal conditions.[30,31] However, it is not widely available, both because of its short half-life and because it is cyclotron produced. ^{111}In-chloride has been suggested as a substitute for ^{52}Fe in marrow scans of humans[32] because ionic indium, like iron, binds to unsaturated transferrin at acid pH. However, the biologic behavior and distribution of transferrin-bound indium are different from those of transferrin-bound iron, and although a good correlation between findings with ^{111}In imaging and the clinical status of patients with aplastic anemia and myelofibrosis has been reported, discrepancies between ^{52}Fe and ^{111}In scans in patients with red cell aplasia also have been described.[33–35] Whether ^{111}In is taken up by erythron or

TABLE 23.5.   The Physical Characteristics of Radiopharmaceuticals Used to Scan Bone Marrow

Class of Agent	Dose*	Physical Half-Life	Photon Energy, *meV*	Liver Dose, *rads*	Bone Marrow Dose, *rads*	Kidney Dose, *rads*
Transferrin-bound metals						
^{59}Fe	40.0 μCi	45.0 days	1.100	—	2.0	—
			1.300	—	2.0	—
^{52}Fe	100.0 μCi†	8.2 hours	0.165	—	2.5	—
			0.511			
^{111}In	2.0 to 5.0 mCi	2.8 days	0.173	6.4 to 16.0	1.3 to 3.3	13.2 to 33.0
			0.247			
Radiocolloids						
^{198}Au colloid	1.0 to 2.5 mCi	2.7 days	0.411	50.0 to 100.0	4.0 to 10.0	—
^{99m}T-sulfur colloid	6.0 mCi	6.0 hours	0.140	1.8	0.2	—

Source: McIntyre 1977[28]

*Average dose administered to an adult patient for a marrow scan.

†This dose is adequate for imaging only with a positron camera; 500 μCi is required if a properly equipped rectilinear scanner is to be used.

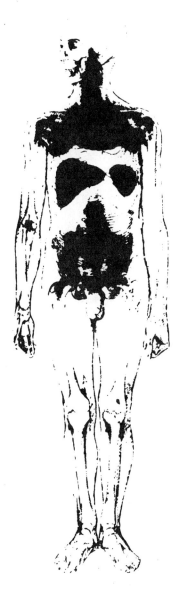

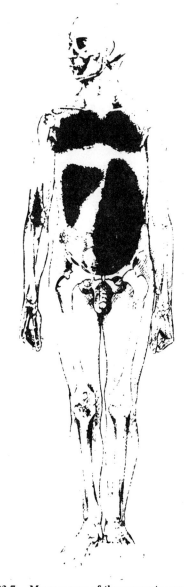

FIGURE 23.6. Marrow scan of the monocyte–macrophage system obtained in a hematologically normal male. A constant dose (12 mCi/60 kg or 12 mCi/1.7 m^2) of ^{99m}Tc-sulfur colloid is given intravenously and multiple camera views obtained of the functional monocyte–macrophage system in the marrow using a preset time for recording the images. This permits both inter- and intrapatient comparisons of the degree of functional monocyte–macrophage system present in the marrow; the technique is then optimized for camera images of the liver and spleen. In normal adults, active marrow is confined to the axial skeleton and the proximal portions of the long bones. *Source:* McIntyre 1971[29] Carol Donner, illustrator.

FIGURE 23.7. Marrow scan of the monocyte–macrophage system obtained in a manner identical to that described in Figure 23.6. This patient, who has myelofibrosis, has no normal monocyte–macrophage system marrow but does have a faint accumulation of ^{99m}Tc in the region of the knees. Note the giant splenomegaly that may be appreciated using this technique. *Source:* McIntyre 1971[29] Carol Donner, illustrator.

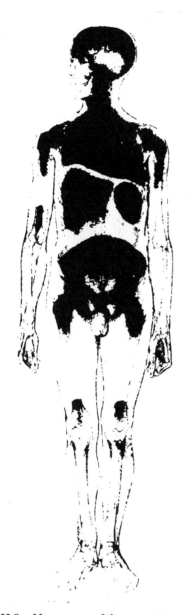

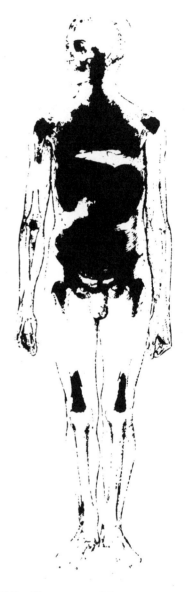

FIGURE 23.8. Marrow scan of the monocyte–macrophage system obtained in a manner identical to that described in Figure 23.6. This patient, who has polycythemia vera, has hyperplasia of the central marrow and marked peripheral expansion. The scan also reveals a significantly enlarged spleen that was not palpable. *Source:* McIntyre 1971[29] Carol Donner, illustrator.

FIGURE 23.9. Marrow scan of the monocyte–macrophage system obtained in a manner identical to that described in Figure 23.6. This young adult had been admitted with symptoms of a viral infection and was noted to have splenomegaly and hemolytic anemia. The initial diagnosis was infectious mononucleosis; however, the marrow scan showed a markedly hyperplastic and expanded marrow, suggesting a more longstanding hemolytic anemia. Laboratory studies failed to confirm the diagnosis of infectious mononucleosis, and his symptoms resolved spontaneously. A subsequent family study confirmed diagnosis of hereditary spherocytosis. *Source:* McIntyre 1971[29] Carol Donner, illustrator.

by the monocyte–macrophage system also remains unclear. Thus, ^{111}In cannot replace iron for scanning erythropoietic activity of the bone marrow.

The readily available, short-lived gamma-emitting isotopes (^{99m}Tc and [113m]In) can be administered as colloids and concentrated by the monocyte–macrophage system of the bone marrow, liver, and spleen and therefore have been evaluated widely as marrow-scanning agents. If ^{99m}Tc is readily available, ^{99m}Tc-sulfur colloid is the agent of choice because of its nearly ideal gamma energy for high-resolution imaging with modern instrumentation. As noted previously, the distribution of this radiocolloid in the marrow of normal subjects is identical to that of transferrin-bound radioiron, and the same is true in the overwhelming majority of disease processes studied. However, there are certain outstanding exceptions; as a general rule, patients with pure red cell aplasia or other severe disorders of erythropoiesis, such as myelodysplasia or hematologic malignancies, may have a paradoxic increase in their monocyte–macrophage system marrow activity, presumably because of increased phagocytic activity that is stimulated by the presence of defective and dying erythroid precursors. Because of the normal uptake of [99m]Tc- or ^{111}In-colloid by the monocyte–macrophage system of the liver and spleen, extramedullary hematopoiesis in these two organs cannot be differentiated by their normal uptakes.

It should be emphasized that the marrow scan pattern alone rarely is diagnostic, but it always should be interpreted according to other clinical and hematologic features of the patient. For instance, some diseases may present with an identical picture of central hyperplasia and peripheral expansion of the marrow on marrow monocyte–macrophage system scans. The [52]Fe scans of the following list (except for the final entry) show the same marrow pattern:

1. Pernicious anemia in relapse,
2. Megaloblastic anemia caused by folate deficiency,
3. Chronic hemolytic anemia,
4. Polycythemia vera (active phase),
5. Essential thrombocytosis,
6. Some patients with leukemia,
7. Some patients with lymphoma, and
8. Any anemia caused by marrow dyserythropoiesis.

The use of monocyte–macrophage system imaging agents has one clear advantage over transferrin-bound [52]Fe: high-resolution images of both the liver and the spleen can be obtained simultaneously with images of the marrow. This frequently provides clinicians with more useful information than that provided by use of an erythroid marrow scan alone; for instance, a typical patient with myeloid metaplasia and myelofibrosis will show essential absence of the normal axial marrow activity (with occasionally faint areas of abnormal expansion in the areas of the knees) and giant splenomegaly. The patient with polycythemia vera also will demonstrate splenomegaly by the use of scanning techniques, and in the active disease phases, there is a characteristic hyperplasia and expansion of the monocyte–macrophage system marrow. Filling defects demonstrated in the normal pelvic marrow areas often provide a guide to the best site for performing a needle biopsy of the marrow. In patients who are known to have a primary tumor with a high incidence of marrow involvement or who show peripheral blood changes that are compatible with myelophthisic process, the monocyte–macrophage system marrow scan may be additive in value to the usual bone scan in "staging" patients preoperatively, and in selected patients, the monocyte–macrophage system marrow scan not infrequently may be abnormal even in those with a normal bone scan. The monocyte–macrophage system marrow scan also can be used both to detect and follow the course of marrow infarction seen in patients with sickle cell anemia.

DISEASES OF THE SPLEEN

Physical examination, even when performed by skilled clinicians, has greater limitations in the detection of diseases involving the spleen than usually are appreciated. A spleen must be grossly enlarged to be detectable by observation. Percussion sometimes is useful in determining the size of the spleen, but modest to marked splenomegaly must be present for a significant increase in splenic dullness to be appreciated. Even then, air within the stomach may obscure this finding. Palpation, the most reliable tool of the clinician, also has significant limitations; in patients with ascites or who are in the later stages of pregnancy, it may be impossible to palpate a significantly enlarged spleen. Furthermore, gastric, pancreatic, and renal tumors often are indistinguishable clinically from an enlarged spleen, and for these reasons, the value of splenic scanning was appreciated quickly.

Three known "filtration" functions of the spleen allow the deliberate design of radiopharmaceuticals that permit the imaging of this organ:

1. the tissue macrophages of the monocyte–macrophage system present in the spleen will ingest radiolabelled colloids;
2. the spleen will sequester selectively the appropriately damaged radiolabelled erythrocytes; and
3. the spleen normally pools one third of the circulating platelets, allowing the imaging of the organ using radiolabelled platelets.

The clearance of radioactive colloids in the tracer doses that are used conventionally in clinical studies predominantly is a function of organ blood flow; accordingly, the liver accumulates the major portion of such radiolabelled colloids. However, a significant proportion of the material also is accumulated by the spleen and the active monocyte–macrophage system in the bone marrow, thus permitting imaging of these organs as well.

A number of methods have been described to damage red cells to the extent required for splenic sequestration and the imaging of this organ:

1. Antibody damage: the incubation of Rh D-positive (Rho) erythrocytes with anti-D isoantibody;
2. Thermal damage;
3. Chemical damage;
   A. Organic mercurials, such as mercurihydroxypropane or N-ethylmaleimide;
   B. Excess acid citrate dextrose solution with or without added stable chromium; and
   C. Excess stannous ion.

It should be emphasized that the type of erythrocyte damage is not the critical factor in determining subsequent clearance into the spleen; rather, it is the degree of damage to the red cells. Too little results in delayed removal from the circulation, but with appropriate selective damage, nearly specific splenic sequestration occurs. If the damage is more severe, clearance of the damaged cells by the liver occurs, and intravascular hemolysis will result from even more damage to the erythrocytes. At present, precise heat treatment of red cells (49.5°C for 20 minutes) followed by ^{99m}Tc labelling appears to be the method of choice for selective spleen scanning.

Approximately one third of injected radiolabelled platelets are pooled in the spleen, while only approximately 10% pool in the liver shortly after injection (30 minutes). Thus, ^{111}In-labelled platelets are an excellent spleen-scanning agent.

In the following clinical situations, splenic scans often make useful and sometimes unique contributions:

1. Detection of splenomegaly;
2. Differential diagnosis of left upper quadrant masses;
3. Detection of hematomas, infarcts, tumors, or other masses involving the spleen;
4. Nonsurgical management of splenic trauma;
5. Demonstration of the absence of functional splenic tissue (functional asplenia);
6. Visualization of one or more accessory spleens after splenectomy;
7. Demonstration of ectopic locations of the spleen; and

8. Visualization of splenosis after splenectomy for splenic rupture.

Clinically, the most important use of the spleen scan is detecting splenomegaly that is not apparent on either physical or conventional radiographic examination. Unfortunately, the state of our knowledge regarding the normal variance in spleen size does not always allow us to determine with certainty in any given patient whether a minimal to modest degree of splenomegaly exists. Normal spleen size varies with both the age and the sex of the patient, and spleen weight decreases from the age of 20 to 29 years, then remains relatively constant until it declines again in those over 60 years of age. Spleen weight also is consistently less in women than in men at all ages.[36]

Various methods have been published both for estimating the size and calculating the weight of the spleen from scan images. Larson et al.[37] suggested a simple and relatively reliable criterion for deciding whether a spleen is enlarged significantly. In 26 normal subjects aged from 20 to 38 years, they found that the mean length of the spleen in posterior view is 10 cm, with a standard deviation of 1.5 cm; thus, any spleen whose posterior scan length is more than 13 cm probably is enlarged. They also found a good correlation of the spleen length in the posterior view with the spleen weight determined at either autopsy or splenectomy in 15 patients regardless of whether the weight was normal or markedly increased. However, it is important to remember that the normal spleen size varies with both age and gender, and using the above criteria, a clinician may find that a normal spleen in an elderly female actually may represent one that is significantly enlarged.

Spleen scans with radioactive colloid also are useful for the differential diagnosis of left upper quadrant masses or the detection of infarction and space-occupying lesions in the spleen. In addition, it has been used to follow patients with traumatic splenic rupture treated nonsurgically.[38] Patients who have had their spleens removed have a markedly increased risk of developing fulminant infection by encapsulated microorganisms such as pneumococcus. The risk of this type of infection is greatest for those patients where an underlying disease necessitates splenectomy, but it also has been documented in otherwise healthy patients who have had their spleens removed because of trauma. Due to the high mortality rate in this type of infection, attempts have been made to avoid splenectomy; in this circumstance, spleen scans are useful not only for the detection of splenic trauma but also during the course of nonsurgical management.

The ready availability of spleen scanning has defined a clinical entity, "functional asplenia."[39] This entity is typified by the older child or adult with sickle cell disease whose spleen anatomically is still present but atrophied (presumably from multiple previous infarctions) and functionally is unable to concentrate either radiolabelled colloids or appropriately damaged radiolabelled erythrocytes.

In certain relatively rare circumstances, the large amount of ^{99m}Tc-sulfur colloid present in the liver may obscure the margins of the spleen or even the presence of ectopic or accessory spleens. In these circumstances, the second, more specific function (sequestering appropriately damaged erythrocytes) should be used to selectively image this organ; for example, in patients with hereditary spherocytosis having a recurrence of clinically significant hemolytic anemia after splenectomy, accessory spleens that were overlooked at the initial surgery may enlarge and assume the function of removing spherocytes from the circulation. They may be located virtually anywhere in the abdomen, and radioactivity of radiocolloid present in the liver may obscure totally the image of such a clinically important accessory spleen.

IN VIVO CROSSMATCHING

In rare instances, blood banks are unable to identify a satisfactory donor for a patient who requires transfusion; in some special instances, the use of ^{51}Cr-labelled donor red cells to perform an in vivo crossmatch may provide an invaluable life-saving service. The major indications for this procedure are when the blood bank serologic test results suggest all donors are incompatible, "cold" antibodies are present and active in vitro at 30°C or higher and a nonreacting donor cannot be found, and the recipient has had a previous unexplained transfusion reaction and requires further transfusions.[3]

The general principle is that no more than 0.5 ml of donor cells, resuspended in saline solution after labelling with and washed free of any unbound ^{51}Cr, is transfused into the patient. Blood samples are then taken from the recipient at timed intervals of 3 and 60 minutes; both whole blood and plasma radioactivity are measured in these samples. Ideally, the recipient's own red cells should be labelled with ^{99m}Tc and used to measure precisely the circulating red cell mass just before infusion of the ^{51}Cr-labelled donor cells. The comparison of the red cell mass measured by the autologous ^{99m}Tc-labelled red cells with that calculated from the sample withdrawn 3 minutes after the infusion of ^{51}Cr-labelled donor cells ensures there has been no rapid removal of the labelled donor cells before the first sampling time.

If there is no significant incompatibility, the red cell mass as measured by the 3-minute sample of the ^{51}Cr-labelled donor cells and by the autologous ^{99m}Tc-labelled donor cells should be identical. Also, the counting rate of the 60-minute whole blood sample should not deviate significantly from that of the 3-minute sample (94% to 104%), and there should be no significant radioactivity present in any plasma sample withdrawn after the infusion of the ^{51}Cr-labelled donor cells. In cases of extreme urgency, however, if the red cell survival at 60 minutes is not less than 70% of the administered labelled donor red cells and no more than 5% of the injected radioactivity is present in the plasma of any sample drawn between 3 and 60 minutes, then 1 unit of packed red cells from the same donor may be infused cautiously; the theory behind this is that if the patient's antibody titer is so low that rapid removal of the small volume (0.5 ml) of donor erythrocytes does not occur, then the amount of antibody available to attach to the erythrocytes in a whole unit of packed red cells obviously will be diluted further and ensure against an immediate and potentially fatal transfusion reaction. However, it should be emphasized that even entirely negative results with this in vivo crossmatch test afford no assurance that the recipient may not have an amnestic response with a delayed "crash" hemolysis of the donor red cells. This response always is a theoretical possibility, even when perfect serologic matches are obtained for patients who have had either multiple transfusions or pregnancies in the past.

THROMBOCYTOPENIA

When evaluating patients with thrombocytopenia, as with anemia, it is useful to consider the rates of both platelet production and removal from the circulation; however, unlike with red blood cells, our ability to quantify this rate of production or destruction is limited. No clinically useful isotopic method similar to that used in ferrokinetics has been developed for evaluating the rate of platelet production. The rate of platelet production can be derived by determining platelet turnover, because at steady state (e.g., stable platelet counts for 1 to 2 weeks), platelet turnover represents the rate of platelet production and destruction; the determination of platelet turnover requires measurements of the mean platelet lifespan, the recovery of platelets in the circulation, and the blood platelet count (turnover = [platelet count/μl $\times$ 90%]/[platelet survival in days $\times$ % of recovery]).[40] Because many patients with thrombocytopenia are not in a steady state and platelet survival studies are not available routinely, morphologic examination of the bone marrow specimen continues to play an important role in the evaluation of patients with thrombocytopenia.

Several methods (including the radiolabelled antiglobulin test) have been used to measure platelet-associated IgG, IgM, or C3,[41,42] and there appears to be a satisfactory correlation between the presence of platelet antibodies and elevated levels of platelet-associated IgG, IgM, or C3. Furthermore, a significant inverse correlation exists between the amount of platelet antibodies and the circulating platelet counts. Thus, elevated levels of platelet-associated IgG, IgM, or C3 would suggest that the patient's thrombocytopenia is caused at least in part by increased immune destruction of platelets.

Kinetic studies using random platelet labels provide important information regarding both the mean platelet lifespan and the recovery of platelets in the circulation, from which the turnover rate can be calculated. However, platelet kinetic studies are not routine procedures, largely because unlike red blood cells, platelets are difficult to isolate in a pure preparation without either activation or damage. In addition, although ^{51}Cr-sodium chromate has been used widely for the study of platelet kinetics in humans, ^{51}Cr as a platelet label has several disadvantages, including low labelling efficiency, long physical half-life (27.8 days), and only 9% of its emissions being gamma photons. Because of the low labelling efficiency, large amounts of blood are required to obtain a limited amount of ^{51}Cr-platelets (10 to 30 μCi) for kinetic studies, and this necessitates the use of homologous platelets for kinetic studies in those with severe thrombocytopenia. The small amounts of ^{51}Cr-labelled platelets injected, coupled with the low emissions of gamma photons, preclude precise in vivo quantification of the distribution and fate of the platelets.[43]

^{111}In-oxine or ^{111}In-tropolone as a platelet label overcomes the disadvantages of ^{51}Cr-chromate. Both have a high labelling efficiency, so only a small amount of blood is sufficient to obtain ^{111}In-platelets for kinetic studies. Thus, even in patients with severe thrombocytopenia, autologous platelets can be used. The 2.8-day physical half-life of ^{111}In also is more suitable for platelet kinetic studies than ^{51}Cr-chromate. In addition, ^{111}In has abundant gamma emissions, with photon energies of 173 (84%) and 247 keV (94%) that are ideal for detection by modern gamma cameras; using a gamma camera interfaced with computer systems, precise in vivo quantification of both the temporal and spatial distribution of ^{111}In-platelets as well as visualization of platelet deposition at sites of thrombus formation and endothelial damage becomes possible.[43]

Studies of the kinetics and distribution of ^{111}In-platelets in the last decade have provided important new information regarding both the platelet physiology and pathophysiology of thrombocytopenic disorders. Computer analysis of platelet kinetics reveals that the multiple-hit model as well as the geographic mean model fit the platelet survival curve better than the linear or the exponential models. With the multiple-hit model, the mean lifespan of human platelets is approximately 8.5 days. The initial recovery of infused ^{111}In-platelets from the circulation is approximately 60% in normal individuals, is reduced markedly in splenomegalic subjects, and is almost 100% in asplenic subjects. At 30 minutes after infusion, 43% and 13% of the infused ^{111}In-platelets are pooled in the spleen and liver, respectively, of normal individuals, and at 10 days postinfusion, when all ^{111}In-platelets have been cleared from the circulation, 37% and 24% were sequestered in the spleen and liver, respectively. Thus, both the spleen and the liver are the primary sites of platelet destruction, accounting for 61% of the infused ^{111}In-platelets. Gamma camera images also reveal ^{111}In activities in areas corresponding to bone marrow distribution, suggesting that bone marrow plays an important role in the sequestration of platelets as well. In asplenic subjects, the liver is the primary site of platelet destruction, accounting for 89%, while the spleen is the major site in splenomegalic subjects, accounting for 71% of the infused ^{111}In-platelets.[43,44]

Immune thrombocytopenia (ITP) is a disorder that is characterized by thrombocytopenia, increased levels of platelet-associated immunoglobulin, and normal to increased numbers of megakaryocytes in the bone marrow. Previous kinetic studies using ^{51}Cr-platelets have shown that the mean platelet lifespan in ITP is reduced markedly and the platelet turnover is either normal or increased, suggesting that thrombocytopenia is primarily due to an increased destruction of circulating platelets.[45] However, recent studies using autologous ^{111}In-platelets demonstrated that a significant portion, (approximately 30%) of patients with ITP have a decreased platelet turnover, especially in patients with severe thrombocytopenia;[46,47] thus, in this group, both increased platelet destruction and reduced platelet production are responsible for the thrombocytopenia. There appears to be an inverse correlation between the levels of platelet-associated antibody and platelet turnover, suggesting that high levels of platelet antibody impair platelet production.[46,47] In vivo quantification of ^{111}In-platelets also reveals two general patterns of platelet sequestration in ITP: those with predominantly splenic sequestration; and those with diffuse sequestration by the monocyte–macrophage system of the liver, spleen, and bone marrow. This latter group of patients have more severe ITP that is reflected by pronounced thrombocytopenia, decreased platelet turnover, and prominent early hepatic sequestration of the platelets.[47]

Using ^{51}Cr-platelets and external counting, researchers have shown that clear-cut splenic sequestration of ^{51}Cr-platelets predicts a successful outcome for splenectomy in ITP; however, some patients with hepatic sequestration also have a good response to splenectomy.[48] This in part may be due to the fact that the spleen is one of the major sites of platelet antibody production in ITP.[49] It also may be a result of the inherent problems associated with the external counting of ^{51}Cr, and the ability of better external quantification using ^{111}In-platelet deposition in the liver and spleen offers an opportunity to reassess the role of splenic sequestration in predicting the response to splenectomy in ITP.

LEUKOPENIA

As with platelets, there is no clinically useful isotopic method for cohort labelling of neutrophils. Although a number of random radiolabels (including ^{32}P-di-isopropyl fluorophosphate [^{32}P-DFP], ^{51}Cr-chromate, and ^{111}In-oxine or -tropolone) have been used to label neutrophils for kinetic studies, the results are difficult to interpret, and they generally are not useful. The major difficulty is the lack of a standardized procedure to obtain a pure preparation of neutrophils without causing either neutrophil activation or damage that leads to altered in vivo behavior; thus, for the evaluation of leukopenia, we continue to rely on the measurement of leukocyte-associated IgG, which correlates well with the presence of leukocyte antibody,[50] and morphologic examination of the bone marrow to determine whether leukopenia is due to an increased destruction or a decreased production from the marrow.

Kinetic studies using ^{32}P-DFP-labelled neutrophils suggest that the neutrophils are distributed evenly between a circulating and a marginating pool. Immediately after injection, no more than 50% of the radiolabelled neutrophils can be recovered from the circulation; when the infusion of neutrophils is followed immediately by exercise or epinephrine injection, up to 80% of those radiolabelled neutrophils can be recovered.[51] This suggests that approximately half the neutrophils in the blood are marginated, probably along the wall of small vessels. The exact location and distribution of this marginated pool is unclear, but the staying time of neutrophils in the circulation is brief, with an exponential disappearance half-life of 6 to 7 hours. With ^{111}In-neutrophils, an immediate concentration of the radioactivity in the liver and the spleen occurs, reaching a plateau by 1 hour after infusion. Some radioactivity also is noted initially in the lungs,[52] but whether the radioactivity noted in the liver, spleen, and lungs (which accounts for approximately 50% of the injected dose) represents the marginated

neutrophil pool and/or sequestration of damaged neutrophils is unclear. The intravascular recovery of ^{111}In-neutrophils is low, approximately 30%, but despite the low initial recovery, ^{111}In-neutrophils are useful in the detection and localization of inflammatory lesions, particularly occult intra-abdominal abscesses.[53]

REFERENCES

1. McIntyre PA. Radioactive tracers in hematologic disease: I. Hosp Pract 1972;7:99–108.
2. Cline MF, Berlin NI. The red cell chromium elution rates in patients with some hematological diseases. Blood 1963;21:63–69.
3. The Panel of Diagnostic Application of Radioisotopes in Hematology, International Committee for Standardization in Hematology. Recommended methods for radioisotope red-cell survival studies. Br J Haematol 1971;21:241–50.
4. The Panel of Diagnostic Application of Radioisotopes in Hematology, International Committee for Standardization in Hematology. Recommended methods for surface counting to determine sites of red-cell destruction. Br J Haematol 1975;30:249–54.
5. Addison GM, Beamish MR, Hales CN, et al. An immunoradiometric assay for ferritin in the serum of normal subjects and patients with iron overload. J Clin Pathol 1972;25:326–9.
6. Jacobs A, Worwood M. The clinical use of serum ferritin estimation. Br J Haematol 1975;31:1–3.
7. Ali MAM, Luxton AW, Walker WHC. Serum ferritin concentration and bone marrow iron stores: a prospective study. Can Med Assoc J 1978;118:945–6.
8. Wands JR, Rowe JA, Mezey SE, et al. Normal serum ferritin concentrations in precirrhotic hemochromatosis. N Engl J Med 1976;294:302–5.
9. Beaumont C, Simon M, Fauchet R, et al. Serum ferritin as a possible marker of the hemochromatosis allele. N Engl J Med 1979;301:169–74.
10. Cooper BA, Whitehead VM. Evidence that some patients with pernicious anemia are not recognized by radiodilution assay for cobalamin in serum. N Engl J Med 1978;299:816–8.
11. Kolhouse JF, Kondo H, Allen NC, et al. Cobalamin analogues are present in human plasma and can mask cobalamin deficiency because current radioisotope dilution assays are not specific for true cobalamin. N Engl J Med 1978;299:785–92.
12. Chu RC, Hall CA. The total serum homocysteine as an indicator of vitamin B[12] and folate status. Am J Clin Pathol 1988;90:446–9.
13. Stabler SP, Allen RH, Savage DG, et al. Clinical spectrum and diagnosis of cobalamin deficiency. Blood 1990;76:871–81.
14. McIntyre PA. Use of radioisotope techniques in the clinical evaluation of patients with megaloblastic anemia. Semin Nucl Med 1975;5:79–94.
15. Glass GBJ, Boyd LJ, Gellin GA. Uptake of radioactive vitamin B[12] by the liver in humans: test for measurement of intestinal absorption of vitamin B[12] and intrinsic factor activity. Arch Biochem 1954;51:251–257.
16. McIntyre PA, Wagner HN. Comparison of the urinary excretion and 8 hour plasma tests for vitamin B-12 absorption. J Lab Clin Med 1966;68:966–971.
17. Hjelt K, Munck O, Hippe E, et al. Vitamin B[12] absorption determined with a double isotope technique employing incomplete stool collection. Acta Med Scand 1977;202:419–22.
18. Briedis D, McIntyre PA, Judisch J, et al. Evaluation of dual isotope method for the measurement of vitamin B[12] absorption. J Nucl Med 1973;14:135–41.

19. Streeter AM, Shum HY, Duncombe M, et al. Vitamin B_{12} malabsorption associated with a normal Schilling test result. Med J Aust 1976;1:54–5.

20. Steinberg WM, King CE, Toskes P. Malabsorption of protein-bound cobalamin but not unbound cobalamin during cimetidine administration. Dig Dis Sci 1980;25:188–91.

21. Streeter AM, Balasubramaniam D, Boyle R, et al. Malabsorption of vitamin B_{12} after vagotomy. Am J Surg 1974;128:340–3.

22. Mahmud K, Ripley D, Doscherholmen A. Vitamin B_{12} absorption tests: their unreliability in postgastrectomy states. JAMA 1971;216:1167–71.

23. Lindenbaum J. Status of laboratory testing in the diagnosis of megaloblastic anemia. Blood 1983;61:624–7.

24. Shane B, Tamura T, Stokstad ELR. Folate assay: a comparison of radioassay and microbiological methods. Clin Chim Acta 1980;100:13–9.

25. Klein BP, Kuo CHY. Comparison of microbiological and radiometric assays for determining total folacin in spinach. J Food Sci 1981;46:552–4.

26. The Panel of Diagnostic Application of Radioisotopes in Hematology, International Committee for Standardization in Hematology. Standard techniques for the measurement of red-cell and plasma volume. Br J Haematol 1973;25:801–14.

27. Conley CL. Polycythemia vera: diagnosis and treatment. Hosp Pract 1987;22:181–212.

28. McIntyre PA. Newer developments in nuclear medicine applicable to hematology. Prog Hematol 1977;10:361–409.

29. McIntyre PA. Visualization of the reticuloendothelial system. Hosp Pract 1971;6:77–87.

30. Van Dyke D, Shkurkin C, Price D, et al. Differences in distribution of erythropoietic and reticuloendothelial marrow in hematologic disease. Blood 1967;30:364–74.

31. Knospe WH, Rayudu GVS, Cardello M, et al. Bone marrow scanning with ^{52}Fe: regeneration and extension of marrow after ablative doses of radiotherapy. Cancer 1976;37:1432–42.

32. Hosain F, McIntyre PA, Poulose KP, et al. Binding of trace amounts of ionic indium to plasma transferrin. Clin Chim Acta 1969;24:69–75.

33. McNeil BJ, Rappeport JM, Nathan DG. Indium chloride scintigraphy: an index of severity in patients with aplastic anemia. Br J Haematol 1976;34:599–604.

34. McNeil BJ, Holman BL, Button LN, et al. Use of indium chloride scintigraphy in patients with myelofibrosis. J Nucl Med 1974;15:647–51.

35. Merrick MV, Gordon-Smith EC, Lavender JP, et al. A comparison of ^{111}In with ^{52}Fe and ^{99m}Tc-sulfur colloid for bone marrow scanning. J Nucl Med 1975;16:66–8.

36. DeLand LH. Normal spleen size. Radiology 1970;94:589–98.

37. Larson SM, Tuell SH, Moores KD, et al. Dimensions of the normal adult spleen scan and prediction of spleen weight. J Nucl Med 1971;12:123–6.

38. Fischer KC, Eraklis AP, Rossello P, et al. Scintigraphy in the follow-up of pediatric splenic trauma treated without surgery. J Nucl Med 1978;19:3–9.

39. Pearson HA, Spencer RP, Cornelius EA. Functional asplenia in sickle-cell anemia. N Engl J Med 1969;281:923–6.

40. Harker LA, Finch CA. Thrombokinetics in man. J Clin Invest 1969;48:963–74.

41. Mueller-Eckhardt C, Schultz G, Sauer KH, et al. Studies on the platelet radioactive anti-immunoglobulin test. J Immunol Methods 1978;19:1–8.

42. Cines DB, Schreiber AD. Immune thrombocytopenia: use of a Coombs antiglobulin test to detect IgG and C_3 on platelets. N Engl J Med 1979;300:106–11.

43. Tsan MF. Kinetics and distribution of platelets in man. Am J Hematol 1984;17:97–104.

44. Hill-Zobel RL, McCandless B, Kang SA, et al. Organ distribution and fate of human platelets: studies of asplenic and splenomegalic patients. Am J Hematol 1986;23:231–8.

45. Harker LA. Thrombokinetics in idiopathic thrombocytopenic purpura. Br J Haematol 1970;19:95–104.

46. Ballem PJ, Segal GM, Stratton JR, et al. Mechanisms of thrombocytopenia in chronic autoimmune thrombocytopenic purpura: evidence of both impaired platelet production and increased platelet clearance. J Clin Invest 1987;80:33–40.

47. Heyns ADP, Badenhorst PN, Lotter MG, et al. Platelet turnover and kinetics in immune thrombocytopenic purpura: results with autologous ^{111}In-labeled platelets and homologous ^{51}Cr-labeled platelets differ. Blood 1986;67:86–92.

48. Aster RH. Platelet sequestration studies in man. Br J Haematol 1972;22:259–62.

49. McMillan R, Longmire RL, Xelenosky R, et al. Quantitation of platelet-binding IgG produced in vivo by spleens from patients with idiopathic thrombocytopenic purpura. N Engl J Med 1974;291:812–6.

50. Cines DB, Passero F, Guerry DIV, et al. Granulocyte-associated IgG in neutropenic disorders. Blood 1982;59:124–32.

51. Athens JW. Neutrophilic granulocyte kinetics and granulopoiesis. In: Gordon AS, ed. Regulation of Hematopoiesis. New York: Appleton-Century-Crofts, 1970:1143–1166.

52. Thaker ML, Lavender JP, Arnot RN, et al. Indium-111 labeled autologous leukocytes in man. J Nucl Med 1977;18:1012–9.

53. Knochel JQ, Koehler R, Lee TG, et al. Diagnosis of abdominal abscesses with computed tomography, ultrasound, and ^{111}In leukocyte scans. Radiology 1980;137:425–32.

Index